Optical Fiber-based Plasmonic Biosensors

This book discusses the history, physics, fundamental principles, sensing technologies, and characterization of plasmonic phenomenon-based fiber-optic biosensors, using optic-plasmonic sensors as a case study. It describes the plasmonic phenomenon and its application in optical fiber-based sensing, presented based on properties and usage of different nanomaterials spread across nine chapters. Content covers advances in nanomaterials, structural designing, and their scope in biomedical applications. Future developments of biosensing devices and related articulate methods are also described.

FEATURES

- Gives a comprehensive view on the nanomaterials used in plasmonic optical fiber biosensors.
- Includes synthesis, characterization, and usage for detection of different analytes.
- Discusses trends in the design of wavelength-based optical fiber sensors.
- Reviews micro- and nanostructured biosensing devices.
- Explores application of plasmonic sensors in the biosensing field.

This book is aimed at researchers and graduate students in Optical Communications, Biomedical Engineering, Optics, Sensors, Instrumentation, and Measurement.

Optical Fiber-based Plasmonic Biosensors

Trends, Techniques, and Applications

Santosh Kumar, Niteshkumar Agrawal,
Chinmoy Saha, and Rajan Jha

CRC **CRC Press**
Taylor & Francis Group
Boca Raton London New York

CRC Press is an imprint of the
Taylor & Francis Group, an **informa** business

Designed cover image: © Shutterstock

First edition published 2023
by CRC Press
6000 Broken Sound Parkway NW, Suite 300, Boca Raton, FL 33487–2742

and by CRC Press
4 Park Square, Milton Park, Abingdon, Oxon, OX14 4RN

CRC Press is an imprint of Taylor & Francis Group, LLC

© 2023 Santosh Kumar, Niteshkumar Agrawal, Chinmoy Saha and Rajan Jha

ISBN: 978-1-032-15237-0 (hbk)
ISBN: 978-1-032-15239-4 (pbk)
ISBN: 978-1-003-24319-9 (ebk)

DOI: 10.1201/9781003243199

Typeset in Times
by Apex CoVantage, LLC

Contents

Author Biographies xi

Preface xiii

Acknowledgments xvii

Chapter 1   Fundamentals of Plasmonics Sensors 1

    1.1   Introduction 1

    1.2   Fundamentals of Fiber-Optic Sensors and Related Concepts 6

        1.2.1   Total Internal Reflection and Evanescent Wave 8

        1.2.2   Surface Plasmons 10

            1.2.2.1   Definition of Surface Plasmon 12

            1.2.2.2   Brief History of Surface Plasmons 13

        1.2.3   Generation of Propagating Surface Plasmons by Light Using Thin Metallic Film 13

    1.3   Kretschmann's Configuration 14

    1.4   Transfer Matrix Method 15

        1.4.1   Calculation of Reflected Intensity 16

            1.4.1.1   Boundary Condition at Interface 1 16

            1.4.1.2   Boundary Condition at Interface 2 17

        1.4.2   Transmitted Power through Optical Fiber 19

    1.5   Plasmon Excitation Using Optical Fiber 20

    1.6   Excitation of Localized Surface Plasmon by Light Using Metallic Nanoparticles 21

        1.6.1   Mie Theory 23

    1.7   Fiber-Optic LSPR Sensor Using Metallic Nanoparticles 27

        1.7.1   Refractive Index Dependence 28

    1.8   Fiber-Optic Plasmonic Biosensing Technique 29

        1.8.1   Surface Plasmon Resonance Sensor 30

    1.9   Performance Parameters of Sensors 32

        1.9.1   Sensitivity 32

        1.9.2   Selectivity 33

        1.9.3   Stability 33

        1.9.4   Limit of Detection 33

        1.9.5   Reproducibility 33

        1.9.6   Response Time 33

        1.9.7   Linearity 33

    1.10   Overview of the Book 34

    References 35

Chapter 2   Important Nanomaterials for Optical Fiber Plasmonic Biosensors 45

    2.1   Introduction 45

    2.2   Basics of Nanomaterial and Its Growing Applications 46

    2.3   Types of Nanomaterial 48

        2.3.1   Metal Nanoparticles 48

        2.3.2   Metal Nanorods and Nanotriangles 52

        2.3.3   Semiconductor Nanoparticles 53

        2.3.4   Carbon-Based Nanoparticles 53

2.3.5   Polymeric Nanoparticles 53
2.3.6   Ceramic Nanoparticles 53
2.3.7   Perovskite Nanoparticles 53
2.3.8   MXene-Based Nanocomposites 54
2.3.9   Lipid-Based Nanoparticles 55
2.4   Synthesis of Nanomaterials 55
2.4.1   Wet Chemical Method 56
2.4.2   Physical Method 56
2.4.3   Exfoliation Method 56
2.5   Characterization of Nanomaterials 56
2.5.1   Morphological Characterizations 56
2.5.2   Structural Characterizations 58
2.5.3   Surface Area and Particle Size Characterization 59
2.5.4   Optical Characterizations 59
2.6   Summary and Conclusion 60
References 61

Chapter 3   Design Methodology 69
3.1   Introduction 69
3.2   Structural Developments 70
3.2.1   Tapered Structure 71
3.2.2   Hetero-Core Structure 73
3.2.3   Other Structures 73
3.3   Nanocoating Process and Characterization 74
3.4   Sensor Development and Applications 75
3.4.1   Biomedical and Diagnostic Applications 75
3.4.1.1   Glucose Detection 76
3.4.1.2   Cholesterol Detection 76
3.4.1.3   Bacteria Detection 78
3.4.1.4   Virus Detection 78
3.4.1.5   Cell Detection 78
3.4.1.6   DNA Biomolecules Detection 81
3.4.2   Environmental Applications 81
3.4.3   Miscellaneous Applications 82
3.5   Summary and Conclusion 83
References 83

Chapter 4   Gold Nanoparticles Assisted Optical Fiber-Based Plasmonic Biosensors 91
4.1   Introduction 91
4.2   Synthesis, Characterization, Properties,
       and Applications of Gold Nanoparticles 91
4.2.1   Turkevich Method 92
4.2.2   Brust Method 95
4.2.3   Seeded Growth Method 95
4.2.4   Electrochemical Method 96
4.2.5   Miscellaneous Methods 96
4.3   Some Biosensor Design Based on AuNPs 97
4.4   Recent Development of Gold Nanoparticles Assisted Plasmonic Biosensors 100
4.4.1   Gold Nanoparticles Assisted Glucose Sensor 100

4.4.2   Gold Nanoparticles Assisted Cholesterol Sensor 100
4.4.3   Gold Nanoparticles Assisted Other Important Biosensors 102
4.4.4   Gold Nanoparticles Assisted Biosensors for Bacteria and
         Virus Detection 103
4.4.5   Gold Nanoparticle-Based Sensor for Dengue Immunoassay 105
4.4.6   Gold Nanoparticles Assisted Biosensors for DNA/RNA
         and Cells Detection 106
4.5   Summary and Conclusion 109
References 109

Chapter 5   Silver Nanoparticles Assisted Optical Fiber-Based Plasmonic Biosensors 113

5.1   Introduction 113
5.2   Synthesis, Characterization, Properties,
       and Applications of Silver Nanoparticles 115
       5.2.1   Synthesis Methods for Silver Nanoparticles and Composites 115
                5.2.1.1   Spherical Silver Nanoparticles 115
                5.2.1.2   Triangular Silver Nanoparticles 119
                5.2.1.3   Synthesis of PVA-AgNPs Composites 120
                5.2.1.4   Green Synthesis of Ag Nanoparticles 120
                5.2.1.5   Synthesis of AgNPs Using Green Route Method 121
5.3   Diverse Usage of Silver Nanoparticles 122
       5.3.1   Silver Nanoparticles Assisted Biosensors for Biomolecules
                Detection 124
5.4   Summary and Conclusion 126
References 127

Chapter 6   Graphene Oxide Coated Gold Nanoparticles-Based Fiber-Optic LSPR Sensor 131

6.1   Introduction 131
6.2   Experimental Section 132
       6.2.1   Synthesis of AuNPs and GO 132
       6.2.2   Preparation of GO Encapsulated AuNPs 133
       6.2.3   Preparation of Fiber Probe 134
6.3   Results and Discussion 135
6.4   Micro-Ball Fiber Sensor Probe Based Uric Acid Biosensor 151
       6.4.1   Fabrication of Micro-Ball Fiber Structure 152
       6.4.2   Experimental Setup 152
       6.4.3   Characterization of Gold Nanoparticles and Graphene
                Oxide 152
       6.4.4   Detection of Uric Acid Solutions 154
       6.4.5   Sensitivity, Linearity, and Detection Limit of Sensor 154
       6.4.6   Selectivity of Sensor 156
       6.4.7   Analysis of Uric Acid in Human Serum 156
6.5   Novel Periodically Tapered Structure-Based Sensor to Detect
       Ascorbic Acid 157
       6.5.1   Design Consideration and Fabrication of Proposed
                Sensors 157
       6.5.2   Detection of Ascorbic Acid 158
6.6   Summary and Conclusion 162
References 162

Chapter 7   Fiber-Optic LSPR Sensor Using Graphene Oxide Coated Silver
               Nanostructures 167

       7.1   Introduction 167
       7.2   Experimental Section 168
               7.2.1   Synthesis of AgNPs, GO, and Preparation of GO-Coated
                       AgNPs 168
               7.2.2   Preparation of Fiber Sensing Probe................................. 168
       7.3   Results and Discussion 168
       7.4   AgNPs and GO-Based Plasmonic Sensor for L-Cysteine Detection 189
               7.4.1   Synthesis of Silver Nanoparticles................................... 190
               7.4.2   Experimental Setup and Results 190
       7.5   Summary and Conclusion 192
       References 193

Chapter 8   Novel Nanomaterials Assisted Optical Fiber-Based Plasmonic Biosensors 197

       8.1   Introduction 197
       8.2   Nanomaterial Synthesis Process 200
               8.2.1   Synthesis Process of AuNPs 200
               8.2.2   Synthesis of AgNPs Solution 201
               8.2.3   Synthesis Process of MXene 201
               8.2.4   Synthesis Process of MoS_2-NPs..................................... 201
               8.2.5   Synthesis Process of CeO_2-NPs 201
               8.2.6   Synthesis Process of GO 202
               8.2.7   Synthesis Process of Colloidal CuO-NPs Solution 202
       8.3   Characterization of Nanoparticles.. 202
       8.4   Immobilization of Nanoparticles Over
               the Optical Fiber Probe 209
               8.4.1   Fabrication of AuNPs/ZnO-NPs-Based Optical Fiber Probe 209
               8.4.2   Fabrication of CuO-NPs-Based Optical Fiber Probe 209
               8.4.3   Fabrication of ZnO-NPs/PVA-AgNPs-Based Optical
                       Fiber Probe 210
               8.4.4   Fabrication of MoS_2-NPs/AuNPs-Based Optical Fiber Probe 210
       8.5   Detection of Various Biomolecules 210
               8.5.1   SMF-MCF-MMF-SMF Structure Based LSPR Biosensor
                       for Creatinine Detection.. 210
               8.5.2   Multicore Tapered Fiber Structure-Based Sensor for
                       Creatinine Detection in Aquaculture 211
               8.5.3   Taper-in-Taper Fiber Structure-Based LSPR Sensor for
                       Alanine Aminotransferase Detection.................................. 213
               8.5.4   Taper Fiber-Based Sensor for Water Pollutants p-Cresol
                       Detection 214
               8.5.5   MPM Fiber Structure Sensor Probe for cTnI 216
               8.5.6   Hetero-Core Fiber Structure-Based Cardiac Troponin I Detection 217
               8.5.7   Multicore Fiber Biosensor for Acetylcholine Detection 219
               8.5.8   Tapered Optical Fiber Based LSPR Biosensor for Ascorbic
                       Acid Detection... 220
               8.5.9   Core Mismatch MPM/SPS Probe-Based Sensor for
                       Cholesterol Detection 223
               8.5.10 CuO and AgNPs Modified SMSMS Structure Probe
                       for Uric Acid Detection 227

8.5.11 Structure of Optical Fiber Mach-Zehnder Interferometer for Collagen IV Detection 228

8.6 Summary and Conclusion 232

References 234

Chapter 9 Optical Sensors for Detection of Microorganisms 241

9.1 Introduction 241
9.2 SPR-Based Sensors 244
9.3 LSPR-Based Sensors 244
9.4 Multicore Fiber Sensor for Cancer Cells Detection 246
  9.4.1 Material and Method 246
    9.4.1.1 Material 246
    9.4.1.2 Fabrication of the Sensor Probe 246
    9.4.1.3 Etching of SMF-MCF Structure 247
    9.4.1.4 Characterization 247
    9.4.1.5 Synthesis of Graphene Oxide/Gold Nanoparticles/ Copper Oxide Nanoflowers 248
    9.4.1.6 Immobilization of GO/AuNPs/CuO-NFs Over SMF-MCF Structure 248
    9.4.1.7 Cell Culture 249
    9.4.1.8 Experimental Setup 249
  9.4.2 Results and Discussion 250
    9.4.2.1 Optimization of Bare Sensor Structure 250
    9.4.2.2 Characterization of Nanomaterials 250
    9.4.2.3 Characterization of Nanoparticles Coated Sensor Probes 254
    9.4.2.4 Detection of Cancerous Cells 254
    9.4.2.5 Analysis of Reusability, Selectivity, and Anti-Interference Ability 258
    9.4.2.6 Performance Comparison 261
9.5 Multicore Fiber Probe for Selective Detection of *Shigella* Bacteria 262
  9.5.1 Materials and Methods 262
    9.5.1.1 Fabrication of Sensor Probe 263
    9.5.1.2 Synthesis of AuNPs and MoS₂-NPs 264
    9.5.1.3 Immobilization of AuNPs and MoS₂-NPs Over MCF-SMF Sensor Probe 264
    9.5.1.4 LSPR Measurements 264
    9.5.1.5 Culture of *Shigella sonnei* Bacteria 264
  9.5.2 Results and Discussion 266
    9.5.2.1 Characterization of Nanoparticles 266
    9.5.2.2 Characterization of a Nanoparticles-Coated Sensor Probe 267
    9.5.2.3 LSPR Sensing Results 267
    9.5.2.4 Comparison with Existing *Shigella* Biosensors 269
9.6 Summary and Conclusions 270
9.7 Future Perspective 270
References 271

Index 277

Author Biographies

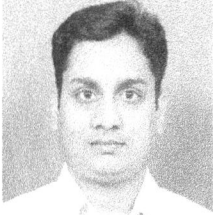

Santosh Kumar earned a doctorate from Indian Institute of Technology (Indian School of Mines) Dhanbad in Dhanbad, India. Currently, he is an associate professor with the School of Physics Science and Information Technology, Liaocheng University, Liaocheng, China. He is ranked in the top 2% of the world's scientists by Stanford University's 2020 data ranking. He has guided eight masters of technology dissertations and six doctoral candidates. Kumar has authored and coauthored more than 220 research articles for national and international Science Citation Index (SCI) journals and conferences and has over 3000 citations and an h-index of 35 in a variety of high-impact journals, including *Biosensors and Bioelectronics*, *Biosensors*, *Journal of Lightwave Technology*, *Optics Express*, and various *IEEE Transactions*. He has also presented many articles at conferences held in India, China, Belgium, and the United States. He authored two books: *Fiber Optic Communication: Optical Waveguides, Devices and Applications* (University Press, India, 2017) and *2D Materials for Surface Plasmon Resonance-Based Sensors* (CRC Press, Taylor & Francis Group, 2021). Kumar recently filed a patent application for optical fiber sensing technology. He has reviewed more than 1200 SCI journals of IEEE, Elsevier, Springer, OPTICA, SPIE, Wiley, and *Nature*. He is a Life Fellow Member of the Optical Society of India (OSI) and a senior member of IEEE, OPTICA, and SPIE and is also a traveling lecturer of OPTICA. He collaborates closely with a number of renowned universities in India, China, Portugal, Brazil, and Italy to conduct scientific research. He is capable of effective teaching and conducting high-quality research in the fields of electronics and communications engineering, as well as physics, with an emphasis on fiber-optic sensors, photonics and plasmonic devices, nano and biophotonics, waveguides, and interferometers. He has been appointed Chair of the Optica Optical Biosensor Technical Group and Associate Editor for *IEEE Sensors Journal*, *IEEE Access*, *IEEE Transactions on NanoBioscience*, *Frontiers in Physics*, and *Biomedical Optics Express*. Recently, he has received the "2022 Best Performing Associate Editor" award from IEEE Sensors Journal.

Niteshkumar Agrawal (S'19—M'22) earned his doctorate from the Indian Institute of Space Science and Technology, Thiruvananthapuram, Kerala, India, and master's of technology degree from the Indian Institute of Technology (IIT-ISM), Dhanbad, Jharkhand, India. He is currently working as an associate professor at Mahatma Education Society's Pillai College of Engineering, Navi Mumbai, Maharashtra, India. He is a former visiting researcher at Shandong Key Laboratory of Optical Communication Science and Technology, Liaocheng University (LCU), Shandong, China. He has delivered more than 20 invited talks at various esteemed institutions and organizations and has more than 20 publications in peer-reviewed national and international journals and conference proceedings. He received an *All India Council for Technical Education-Indian National Academy of Engineering/Department of Space-TRF* fellowship during his doctoral degree. He is an industry coordinator of *IEEE EMBS Chapter*, Kerala State, India and serves as an active member of various technical societies like IEEE, OSA, and SPIE. He is also on the board of reviewers of *IEEE Transactions on NanoBioscience* and *IEEE Sensors Journal*. His current research interests include optical/plasmonic/biosensors, nanomaterials, nanotechnology, optical communication, avionics, and space communication.

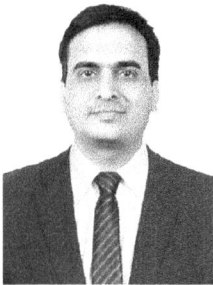

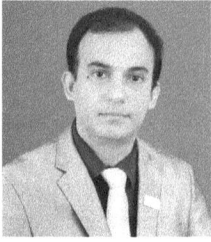

Chinmoy Saha (MIEEE'06—SMIEEE'15, SM URSI) earned his bachelor technology, master's of technology, and doctoral degrees in Radio Physics and Electronics, University of Calcutta, Kolkata, India, in 2002, 2005, and 2012, respectively. He is currently working as an associate professor in the Department of Avionics, Indian Institute of Space Science and Technology, Department of Space, Government of India. He has visited several international universities of repute, such as Royal Military College of Canada (RMC), Queens University, Ontario, Canada, from 2015 to 2018 in various capacities and having collaborative research with RMC Canada, Kingston, Ontario, and Queens University, Canada. He is a senior member of the IEEE, senior member of International Union of Radio Science, and a life member of IETE. He is the founding chairman of IEEE MTT-S Kerala chapter and has served as the chairman of the Antennas and Propagation Chapter of the IEEE Kerala section from 2018 to 2019. Saha has received several prestigious awards, including the national award *AICTE Visvesvaraya Best Teacher Award 2021* received from Union Education minister, Government of India; *IETE Prof. SN Mitra Memorial Award 2021, Outstanding Teacher Award* in 2019 from Department of Avionics, IIST; *National Scholarship from Ministry of Human Resource Development* from Government of India; *Outstanding Contribution Award* from the AP-MTT Kolkata chapter; *Best Contribution Award for Notable Services and Significant Contributions towards the Advancements of IEEE and the Engineering Profession* from IEEE Kolkata section; and several best paper awards at various international conferences. His current research interest includes wireless power transfer (WPT) and energy harvesting, channel modeling for WB/UWB systems, microwave circuits, engineered materials, metamaterial inspired antennas and circuits, reconfigurable and multifunctional antennas for modern wireless applications, mm-wave THz antennas, and antennas and components for space applications. He has published in more than 150 publications, including 40 journal papers in peer-reviewed national and international journals and conference proceedings and authored two books: *Basic Electronics: Principles and Applications* (2021, Cambridge University Press, UK) and *Multifunctional Ultrawideband Antennas* (2019, CRC Press, Taylor and Francis Group, Boca Raton, FL). He is on the board of reviewers of several international journals of repute including *IEEE Transaction in Microwave Theory and Techniques*; *IEEE Transaction in Antennas and Propagation*; *IEEE Antennas and Wireless Propagation Letters*; *IET Microwaves, Antennas and Propagation*; *Electronic Letters*; *Nature Scientific Reports*; and more. He is an associate editor of *IEEE Access* and *International Journal of RF and Microwave Computer Aided Engineering* and guest editor in chief for a special issue in the same journal.

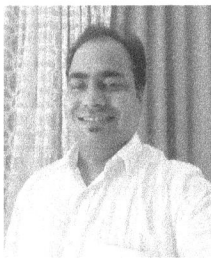

Rajan Jha earned his master of science degree and doctorate from IIT Delhi in 2001 and 2007, respectively; was a postdoctoral fellow at ICFO Barcelona from 2009 to 2010; and was a visiting scientist at TU Berlin in 2013. Currently, he is an associate professor at the Discipline of Physics, School of Basics Sciences at IIT Bhubaneswar, India. His research includes high-resolution interferometers and their combinations based multiparameter interrogation systems, flexible/wearable photonic systems, cavity resonator sensors, plasmon coupled configurations and nanoscale interaction platforms for quantum technologies. He is an inventor with eight patents and has published more than 110 international research articles and 75 conference papers. He was selected as an Optica (formerly OSA) ambassador and senior member in 2017. He was awarded DAAD Fellowship (2013) and the JSPS Fellowship (2009). He was a regular associate of the International Centre for Theoretical Physics, Italy (2016–2021) and young associate/member of all the science academies of India. For his breakthrough contribution in design and development of photonics devices and promotion of research activities in India, he is a recipient of the 2015 ICO/ICTP Gallieno Denardo award. Recently, he was awarded a SERB-STAR Fellowship (Physical Sciences) from the Government of India.

Preface

In the past decade, rapid development and globalization have brought healthcare issues to the fore. To date, healthcare problems have become the most essential and challenging issue worldwide. Demands for fast, reliable, accurate, and low-cost detecting methods and devices in biomedical industries have been growing rapidly in recent years, particularly in underdeveloped areas. In the field of health monitoring and diagnosis, plasmonic optical fiber sensors (P-OFSs) have shown extraordinary capabilities as highly sensitive and accurate sensors for the measurement of biological analytes. These sensors offer a unique capacity for real-time monitoring of molecular binding events. Plasmonics, thanks to various alluring features and applications, is a highly dynamic field catering to multifaceted research domains and naturally involves researchers, scientists, and engineers from diversified areas. Unprecedented acceleration in the realization of plasmonic nanostructures, deposition of thin films, and development of highly sensitive optical characterization techniques have been mainly propelled by advances in nanoscience and nanotechnology. Different approaches to nanostructuring metals have led to a wealth of interesting optical properties and functionality via manipulation of the plasmon modes that such structures support. The sensitivity of plasmonic structures to the changes in their local dielectric environment has led to the development of new sensing strategies and systems. Fiber-optic sensors/communications are necessary subjects that need to be deciphered by students and practitioners in electrical, electronics, and communication engineering. Linking plasmonic sensors with their applications in the biomedical field forms the basis of our book. This book presents the most widely employed approaches to sensing based on P-OFSs and the numerous biomedical applications associated with them.

ORGANIZATION OF THE BOOK

This book deals with recent advances in various plasmonics sensing techniques, detection schemes, their realization, configuration, components employed, and application of sensors. The coverage of the book encompasses the plasmonic phenomenon and its application in optical fiber-based sensing, broadly distributed over nine chapters. These chapters are systematically presented based on the use of nanomaterials (NMs), types of nanoparticles (NPs), and their size, shape, and composition. These chapters' overall focus on advances in NMs and structural designing extends the scope and expertise of rapid growth in biomedical applications. It also covers the synthesis, characterization, properties, and applications of NMs. The potential for optical technology to function as a basic phenomenon used for the development of highly sensitive optical fiber sensors is analyzed. The overall aim is to consider issues about future developments of biosensing devices and articulate methods through studies. Brief descriptions of each of the chapters follow.

Chapter 1 presents a brief overview and identifies the existing challenges in the plasmonic-based sensor for biomedical applications in the new millennium. Further, fundamentals of optical fiber-based plasmonic biosensors, plasmonic theory, different plasmonic sensing techniques, the development of fiber-optic plasmonic sensors, and applications of these sensors in different fields are presented in this study. In particular, the chapter identifies the major challenges and problems and discusses possible solutions. The purpose of this chapter is to discuss in depth the history, physics, fundamental principles, sensing technologies, and characterization of P-OFSs, which are primarily used for biosensing. This chapter provides a broad overview of biosensors, optical fiber sensors (OFSs) and surface plasmons, plasmon excitation using optical fiber, fiber-optic plasmonic techniques, and sensing parameters. Also discussed in this chapter are several of the most significant contributions that have been made in the field of P-OFSs.

Chapter 2 deals with the major development of synthesis methods and characterization of gold nanoparticles (AuNPs)-based P-OFSs. It also discusses the emphasis on recent advances, approaches to overcome the limitations, and future possibilities in the sensing field. The latest challenges in engineering and the role of AuNPs to enhance the performance of optical biosensors are discussed herein. Description of NMs and their potential for use in biosensing devices are provided in this chapter. Focus is placed on the use of nanoplasmonics in biosensors. Since the localized surface plasmonic resonance (LSPR) band is sensitive to particle size, shape, composition, and the surrounding medium, we present some innovative designs for label-free biosensors by modulating the parameters of NPs. This chapter also focuses on the process of fabricating, propagating, converting, and generating optical energy from metallic NPs, nanowires, nanorods, and other nonmetallic materials. Also described is the chronological progression of the various NMs used in the P-OFS development process. This chapter concludes by summarizing the current state of novel NMs and their role in the development of P-OFSs as well as possible future developments.

Chapter 3 describes the optical transduction mechanisms of P-OFSs with a variety of geometrical structures, as well as the photonic properties of the geometries. Brief literature reviews on the design and development of P-OFSs are presented. The focus here is on the structural, nanocoating, and characterization processes of P-OFSs, as well as the many applications, functions, and performance parameters. The fabrication methods and protocols used to produce P-OSF biosensors have been described. P-OFSs and a variety of related sensors are covered both in theory and in practice in this chapter. Furthermore, this part discusses innovative methods developed to improve the sensitivity, selectivity, and detection limit. As a result of advances in novel NMs, probe designs, and based sensing devices, rapid growth in biomedical applications are extending its scope and expertise.

Chapters 4 and 5 are dedicated to the gold nanoparticles (AuNPs) and silver nanoparticles (AgNPs) based P-OFSs, respectively. These NPs are attractive in the biosensing field due to their physicochemical properties and biological functionalities, including their high antimicrobial activity and nontoxic nature.

Graphene oxide (GO) and graphene derivatives, such as fluorinated graphene (fluorographene), oxidized graphene (graphene oxide), reduced graphene oxide (rGO), and graphene introduced by acetylenic chains, such as graphene and graphdiyne, are the novel NMs broadly used in development of various P-OFSs, which is discussed in Chapters 6 and 7. These new carbon materials, evolved from analytical and experimental investigations, can enhance properties of composite materials like elasticity, tensile strength, and conductivity. Further, such materials can be mixed with different polymers and other functional materials to realize various new phenomena.

The performance of the fiber-based tip sensor using GO-encapsulated AuNPs (GOE-AuNPs) is studied in Chapter 6. The tip sensor is easy to handle, can detect a small amount of analyte due to the small size of the sensing tip, can work in harsh environmental conditions, and provides a miniaturized, simplified solution. It has been found in our study that agglomeration of AuNPs broadens the absorbance spectra by more than 25%. Further, theoretically obtained absorbance spectra have been compared using Mie theory, and it is in agreement with experimental results. Therefore, GO has been used for its encapsulation. GOE-AuNPs have been deposited around the tip of plastic-cladded silica (PCS) fiber. The performance has been studied, and it was found that such a sensing system has a poor signal-to-noise ratio. To address the poor signal-to-noise ratio, GO-coated AuNPs have been studied in transmission mode. In fiber cladding, 1 cm in the middle of the 10-cm-long fiber is removed. The decladded site of the probe is treated with silane and is dipped in the GO-coated AuNP solution in order to immobilize these nanoparticles. The performance of the sensor has been studied in terms of sensitivity and resolution using a sucrose solution of different refractive indexes. Further, the work has been extended for biosensing, where the interaction of bovine serum albumin (BSA) with GO using AuNPs on optical fiber has been studied. The AuNPs are immobilized around the core of processed and functionalized optical fiber and then GO has been immobilized with the help of cysteamine. Further, to activate the –COOH functional group in GO, the GO-coated probe is dipped in EDC (1-ethyl-3-[3-dimethylaminopropyl]carbodiimide)/NHS (*N*-hydroxy-succinimide) solution. Further, a uric acid biosensor using AuNPs and GO functionalized micro-ball fiber sensor has been shown. The linearity response is in the range of 10 μM^{-1} mM UA concentrations.

The reflectance of the sensor linearly decreases with the increasing UA concentrations. To test the accuracy of the proposed sensor, the UA concentrations in serum samples have been compared with the automatic biochemical analyzer. Also, a novel periodically tapered structure-based AuNPs and GO-immobilized optical fiber sensor to detect ascorbic acid is reported.

Chapter 7 deals with the design and development of an optical fiber-based sensor using GOE-AgNPs. AgNPs are encapsulated with a very thin layer of GO, as it controls the interparticle distance, thereby preventing aggregation and oxidation. The high-resolution transmission electron microscopy (HRTEM) results support the formation of a very thin layer (~1 nm) of GO around AgNPs of average size 35 nm. Further, the GOE-AgNPs are immobilized on the core of the fiber for refractive index sensing. The theoretical calculation using Mie theory is in agreement with experimental results. Also, the work has been extended from single metallic to bimetallic NPs coated with GO. The absorbance obtained using an ultraviolet-visible (UV-Vis) spectrometer is compared theoretically and is in agreement with the experimental results. The electric field distribution for different NPs has been studied. Further, two distinct and well-separated plasmon bands at around 420 nm and 530 nm for AgNPs and AuNPs, respectively, are observed. To address the aggregation and stability of the mixture of AuNPs and AgNPs, and to prevent the AgNPs from oxidation, they are encapsulated with GO. Here two absorbance peaks increase with the analyte refractive index. The uniform and reproducible coating of metallic nanoparticles around the core of the optical fiber using a chemical method is difficult. Also, some of the limitations of intensity fluctuations can be addressed by a wavelength-based LSPR sensor using GO-coated Ag-island. The Ag-island is coated using a thermal evaporation technique to excite the LSPR field that is responsible for the analyte sensing through a shift in resonance wavelength. The usage of GO helps to protect the Ag-island from oxidation along with opening a new window for biosensing due to its structural compatibility with the biosensing system. In the last section, a GO-assisted AuNPs LSPR sensor is developed for detection of L-cysteine.

Chapter 8 describes the role of novel nanomaterials in the development of plasmonic optical fiber biosensors, major findings, and future trends in this area. Further, innovative methodologies that have been established to improve the sensitivity, selectivity, and detection limit are highlighted in this part. The overall focus on advances in novel nanomaterials, and based sensing devices, extends the scope and expertise of rapid growth in biomedical applications. This chapter presents the major development of zinc-oxide nanoparticles (ZnO-NPs) and copper-oxide nanoparticles (CuO-NPs) based on P-OFSors. These two chapters examine the ZnO and CuO-NP-based advanced developments and major challenges in the biosensing field. Chapter 8 discusses the recently developed variety of optical fiber-based biosensors for the detection and measurement of biomolecules such as creatinine, alanine aminotransferase enzyme, p-cresol, cardiac troponin I, acetylcholine, ascorbic acid, cholesterol, uric acid, and L-cysteine. The sensors have been fabricated using a variety of special fibers, including tapered optical fibers, fiber ball structures, single mode-multimode mismatch fibers, multicore fiber, photosensitive fiber, and tapered-in-tapered fiber structures. The tapered fiber/tapered-in-tapered structure is fabricated using a plasma technique-based combiner manufacturing machine. The remaining fiber sensor structures are developed using an advanced fusion splicer machine. To increase sensor sensitivity, a variety of novel nanoparticles are used, including AuNPs, AgNPs, MXene, molybdenum disulfide NPs, cerium oxide NPs, GO, CuO-NPs, and ZnO-NPs. Its synthesis and characterization are also discussed. After that, several specific enzymes are used to incorporate the selectivity property of the biosensors. An HRTEM, a scanning electron microscope (SEM), energy-dispersive spectroscopy (EDS), a UV-Vis spectrophotometer, and atomic force microscopy (AFM) are used to characterize the sensor structure. The sensor is based on the phenomenon of localized surface plasmon resonance that is caused by the immobilization of nanoparticles on the fiber structure. This chapter discusses the fabrication and development of optical fiber-based biosensors for clinical and everyday applications.

Chapter 9 discusses plasmonic fiber-optic biosensors that combine the flexibility and compactness of optical fibers with the high sensitivity of NMs and are applied in the environment to detect biological species such as cells and bacteria. Because of their small size, accuracy, low cost, and ability to perform remote and distributed sensing, plasmonic fiber-optic biosensors are promising alternatives to conventional biomolecule detection methods. They have the potential to benefit clinical diagnostics, drug discovery, food process control, disease detection, and environmental monitoring. Recent advances in cancer cell detection have resulted in the development of multi-core optical fiber-based biosensors. The culture process of six distinct normal and cancer cells is investigated, as is the detection of these cells using a newly developed sensor. *Shigella* bacteria that cause bacillary dysentery in developing countries are being detected using optical fiber biosensors. Additionally, this chapter discusses the fabrication of optical fiber sensors and the development of biosensors for the detection of cancer cells and other microorganisms through a cell culture process. The discussion will benefit researchers working in optical fiber technology and biosensing. The prospects of these studies are summarized in Chapter 9. The latest challenges in engineering and the role of different NMs (metallic, magnetic, carbon-based NMs, novel NPs, etc.) to enhance the performance of optical sensors are discussed herein; such information is possible in the context of providing a useful platform for the development of future plasmonic biosensors. The chapter's results are well verified, and it will be helpful for industry and academic concerns in better understanding and prototype development.

The authors thank CRC Press and, in particular, the editor who meticulously edited the book for publication.

Santosh Kumar
Niteshkumar Agrawal
Chinmoy Saha
Rajan Jha

Acknowledgments

The authors would like to express their most sincere gratitude and thanks to CRC Press, in particular the editor who meticulously edited the book for the publication. It has been extremely rewarding.

We are grateful to our colleagues for their wonderful input, both directly as contributors in this book or indirectly through discussions and suggestions. It has been a great pleasure working with them, and we trust they feel the same, too.

Santosh Kumar gratefully acknowledges the support from the Double-Hundred Talent Plan of Shandong Province, China. SK also thanks his students, Mr. Zhi Wang and Mr. Muyang Li, without whom this book would not have been compiled. SK would also like to express his heartfelt gratitude to his wife, Dr. Ragini Singh, and son, Ayaansh Singh, for their unwavering support, encouragement, and cooperation, as well as to his loving parents.

Dr. Agrawal thanks all the research scholars for their contributions generally. Moreover, Dr. Agrawal would like to express his heartfelt gratitude for the supportive, encouraging, and cooperative spirit of his wife Nitisha, daughter Erica, as well as his loving parents (Shri Subhashchandra Agrawal and Smt. Santoshi Agrawal) and all the other members of his family.

Rajan Jha gratefully acknowledges support from the SPARC fellowship and SERB STAR fellowship from the Government of India. RJ would like to thank all his research scholars for their research contributions and especially Dr. Pradeep Maharana and Dr. Jeeban Kumar Nayak who worked on plasmonics-based sensing systems. Further, RJ expresses his deep sense of appreciation for his wife Archana and children Samarth and Advika for their constant support and cooperation and gratitude to his loving parents (Shri Shambhu Nath Jha and Smt. Pramila Jha), in-laws (Shri Namonath Mishra and Smt. Kanti Devi), and all other family members.

Dr. Saha gratefully acknowledges support from the DST-SERB project and all the research scholars for their research contributions in general. Dr. Saha also would like to express his deep sense of appreciation for his wife Debarati and daughter Chitraupa (Rai) for their constant support, encouragement, and cooperation and gratitude to his loving parents (Shri Chittaranjan Saha and Smt. Shikha Saha) and caring mother-in-law (Smt. Chandrima Adhikari).

We hope that this book serves as a foundation for future advancements in the field and serves as a valuable reference for engineers, researchers, and students working in the fields of nano-optics, nanophotonics, plasmonics, and optical fiber biosensors.

Santosh Kumar, Niteshkumar Agrawal, Chinmoy Saha, and Rajan Jha

1 Fundamentals of Plasmonics Sensors

1.1 INTRODUCTION

The biosensor as a fantastic bridge can establish a connection between biological responses to electrical signals. It is a promising tool useful to detect and monitor the presence or interaction of active biomolecular substances: biomolecules, microorganisms, genetic structures, or insects (Mazhari, Agsar, and Prasad 2017; Mohanty and Kougianos 2006; Su et al. 2011). Biosensors are currently used exclusively in healthcare applications, as well as in many other areas like point-of-care (PoC) monitoring, disease progression in healthcare delivery, environmental testing, forensics, water management, food quality, medicine, drug discovery, and technical assessment (Srivastava and Khare 2021; Bhatt and Bhattacharya 2019; Gräwe et al. 2019). The major areas of applications for biosensors are presented in Figure 1.1. Charles Clark Jr., father of biosensors, first describes biosensor components for measuring blood oxygen density in his 1956 report (Thakur and Ragavan 2013). Further, he also proposed the experimental study over glucose sensors based on ampere-metric enzyme electrodes in 1962 (Yoo and Lee 2010). Figure 1.2 illustrates three generations of biosensors (Naresh and Lee 2021a). In its third generation, the biosensor molecule emerged as a vital part of the primary receptor element (i.e., biosensors continue to use enzymes and mediators on the same electrode). Between the enzyme and the electrode, the direct transfer is established by the movement of the electrons (Matthews, Andrews, and Patrick 2021). In addition, design cost and repeatability are likely the benefits of this generation of biosensors (Vigneshvar et al. 2016). In 1983, Lidberg identified real-time dependency reactions using SPR (Schasfoort 2017). At the next level, blood glucose levels were measured with a pen-size detector, proposed by Cambridge University, United States, in 1987 (Newman and Turner 2005). Typical biosensors development includes transducers (transform energy from one form to another—optically, electrochemically, thermally, or electronically), bioreceptors (that identify the analyte), electronics systems (processors and amplifiers), display, and analyte (i.e., substance or system to be detected), as shown in Figure 1.3. The well-known electrochemical transducer is most commonly applied in the detection of biomolecules, proteins, and cells (Anik 2017). Electrochemical biosensors are used in conjunction with high testing demand to perform electrochemical analysis (da Silva et al. 2017). But this electrochemical sensing system has limitations, such as short shelf life, sensory communication issues, and short life span (Grieshaber et al. 2008). Other biosensors viz. microelectrode (Llaudet et al. 2005), immunosensors (Luppa, Sokoll, and Chan 2001), magnetic (Llandro et al. 2010), thermometric (Zhou et al. 2013), piezoelectric (Narita et al. 2021), magneto-elastic (Guo et al. 2017), acoustic (Lakshmanan et al. 2020), quartz crystal microbalance (Lim et al. 2020), and optical biosensors (Naresh and Lee 2021b) have been reported along with some of the hybrid concepts of magneto-elastic, piezoelectric, and quartz crystal microbalance-based biosensors as shown in Figure 1.4. The different kinds of biosensors and common techniques employed are summarized in Table 1.1. These biosensors are diffusely used in multifarious significant fields like environmental studies, physical parameter measurements, clinical diagnostics (detection of bacteria/virus/DNA/RNA/cells), telemedicine, and bio-imaging (Castillo-Henríquez et al. 2020; Brooks and Alper 2021; Chen and Wang 2020). The diverse uses of plasmonic optical fiber sensors (OFSs) are presented in Figure 1.5.

DOI: 10.1201/9781003243199-1

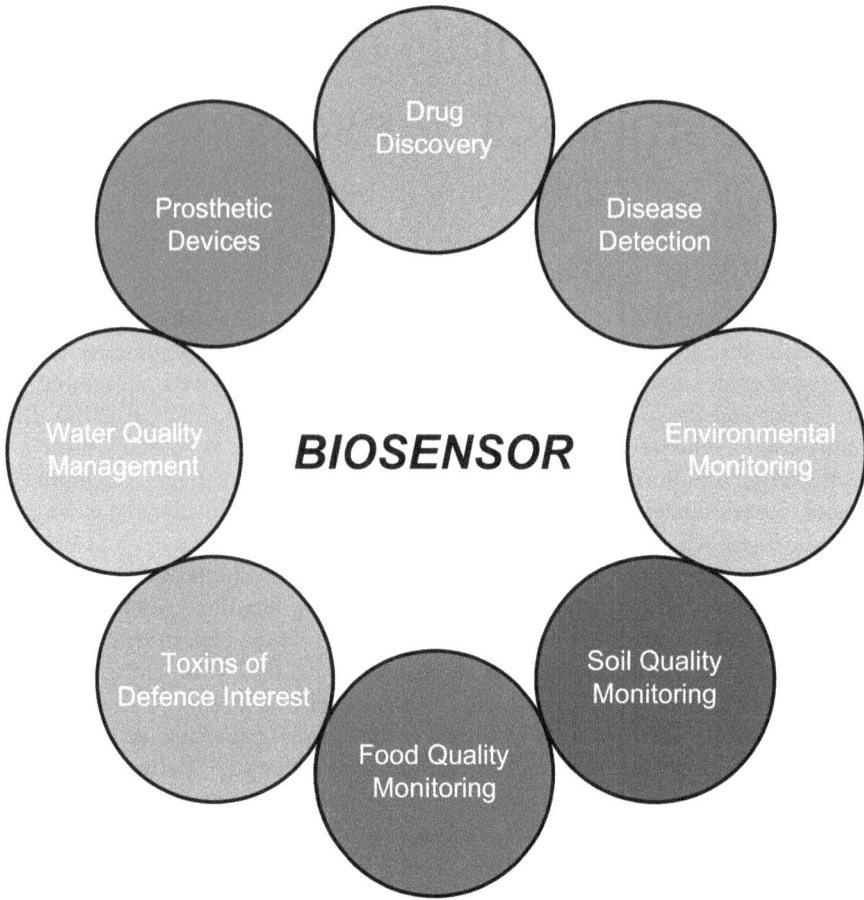

FIGURE 1.1   Major areas of applications for biosensors.

Source: Reprinted with permission from *Essays in Biochemistry*, Copyright 2021, Portland Press (Bhalla et al. 2016).

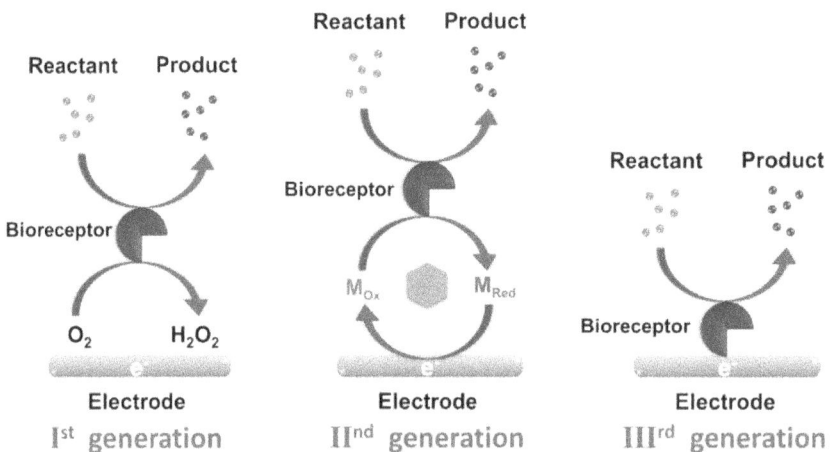

FIGURE 1.2   Three generations of the biosensor (Naresh and Lee 2021a).

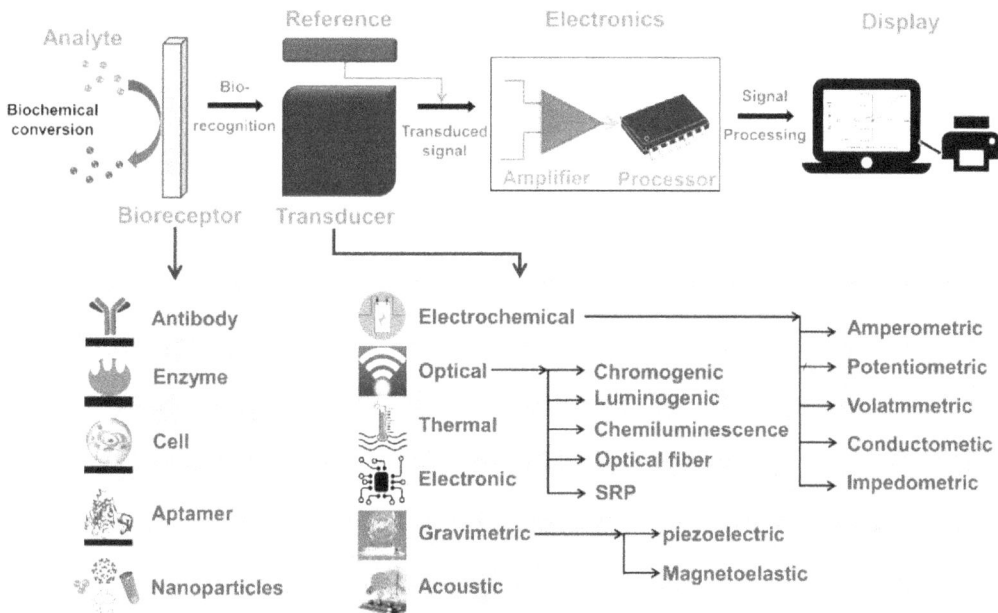

FIGURE 1.3   Typical biosensors (Naresh and Lee 2021a).

Various optical techniques have been used for biosensing: Raman (Tyler et al. 2009), evanescent wave absorption (Ruddy, MacCraith, and Murphy 1990), luminescence (Demas, DeGraff, and Coleman 1999), fluorescence (MacCraith et al. 1993), phosphorescence (Hase et al. 2002), interferometry (modal interferometry [Gu et al. 2009], white light interferometry [Totsu, Haga, and Esashi 2004]), and SPR (Sharma, Jha, and Gupta 2007). Out of these mentioned techniques, SPR has achieved more attention during the last few decades due to its label-free nature and enhanced performance (Homola 2008). SPR has broadly divided into propagating SPR (PSPR, commonly known as SPR) and localized SPR (LSPR). In both cases, the plasmonic field is very sensitive to the analyte present around it. Therefore, these label free systems are used for the refractive index (RI) sensing of a given analyte as it also offers advantages of overall high performance with real-time monitoring and fast response time.

In later years, the strange challenges of pandemics and diseases invaded like back-to-back storms around the world, and healthcare played an indispensable role and became an inescapable topic. Therefore, researchers must study, optimize, and develop new methods of early discovery and treatment that are fast, availably sensitive, transferable, and economical. This chapter presents an overview of biosensors, different biosensors reported in the past, along with the drawbacks and merits of different biosensors. In further sections, special emphasis is given on optic-plasmonic biosensors (i.e., basics of optics and plasmonic, the necessity of optic-plasmonic biosensors, different optic-plasmonic biosensing techniques, and various sensing parameters).

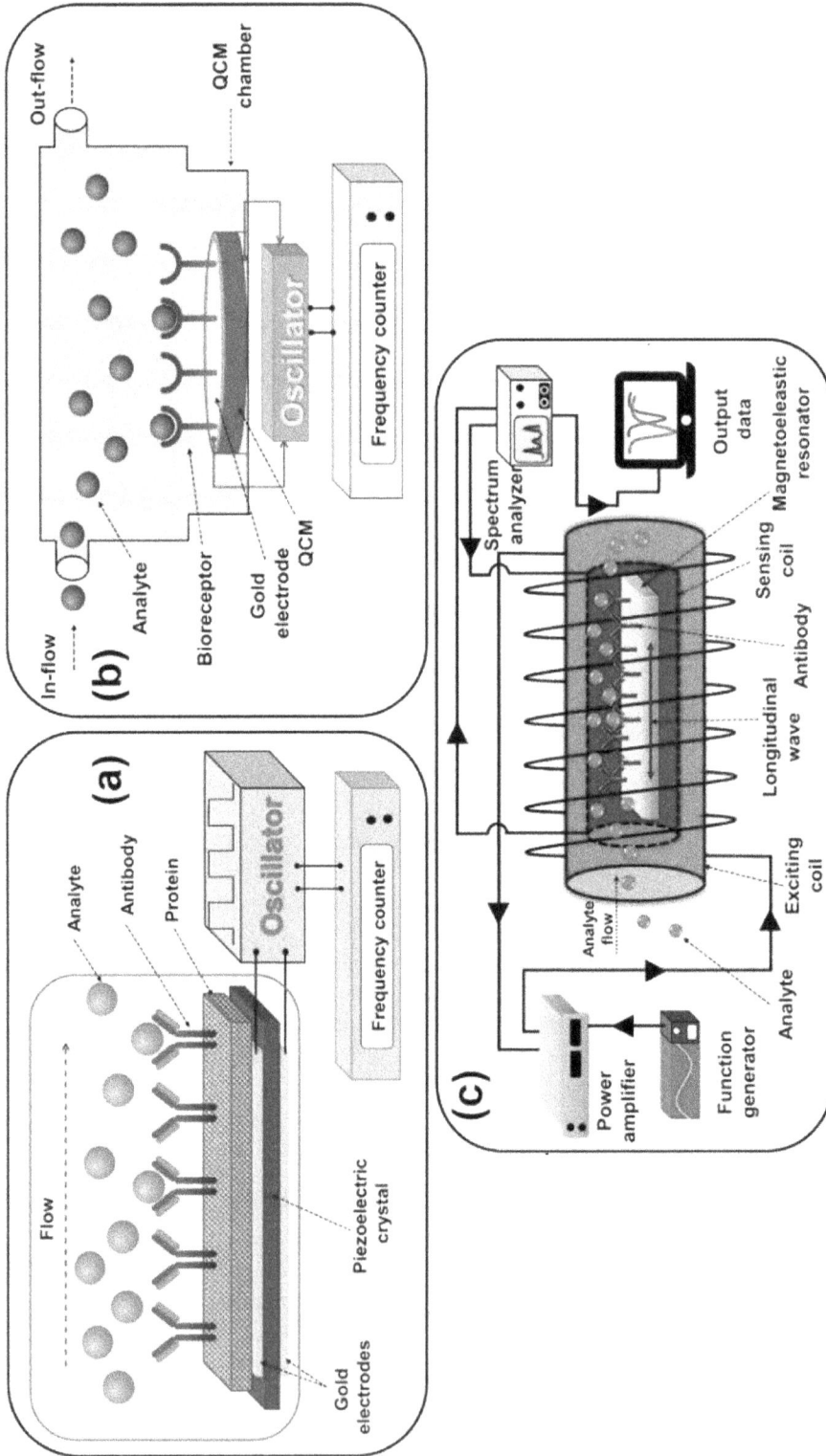

FIGURE 1.4 Experimental setup for magneto-elastic, piezoelectric, and quartz crystal microbalance-based biosensors (Naresh and Lee 2021a).

TABLE 1.1
Types of Biosensors and Common Techniques Employed

Type of biosensor	Common techniques employed	Change monitored	Bio-element	Detection element	Ref.
Electrochemical based system	Amperometric Potentiometric Conductometric	Ion concentration (electrical conductivity)	Enzyme Antibody Microbial cells Nucleic acid Others	Glucose (enzyme) CA 15-3 Antibody (breast cancer detection) *Pseudomonas putida* (microbial cells) SARS-CoV-2 (virus) RNA (nucleic acid) FAM134B protein Pesticides and heavy metal toxicants in water Environmental contaminants	Zhu et al. 2015 Selwyna, Loganathan, and Begam 2013 Kim et al. 2003 Mojsoska et al. 2021 Ellington and Szostak 1990 Islam et al. 2017 Hara and Singh 2021 Khanmohammadi et al. 2020
Calorimetric-based system	Thermistors	Temperature	Enzyme Others	Glucose, hydrogen peroxide, and urea (enzyme) Toxic industrial chemicals	Zhang and Tadigadapa 2004 Feng et al. 2010
Piezoelectric-based system	Resonance frequency Surface transverse and acoustic wave	Resonant frequency	Nucleic acid like DNA and RNA Antibodies Others	Albuminuria (antibody) *Francisella tularensis* (antibody) *Escherichia coli* (bacteria) DNA (nucleic acid) Dengue (virus)	Pohanka 2018 Pohanka and Skládal 2007 Guo et al. 2012 Kirimli, Shih, and Shih 2014 Chen et al. 2009
Optical	SPR LSPR Potentiometric Interferometric Fluorescent	Absorbance/ optical parameters	Enzymes Antibody Cells Aptamer Nucleic acid Others	Ascorbic acid (enzyme) IgG (antibody) Cancel cells (cells) Mycotoxins (aptamer) Nucleic acid Collagen-IV Malaria	Zhu, Singh, et al. 2020 Tran et al. 2020 Singh et al. 2020 Guo et al. 2020 Bonyár 2020 Kaushik et al. 2020 Chaudhary, Kumar, and Kumar 2021

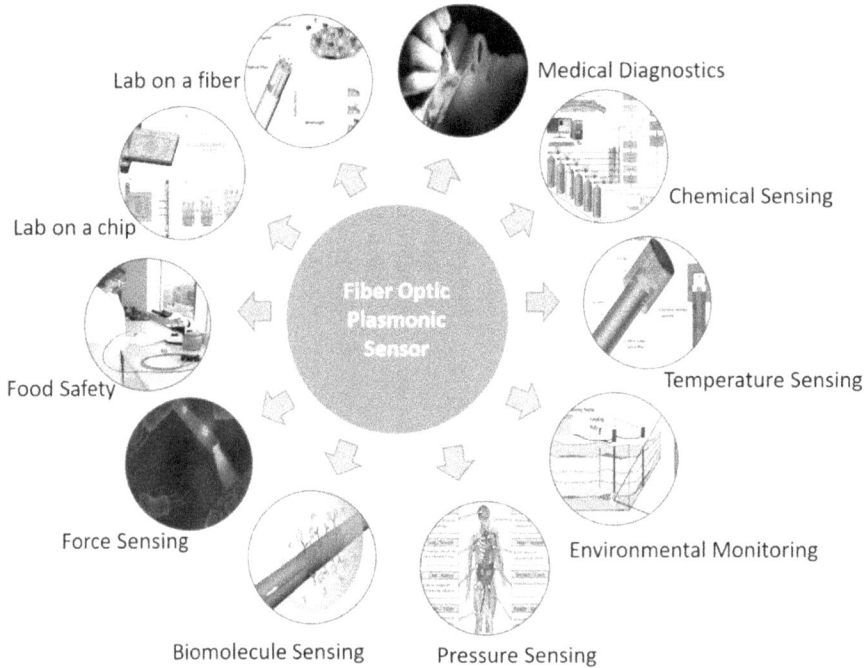

FIGURE 1.5   Diverse applications of plasmonic fiber-optic sensors (Aruna Gandhi et al. 2019).

1.2   FUNDAMENTALS OF FIBER-OPTIC SENSORS AND RELATED CONCEPTS

The gradual success of optical fibers has been possible through a series of discoveries. The different phenomena that gave rise to the milestones of optical fibers involve the demonstration of the optical telegraph in the eighteenth century, light guidance using total internal reflectance (TIR) by Jean-Daniel Colladon in 1840, optical photo phone by Graham Bell in 1880, and fiberscope in 1950 (Goff 2003). The scope of application of optical fiber took a quantum jump after the invention of lasers and light-emitting diodes. The modern era of optical fibers began with the development of fiber with lower index cladding (Goff 2003). This was followed by invention of a low loss fiber (20 dB/Km) as proposed by Charles K. Kao (Goff 2003; Kao and Hockham 1966; Chack, Agrawal, and Raghuwanshi 2014). Since this invention, the use of optical fibers has created a new era not only in the field of telecommunications but also in optical sensors networks (Perez-Herrera and Lopez-Amo 2013). Optical fiber research and applications increased during the 1970s. Fiber-optic sensors (OFSs) with widespread numerous applications appeared due to their exclusive characteristics like chemical inertness, multiplexing, immunity to electromagnetic (EM) fields, and increased efficiency (Roriz et al. 2020a). Due to all these advantages, the use of OFSs is becoming very popular in the real world, especially in the medical diagnostics field (Angelov et al. 2019). The various advantages of OFSs are broadly categorized in three sections as summarized in Table 1.2. The OFSs are classified largely based on their function, working principle, modulation method, and measurable spatial scope (Roriz et al. 2020b). The main applications of OFSs such as temperature (Drusová et al. 2021), flow (Ganguly and Mondal 2011), torsion (Budinski and Donlagic 2017), bending (Niu et al. 2021), vibration (García, Corres, and Goicoechea 2010), pressure (Paulo et al. 2013), chemical (Pospíšilová, Kuncová, and Trögl 2015; Wolfbeis and Weidgans 2006), humidity (Mitschke 1989), RI (Takeo and Hattori 1982), magnetic field (Alberto et al. 2018), and biomolecular detection (Agrawal, Zhang, Saha, Kumar, Kaushik et al. 2020) have been carefully studied and combined with different research groups (Fidanboylu and Efendioglu 2009). Different

TABLE 1.2

Summary of Advantages of Optical Fiber System With Respect to Design, Environment, and Others

Design	Environment	Others
Chemical inertness	Chemical resistant	Biocompatible and sterilization
Robust packaging	Cryogenic to high temperature	Lightweight
Light power	Immunity to EM fields	Intrinsically safe
Small dimensions	In situ monitoring	Cheaper
Less attenuation	Remote monitoring	Capability of multiplexing

TABLE 1.3

Categorization of Optical Fiber Systems Under Different Categories

Applications	Measurable spatial scope	Modulation process	Working principle
Temperature	Point sensors	Intensity	Interferometry
Strain	Quasi-distributed sensors	Phase	Fluorescence
Displacement	Distributed sensors	Polarization	Plasmonics
Current		Wavelength shift	Raman scattering, Rayleigh
Torsion			scattering, and Brillouin
Vibration			scattering
Pressure			
Humidity			
Bending			
RI			
Magnetic fields Chemicals and biomolecules			

types of sensors measuring at a point sensor or are quasi-distributed or full distributed are classified in measurable spatial scope-based OFSs (Joe et al. 2018), whereas changes in phase, polarization, and wavelength are classified in modulation process-based OFSs (Fidanboylu and Efendioglu 2009). The fiber designs have been modified and processed to develop different, new classes of of fiber-based structures like fiber Bragg grating (FBG) (Jin et al. 2006), long period grating (LPG) (Mishra, Lohia, and Dwivedi 2020), tilted FBG (TFBG) (Guo et al. 2016), Fabry-Pérot interferometer (FPI), Sagnac interferometer (SI), chirped FBG (CFBG) (Tosi 2018), Michelson interferometer, high birefringence loop mirror, Mach-Zehnder, U-shaped (Tan et al. 2020), D-shaped (Melo et al. 2018), plus-shaped cavity (Singh, Agrawal, Saha, Singh, et al. 2022; Singh, Agrawal, Saha, and Kaushik 2022), hetero-core (Agrawal, Zhang, Saha, Kumar, Pu et al. 2020), and tapered probe (Zhu, Agrawal et al. 2020) OFSs to name some of the major systems. Various OFSs are widely employed in biosensing applications and are divided based on their application, modulation process, working principle, and measurable spatial scope, which are presented in tabular form in Table 1.3. Above all mentioned biosensors, P-OFSs have had a significant impact in both laboratory research and clinical diagnostics due to their fast and consistent detection characteristics (Shrivastav, Cvelbar, and Abdulhalim 2021). Several researchers, scientists, and people from multidisciplines are involved in the development of P-OFSs for biosensing applications. To understand the process involved in the working of P-OFSs for biosensing, lets us first understand the fundamental concepts related to optical fiber and evanescent wave in the next section.

1.2.1 Total Internal Reflection and Evanescent Wave

The confinement or availability of an optical field near current or oscillating charges forms the genesis of an evanescent wave. Evanescent is derived from *evanescere*, the Latin word, and it means "vanishing." According to the form $E_0\exp[i(k.r\text{-}\omega t)]$ of plane waves, these mentioned fields can be well described and at least one part of the wave vector indicates the direction of propagation (k) as an imaginary portion. This means the wave is not propagating but rather decays exponentially as shown in Figure 1.6. This section discusses in detail the fundamental principle of evanescent waves (EWs) and its application in experiments.

Let's consider a transverse magnetic (TM) polarized light traveling from a denser medium (n_1) to an optically rarer medium (n_2) as shown in Figure 1.6. The plane of incidence is lying on the XZ plane, and the two semi-infinite mediums form an interface along the X-axis at Z = 0. In Figure 1.6, θ_i represents the incidence angle, θ_r represents the reflection angle, and θ_t is the angle of transmission with the normal. Snell's law allows us to calculate the angle of transmission of light from one medium to another medium. In our case, light is traveling from an optically denser (n_1) to a rarer medium (n_2). From Snell's law,

$$n_1 \sin\theta_i = n_2 \sin\theta_t \tag{1.1}$$

$$\theta_t = \sin^{-1}\left(\frac{n_1}{n_2}\sin\theta_i\right) \tag{1.2}$$

As $n_1 > n_2$, then n_1/n_2 is more than one. According to Eq. (1.1), if θ_i increases, then θ_t also increases, and finally it becomes 90° corresponding to an incident angle, which is called a critical angle (θ_c) as given in Eq. (1.3). At critical angle of incidence, the angle of transmission is 90° and the transmitted light grazes the interface.

$$\theta_i = \theta_{critical} = \sin^{-1}\left(\frac{n_2}{n_1}\right) \tag{1.3}$$

As angle of incidence increases gradually from 0° to θ_c, the transmitted light becomes dimmer and dimmer and finally it becomes zero and the reflected light becomes maximum intense (i.e., 100%). This phenomenon is called total internal reflection (TIR). When θ_i increases beyond θ_c then $n_1\sin\theta_i/n_2$ in Eq. (1.2) becomes greater than one and $\sin\theta_t$ becomes greater than one, which shows that $\cos\theta_t$ becomes a complex quantity. Hence, the reflection coefficient for perpendicular (r_s) and parallel (r_p) component of electric fields (for a TM polarized light) become complex quantity as observed from below Eq. (1.4).

$$r_s = \frac{n_1 \cos\theta_i - n_2 \cos\theta_t}{n_1 \cos\theta_i + n_2 \cos\theta_t} \text{ and } r_p$$
$$= \frac{n_2 \cos\theta_i - n_1 \cos\theta_t}{n_2 \cos\theta_i + n_1 \cos\theta_t} \tag{1.4}$$

Beyond critical angle, all values of incident angle $\cos\theta_t$ become complex, and the reflectances ($R_s = r_s.r_s^* = 1$ and $R_p = r_p.r_p^* = 1$) become unity giving rise to 100% reflectance as shown in Figure 1.7. So, all the power gets reflected, and there exists no transmitted light in the rarer medium. But this boundary condition is in the color of violets (i.e., the tangential component of electric field across boundary of two media should be continuous). So, there should be a tangential component of the electric field in the rarer medium at the interface corresponding to the tangential component of the electric field in the denser medium at the interface for the boundary condition to be valid. Hence, for the validity of the boundary condition, there must be transmitted light in the rarer medium beyond critical angle. As soon in Figure 1.6, the wave vector (K_t) of transmitted light must have X- and Z-components and are given by $k_t \sin\theta_t$ and $k_t \cos\theta_t$, respectively, where $k_t \cos\theta_t$ is purely imaginary and $k_t \sin\theta_t$ is purely real. Hence, the wave vector of transmitted light is as shown in Figure 1.7.

$$\overline{K_t} = k_t \sin\theta_t \hat{x} + k_t \cos\theta_t \hat{z} = k_x \hat{x} + ik_z \hat{z} \tag{1.5}$$

Here, $k_t = 2\pi n_2/\lambda$, $k_x = k_t \sin\theta_t$, $ik_z = k_t \cos\theta_t$, and k_z is a real number. This shows that the wave vector of the transmitted light beyond the critical angle of incidence is a complex quantity, and the transmitted wave in the rarer medium is given by

$$E_t(x,z,t) = tE_{0i} \exp\left[i(K_t r - \omega t)\right] = tE_{0i} \exp\left[i\left\{(k_x \hat{x} + ik_z \hat{z}) \times (x\hat{x} + z\hat{z}) - \omega t\right\}\right]$$
$$\Rightarrow E_t(x,z,t) = tE_{0i} \exp(-k_z z) \exp\left[i(k_x x - \omega t)\right] \tag{1.6}$$

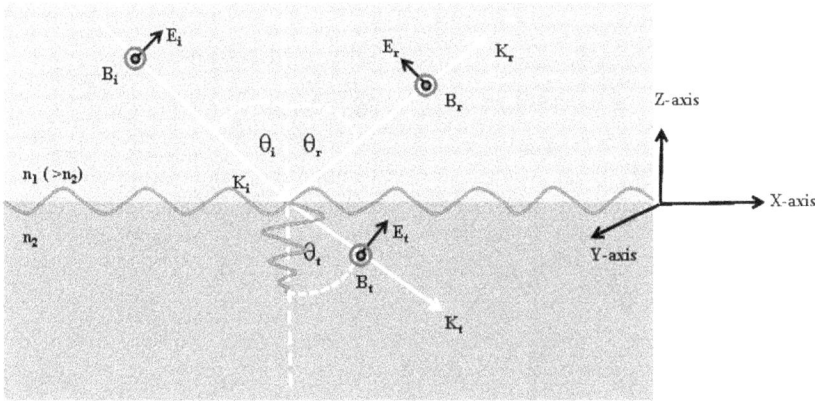

FIGURE 1.6 Total internal reflection and formation of an evanescent wave at and beyond a critical angle of incidence.

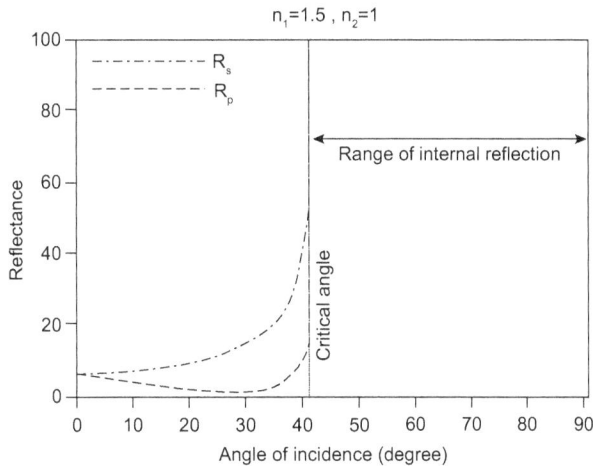

FIGURE 1.7 Variation of reflectance for the parallel component (also called "p" type) and the perpendicular component (also called "s" type) of electric field with angle of incidence at the interface for TM polarized light passing from denser (of refractive index 1.5) to rarer medium (air).

From Eq. (1.6), one can observe that the transmitted wave exponentially decays from the interface and is a free propagating wave along the interface (*x*-direction). Therefore, the transmitted wave (the evanescent wave) does not carry any energy from the interface. By placing a high RI material in the presence of an evanescent wave, power can be coupled through a low RI gap by the phenomenon of Fourier transform infrared. In order to understand how these evanescent fields excite surface plasmons (SPs), the following sections deal with the dispersion characteristics of SPs.

1.2.2 SURFACE PLASMONS

SPs are TM polarized. The field distribution of SPs is shown in Figure 1.8. Mathematically, the electric fields and magnetic fields in any of the given medium Z > 0 (sensing layer) and Z < 0 (metal) are given by

$$Z>0, \begin{cases} H_s = \left(0, H_{ys}, 0\right)\exp\ i\left(K_{xs}x + K_{zs}z - \omega t\right) \\ E_s = \left(E_{xs}, 0, E_{zs}\right)\exp\ i\left(K_{xs}x + K_{zs}z - \omega t\right) \end{cases} \tag{1.7}$$

$$Z<0 \begin{cases} H_m = \left(0, H_{ym}, 0\right)\exp\ i\left(K_{xm}x + K_{zm}z - \omega t\right) \\ E_d = \left(E_{xm}, 0, E_{zm}\right)\exp\ i\left(K_{xm}x + K_{zm}z - \omega t\right) \end{cases} \tag{1.8}$$

Here, E_{xs} and E_{zs} are electric fields along *X*- and *Z*-directions in the sensing layer, and H_{ys} is the magnetic field intensity along the *Y*-direction in the sensing layer. Similarly, E_{xm} and E_{zm} are electric fields along the *X*- and *Z*-directions in the metal, and H_{ym} is the magnetic field intensity along *Y*-direction in the metal. Maxwell's equations in medium $i(i$ = metal [*m*] or sensing layer [*s*]) are given by

$$\begin{cases} \nabla.\varepsilon_i\,E = 0 \\ \nabla.H = 0 \\ \nabla \times E = -\mu_0 \dfrac{\partial H}{\partial t} \\ \nabla \times H = \varepsilon_i \dfrac{\partial E}{\partial t} \end{cases} \tag{1.9}$$

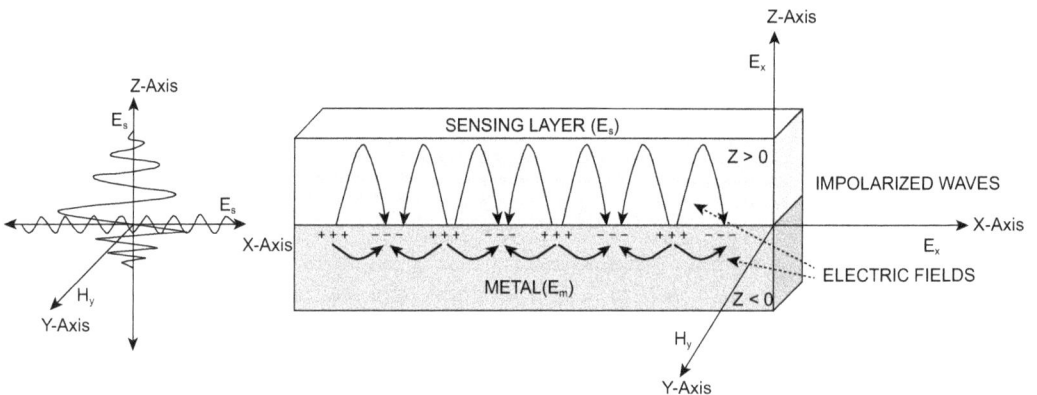

FIGURE 1.8   Surface plasmon field distribution in the *XZ*-plane at the metal-sensing layer interface.

where the tangential component of E_x, H_y are in forms of continuity at the boundary ($z=0$). Therefore, the normal component of D_z demands that $E_{xm} = E_{xs}$, $H_{ym} = H_{ys}$ and $\varepsilon_m E_{zm} = \varepsilon_s E_{zs}$. Evaluating curl of H_i, one can obtain,

$$\left(\frac{\partial H_{zi}}{\partial y} - \frac{\partial H_{yi}}{\partial z}, \frac{\partial H_{xi}}{\partial z} - \frac{\partial H_{zi}}{\partial x}, \frac{\partial H_{yi}}{\partial x} - \frac{\partial H_{xi}}{\partial y} \right) = \left(-iK_{zi}H_{yi}, 0, iK_{xi}H_{yi} \right) = \left(-i\omega\varepsilon_i E_{xi}, 0, -i\omega\varepsilon_i E_{zi} \right)$$

$$\Rightarrow K_{zi}H_{yi} = \omega\varepsilon_i E_{xi}$$

$$\Rightarrow \begin{cases} K_{zm}H_{ym} = \omega\varepsilon_m E_{xm} \\ K_{zs}H_{ys} = \omega\varepsilon_d E_{xs} \end{cases}$$

$$\Rightarrow \frac{K_{zm}}{\varepsilon_m}H_{ym}$$

$$= \frac{K_{zs}}{\varepsilon_s}H_{ys}$$

(1.10)

Taking the continuity of tangential components E_x (i.e., $E_{xm} = E_{xs}$) and H_y (i.e., $H_{ym} = H_{ys}$) across the boundary ($z = 0$) along with Eq. (1.10), one can obtain,

$$\frac{K_{zm}}{\varepsilon_m} = \frac{K_{zs}}{\varepsilon_s}$$

(1.11)

Eq. (1.10) fulfills the surface plasmon condition to exist at a metal-dielectric interface. Using the continuity of tangential components E_x and H_y at metal-interface ($z = 0$) results in $K_{xm} = K_{xs}$. So for any medium i, the propagation vector of the electromagnetic wave will be given by

$$K^2 = \varepsilon_i \left(\frac{\omega}{c} \right)^2 = K_x^2 + K_{zi}^2, \quad \text{where,} \quad K_{xm} = K_{xs} = K_x$$

(1.12)

$$K_x^2 = \varepsilon_i \left(\frac{\omega}{c} \right)^2 - K_{zi}^2$$

(1.13)

where K_x is the surface plasmon propagation constant value (PC-value) along the x-direction, inside both the metal and sensing layers. With the help of Eq. (1.13), one can write

$$\varepsilon_m \left(\frac{\omega}{c} \right)^2 - K_{zm}^2 = \varepsilon_s \left(\frac{\omega}{c} \right)^2 - K_{zs}^2$$

(1.14)

Solving Eq. (1.14) with the help of Eq. (1.11), one can have

$$K_x = \frac{\omega}{c} \sqrt{\frac{\varepsilon_m \varepsilon_s}{\varepsilon_m + \varepsilon_s}}$$

(1.15)

and

$$K_{zm} = \frac{\omega}{c} \sqrt{\frac{\varepsilon_m^2}{\varepsilon_m + \varepsilon_s}}, K_{zs} = \frac{\omega}{c} \sqrt{\frac{\varepsilon_s^2}{\varepsilon_m + \varepsilon_s}}$$

(1.16)

Surface plasmon waves (SPWs) are characterized by free propagating nature along the interface (i.e., along x-axis) and decaying nature along normal to interface (i.e., along z-axis). The propagating nature of SPW forces K_x to be positive real number for which,

$$\frac{\varepsilon_m \varepsilon_s}{\varepsilon_m + \varepsilon_s} = +ve \tag{1.17}$$

The decaying nature of SPW forces K_{zm} and K_{zs} to be purely imaginary for which,

$$\begin{cases} \dfrac{\varepsilon_m^{\,2}}{\varepsilon_m + \varepsilon_s} = -ve \\[3mm] and \ \dfrac{\varepsilon_s^{\,2}}{\varepsilon_m + \varepsilon_s} = -ve \end{cases} \tag{1.18}$$

Eqs. (1.17) and (1.18) can only be satisfied if and only if the numerical values of $\varepsilon_m \varepsilon_s$ and $\varepsilon_m + \varepsilon_s$ are both negative, simultaneously. This restricts ε_m to be large negative (i.e., $\varepsilon_m \ll 0$) and ε_s to be small positive (i.e., $\varepsilon > 0$). Therefore, K_{sp} (surface plasmon wave vector) can be represented as

$$K_{sp} = \left[\frac{\omega}{c} \left(\frac{\varepsilon_m \varepsilon_s}{\varepsilon_m + \varepsilon_s} \right)^{1/2} \right] = Re\left(K_{sp} \right) + Im\left(K_{sp} \right) = K_x + Im\left(K_{sp} \right)$$

where

$$Re\left(K_{sp} \right) = \left[\frac{\omega}{c} \left(\frac{\varepsilon_{mr} \varepsilon_s}{\varepsilon_{mr} + \varepsilon_s} \right)^{1/2} \right]$$

$$Im\left(K_{sp} \right) = \left[\frac{\omega}{c} \left(\frac{\varepsilon_{mr} \varepsilon_s}{\varepsilon_{mr} + \varepsilon_s} \right)^{3/2} \right] \left(\frac{\varepsilon_{mi}}{2\varepsilon_{mr}^2} \right) \tag{1.19}$$

1.2.2.1 Definition of Surface Plasmon

Surface plasmons are defined as a collective oscillation of the free electrons (COFE) propagating at the boundary among a metal and a dielectric, which is dwindling and indicated in the orientation perpendicular to the boundary (Maier 2007). A metal (charge neutral) is consisting of a collection of lattice ions surrounded by free electrons. By applying an electric field, a density of free electrons tries to stretch off the lattice ion in an orientation opposite to that of electric vector, creating a dipole. The lattice ion with heavier mass and positive charge tries to pull the negatively charged free electron density toward it. The repetition of pulling and stretching of a free electron cloud from the lattice ion with an incident-controlled electric field leads to the COFE in a metal, which is known as plasmon. Plasmon can be surface plasmon or bulk/volume plasmon, depending on the dimension of the plasmon active metal. Bulk plasmon occurs when the dimensions of the plasmon active metal in all three directions are larger as compared to the wavelength of incident light. However, the surface plasmon occurs for the semi-infinite metal for which one dimension is suitable, compared to the incident light wavelength in which the surface plasmon wave propagates. In the case of bulk plasmon, the plasmon wave propagates throughout the metal volume. For bulk plasmons, the plasmon oscillations take place at the plasma frequency,

$$E_p = \hbar \sqrt{\frac{ne^2}{m\varepsilon_0}} \tag{1.20}$$

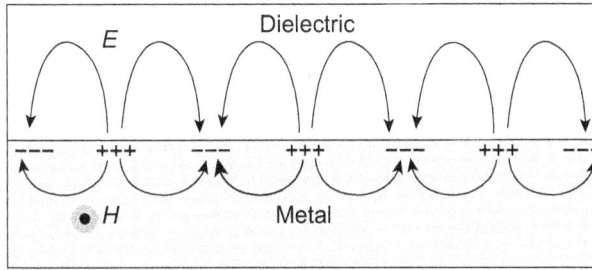

FIGURE 1.9 Surface plasmons at the interface of a metal and dielectric, the curve shows the electric field.

Here, E_p is the energy of plasmons, n is the density of electron, ε_0 is the permittivity of free space, e is the charge of the electron, and m is the mass of electron. At the metal SPs take the form of an SPs wave as shown in Figure 1.9, also simply called SPs.

1.2.2.2 Brief History of Surface Plasmons

In 1957, Ritchie predicted that collective excitations of electrons can be self-sustained at metal surfaces, if fast electrons penetrate into thin metal films (Ritchie 1957). Pines and Bohm (Pines 1956; Pines and Bohm 1952) mentioned that the physical laws of the Coulomb interaction among valence electrons within metals that cause the collective plasma oscillations and the proposed phenomenon here were similar to Tonks and Langmuir's predication about the electron-density oscillations in electrical discharges in gases (Fried and Gould 1961). This explained the early experimental demonstration by Ruthemann and Lang (Ruthemann 1948, 1942), when they bombarded the thin metallic films by fast moving electrons. Further, by conducting experiments related to electron energy loss, Powell and Swan (Ruthemann 1942; Powell and Swan 1959) mentioned the collective electron oscillations. However, it was Stern and Ferrell who gave a new term to quanta of collective excitations as the surface plasmon (Stern and Ferrell 1960).

1.2.3 GENERATION OF PROPAGATING SURFACE PLASMONS BY LIGHT USING THIN METALLIC FILM

SPs in metal were engendered by photons (electromagnetic radiation) or electrons (electron beam). By moving the electron beam parallel and perpendicular toward the metallic outer layer, one can excite the SP. Using the high-quality scanning electron microscope (SEM), perpendicular excitation of SPs has been widely studied, and this has helped in enriching the application of SEM further. However, parallel excited SPs, here, were applied to build coherent and tunable radiation. A SPs coupling to a photon is known as surface plasmon polariton (SPP).

To generate SPs or PSP at the metal dielectric interface, a suitable condition (i.e., the conservation of momentum [$p = \hbar k$] between the incident light and surface plasmon is required). Further, the generation of SPs wave is meaningless if the surface plasmon field cannot be investigated for different applications. Therefore, single interface geometry is required to modify. The simplest approach is to introduce a second interface, and the configurations are known as well-known Otto (Otto 1968) and Kretschmann's (Kretschmann and Raether 1968) configurations. In both configurations, the momentum matching condition is given by

$$\frac{\omega}{c}\sqrt{\varepsilon_p}\sin\theta_{res} = \frac{\omega}{c}\sqrt{\frac{\varepsilon_m\varepsilon_s}{\varepsilon_m + \varepsilon_s}} \tag{1.21}$$

where ε_p represents the prism dielectric constant, ε_s represents the dielectric constant in the sensing area, c is the velocity of light in air, ω represents the angular frequency of incident light, and θ_{res}

describes the resonance angle. In the left side of Eq. (1.21), this part represents the momentum of the incident light, and momentum of SPs is given on the right-hand side of Eq. (1.21). However, these momentum matching requires some high-index material like a prism. To understand how plasmons can be excited, here we discuss briefly a widely used Kretschmann's configuration.

1.3 KRETSCHMANN'S CONFIGURATION

In the beginning, the SPR sensing system was discussed and studied by coating a suitable metal film of plasmon active metal (mostly silver/gold) on the prism base (Kumar et al. 2022). However, if a small interstice exists on the metal film to the optical prism as proposed by Otto, and named the Otto configuration (Otto 1968), it is not suitable from a practical point of view. Therefore, in 1971, a modified Otto configuration, also known as a Kretschmann configuration, was proposed where a metallic layer was deposited on the prism base and the system under investigation called an analyte/sample/dielectric medium/sensing medium is in direct touch with the optimized thin metal films. Here, the schematic diagram of the modified Otto configuration (i.e., Kretschmann configuration) is shown in Figure 1.10, where ~50-nm metallic layer is deposited on a prism base of a higher RI. Here, the prism is used as a coupling medium, and the metallic layer is used to generate using a form of EWs that get leakage at the interface of prism-metal (P-M) active through attenuated total reflection (ATR). However, the property of the incident light is important, and one requires transverse magnetic polarization applied to the vibrancy of the surface plasmon. Here, at the condition that the incident light is TM polarized, the magnetic field vector of the incident electromagnetic radiation should be normal (in Z-direction) to the plane of incidence (in XY-plane), as shown in Figure 1.10.

If the angle of TM-polarized light at the juncture is equal to or greater than the angle $\theta_{critical}$, the EWs here are generated at the P-M layer juncture that penetrates the metal film and generates SPs from the metal-sensing layer (analyte) border. The manifestation of the SPs from this analyte border

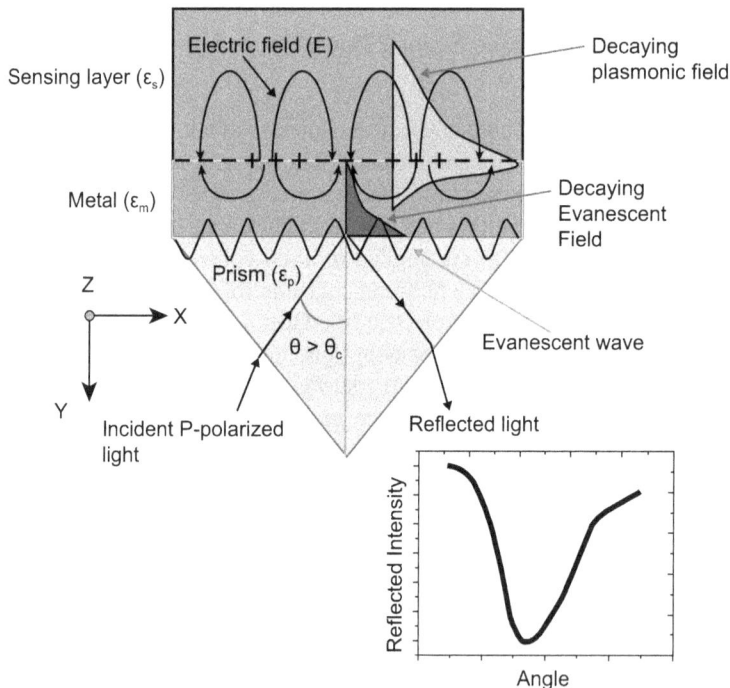

FIGURE 1.10 Kretschmann's configuration.

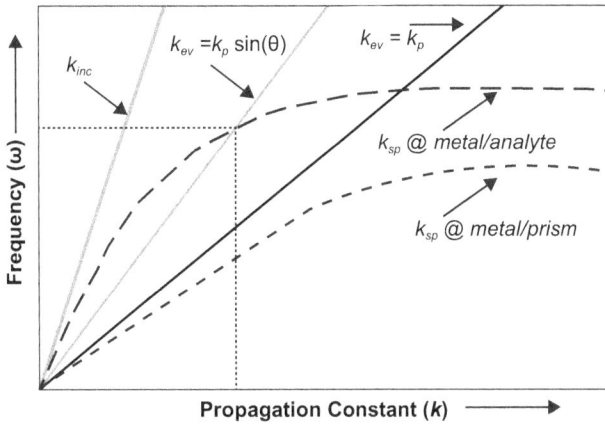

FIGURE 1.11 Dispersion curves for direct light wave in dielectric (k_{inc}), evanescent wave (k_{ev}), and surface plasmon (k_{sp}) at the metal/analyte layer border and at the metal/prism border.

by coupling element can be best understood from the propagation constant (PC)-value dispersion relation for SPs and direct light through the coupling element as shown in Figure 1.11.

The PC-value curves corresponding to SPs (K_{sp} at the metal-analyte interface) and wave vector of evanescent wave (K_{ev}) lie between $K_{ev} = K_p sin\theta$ and $K_{ev} = K_p$ (i.e., as discriminative incidence angle and frequency [θ, ω]), where K_p refers to the PC-value in the prism. Further, no incitement of SPs at the P-M border appeared here as the surface plasmon wave (SPW) PC-value for the M-P border is situated at the right side of the maximum PC-value of EWs ($Kev = K_p$), and the curves do not overlap. As can be observed in Figure 1.11, the existence of SPs is subject to equalization of the PC-value of EWs with that of SPs. This situation can be called SPR and is characterized by recession of RI of the reflected light in Figure 1.11. Through Fresnel's equations, the relationship between the minimum normalized RI of the three-layer system (P-M-sensing layer) can be clearly qualitatively analyzed. At the particular wavelength of incident light and dielectric function of metal along with the sensing layer, at a certain angle, the resonance condition is reached and is called the resonance angle (θ_{spr}). Here, it may be emphasized that the resonance angle (θ_{spr}) is sensitive to sensing layer RI ($n_s = \sqrt{\varepsilon_s}$). Therefore, one can sense the medium placed close to the surface of metal films. This is the basis for sensing in an SPR-based sensor. In 1983, Liedberg et al. (Liedberg, Nylander, and Lunström 1983) first presented an SPR sensor in the field of chemical, gas, and biosensing in the Kretschmann configuration, using angular interrogation. They used a thin layer of Ag as an SPR active metal. However, the prism-based SPR sensors are bulky, and its commercial development has been hampered due to the many sophisticated components related to optics and mechanical kinematics in its interior. In addition, remote sensing cannot be realized by the prism-based SPR sensing device. After the introduction of the phenomenon of SPR in sensing by Kretschmann, various efforts were made toward the development of optical fiber using the SPR sensing system, where the core of the fiber-optic plays the same role of a prism (i.e., the coupling phenomenon of the light into the interface of metal layer and dielectric). Further, the miniaturization of the SPR probe is developed by employing an optical fiber, benefiting from its small core diameter. Moreover, a fiber-optic SPR sensing system offers a design concept with the extra feature of remote sensing and momentum to the incident field that can be imparted by using optical fibers.

1.4 TRANSFER MATRIX METHOD

There are various computational methods in photonics to analyze the propagation of light through different layered mediums. These methods are transferred matrix method (TMM), finite difference

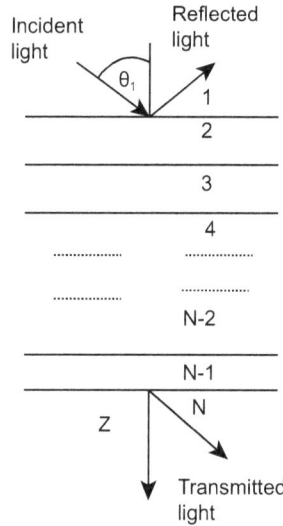

FIGURE 1.12 Transfer matrix for each layer.

time-domain (FDTD), scattering matrix method (SMM), beam propagation method (BPM), and finite element method (FEM). TMM is adapted in numerous areas of engineering and technology to find resultant energies due to the propagation of light through a layered medium (Kaur, Kumar, and Kaushik 2021, 2022). TMM gives accurate results due to the absence of approximations. In optics, Fresnel equations are used to analyze light from a single interface. However, when there are multiple interfaces, the calculation becomes very cumbersome to calculate solutions for each interface. The TMM is based on continuity conditions (i.e., if the field is known at the first layer, the transmitted field at the end of the layer can be derived using a simple matrix operation). For N-layer systems, there will be N-1 interfaces, as shown in Figure 1.12. By the product of N-1 matrices, the N-layers stack is then, in here, emblematic as a system matrix.

1.4.1 CALCULATION OF REFLECTED INTENSITY

Here, for the calculation of reflected intensity, a linearly polarized light is incident on stacks of dielectric layers. At the interfaces of the layers, both magnetic ($V = B/\mu$) fields and electric (U) are continuous. For simplicity, let us consider the three-layered system, which has two interfaces. Here, U_1, V_1, U_2, V_2, and U_3, V_3 are the electric and magnetic field associated with layer 1, layer 2, and layer 3, respectively, as shown in Figure 1.13. The subscripts i, r, and t of U/V stand for the incident, reflected, and transmitted light, respectively.

The boundary conditions that are the magnetic and electric fields are continuous through interface 1 and interface 2.

1.4.1.1 Boundary Condition at Interface 1

Here, boundary condition applying i.e., the electric field is successively obtained through the interface 1. At interface 1, the electric field is given as

$$U_1 = \left(U_{i1} - U_{r1}\right)\cos\left(\theta_{i1}\right) = \left(U_{t1} - U'_{r2}\right)\cos\left(\theta_{i2}\right) \tag{1.22}$$

Here, U describe the wave amplitudes of electric fields at boundary 1. Thus, U_{i1} represents that of the incident wave, U_{r1} is relate to the reflected wave, and U_{t1} is defined as that of the transmitted

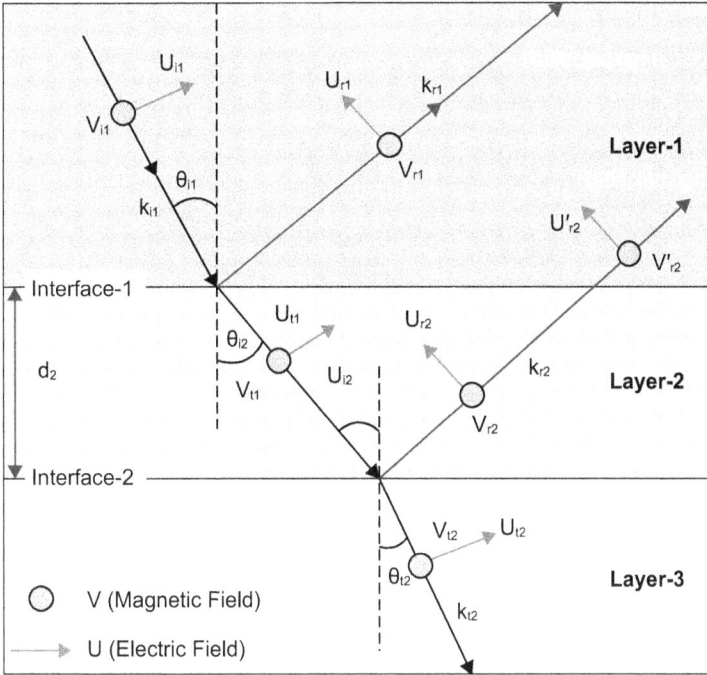

FIGURE 1.13   Transfer matrix for three-layer system.

wave; U'_{r2} describes the reflected wave with the incidence direction from boundary 2 to boundary 1. Similarly, going for the boundary condition of the magnetic field at boundary 1,

$$V_1 = \sqrt{\varepsilon_0 / \mu_0} \left(U_{i1} + U_{r1} \right) n_1 = \sqrt{\varepsilon_0 / \mu_0} \left(U_{t1} + U'_{r2} \right) n_2 \tag{1.23}$$

In Eq. (1.23), U and V can be converted as

$$V = \sqrt{\varepsilon_0 / \mu_0} U n \tag{1.24}$$

where n represents the RI of the medium, and θ_{i1} and θ_{i2} are the angles of incidence lights at interfaces 1 and 2, separately.

1.4.1.2   Boundary Condition at Interface 2

Here, applying the boundary condition i.e., the electric field is through interface 2 in succession state. At interface 2, the electric and magnetic fields are given as

$$U_2 = \left(U_{i2} - U_{r2} \right) \cos\left(\theta_{i2} \right) = U_{t2} \cos\left(\theta_{t2} \right) \tag{1.25}$$

and

$$V_2 = \sqrt{\varepsilon_0 / \mu_0} \left(U_{i2} - U_{r2} \right) n_2 = \sqrt{\varepsilon_0 / \mu_0} U_{t2} n_2 \tag{1.26}$$

Similar to U, here at interface 2, θ_{t2} can be defined as the angle of the refracted ray. U_{i2}, U_{r2}, and U_{t2} are the amplitudes related to the incident, reflected, and transmitted waves, separately.

As a wave crosses a very short distance d_2, then the phase shift is represented as

$$\beta_2 = (2\pi d_2 / \lambda)\sqrt{\varepsilon_2 - n_1^2 \sin^2\theta_1} \qquad (1.27)$$

The field equations at interface 2 can be given

$$U_{i2} = U_{t1}e^{-i\beta_2} \qquad (1.28)$$

$$U_{r2} = U'_{r2}e^{i\beta_2} \qquad (1.29)$$

It can be also written as

$$U_2 = (U_{t1}e^{-i\beta_2})\cos(\theta_{t2}) - U'_{r2}e^{i\beta_2}\cos(\theta_{t2}) \qquad (1.30)$$

$$V_2 = \sqrt{\varepsilon_0 / \mu_0}\left(U_{t1}e^{-i\beta_2} + U'_{r2}e^{i\beta_2}\right)n_2 \qquad (1.31)$$

After solving, toward U_{t1} and $U'r_2$, one can obtain

$$U_1 = U_2 \cos\beta_2 - V_2\left(i\sin\beta_2\right)/q_2 \qquad (1.32)$$

$$V_1 = -U_2 q_2\left(i\sin\beta_2\right) + V_2\left(\cos\beta_2\right) \qquad (1.33)$$

where

$$q_2 = \sqrt{\varepsilon_2 - n_1^2 \sin^2\theta_{i1}} \ / \varepsilon_2 \qquad (1.34)$$

In matrix notation, it can be given as

$$\begin{bmatrix} U_1 \\ V_1 \end{bmatrix} = \begin{bmatrix} \cos(\beta_2) & -\dfrac{i}{q_2}\sin(\beta_2) \\ -iq_2\sin(\beta_2) & \cos(\beta_2) \end{bmatrix}\begin{bmatrix} U_2 \\ V_2 \end{bmatrix} \qquad (1.35)$$

$$\begin{bmatrix} U_1 \\ V_1 \end{bmatrix} = m_2 \begin{bmatrix} U_2 \\ V_2 \end{bmatrix} \qquad (1.36)$$

where

$$m_2 = \begin{bmatrix} \cos(\beta_2) & -\dfrac{i}{q_2}\sin(\beta_2) \\ -iq_2\sin(\beta_2) & \cos(\beta_2) \end{bmatrix} \qquad (1.37)$$

In general, the magnetic field and electric at interface 1, $Z = Z_1$ can be linked to those at the last interface $Z = Z_{N-1}$ by

$$\begin{bmatrix} U_1 \\ V_1 \end{bmatrix} = M \begin{bmatrix} U_{N-1} \\ V_{N-1} \end{bmatrix} \qquad (1.38)$$

Here U_1 and V_1 can be described as the magnetic fields and tangential components of electric at interface 1, as U_{N-1} and V_{N-1} defined the matchup fields at the interface $N - 1$. The characteristic matrix (M) for the whole platform is obtained as

$$m_2 = \prod_{k=2}^{N-1} m_k = \begin{bmatrix} M_{11} & M_{12} \\ M_{21} & M_{22} \end{bmatrix} \tag{1.39}$$

Here k represents the count of layers ranging from 1 to N. For $N - 1$ interfaces, characteristic matrices can be found from the following general matrix:

$$m_k = \begin{bmatrix} \cos(\beta_k) & -\dfrac{i}{q_k}\sin(\beta_k) \\ -iq_k \sin(\beta_k) & \cos(\beta_k) \end{bmatrix} \tag{1.40}$$

where

$$q_k = \sqrt{\varepsilon_0 / \mu_0}\, n_k \cos(\theta_k) = \sqrt{\varepsilon_k - n_1^2 \sin^2\theta_1}\,/\,\varepsilon_k \tag{1.41}$$

and

$$\beta_k = (2\pi / \lambda) n_k \cos(\theta_k)(z_k - z_{k-1}) = (2\pi d_k / \lambda)\sqrt{\varepsilon_k - n_1^2\sin^2\theta_1} \tag{1.42}$$

Here $\varepsilon = n^2$, and $\theta_1 = \theta_{i1}$.

Then, from Fresnel equations, reflected amplitude of the light at incident angle θ is given by

$$r_p = \frac{(M_{11} + M_{12}q_N)q_1 - (M_{21} + M_{22}q_N)}{(M_{11} + M_{12}q_N)q_1 + (M_{21} + M_{22}q_N)} \tag{1.43}$$

Then, reflectance is the square of reflected amplitude given by

$$R_p = |r_p|^2 \tag{1.44}$$

1.4.2 Transmitted Power through Optical Fiber

For the transmitted power calculations, all incidence rays can be considered to be propagated into the fiber core. It is considered that, using a suitable microscopic objective, the guide ray from a collimated source will be limited to one terminate surface of the fiber. To calculate the angular power distribution,

$$dp \propto \frac{n_1^2 \sin\theta \cos\theta}{(1 - n_1^2 \cos^2\theta)^2}\, d\theta \tag{1.45}$$

According to the equation, n_1 represents the RI of fiber core. The P_{trans} as normalized transmitted power in a SPR-based fiber sensor can then be calculated as

$$P_{trans} = \int_{\theta_{cr}}^{\pi/2} R_p^{N_{ref}(\theta)} \frac{n_1^2 \sin\theta \cos\theta}{(1 - n_1^2 \cos^2\theta)^2}\, d\theta \,/\, \int_{\theta_{cr}}^{\pi/2} \frac{n_1^2 \sin\theta \cos\theta}{(1 - n_1^2 \cos^2\theta)^2}\, d\theta \tag{1.46}$$

where

$$N_{ref}\left(\theta\right) = l / \left(D_C \tan\theta\right) \tag{1.47}$$

and

$$\theta_{cr} = \sin^{-1}\left(n_{cl} / n_1\right) \tag{1.48}$$

N_{ref} can be performed as the total number of reflections that is dependent upon the core diameter of fiber D_C and effective length of sensing region l. θ is the angle of rays normal to the metal-core boundary. The calculated output spectrum for multimode fiber correlates with the experimental results of optical fiber-based plasmonic systems. Let's consider how plasmon excitation happens using suitable optical fiber and its advantages.

1.5 PLASMON EXCITATION USING OPTICAL FIBER

A fiber-based SPR sensor has a compact, disposable, label-free, simplified optical design and is low cost, easy to handle, can be used for remote sensing, and can detect a small volume sample as the sensing region is very small. Therefore, fiber has been used as a coupling element. The TIR phenomena and therefore the causing of EWs form the basis behind the excitation of SPs as shown in Figure 1.14.

Inside the fiber-optic core, the light propagates using a principle of TIR. However, an EWs, as discussed earlier, propagates along the interface of core cladding of the fiber. In an optical fiber-based SPR sensor, mostly multimode plastic cladded optical fiber is used where from the center proportion of the fiber, a small proportion of cladding around fiber core is removed, and a thin metallic layer such as Au or Ag (as a plasmon active metal) is coated around the bare core using a customized deposition system; it also acts as a cladding. The EWs appeared at the interface of metal layer and fiber core and penetrates the thin metallic layer; this evanescent field generates the SPs at the boundary of the metallic thin film and sensing layer. The proposed SPs field evanescently decays into the sensing region. The test sample is in direct contact with metallic thin films as shown in Figure 1.14, where the EWs interact with analytes present in the sensing region. The sensor element will be a strip of bare fiber without a cladding layer, and a 500 angstroms SPR active symmetrical metal film will be evenly deposited on the surface of the fiber core, via a customized rotating metal deposition system. By changing the length of the bare fiber, the average number of reflections of the light propagating inside the fiber will be adjusted. The range of the incident angle depends on the propagation angle in the fiber. Here, one of the differences between the SPR optical fiber sensing system

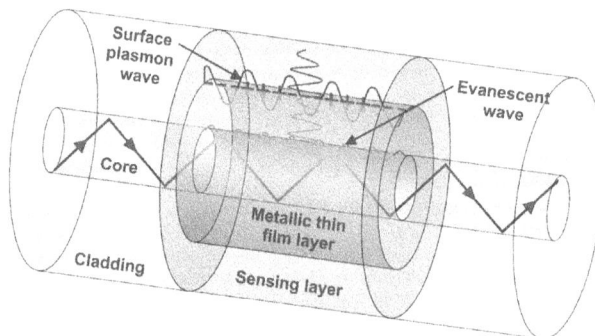

FIGURE 1.14   Surface plasmon excitation at the interface of metal-dielectric in an optical fiber.

and the traditional SPR measurement is the choice of light sources, for this, the former using a wide range of excitation wavelengths and the latter with discrete excitation wavelength. The output light will be collected using suitable optics and will be fed to a highly sensitive spectrometer. The sensing parameters will be obtained by calculating the intensity distribution of the resonance spectrum described to the transmission spectrum. The sensed parameters can then be determined from the measured resonance spectrum in the transmitted spectral intensity distribution. Optical fiber-based SPR sensors have better sensitivity than LSPR-based sensors, but LSPR has its own advantages. It has advantages over SPR sensors for the ease of fabrication and for its better linear performance. The sensitivity of LSPR sensors is controlled by limiting the size and shape of the NPs, which is not the case for SPR sensors.

For the coating of thin film, a costly coating instrument is required. But the coating of NPs on the core of the fiber by the chemical method is very easy and cost-effective. So, the nanoparticle-based fiber sensor may be cost-effective. However, surface-enhanced Raman scattering (SERS) is a typical example of unique optical characteristics of known metal NPs (Chen, de Castro, and Shen 1981). One can use a nanoparticle deposited fiber sensor based on SERS for the development of a compact system that may be helpful in addressing the selectivity issue. Moreover, advancement in fabrication techniques (lithographic and synthetic) helps to tune the SPR wavelength due to the NPs with the EM spectrum in monitoring limitation ranging from the visible to the infrared region, using the shape, size, and material properties of the NPs that are plasmon active, contrary to a thin film-based sensor (Sherry et al. 2005; Nehl, Liao, and Hafner 2006; Xia and Halas 2005; Wiley et al. 2005; Zhang et al. 2005; Jin et al. 2003). This offers additional flexibility when designing SPR with NPs for sensing experiments, and this is elaborated in the next section along with the origin of SPs in metallic NPs.

1.6 EXCITATION OF LOCALIZED SURFACE PLASMON BY LIGHT USING METALLIC NANOPARTICLES

Ordinary light cannot excite plasmons due to momentum mismatch of the dispersion relation among the photon and the plasmon. When the size of the bulk material is reduced to a particle with spherical dimension, a new physics arises as a solution after solving the Maxwell equations at the interface of the NPs surrounded by a dielectric. For numerous metals, like cadmium, tin, lead, mercury, and indium, the plasma frequency is at the ultraviolet part of the spectrum; hence, such NPs do not have any conspicuous color tendency visible to our eyes. These teeny metallic particles lightly get oxidized; thereby, its usage for SPs applications is difficult. Therefore, noble metals are used for plasmons, this is existing in a colloidal state in the air. Under this condition, the frequency of this plasmon is in the visible light region owing to d-d band transitions. Further, the nonmail value of the imaginary part of the dielectric constant about the plasmon frequency makes it more useful and interesting for the near-field absorptive effect. Therefore, gold, the NPs like silver, and copper are popular and suitable for SPs experiments. Similar to the generation of SPs at the boundary of metallic films and the dielectric layer, SPs at the interface of these metallic NPs surrounded with a dielectric can be realized. The resonance in the former case is known as PSPR, whereas the resonance in the latter case is known as LSPR. LSPR is a phenomenon limited in NPs, which is confined to the chromophore collective oscillation of conducting electrons stimulated by the incident electromagnetic radiation. Metallic NPs is similar to the lattice of an ion nucleus (ionic core is heavier with respect to conduction electron), providing a big stage for the conducting electron to move freely within, as shown in Figure 1.15. Under the illumination, the incident light with the EM field puts to use a force on the conduction electrons of a metallic NPs and allows them to drift toward the outer edge of the NPs. Due to these electrons being restrained within the NPs, positive and negative charges converge to the opposite side, thereby forming a separation between the charges to form an electric dipole, with an electric field (E_{RES}) within the NPs for the dynamic equilibrium state. This specific field, in the opposite direction to the incident light, causes the internal electrons to return to their equilibrium position (Figure 1.15).

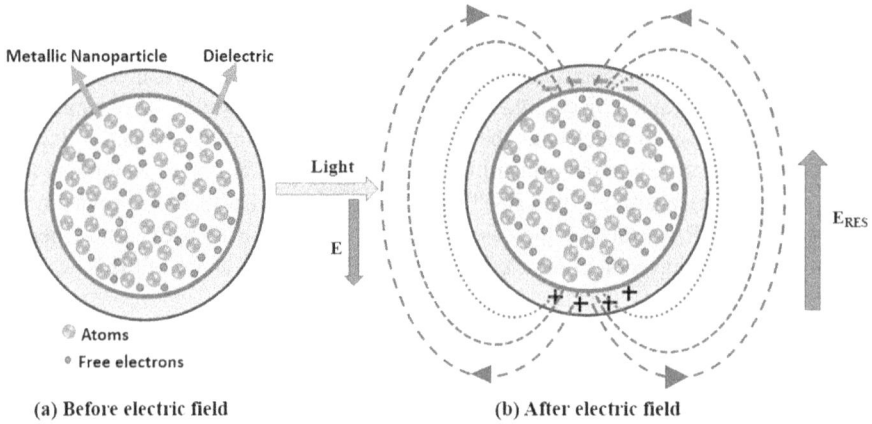

FIGURE 1.15   The generation of surface plasmon in metallic nanoparticles due to the interaction of electromagnetic radiation with the metal sphere.

This dynamic equilibrium state is that for different electrons, the restoring force is proportional to the displacement from the equilibrium position, which is similar to a linear oscillator. In particular, when the electron is shifted and not affected by the electric field in SPs, it will be in a certain frequency oscillation state, which is called the resonance frequency of plasma. This plasmonic frequency depends on four factors: the shape and size, charge distribution, density of electrons, as well as effective mass of the electron. Change in one of these factors alters the NP's performances and determines its usage for many electronic and optical applications (Shipway, Katz, and Willner 2000) and chemical and biological sensors (Hainfeld et al. 2006; Niemeyer 2001). Further, the electric field near the particle surface is enormously heightened, and the effect rapidly decays outward from the surface (in the nanometer range). The resonance frequency of LSPR with maximum optical extinction is affected by many factors, such as dielectric properties, surrounding environment, morphology including shape and size, and interactions between different interparticles (Mock et al. 2002; Smitha et al. 2008). This extinction peak rests with the RI of the ambient environment, and this is the basis for the sensing applications. The energy of bulk plasmons can be calculated as

$$E_p = \frac{h}{2\pi} \sqrt{\frac{ne^2}{m\epsilon_0}} \tag{1.49}$$

where m, e, n, and ϵ_0 represent the electron mass, electron charge, electron density, and permittivity of free space, respectively. Surface plasmons are optically excited by the effect of an oscillating electric field from an incoming plane wave. Local surface plasmons (LSPs) occur only on the surface of particles whose oscillatory frequency is equal to the wavelength of light. The LSPs has many properties, such as the strong surface electric field and the strong extinction ability of the particles. This specific optical extinction can be observed at visible wavelengths. Here, the extinction peak in spectrum related to the surrounding RI is the basis for sensing applications.

When an EM field comes into contact with an object, the field is scattered. The incident fields are distinct to the scattered fields, influenced by the geometry and physical property of surroundings and object. According to the Mie theory, the most usual tool to observe electromagnetic scattering is a sphere. Let us assume the radius of the sphere is R. It is illuminated by a plane wave when embedded in a medium that is isotropic and homogeneous (Goss et al. 1980).

1.6.1 MIE THEORY

An EM field in a time harmonic form presented by $\left[\vec{E}\left(\vec{r},t\right)\right], \left[\vec{H}\left(\vec{r},t\right)\right]$ is incident. Let us assume the medium is homogeneous, isotropic, and linear, with the help of the wave equation:

$$\nabla^2 \vec{E} + k^2 \vec{E} = 0 \qquad \nabla^2 \vec{H} + k^2 \vec{H} = 0 \qquad (1.50)$$

where $k^2 = \omega^2 \varepsilon \mu$: μ is the the magnetic permeability, ε is the electric permittivity, and ω is the frequency of the incident field.

As $\vec{E}$ and $\vec{H}$ are divergence free, and the charge density is zero,

$$\nabla.\vec{E} = 0 \qquad \nabla.\vec{H} = 0 \qquad (1.51)$$

As the field is time harmonic, Faraday's and Ampere's laws become

$$\nabla \times \vec{E} = i\omega\mu\vec{H} \qquad \nabla \times \vec{H} = -i\omega\varepsilon E \qquad (1.52)$$

M, an intermediate vector function, is introduced.

$$\vec{M} = \nabla \times \left(\vec{c}\psi\right) \qquad (1.53)$$

where $\vec{c}$ is the constant vector and ψ is the scalar function.

As the divergence of the curl of any vector is zero,

$$\nabla.\vec{M} = 0 \qquad (1.54)$$

So, from Eq. (1.53),

$$\nabla^2 \vec{M} + k^2 \vec{M} = \nabla \times \left[\vec{c}\left(\nabla^2 \overline{\Psi} + k^2 \overline{\Psi}\right)\right] \qquad (1.55)$$

From Eqs. (1.50) and (1.55), $\vec{M}$ verifies that the wave function $\overline{\Psi}$ satisfies the scalar equation:

$$\left(\nabla^2 \overline{\Psi} + k^2 \overline{\Psi}\right) = 0 \qquad (1.56)$$

So $\vec{M}$ can also mean the magnetic field or electric. Hence, according to another divergence-free vector function which examine the equation of vector wave, it represents the other field

$$\vec{N} = \frac{\nabla \times \vec{M}}{k} \qquad (1.57)$$

or, equivalently,

$$\nabla \times \vec{N} = k\vec{M} \qquad (1.58)$$

$\vec{N}$ and $\vec{M}$ are called vector spherical harmonics (VSH). They both are the solution to the wave equation.

  I. Both are divergence-free.
  II. $\vec{M}$ is proportional to the curl of $\vec{N}$ and vice versa.

But only if Eq. (1.56) has a solution will this be true. Therefore, the solution of the vector wave equation (1.50) can be obtained only by solving the scalar wave equation.

To solve the scalar equation (1.55), we use spherical coordinate (r, θ, φ), here $\vec{r}$ indicates the vector position. As an alternative, we can choose $\vec{c} = \vec{r}$.

In the spherical coordinate, Eq. (1.56) is expressed as

$$\frac{1}{r^2}\frac{\partial}{\partial r}\left(r^2\frac{\partial \Psi}{\partial r}\right) + \frac{1}{r^2\sin\theta}\frac{\partial}{\partial \theta}\left(\sin\theta\frac{\partial \Psi}{\partial \theta}\right) + \frac{1}{r^2\sin\theta}\frac{\partial}{\partial \varphi}\left(r^2\frac{\partial^2 \Psi}{\partial \varphi^2}\right) \tag{1.59}$$

The scalar function Ψ is given by

$$\Psi(r, \theta, \varphi) = R(r)\theta(\theta)\Phi(\varphi) \tag{1.60}$$

Thus, the complete solution of the scalar wave in Eq. (1.56) can be obtained:

$$\Psi_{emn}(r, \theta, \varphi) = \cos m\varphi P_n^m(\cos\theta)z_n(kr) \tag{1.61}$$

$$\Psi_{omn}(r, \theta, \varphi) = \sin m\varphi P_n^m(\cos\theta)z_n(kr) \tag{1.62}$$

Here, e and o in scalar function Ψ mean even and odd, separately. On the right-hand side of the equation, z_n indicates any of the four Bessel functions. P_n^m are the associated Legendre functions of first kind of order m and degree n. Each solution of the scalar equation (1.56) can be expressed as an infinite series of the functions (1.61) and (1.62). Therefore, VSH can be calculated as

$$\vec{M}_{emn} = \nabla \times \left(\vec{r}\,\Psi_{emn}\right)$$
$$\vec{M}_{omn} = \nabla \times \left(\vec{r}\,\Psi_{omn}\right) \tag{1.63}$$

$$\vec{N}_{emn} = \frac{\nabla \times \left(\vec{r}\,\Psi_{emn}\right)}{k}$$

$$\vec{N}_{omn} = \frac{\nabla \times \left(\vec{r}\,\Psi_{emn}\right)}{k} \tag{1.64}$$

It can be concluded that according to Eqs. (1.63) and (1.64), we can use an infinite series of the vector harmonics to express any solution of the wave equation (1.50).

Now the incident and scattered fields will be found using Mie theory.

As shown in Figure 1.16, the incident field is a linearly polarized plane wave that propagates along the z-direction and is parallel to the X-axis.

The incident field is considered to be a plane wave linearly polarized parallel to the x-axis and propagating in the z-direction, and the spherical coordinates are listed as

$$\vec{E}_i = E_0 e^{ikr\cos\theta}\,\widehat{e}_x \tag{1.65}$$

where E_0 is the amplitude of the electric field, k is the wave number, and $\widehat{e}_x$ is the unit vector in the polarization direction.

Then, use the infinite series of VSH to express the incident field as follows:

$$\vec{E}_i = \sum_{m=0}^{\infty}\sum_{n=0}^{\infty}\left(B_{emn}\vec{M}_{emn} + B_{omn}\vec{M}_{omn} + A_{emn}\vec{N}_{emn} + A_{omn}\vec{N}_{omn}\right) \tag{1.66}$$

where B_{emn}, B_{omn}, A_{emn}, and A_{omn} are the expansion coefficients. With the help of the orthogonality of the vector harmonics and the finite value of the incident field at the origin, the expansion reduced to

$$\vec{E}_i = \sum_{n=1}^{\infty}\left(B_{oln}\vec{M}_{oln}^{(1)} + A_{eln}\vec{N}_{eln}^{(1)}\right) \tag{1.67}$$

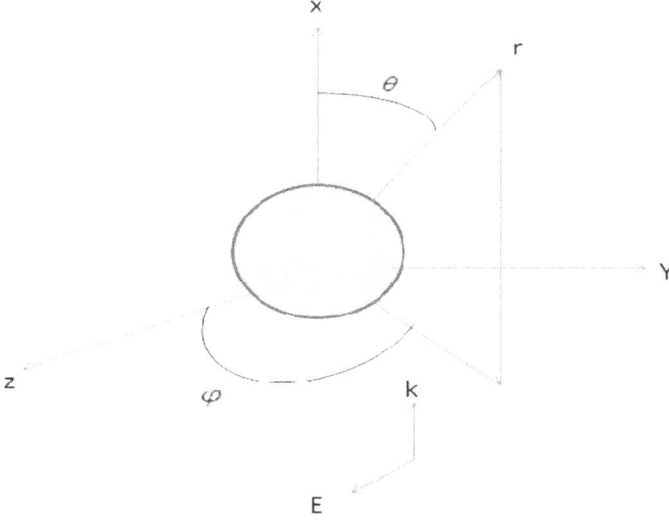

FIGURE 1.16 The geometry of the scattering problem along with the spherical coordinates is included.

Here the superscript (1) can be related to the spherical Bessel function $j_n(kr)$, employed for the radial part of the generating function.

After some calculations, the final form of the expansion coefficients is

$$B_{oln} = i^n E_0 \frac{2n+1}{n(n+1)} \tag{1.68}$$

$$A_{eln} = -E_0 i^n \frac{2n+1}{n(n+1)} \tag{1.69}$$

Putting these values in Eq. (1.67), the incident electric field is as follows:

$$\vec{E}_i = E_0 \sum_{n=1}^{\infty} \left(i^n \frac{2n+1}{n(n+1)} \left(\vec{M}_{oln}^{(1)} - \vec{N}_{eln}^{(1)} \right) \right) \tag{1.70}$$

and the corresponding magnetic field becomes

$$\vec{H}_i = \frac{-k}{\varepsilon\mu} E_0 \sum_{n=1}^{\infty} \left(i^n \frac{2n+1}{n(n+1)} \left(\vec{M}_{eln}^{(1)} + \vec{N}_{oln}^{(1)} \right) \right) \tag{1.71}$$

With the substitution of boundary conditions between the surrounding medium and sphere, the scattered field $(\overrightarrow{E_S}, \overrightarrow{H_S})$ and the field inside the particle $(\overrightarrow{E_I}, \overrightarrow{H_I})$ can be obtained:

$$\left(\overrightarrow{Ei} + \overrightarrow{Es} - \overrightarrow{EI} \right) \times \hat{e}_r = \left(\overrightarrow{Hi} + \overrightarrow{Hs} - \overrightarrow{HI} \right) \times \hat{e}_r = 0 \tag{1.72}$$

The scattered films are then given by

$$\vec{E}_s = \sum_{n=1}^{\infty} \left(E_n \left(ia_n \vec{N}_{eln}^{(3)} - b_n \vec{M}_{oln}^{(3)} \right) \right) \tag{1.73}$$

$$\vec{H}_s = \sum_{n=1}^{\infty} \left(E_n \left(ib_n \vec{N}_{oln}^{(3)} + a_n \vec{M}_{eln}^{(3)} \right) \right) \tag{1.74}$$

Here the superscript (3) reveals the radial dependence of the generating function, Ψ, that can be obtained with the help of the spherical Hankel function that is presented as $h_n^{(1)}$. Then a_n and b_n are called Mie coefficients of the scattered field.

When we apply the boundary conditions of Eq. (1.72), the analytical expression for the Michaelis coefficient will be obtained from the following four equations:

$$a_n = \frac{\mu m^2 j_n(mx)\left[xj_n(x)\right]' - \mu_l j_n(x)\left[mxj_n(mx)\right]'}{\mu m^2 j_n(mx)\left[xh_n^{(1)}(x)\right]' - \mu_l h_n^{(1)}(x)\left[mxj_n(mx)\right]'} \qquad (1.75)$$

$$b_n = \frac{\mu_l j_n(mx)\left[xj_n(x)\right]' - \mu j_n(x)\left[mxj_n(mx)\right]'}{\mu_l j_n(mx)\left[xh_n^{(1)}(x)\right]' - \mu h_n^{(1)}(x)\left[mxj_n(mx)\right]'} \qquad (1.76)$$

where μ_l is the magnetic permeability of the sphere; μ is the magnetic permeabilities of the surrounding medium; $x = kR = \dfrac{2\pi R n}{\lambda}$ is the size parameter; $m = \dfrac{n_l}{n_m}$ is the relative RI among the embedded medium and sphere; λ indicates the incident wavelength; R is the radius of the sphere; $n_l = n_R + in_l$ is the sophisticated RI of the metal; n_R describes the real RI of the sphere; and n_R is the RI of the surrounding medium.

Using Ricatti-Bessel functions, we can simplify the Mie coefficients for the scattered field:

$$\psi_n(\rho) = \rho j_n(\rho) \quad \xi_n(\rho) = \rho h_n^1(\rho) \qquad (1.77)$$

As the magnetic permeability of the surrounding medium and particle equals 1, the Mie coefficients can be expressed as

$$a_n = \frac{m\psi_n(mx)\psi_n'(x) - \psi_n(x)\psi_n'(mx)}{m\psi_n(mx)\xi_n'(x) - \xi_n(x)\psi_n'(mx)} \qquad (1.78)$$

$$b_n = \frac{\psi_n(mx)\psi_n'(x) - m\psi_n(x)\psi_n'(mx)}{\psi_n(mx)\xi_n'(x) - m\xi_n(x)\psi_n'(mx)} \qquad (1.79)$$

Here, the electromagnetic energy is scattered (W_{sca}) or absorbed (W_{abs}) by the diffuser, and scattering cross sections (C_{sca}) and the absorption (C_{abs}) are calculated for the sake of analyzing the ratio of the energy.

$$C_{abs} = \frac{W_{abs}}{I_i} \quad C_{sca} = \frac{W_{sca}}{I_i} \qquad (1.80)$$

The extinction cross section can be calculated as $C_{ext} = C_{abs} + C_{sca}$.

As a function of the Mie coefficients, these parameters are listed as

$$C_{sca} = \frac{W_{sca}}{I_i} = \frac{2\pi}{k^2}\sum_{n=1}^{\infty}(2n+1)\left(|a_n|^2 + |b_n|^2\right) \qquad (1.81)$$

$$C_{ext} = \frac{W_{ext}}{I_i} = \frac{2\pi}{k^2}\sum_{n=1}^{\infty}(2n+1)Re\left(a_n + b_n\right) \qquad (1.82)$$

$$C_{abs} = C_{sca} - C_{ext} \qquad (1.83)$$

Now we have the values of coefficients a_n and b_n. At this point, let us assume the size of the NP is considered as the relationship $(x \ll 1)$. For this condition, use a power series and keep only terms to order x^3, to gain ground upon the Riccati-Bessel functions. Thus, Eqs. (1.78) and (1.79) can be written as

$$a_1 \approx \frac{-i2x^3}{3} \frac{m^2 - 1}{m^2 + 2} \tag{1.84}$$

$$b_1 \approx 0 \tag{1.85}$$

Putting $m = \dfrac{n_R + in_I}{n}$ in Eq.(1.82),

$$a_1 = -i\frac{2x^3}{3} \frac{n_R^2 - n_I^2 + i2n_Rn_I - n_m^2}{n_R^2 - n_I^2 + i2n_Rn_I + 2n_m^2} \tag{1.86}$$

$$\tilde{\varepsilon} = \varepsilon_1 + \varepsilon_2 \tag{1.87}$$

$$\varepsilon_1 = n_R^2 - n_I^2 \tag{1.88}$$

$$\varepsilon_2 = 2n_Rn_I \tag{1.89}$$

$$\varepsilon_m = n_m^2 \tag{1.90}$$

Using the relations (1.87) to (1.90) in Eq. (1.86),

$$a_1 = \frac{2x^3}{3} \frac{-i\varepsilon_1^2 - i\varepsilon_1\varepsilon_m + 3\varepsilon_2\varepsilon_m - i\varepsilon_2^2 + i2\varepsilon_m^2}{(\varepsilon_1 + 2\varepsilon_m)^2 + (\varepsilon_2)^2} \tag{1.91}$$

Substituting Eq. (1.91) into Eq. (1.82), the expression for NPs plasmon resonances can then be obtained by taking the dipole term:

$$C_{ext} = \frac{18\pi\varepsilon_m^{3/2}V}{\lambda} \frac{\varepsilon_2(\lambda)}{[\varepsilon_1(\lambda) + 2\varepsilon_m^2]^2 + \varepsilon_2(\lambda)^2} \tag{1.92}$$

$$C_{sca} = \frac{32\pi^4\varepsilon_m^2V}{\lambda^4} \frac{(\varepsilon_1 - \varepsilon_m)^2 + (\varepsilon_2)^2}{(\varepsilon_1 + 2\varepsilon_m)^2 + (\varepsilon_2)^2} \tag{1.93}$$

When $\varepsilon_1 = -2\varepsilon_m$ in Eq. (1.92), the extinction cross section will be maximized. It reveals the substantial connection between the surrounding dielectric environment and the LSPR extinction peak.

However, using the optical property of NPs, one can design an optical fiber-based RI sensor by immobilizing the metallic NPs on the core of the plastic cladded silica multimode optical fiber. Details about the design of the optical fiber-based RI sensor using metallic NPs are presented in the next section.

1.7 FIBER-OPTIC LSPR SENSOR USING METALLIC NANOPARTICLES

Similar to the fiber-based SPR sensor, one can design a fiber-based LSPR sensor using metallic NPs instead of a metallic membranaceous layer on the core of an optical fiber. Here, these metal NPs are coated around the silica core to generate SPs as illustrated in Figure 1.17. The field of EWs created at the core and the metallic NPs interface interact with the NPs, which excites the SPs inside the metallic NPs; hence, the high field at the surface will be generated as described in Section 1.6.

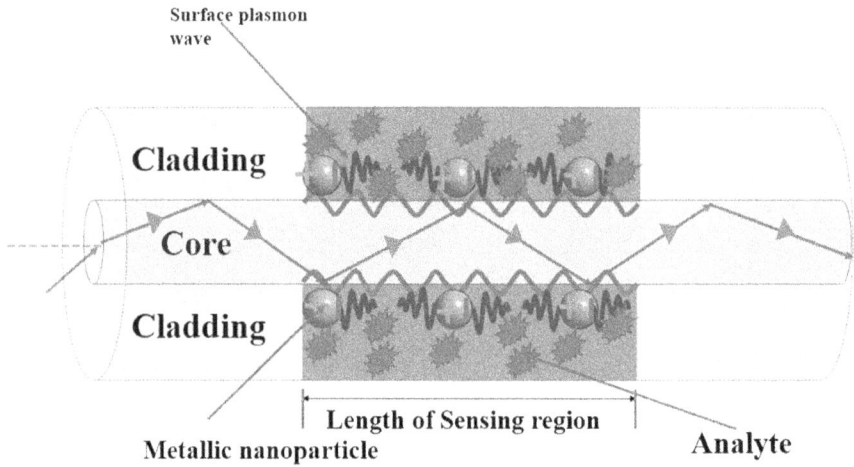

FIGURE 1.17 Excitation of surface plasmons due to metal nanoparticles in a multimode optical fiber.

This field will be used for sensing by placing the analyte to be sensed in direct contact with metal NPs films.

During the experiment, the light is launched at the terminal plane of the optical fiber using a broadband source, and the light is collected through a spectrometer at the other terminal part. The light collected by the spectrometer can be interpreted in transmittance or absorbance mode. As the metallic NPs show strong absorbance to the incident visible light, the absorbance mode is preferred during the experiments. As mentioned earlier, the fields developed on the surface of the NPs are sensitive to the surrounding RI. By changing the RI of the analyte, the output absorbance spectra will change. From the peak absorbance variation with analyte RI, the performance of the fiber sensor can be studied.

1.7.1 REFRACTIVE INDEX DEPENDENCE

In Drude model, the frequency ε_1 of the electronic structure of bulk metals can be written as

$$\varepsilon_1 = 1 - \frac{\omega_p^2}{\omega^2 + \gamma^2} \tag{1.94}$$

where the damping parameter of the bulk metal is defined as γ, and ω_p represents the plasma frequency. In the range of visible and near-infrared frequencies, $\gamma \ll \omega_p$. Thus, the equation can be converted to

$$\varepsilon_1 = 1 - \frac{\omega_p^2}{\omega^2} \tag{1.95}$$

By forming $\varepsilon_1 = -2\varepsilon_m$, we get the following:

$$\omega_{max} = \frac{\omega_p}{\sqrt{2\varepsilon_m + 1}} \tag{1.96}$$

Here, the frequency of the LSPR peak can be described as ω_{max}.

Expressing the wavelength as $\lambda = 2\pi c / \omega$ and then expressing the dielectric constant as $\varepsilon_m = n^2$, the following relation is obtained:

$$\lambda_{max} = \lambda_p \sqrt{2n_m^2 + 1} \qquad (1.97)$$

where λ_{max} and λ_p are the LSPR peak wavelength and wavelength related to plasma frequency, respectively. From these, we can easily understand the relation between the RI of the surrounding medium and the resonance peak wavelength of LSPR (Haidekker et al. 2006; Choi et al. 2008; Sun et al. 2008).

1.8 FIBER-OPTIC PLASMONIC BIOSENSING TECHNIQUE

The main goals behind the development of novel sensing devices are (i) to improve the performance of the transducer (i.e., enhance the sensitivity performance, fasten the response rater), reusability, and lower value of limit of detection (*LoD*), as well as (ii) to miniaturize the sensing platform using micro- and nanotechnology (Purohit et al. 2020; Singh et al. 2020). Emerging NMs with developments over sensing technology could address these unmet challenges (Yang and Duncan 2021), and optic-plasmonic biosensors could contribute significantly to achieve these objectives. Optic-plasmonic biosensors take advantage of integration of the fiber optics' flexibility and durability with the sensitivity of NMs for the detection of biomolecules including several analytes, proteins, bacteria, viruses, RNA, and DNA (Esfahani Monfared 2020; Xavier et al. 2018). Accounting for its multiple advantages such as small size, chemically inert nature, cost-effectiveness, good linearity and manageability, and real-time monitoring, optic-plasmonic biosensors are preferred over conventional methods for biomolecule recognition and associated applications (Masson 2017). These sensors are widely applicable in healthcare with biomedical instrumentation and monitoring, attributed to their unique features like higher sensitivity and selectivity, multiplexing, no EM interference, and distributed sensing (Roriz et al. 2020b). The basic working principle of optical fiber biosensors is displayed in Figure 1.18.

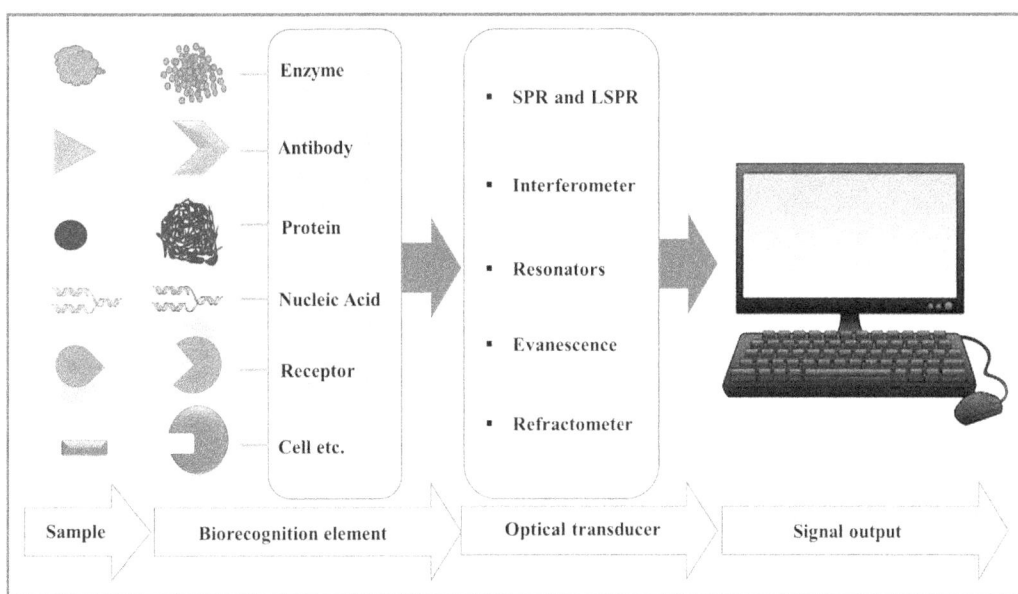

FIGURE 1.18 Principle of optical fiber biosensors.

Source: Reprinted with permission from *Optics & Laser Technology*, Copyright 2021, Elsevier (Shukla et al. 2019).

1.8.1 SURFACE PLASMON RESONANCE SENSOR

There was a pivotal development in SPR sensing that inspired, as discussed in the report by Liedberg and Nylander, the initial practical milepost of SPR in biomolecular detection (Liedberg, Nylander, and Lunström 1983) in 1983. Since the potential of SPR sensing was first recognized, there has been a significant advancement in the development of SPR biosensors. Now, it reached to be a promising stage for quantify monitoring and detecting analysis of biomolecular interactions in both qualitative and quantitative ways (Helmerhorst et al. 2012). SPR biosensors thus exhibit a wild field of applications, especially in food quality and medical diagnostics (Nguyen et al. 2015), correlating with their sensing applicability in biology, chemistry, and physics (Yu et al. 2019; Wang et al. 2021). SPR or LSPR phenomenon-based OFSs have been gradually replaced by plastic optical fiber (POF) in recent years due to their high cost and fragility (Jiang et al. 2017). Biacore instrument in 1990 was the first to introduce a commercial SPR sensor (Schasfoort 2017).

Surface plasmon polariton (SPP) can be widely used to monitor the changes of RI near the sensing layer. In this region, the change in RI is usually due to a specific binding of the target molecules. SPR excitation is possible, if a particular waveguide structure is used as the couple medium. Examples of such structures include optical fiber, grating, and high-index prism. These structures provide the required photon momentum along the boundary.

Figure 1.19 shows the schematics of several major SPR sensing devices. The prism-based SPR sensor, shown in Figure 1.19(a), was first proposed by Kretschmann and Reather in 1968 and first

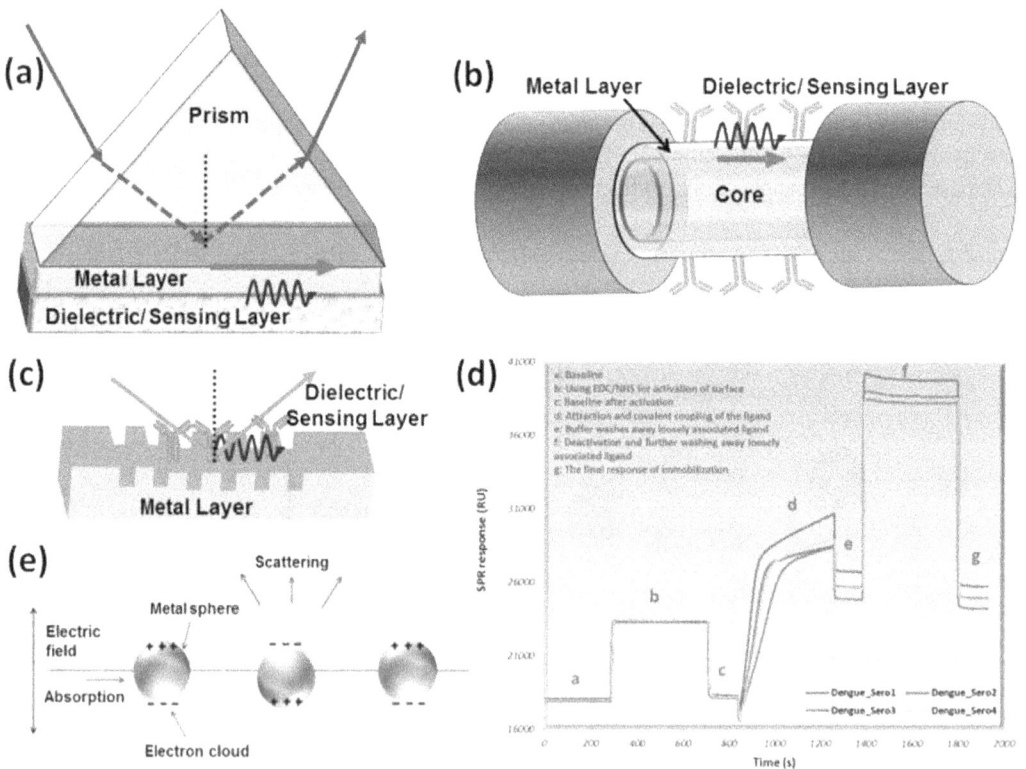

FIGURE 1.19 (a) Prism based, (b) optical fiber based, and (c) grating based. (d) Surface plasmon resonance response during sensor fabrication using immobilization of four serotypes of dengue antigen at each step used for the detection of dengue virus (DENV)-specific IgM antibodies (Jahanshahi et al. 2014). (e) Localized surface plasmon resonance, the behavior of metallic nanosphere in an external electromagnetic field (Roh, Chung, and Lee 2011).

successfully applied to sensing experiments by Liedberg. This sensational report greatly stimulated the research upsurge of SPR and promoted the development of PoC application. Today, the development of chip-based PoC sensors is still in full swing, and companies like Biacore, PhotonicSys, Plasmetrix, and others are investing significantly in research and development. They form a microfluidic channel for quantitative analysis of liquid analytes by uniformly depositing a thin metal (~50 nm) coating onto a glass substrate. These types of sensing systems have unique advantages over traditional methods. For instance, (i) label-free test methods such as ELISA have saved production costs, (ii) dynamic measurements of binding and nonbinding kinetics enable real-time monitoring of the interaction between analyte and receptor, and (iii) they have higher sensitivity. In particular, the limitation of TM polarized light and the decrease of selectivity and transmission depth (200–300 nm) are the unavoidable problems of standard SPR chips. However, subsequent modifications to the chip, like long-range SPR chips, can be used to detect larger biological entities such as bacteria or cells.

In this section, the recently reported fundamental spectroscopic studies, indicating the essential relationships involved in the spectral location of LSPR along with their environmental sensitivity governed by the shape and size of NPs, are described (Kumar et al. 2021). Reports illustrating the sensing distance dependence about enhanced activating energy, EM field, and plasmon resonance are also described here (Jia et al. 2012). Detection of biomolecular interactions employing LSPR-based nano-biosensors has been developed with utilization of this technique as a highly sensitive, flexible, and label-free sensing tool (Bonyár 2020; Kaushik et al. 2020). This helps in sensitive detection and quantification of biomolecules for a better disease diagnosis, and reliable prognoses are made achievable with this technology (Kelley et al. 2014; Soler et al. 2020). The schematic presentation demonstrating the LSPR phenomenon is shown in Figure 1.20. LSPR spectroscopy about the metal NPs is potentially used for sensing experimentation in the fields of chemistry and biology (Hong et al. 2012). Moreover, LSPR is responsible for surface-enhanced processes and EM field improvement (Willets and Van Duyne 2007). LSPR phenomenon-based sensors have several advantages for biomolecules detection: (i) high sensitivity with an assessment of alteration in RI, (ii) label-free detection, (iii) real-time accessibility, (iv) good reusability and reproducibility, and (v) easy assembling and cost-effectiveness (Jiang et al. 2018; Unser et al. 2015; Agrawal, Zhang, Saha, Kumar, Pu et al. 2020). Due to these advantages, LSPR-based nano-biosensors are emerging as better and more potent tools in the field of biotechnology and biosensors, over other available nano-biosensors (Malik et al. 2013). The LSPR technique, as a label-free detection method, makes use of the optical phenomenon of the collective oscillation of the valence electrons of noble metal NPs, that caused by the incident light field. With the help of this method, the absorption spectral detection is well realized in the ultraviolet-visible (UV-Vis) band.

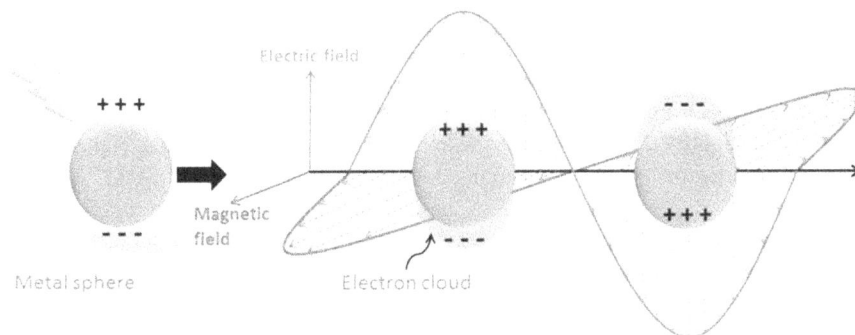

FIGURE 1.20 Localized surface plasmon resonance phenomenon (Qi et al. 2020).

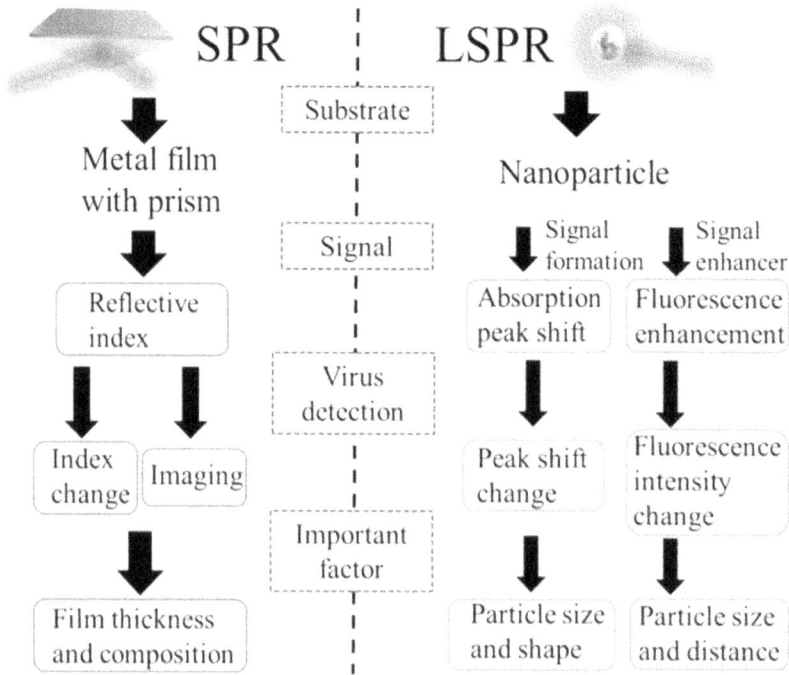

FIGURE 1.21 Summary of the comparative study, foundation, signal measurement methods, and critical factors of major plasmonic techniques (i.e., SPR and LSPR).

The use of LSPR techniques has recently emerged as an important label-free sensing technique: it is an optical phenomenon that causes a collective oscillation of valence electrons and subsequent absorption within the UV-Vis band of the light spectrum, due to interactions between the incident photons and the conduction band of a noble metal nanostructure.

We know that the sensitivity of biosensor systems based on the LSPR is evaluated by the quantitative analysis of the RI near the coating. In order to improve the sensing performance, people focus on the nanocoating materials, and its nano-size and shape were studied in depth. AuNPs are the most common coating materials because of their excellent stability, and many methods have been proposed to synthesize stable Au NMs rapidly. However, its poor molecular affinity cannot provide enough molecular attachment sites, which is an inevitable problem. In comparison, AgNPs have better molecular affinity and stronger sensing performance but poorer physical stability, which severely limits their application environment. Therefore, some researchers have proposed using other biocompatible two-dimensional materials, such as GO, to compensate for these shortcomings. For example, we coated a layer of GO on the surface of the sensor to study its effect on sensitivity, and the results show that sensitivity increased by about 20%. In recent years, various synthesis methods have emerged in the development of nanotechnology. Among them, silver triangle plate NPs have attracted much attention because of their unique structure, which can excite stronger local electric fields. Figure 1.21 summarizes the comparative study, foundation, signal measurement methods, and critical factors of major plasmonic techniques (i.e., SPR and LSPR).

1.9 PERFORMANCE PARAMETERS OF SENSORS

1.9.1 SENSITIVITY

As the most important characteristic of a biosensor, sensitivity defines the correlation between the signal intensity and variation in biomolecule concentration (Liu et al. 2019). The concentration of the target analyte is captured with accuracy even considering the minute changes in it, by a biosensor in the form of an optical signal (Qazi and Raza 2020). With a widespread requirement of medical utilization and significance in environmental monitoring, biosensors as per requirement, quantify the alterations in analyte concentrations (Song, Xu, and Fan 2006).

1.9.2 SELECTIVITY

Selectivity means that the biosensor can only respond to a selective analyte in the presence of other biomolecules (Mehrotra 2016). In selectivity, a signal or response is generated from interactions with a biomolecule that is different from the target biomolecule (Morales and Halpern 2018a). Biosensors with poor selectivity have such responses and are thus not suitable for clinical applications. Hence, selectivity is a crucial feature for biomedical applications. The test sample might contain several molecules with similarity to the target analyte and show competitive binding with the biological receptor (Morales and Halpern 2018b; Vasylieva 2012).

1.9.3 STABILITY

The stability of the biosensors is one of the most important attributes, especially when used for real-time monitoring processes (Tric et al. 2017). This measures the ability of a biosensor to withstand changes in performance variation due to interruptions arising from external factors such as temperature, humidity, or any other environmental constraints (McGrath and Scanaill 2013). The precision and accuracy of the biosensor device depend on these factors, and the signal generated could get corrupt if such variations are present (Marinesco 2018). The temperature sensitivity of the transducers used in biosensor devices also affects the stability. Further, interruptions in temperature also influence the integrity of the biological receptor (Patel et al. 2016).

1.9.4 LIMIT OF DETECTION

LoD describes the lowest concentration of the target analyte that can elicit a measurable signal (Armbruster and Pry 2008). Considering the imperceptible analyte content, a low *LoD* is a necessary feature for a biosensor, especially for medical purposes (Agrawal, Zhang, Saha, Kumar, Kaushik et al. 2020).

1.9.5 REPRODUCIBILITY

Reproducibility defines the capability of the sensing device to produce matching output signals or the results obtained in duplicate experiments (Agrawal, Saha, et al. 2020). It is one of the most essential features in biosensing, and the capabilities of the biosensor depend on the transducer performing with full precision and accuracy (Bhalla et al. 2020).

1.9.6 RESPONSE TIME

Response time is the time elapsed by the sensing system to produce a response signal after it has been tested by a biomarker with in-depth analysis (i.e., interaction of the biological receptor with the target biomolecule) (Pearson, Gill, and Vadgama 2000).

1.9.7 LINEARITY

Linearity determines the accuracy of a signal obtained in response to a series of measurements by varying analyte concentrations (Gauglitz 2018). This process provides an understanding of biosensor modification, describing a change in the targeting test that reveals the biosensor response (Portaccio and Lepore 2017). This is a crucial feature for a biosensor to obtain effective measurements of a target analyte with varying concentrations (Szunerits and Boukherroub 2018).

1.10   OVERVIEW OF THE BOOK

This book broadly covers the technologies and advancements associated with P-OFSs. It outlines the major developments seen over the last five years in the biomedical field. It also encompasses both theoretical and experimental approaches adopted for the development of P-OFSs. Further, several methods in biosensing technology involving an interdisciplinary approach are introduced. Overall, this book provides an overview of current advances in this area with a future perspective. Including real-life incidents and current developments over plasmonic biosensing devices would generate interest in readers and an inclination toward this subject. The future directions of PoC platforms toward improving capabilities and integrabilities are also presented. Several researchers from different disciplines have become involved in plasmonic sensing, considering it one of the most dynamic and promising fields of research. This book highlights the technologies involved in plasmonic sensing and their associated applications. It overviews the core ideology in the design of fiber-optic biosensors, as well as the kernel conception using traditional optical fibers, such as tapered, unclad, U-shaped fiber, hetero-core, side-polished, core, mismatched, bending, and hollow core. Meanwhile, other designs using characteristic optical fibers like photonic crystal fiber (PCF), photosensitive fiber (PSF), TFBG, and other special fiber. These sensors enable real-time observation of molecular binding with flying colors. Advances in nanoscience and nanotechnology have made it possible to develop plasmon NPs, thin films, and a highly sensitive optical characterization technique (Malekzad et al. 2017). This book also deals with recent advances in various plasmonic sensing techniques based on SERS and SPR phenomena. These phenomena are based on plasmonic sensors, detection schemes, their realization at the surface of NSs, configuration, components employed, and application of sensors are reported. To present the plasmonic phenomenon and based on OFSs, this write-up is broadly distributed over 9 chapters including this chapter. Book is mainly divided based on the use of NMs. The types of NPs, size, shape, and composition of metallic NPs are great effects on the sensitivity of sensors.

Chapters 1–3 covers the basics of optics and plasmonic, NMs, structural developments, and design methodology P-OFSs. This study will be of benefit to students, academicians, engineers, and researchers in the study area of optical fiber technology, nanotechnology, and biosensing. Chapter 2 involves the fundamentals of different NMs in the research course of the plasmonic phenomenon-based biosensing platform. The original intention of this write-up is to cover the development and future of the plasmonic NMs-based biosensing system and to account for the key knowledge of various NMs in distinct genres of the biosensing system. It also covers the basics of NPs, types of NMs, synthesis, characterization, and properties of NMs and their growing applications. Chapter 3 describes the major structure developments and design methodology over P-OFSs. To improve the sensitivity performance of sensors, various structural advancements are proposed that are briefly covered in this chapter. The process such as nanocoating and functionalization, along with a characterization of NMs and probe and measurement techniques are also widely covered in this chapter.

Chapter 4–8 categorizes the different P-OFSs used in biosensing applications. Chapter 4 covers the use of AuNPs in the development of P-OFSs. It discusses recent advances, as well as methods with definite value to solve the key obstacles and future possibilities in the sensing field. This also discusses the synthesis of AuNPs and associated novel NMs, characterization, and various applications of AuNPs. Chapter 5 is dedicated to the AgNPs-based P-OFSs. Synthesis, characterization, and applications of AgNPs are briefly discussed in this chapter. The employment of AgNPs for the quantity detection of glucose, cholesterol, bacteria detection, virus, DNA/RNA, and cells are covered herein. Graphene and its derivatives (GO/rGO) are one of the innovative NMs broadly used in the development of various P-OFSs, which is well discussed in Chapters 6 and 7. It will cover a vast surface area and higher conductivity. Different GO/rGO-based studies are summarized in this part, and future trends are presented. Similarly, major developments over novel NMs based P-OFSs are discussed briefly in Chapter 8. This chapter focuses on advances in novel materials-based sensor structural designing and extends the scope and expertise of rapid growth in biomedical applications. Chapter 9 summarizes the study over novel NMs based on P-OFSs for microorganism detection. It describes the role of novel NMs in the development of P-OFSs, future trends, and major findings. It also covers the synthesis, characterization, properties, and applications of novel NMs for cancer cell detection and bacterial detection. Future perspectives of the above studies are well summarized in Chapter 9. The potential for optical technology to function as a basic phenomenon used for the development of highly sensitive OFSs is analyzed and summarized in this chapter. Moreover, benefits and challenges associated with several experimental aspects, synthesis of NPs, and mechanisms of quantity analysis, besides the innovative methodologies that have been established to enhance the sensitivity, selectivity, as well as *LoD* are underlined.

The book also discusses the latest challenges correlated with engineering and the role of different NMs (metallic, magnetic, carbon-based NMs, and novel NPs) in advancement of the P-OFSs and provides a suitable platform for future enhancements in plasmonic biosensors. With healthcare issues emerging as challenging and crucial all over the world, there is an urgent demand for rapid and cost-effective measures and devices in biomedical industries, especially in underdeveloped countries.

REFERENCES

Agrawal, N., C. Saha, C. Kumar, R. Singh, B. Zhang, and S. Kumar. 2020. "Development of uric acid sensor using copper oxide and silver nanoparticles immobilized SMSMS fiber structure-based probe." *IEEE Transactions on Instrumentation and Measurement* 69 (11):9097–9104. DOI: 10.1109/TIM.2020.2998876.

Agrawal, N., B. Zhang, C. Saha, C. Kumar, B. K. Kaushik, and S. Kumar. 2020. "Development of dopamine sensor using silver nanoparticles and PEG-functionalized tapered optical fiber structure." *IEEE Transactions on Biomedical Engineering* 67 (6):1542–1547. DOI: 10.1109/TBME.2019.2939560.

Agrawal, Niteshkumar, Bingyuan Zhang, Chinmoy Saha, Chandrakanta Kumar, Xipeng Pu, and Santosh Kumar. 2020. "Ultra-sensitive cholesterol sensor using gold and zinc-oxide nanoparticles immobilized core mismatch MPM/SPS probe." *Journal of Lightwave Technology* 38 (8):2523–2529.

Alberto, Nélia, Maria F. Domingues, Carlos Marques, Paulo André, and Paulo Antunes. 2018. "Optical fiber magnetic field sensors based on magnetic fluid: A review." *Sensors* 18 (12). DOI: 10.3390/s18124325.

Angelov, George Vasilev, Dimitar Petrov Nikolakov, Ivelina Nikolaeva Ruskova, Elitsa Emilova Gieva, and Maria Liubomirova Spasova. 2019. "Healthcare sensing and monitoring." In *Enhanced Living Environments: Algorithms, Architectures, Platforms, and Systems*, edited by Ivan Ganchev, Nuno M. Garcia, Ciprian Dobre, Constandinos X. Mavromoustakis and Rossitza Goleva, 226–262. Cham: Springer International Publishing.

Anik, Ü. 2017. "12—Electrochemical medical biosensors for POC applications." In *Medical Biosensors for Point of Care (POC) Applications*, edited by Roger J. Narayan, 275–292. Duxford: Woodhead Publishing. https://www.sciencedirect.com/science/article/pii/B9780081000724000125.

Armbruster, David A., and Terry Pry. 2008. "Limit of blank, limit of detection and limit of quantitation." *The Clinical Biochemist: Reviews* 29 (Suppl 1):S49–S52.

Aruna Gandhi, M. S., Suoda Chu, K. Senthilnathan, P. R. Babu, K. Nakkeeran, and Qian Li. 2019. "Recent advances in plasmonic sensor-based fiber optic probes for biological applications." *Applied Sciences* 9:949. DOI: 10.3390/app9050949.

Bhalla, Nikhil, Pawan Jolly, Nello Formisano, and Pedro Estrela. 2016. "Introduction to biosensors." *Essays in Biochemistry* 60 (1):1–8. DOI: 10.1042/EBC20150001.

Bhalla, Nikhil, Yuwei Pan, Zhugen Yang, and Amir Farokh Payam. 2020. "Opportunities and challenges for biosensors and nanoscale analytical tools for pandemics: COVID-19." *ACS Nano* 14 (7):7783–7807. DOI: 10.1021/acsnano.0c04421.

Bhatt, Geeta, and Shantanu Bhattacharya. 2019. "Biosensors on chip: A critical review from an aspect of micro/nanoscales." *Journal of Micromanufacturing* 2 (2):198–219. DOI: 10.1177/2516598419847913.

Bonyár, Attila. 2020. "Label-free nucleic acid biosensing using nanomaterial-based localized surface plasmon resonance imaging: A review." *ACS Applied Nano Materials* 3 (9):8506–8521. DOI: 10.1021/acsanm.0c01457.

Brooks, Sierra M., and Hal S. Alper. 2021. "Applications, challenges, and needs for employing synthetic biology beyond the lab." *Nature Communications* 12 (1):1390. DOI: 10.1038/s41467-021-21740-0.

Budinski, Vedran, and Denis Donlagic. 2017. "Fiber-optic sensors for measurements of torsion, twist and rotation: A review." *Sensors (Basel, Switzerland)* 17 (3):443. DOI: 10.3390/s17030443.

Castillo-Henríquez, Luis, Mariana Brenes-Acuña, Arianna Castro-Rojas, Rolando Cordero-Salmerón, Mary Lopretti-Correa, and José Roberto Vega-Baudrit. 2020. "Biosensors for the detection of bacterial and viral clinical pathogens." *Sensors (Basel, Switzerland)* 20 (23):6926. DOI: 10.3390/s20236926.

Chack, Devendra, Niteshkumar Agrawal, and S. K. Raghuwanshi. 2014. "To analyse the performance of tapered and MMI assisted splitter on the basis of geographical parameters." *Optik* 125 (11):2568–2571. https://doi.org/10.1016/j.ijleo.2013.11.019.

Chaudhary, V. S., D. Kumar, and S. Kumar. 2021. "Gold-immobilized photonic crystal fiber-based SPR biosensor for detection of malaria disease in human body." *IEEE Sensors Journal* 1–1. DOI: 10.1109/JSEN.2021.3085829.

Chen, C. K., A. R. B. de Castro, and Y. R. Shen. 1981. "Surface-enhanced second-harmonic generation." *Physical Review Letters* 46 (2):145–148. DOI: 10.1103/PhysRevLett.46.145.

Chen, Chen, and Junsheng Wang. 2020. "Optical biosensors: An exhaustive and comprehensive review." *Analyst* 145 (5):1605–1628. DOI: 10.1039/C9AN01998G.

Chen, S. H., Y. C. Chuang, Y. C. Lu, H. C. Lin, Y. L. Yang, and C. S. Lin. 2009. "A method of layer-by-layer gold nanoparticle hybridization in a quartz crystal microbalance DNA sensing system used to detect dengue virus." *Nanotechnology* 20 (21):215501. DOI: 10.1088/0957-4484/20/21/215501.

Choi, Hae Young, Kwan Seob Park, Seong Jun Park, Un-Chul Paek, Byeong Ha Lee, and Eun Seo Choi. 2008. "Miniature fiber-optic high temperature sensor based on a hybrid structured Fabry: Perot interferometer." *Optics Letters* 33 (21):2455–2457. DOI: 10.1364/OL.33.002455.

da Silva, Everson T. S. G., Dênio E. P. Souto, José T. C. Barragan, Juliana de F. Giarola, Ana C. M. de Moraes, and Lauro T. Kubota. 2017. "Electrochemical biosensors in point-of-care devices: Recent advances and future trends." *ChemElectroChem* 4 (4):778–794. https://doi.org/10.1002/celc.201600758.

Demas, James N., B. A. DeGraff, and Patricia B. Coleman. 1999. "Peer reviewed: Oxygen sensors based on luminescence quenching." *Analytical Chemistry* 71 (23):793A–800A.

Drusová, Sandra, Wiecher Bakx, Pieter J. Doornenbal, R. Martijn Wagterveld, Victor F. Bense, and Herman L. Offerhaus. 2021. "Comparison of three types of fiber optic sensors for temperature monitoring in a groundwater flow simulator." *Sensors and Actuators A: Physical*:112682. https://doi.org/10.1016/j.sna.2021.112682.

Ellington, A. D., and J. W. Szostak. 1990. "In vitro selection of RNA molecules that bind specific ligands." *Nature* 346 (6287):818–822. DOI: 10.1038/346818a0.

Esfahani Monfared, Yashar. 2020. "Overview of recent advances in the design of plasmonic fiber-optic biosensors." *Biosensors* 10 (7):77. DOI: 10.3390/bios10070077.

Feng, Liang, Christopher J. Musto, Jonathan W. Kemling, Sung H. Lim, Wenxuan Zhong, and Kenneth S. Suslick. 2010. "Colorimetric sensor array for determination and identification of toxic industrial chemicals." *Analytical Chemistry* 82 (22):9433–9440. DOI: 10.1021/ac1020886.

Fidanboylu, Kemal, and Hasan Efendioglu. 2009. "Fiber optic sensors and their applications." 5th International Advanced Technologies Symposium (IATS'09), 13–15 May, Karabuk, Turkey.

Fried, Burton D., and Roy W. Gould. 1961. "Longitudinal ion oscillations in a hot plasma." *The Physics of Fluids* 4 (1):139–147. DOI: 10.1063/1.1706174.

Ganguly, Amar, and Bikas Mondal. 2011. *Fluid Flow Measurement Using Bending Loss of Optical Fiber.*

García, Yoany, Jesus Corres, and Javier Goicoechea. 2010. "Vibration detection using optical fiber sensors." *Journal of Sensors* 2010. DOI: 10.1155/2010/936487.

Gauglitz, Günter. 2018. "Analytical evaluation of sensor measurements." *Analytical and Bioanalytical Chemistry* 410 (1):5–13. DOI: 10.1007/s00216-017-0624-z.

Goff, David R., Kimberly S. Hansen, and Michelle K. Stull. 2003. *Fiber Optic Video Transmission: The Complete Guide.* Oxford; Boston: Focal Press.

Goss, W. C., R. Goldstein, M. D. Nelson, H. T. Fearnehaugh, and O. G. Ramer. 1980. "Fiber-optic rotation sensor technology." *Applied Optics* 19 (6):852–858. DOI: 10.1364/AO.19.000852.

Gräwe, Alexander, Anna Dreyer, Tobias Vornholt, Ursela Barteczko, Luzia Buchholz, Gila Drews, Uyen Linh Ho, Marta Eva Jackowski, Melissa Kracht, Janina Lüders, Tore Bleckwehl, Lukas Rositzka, Matthias Ruwe, Manuel Wittchen, Petra Lutter, Kristian Müller, and Jörn Kalinowski. 2019. "A paper-based, cell-free biosensor system for the detection of heavy metals and date rape drugs." *PLoS One* 14 (3):e0210940. DOI: 10.1371/journal.pone.0210940.

Grieshaber, Dorothee, Robert MacKenzie, Janos Vörös, and Erik Reimhult. 2008. "Electrochemical biosensors: Sensor principles and architectures." *Sensors (Basel, Switzerland)* 8 (3):1400–1458. DOI: 10.3390/s80314000.

Gu, Bobo, Ming-Jie Yin, A. Ping Zhang, Jin-Wen Qian, and Sailing He. 2009. "Low-cost high-performance fiber-optic pH sensor based on thin-core fiber modal interferometer." *Optics Express* 17 (25):22296–22302. DOI: 10.1364/OE.17.022296.

Guo, Tuan, Fu Liu, Bai-Ou Guan, and Jacques Albert. 2016. "[INVITED] tilted fiber grating mechanical and biochemical sensors." *Optics & Laser Technology* 78:19–33. https://doi.org/10.1016/j.optlastec.2015.10.007.

Guo, X., C. S. Lin, S. H. Chen, R. Ye, and V. C. Wu. 2012. "A piezoelectric immunosensor for specific capture and enrichment of viable pathogens by quartz crystal microbalance sensor, followed by detection with antibody-functionalized gold nanoparticles." *Biosens Bioelectron* 38 (1):177–183. DOI: 10.1016/j.bios.2012.05.024.

Guo, Xiaodong, Fang Wen, Nan Zheng, Matthew Saive, Marie-Laure Fauconnier, and Jiaqi Wang. 2020. "Aptamer-based biosensor for detection of mycotoxins." *Frontiers in Chemistry* 8. DOI: 10.3389/fchem.2020.00195.

Guo, Xing, Shengbo Sang, Jinyu Guo, Aoqun Jian, Qianqian Duan, Jianlong Ji, Qiang Zhang, and Wendong Zhang. 2017. "A magnetoelastic biosensor based on E2 glycoprotein for wireless detection of classical swine fever virus E2 antibody." *Scientific Reports* 7 (1):15626. DOI: 10.1038/s41598-017-15908-2.

Haidekker, Mark A., Walter J. Akers, Derek Fischer, and Emmanuel A. Theodorakis. 2006. "Optical fiber-based fluorescent viscosity sensor." *Optics Letters* 31 (17):2529–2531. DOI: 10.1364/OL.31.002529.

Hainfeld, J. F., D. N. Slatkin, T. M. Focella, and H. M. Smilowitz. 2006. "Gold nanoparticles: A new X-ray contrast agent." *Br J Radiol* 79 (939):248–253. DOI: 10.1259/bjr/13169882.

Hara, Tony O., and Baljit Singh. 2021. "Electrochemical biosensors for detection of pesticides and heavy metal toxicants in water: Recent trends and progress." *ACS ES&T Water* 1 (3):462–478. DOI: 10.1021/acsestwater.0c00125.

Hase, K., S. Sakai, K. Tsukada, E. Sekizuka, C. Oshio, and H. Minamitani. 2002. "Continuous measurement of blood oxygen pressure using a fiber optic sensor based on phosphorescence quenching." Proceedings of the Second Joint 24th Annual Conference and the Annual Fall Meeting of the Biomedical Engineering Society, Engineering in Medicine and Biology, 23–26 Oct.

Heller, Adam, and Ben Feldman. 2008. "Electrochemical glucose sensors and their applications in diabetes management." *Chemical Reviews* 108 (7):2482–2505. DOI: 10.1021/cr068069y.

Helmerhorst, Erik, David J. Chandler, Matt Nussio, and Cyril D. Mamotte. 2012. "Real-time and label-free bio-sensing of molecular interactions by surface plasmon resonance: A laboratory medicine perspective." *The Clinical Biochemist: Reviews* 33 (4):161–173.

Homola, Jiří. 2008. "Surface plasmon resonance sensors for detection of chemical and biological species." *Chemical Reviews* 108 (2):462–493. DOI: 10.1021/cr068107d.

Hong, Yoochan, Yong-Min Huh, Dae Sung Yoon, and Jaemoon Yang. 2012. "Nanobiosensors based on localized surface plasmon resonance for biomarker detection." *Journal of Nanomaterials* 2012:759830. DOI: 10.1155/2012/759830.

Islam, Farhadul, Md Hakimul Haque, Sharda Yadav, Md Nazmul Islam, Vinod Gopalan, Nam-Trung Nguyen, Alfred K. Lam, and Muhammad J. A. Shiddiky. 2017. "An electrochemical method for sensitive and rapid detection of FAM134B protein in colon cancer samples." *Scientific Reports* 7 (1):133. DOI: 10.1038/s41598-017-00206-8.

Jahanshahi, Peyman, Erfan Zalnezhad, Shamala Devi Sekaran, and Faisal Rafiq Mahamd Adikan. 2014. "Rapid immunoglobulin M-based dengue diagnostic test using surface plasmon resonance biosensor." *Scientific Reports* 4 (1):3851. DOI: 10.1038/srep03851.

Jia, Kun, Jean L. Bijeon, Pierre M. Adam, and Rodica E. Ionescu. 2012. "Sensitive localized surface plasmon resonance multiplexing protocols." *Analytical Chemistry* 84 (18):8020–8027. DOI: 10.1021/ac301825a.

Jiang, Jing, Xinhao Wang, Shuang Li, Fei Ding, Nantao Li, Shaoyu Meng, Ruifan Li, Jia Qi, Qingjun Liu, and Gang Logan Liu. 2018. "Plasmonic nano-arrays for ultrasensitive bio-sensing." *Nanophotonics* 7 (9):1517–1531. DOI: 10.1515/nanoph-2018-0023.

Jiang, Shouzhen, Zhe Li, Chao Zhang, Saisai Gao, Zhen Li, Hengwei Qiu, Chonghui Li, Cheng Yang, Mei Liu, and Yanjun Liu. 2017. "A novel U-bent plastic optical fibre local surface plasmon resonance sensor based on a graphene and silver nanoparticle hybrid structure." *Journal of Physics D: Applied Physics* 50 (16):165105. DOI: 10.1088/1361-6463/aa628c.

Jin, Rongchao, Y. Charles Cao, Encai Hao, Gabriella S. Métraux, George C. Schatz, and Chad A. Mirkin. 2003. "Controlling anisotropic nanoparticle growth through plasmon excitation." *Nature* 425 (6957):487–490. DOI: 10.1038/nature02020.

Jin, Wei, T. K. Y. Lee, S. L. Ho, H. L. Ho, K. T. Lau, L. M. Zhou, and Y. Zhou. 2006. "CHAPTER 25: Structural strain and temperature measurements using fiber Bragg grating sensors." In *Guided Wave Optical Components and Devices*, edited by Bishnu P. Pal, 389–400. Burlington: Academic Press.

Joe, Hang-Eun, Huitaek Yun, Seung-Hwan Jo, Martin B. G. Jun, and Byung-Kwon Min. 2018. "A review on optical fiber sensors for environmental monitoring." *International Journal of Precision Engineering and Manufacturing-Green Technology* 5 (1):173–191. DOI: 10.1007/s40684-018-0017-6.

Kao, K. C., and G. A. Hockham. 1966. Dielectric-fibre surface waveguides for optical frequencies. *Proceedings of the Institution of Electrical Engineers* 113 (7): 1151–1158.

Kaur, B., S. Kumar, and B. K. Kaushik. 2021. "2D materials-based fiber optic SPR biosensor for cancer detection at 1550 nm." *IEEE Sensors Journal* 21 (21):23957–23964. DOI: 10.1109/JSEN.2021.3110967.

Kaur, B., S. Kumar, and B. K. Kaushik. 2022. "MXenes-based fiber-optic SPR sensor for colorectal cancer diagnosis." *IEEE Sensors Journal* 22 (7):6661–6668. DOI: 10.1109/JSEN.2022.3154385.

Kaushik, B. K., L. Singh, R. Singh, G. Zhu, B. Zhang, Q. Wang, and S. Kumar. 2020. "Detection of collagen-IV using highly reflective metal nanoparticles: Immobilized photosensitive optical fiber-based MZI structure." *IEEE Transactions on NanoBioscience* 19 (3):477–484. DOI: 10.1109/TNB.2020.2998520.

Kelley, Shana O., Chad A. Mirkin, David R. Walt, Rustem F. Ismagilov, Mehmet Toner, and Edward H. Sargent. 2014. "Advancing the speed, sensitivity and accuracy of biomolecular detection using multi-length-scale engineering." *Nature Nanotechnology* 9 (12):969–980. DOI: 10.1038/nnano.2014.261.

Khanmohammadi, Akbar, Arash Jalili Ghazizadeh, Pegah Hashemi, Abbas Afkhami, Fabiana Arduini, and Hasan Bagheri. 2020. "An overview to electrochemical biosensors and sensors for the detection of environmental contaminants." *Journal of the Iranian Chemical Society* 17 (10):2429–2447. DOI: 10.1007/s13738-020-01940-z.

Kim, Byung Hong, In Seop Chang, Geun Cheol Gil, Hyung Soo Park, and Hyung Joo Kim. 2003. "Novel BOD (biological oxygen demand) sensor using mediator-less microbial fuel cell." *Biotechnology Letters* 25 (7):541–545. DOI: 10.1023/A:1022891231369.

Kirimli, C. E., W. H. Shih, and W. Y. Shih. 2014. "DNA hybridization detection with 100 zM sensitivity using piezoelectric plate sensors with an improved noise-reduction algorithm." *Analyst* 139 (11):2754–2763. DOI: 10.1039/c4an00215f.

Kretschmann, E., and H. Raether. 1968. "Notizen: Radiative decay of nonradiative surface plasmons excited by light." *Zeitschrift für Naturforschung A* 23 (12):2135–2136. DOI: DOI: 10.1515/zna-1968-1247.

Kumar, R., S. Pal, Y. K. Prajapati, S. Kumar, and J. P. Saini. 2022. "Sensitivity improvement of a MXene-immobilized SPR sensor with Ga-Doped-ZnO for biomolecules detection." *IEEE Sensors Journal* 22 (7):6536–6543. DOI: 10.1109/JSEN.2022.3154099.

Kumar, S., Z. Guo, R. Singh, Q. Wang, B. Zhang, S. Cheng, F. Z. Liu, C. Marques, B. K. Kaushik, and R. Jha. 2021. "MoS$_2$ functionalized multicore fiber probes for selective detection of *Shigella* bacteria based on localized plasmon." *Journal of Lightwave Technology* 39 (12):4069–4081. DOI: 10.1109/JLT.2020.3036610.

Lakshmanan, Anupama, Zhiyang Jin, Suchita P. Nety, Daniel P. Sawyer, Audrey Lee-Gosselin, Dina Malounda, Mararet B. Swift, David Maresca, and Mikhail G. Shapiro. 2020. "Acoustic biosensors for ultrasound imaging of enzyme activity." *Nature Chemical Biology* 16 (9):988–996. DOI: 10.1038/s41589-020-0591-0.

Liedberg, Bo, Claes Nylander, and Ingemar Lunström. 1983. "Surface plasmon resonance for gas detection and biosensing." *Sensors and Actuators* 4:299–304. https://doi.org/10.1016/0250-6874(83)85036-7.

Lim, Hui Jean, Tridib Saha, Beng Ti Tey, Wen Siang Tan, and Chien Wei Ooi. 2020. "Quartz crystal microbalance-based biosensors as rapid diagnostic devices for infectious diseases." *Biosensors & Bioelectronics* 168:112513–112513. DOI: 10.1016/j.bios.2020.112513.

Liu, Haoran, Jun Ge, Eugene Ma, and Lei Yang. 2019. "10—Advanced biomaterials for biosensor and theranostics." In *Biomaterials in Translational Medicine*, edited by Lei Yang, Sarit B. Bhaduri, and Thomas J. Webster, 213–255. Cambridge, MA: Academic Press.

Llandro, J., J. J. Palfreyman, A. Ionescu, and C. H. W. Barnes. 2010. "Magnetic biosensor technologies for medical applications: A review." *Medical & Biological Engineering & Computing* 48 (10):977–998. DOI: 10.1007/s11517-010-0649-3.

Llaudet, Enrique, Sonja Hatz, Magali Droniou, and Nicholas Dale. 2005. "Microelectrode biosensor for real-time measurement of ATP in biological tissue." *Analytical Chemistry* 77 (10):3267–3273. DOI: 10.1021/ac048106q.

Luppa, P. B., L. J. Sokoll, and D. W. Chan. 2001. "Immunosensors: Principles and applications to clinical chemistry." *Clin Chim Acta* 314 (1–2):1–26. DOI: 10.1016/s0009-8981(01)00629-5.

MacCraith, Brian D., Colette M. McDonagh, Gerard O'Keeffe, Emmetine T. Keyes, Johannes G. Vos, Brendan O'Kelly, and John F. McGilp. 1993. "Fibre optic oxygen sensor based on fluorescence quenching of eva-nescent-wave excited ruthenium complexes in sol:gel derived porous coatings." *Analyst* 118 (4):385–388. DOI: 10.1039/AN9931800385.

Maier, Stefan A. 2007. *Plasmonics: Fundamentals and Applications*. Vol. 1. New York: Springer.

Malekzad, Hedieh, Parham Sahandi Zangabad, Hamed Mirshekari, Mahdi Karimi, and Michael R. Hamblin. 2017. "Noble metal nanoparticles in biosensors: Recent studies and applications." *Nanotechnology Reviews* 6 (3):301–329. DOI: 10.1515/ntrev-2016-0014.

Malik, Parth, Varun Katyal, Vibhuti Malik, Archana Asatkar, Gajendra Inwati, and Tapan K. Mukherjee. 2013. "Nanobiosensors: Concepts and variations." *ISRN Nanomaterials* 2013:327435. DOI: 10.1155/2013/327435.

Marinesco, S. 2018. "Microelectrode biosensors for in vivo functional monitoring of biological molecules." In *Encyclopedia of Interfacial Chemistry*, edited by Klaus Wandelt, 350–363. Oxford: Elsevier.

Masson, Jean-Francois. 2017. "Surface plasmon resonance clinical biosensors for medical diagnostics." *ACS Sensors* 2. DOI: 10.1021/acssensors.6b00763.

Matthews, Christopher J., Emma S. V. Andrews, and Wayne M. Patrick. 2021. "Enzyme-based amperometric biosensors for malic acid: A review." *Analytica Chimica Acta* 1156:338218. https://doi.org/10.1016/j.aca.2021.338218.

Mazhari, Bi Bi Zainab, Dayanand Agsar, and M. V. N. Ambika Prasad. 2017. "Development of paper bio-sensor for the detection of phenol from industrial effluents using bioconjugate of tyr-AuNps medi-ated by novel isolate *Streptomyces tuirus* DBZ39." *Journal of Nanomaterials* 2017:1352134. DOI: 10.1155/2017/1352134.

McGrath, Michael J., and Cliodhna Ní Scanaill. 2013. "Sensing and sensor fundamentals." In *Sensor Technologies: Healthcare, Wellness, and Environmental Applications*, edited by Michael J. McGrath and Cliodhna Ní Scanaill, 15–50. Berkeley, CA: Apress.

Mehrotra, Parikha. 2016. "Biosensors and their applications: A review." *Journal of Oral Biology and Craniofacial Research* 6 (2):153–159. DOI: 10.1016/j.jobcr.2015.12.002.

Melo, Arthur A., Márcia F. S. Santiago, Talita B. Silva, Cleumar S. Moreira, and Rossana M. S. Cruz. 2018. "Investigation of a D-shaped optical fiber sensor with graphene overlay." *IFAC-PapersOnLine* 51 (27):309–314. https://doi.org/10.1016/j.ifacol.2018.11.623.

Mishra, A. C., P. Lohia, and D. K. Dwivedi. 2020. "Long period grating based optical fiber sensors: Fabrication techniques and characteristics." 2020 International Conference on Electrical and Electronics Engineering (ICE3), 14–15 Feb.

Mitschke, Fedor. 1989. "Fiber-optic sensor for humidity." *Optics Letters* 14 (17):967–969. DOI: 10.1364/OL.14.000967.

Mock, J. J., M. Barbic, D. R. Smith, D. A. Schultz, and S. Schultz. 2002. "Shape effects in plasmon reso-nance of individual colloidal silver nanoparticles." *Journal of Chemical Physics* 116 (15):6755–6759. DOI: 10.1063/1.1462610.

Mohanty, S. P., and E. Kougianos. 2006. "Biosensors: A tutorial review." *IEEE Potentials* 25 (2):35–40. DOI: 10.1109/MP.2006.1649009.

Mojsoska, Biljana, Sylvester Larsen, Dorte A. Olsen, Jonna S. Madsen, Ivan Brandslund, and Fatima A. Alatraktchi. 2021. "Rapid SARS-CoV-2 detection using electrochemical immunosensor." *Sensors* 21 (2). DOI: 10.3390/s21020390.

Morales, Marissa A., and Jeffrey Mark Halpern. 2018a. "Guide to selecting a biorecognition element for bio-sensors." *Bioconjugate Chemistry* 29 (10):3231–3239. DOI: 10.1021/acs.bioconjchem.8b00592.

Morales, Marissa A., and Jeffrey Mark Halpern. 2018b. "Guide to selecting a biorecognition element for bio-sensors." *Bioconjugate Chemistry* 29. DOI: 10.1021/acs.bioconjchem.8b00592.

Naresh, Varnakavi, and Nohyun Lee. 2021a. "A review on biosensors and recent development of nanostruc-tured materials-enabled biosensors." *Sensors (Basel, Switzerland)* 21 (4):1109. DOI: 10.3390/s21041109.

Naresh, Varnakavi, and Nohyun Lee. 2021b. "A review on biosensors and recent development of nanostruc-tured materials-enabled biosensors." *Sensors* 21 (4). DOI: 10.3390/s21041109.

Narita, Fumio, Zhenjin Wang, Hiroki Kurita, Zhen Li, Yu Shi, Yu Jia, and Constantinos Soutis. 2021. "A review of piezoelectric and magnetostrictive biosensor materials for detection of COVID-19 and other viruses." *Advanced Materials* 33 (1):2005448. https://doi.org/10.1002/adma.202005448.

Nehl, Colleen L., Hongwei Liao, and Jason H. Hafner. 2006. "Optical properties of star-shaped gold nanoparticles." *Nano Letters* 6 (4):683–688. DOI: 10.1021/nl052409y.

Newman, Jeffrey D., and Anthony P. F. Turner. 2005. "Home blood glucose biosensors: A commercial perspective." *Biosensors and Bioelectronics* 20 (12):2435–2453. https://doi.org/10.1016/j.bios.2004.11.012.

Nguyen, Hoang Hiep, Jeho Park, Sebyung Kang, and Moonil Kim. 2015. "Surface plasmon resonance: A versatile technique for biosensor applications." *Sensors (Basel, Switzerland)* 15 (5):10481–10510. DOI: 10.3390/s150510481.

Niemeyer, Christof M. 2001. "Nanoparticles, proteins, and nucleic acids: Biotechnology meets materials science." *Angewandte Chemie International Edition* 40 (22):4128–4158. https://doi.org/10.1002/1521-3773(20011119)40:22<4128::AID-ANIE4128>3.0.CO;2-S.

Niu, Y. D., Q. Chen, Chunliu Zhao, and D. N. Wang. 2021. "Highly sensitive optical fiber bending sensor based on hollow core fiber and single mode fiber." *Optik* 228:166209. https://doi.org/10.1016/j.ijleo.2020.166209.

Otto, Andreas. 1968. "Excitation of nonradiative surface plasma waves in silver by the method of frustrated total reflection." *Zeitschrift für Physik a Hadrons and Nuclei* 216 (4):398–410. DOI: 10.1007/BF01391532.

Patel, Suprava, Rachita Nanda, Sibasish Sahoo, and Eli Mohapatra. 2016. "Biosensors in health care: The milestones achieved in their development towards lab-on-chip-analysis." *Biochemistry Research International* 2016:3130469. DOI: 10.1155/2016/3130469.

Paulo, Roriz, Frazão Orlando, B. Lobo-Ribeiro Antonio, L. Santos José, and A. Simoes Jose. 2013. "Review of fiber-optic pressure sensors for biomedical and biomechanical applications." *Journal of Biomedical Optics* 18 (5):1–19. DOI: 10.1117/1.JBO.18.5.050903.

Pearson, J. E., A. Gill, and P. Vadgama. 2000. "Analytical aspects of biosensors." *Annals of Clinical Biochemistry* 37 (Pt 2):119–145. DOI: 10.1258/0004563001899131.

Perez-Herrera, R. A., and M. Lopez-Amo. 2013. "Fiber optic sensor networks." *Optical Fiber Technology* 19 (6, Part B):689–699. https://doi.org/10.1016/j.yofte.2013.07.014.

Pines, David. 1956. "Collective energy losses in solids." *Reviews of Modern Physics* 28 (3):184–198. DOI: 10.1103/RevModPhys.28.184.

Pines, David, and David Bohm. 1952. "A collective description of electron interactions: II. Collective vs individual particle aspects of the interactions." *Physical Review* 85 (2):338–353. DOI: 10.1103/PhysRev.85.338.

Pohanka, M. 2018. "Overview of piezoelectric biosensors, immunosensors and DNA sensors and their applications." *Materials (Basel, Switzerland)* 11 (3):448. DOI: 10.3390/ma11030448.

Pohanka, M., and P. Skládal. 2007. "Piezoelectric immunosensor for the direct and rapid detection of *Francisella tularensis*." *Folia Microbiol (Praha)* 52 (4):325–330. DOI: 10.1007/bf02932086.

Portaccio, Marianna, and Maria Lepore. 2017. "Determination of different saccharides concentration by means of a multienzymes amperometric biosensor." *Journal of Sensors* 2017:7498945. DOI: 10.1155/2017/7498945.

Pospíšilová, Marie, Gabriela Kuncová, and Josef Trögl. 2015. "Fiber-optic chemical sensors and fiber-optic bio-sensors." *Sensors (Basel, Switzerland)* 15 (10):25208–25259. DOI: 10.3390/s151025208.

Powell, C. J., and J. B. Swan. 1959. "Origin of the characteristic electron energy losses in magnesium." *Physical Review* 116 (1):81–83. DOI: 10.1103/PhysRev.116.81.

Purohit, Buddhadev, Pramod R. Vernekar, Nagaraj P. Shetti, and Pranjal Chandra. 2020. "Biosensor nanoengineering: Design, operation, and implementation for biomolecular analysis." *Sensors International* 1:100040. https://doi.org/10.1016/j.sintl.2020.100040.

Qazi, Sahar, and Khalid Raza. 2020. "Chapter 4: Smart biosensors for an efficient point of care (PoC) health management." In *Smart Biosensors in Medical Care*, edited by Jyotismita Chaki, Nilanjan Dey, and Debashis De, 65–85. Cambridge, MA: Academic Press.

Qi, Miao, Nancy M. Zhang, Kaiwei Li, Swee C. Tjin, and Lei Wei. 2020. "Hybrid plasmonic fiber-optic sensors." *Sensors* 20 (11). DOI: 10.3390/s20113266.

Ritchie, R. H. 1957. "Plasma losses by fast electrons in thin films." *Physical Review* 106 (5):874–881. DOI: 10.1103/PhysRev.106.874.

Roh, Sookyoung, Taerin Chung, and Byoungho Lee. 2011. "Overview of the characteristics of micro- and nano-structured surface plasmon resonance sensors." *Sensors (Basel, Switzerland)* 11 (2):1565–1588. DOI: 10.3390/s110201565.

Roriz, Paulo, Susana Silva, Orlando Frazão, and Susana Novais. 2020a. "Optical fiber temperature sensors and their biomedical applications." *Sensors* 20:2113. DOI: 10.3390/s20072113.

Roriz, Paulo, Susana Silva, Orlando Frazão, and Susana Novais. 2020b. "Optical fiber temperature sensors and their biomedical applications." *Sensors (Basel, Switzerland)* 20 (7):2113. DOI: 10.3390/s20072113.

Ruddy, V., B. D. MacCraith, and J. A. Murphy. 1990. "Evanescent wave absorption spectroscopy using multi-mode fibers." *Journal of Applied Physics* 67 (10):6070–6074.

Ruthemann, Gerhard. 1942. "Elektronenbremsung an Röntgenniveaus." *Die Naturwissenschaften* 30 (9):145–145. DOI: 10.1007/BF01475385.

Ruthemann, Gerhard. 1948. "Diskrete Energieverluste mittelschneller Elektronen beim Durchgang durch dünne Folien." *Annalen der Physik* 437:113–134.

Schasfoort, Richard B. M. 2017. "Chapter 1: Introduction to surface plasmon resonance." In *Handbook of Surface Plasmon Resonance (2)*, 1–26. Piccadilly, London: The Royal Society of Chemistry.

Selwyna, P. G. C., P. R. Loganathan, and K. H. Begam. 2013. "Development of electrochemical biosensor for breast cancer detection using gold nanoparticle doped CA 15–3 antibody and antigen interaction." 2013 International Conference on Signal Processing, Image Processing & Pattern Recognition, 7–8 Feb.

Sharma, A. K., R. Jha, and B. D. Gupta. 2007. "Fiber-optic sensors based on surface plasmon resonance: A comprehensive review." *IEEE Sensors Journal* 7 (8):1118–1129. DOI: 10.1109/JSEN.2007.897946.

Sherry, Leif J., Shih-Hui Chang, George C. Schatz, Richard P. Van Duyne, Benjamin J. Wiley, and Younan Xia. 2005. "Localized surface plasmon resonance spectroscopy of single silver nanocubes." *Nano Letters* 5 (10):2034–2038. DOI: 10.1021/nl0515753.

Shipway, A. N., E. Katz, and I. Willner. 2000. "Nanoparticle arrays on surfaces for electronic, optical, and sensor applications." *Chemphyschem* 1 (1):18–52. DOI: 10.1002/1439-7641(20000804)1:1<18::aid-cphc18>3.0.co;2-l.

Shrivastav, Anand M., Uroš Cvelbar, and Ibrahim Abdulhalim. 2021. "A comprehensive review on plasmonic-based biosensors used in viral diagnostics." *Communications Biology* 4 (1):70. DOI: 10.1038/s42003-020-01615-8.

Shukla, S. K., Chandra Shekhar Kushwaha, Tugrul Guner, and Mustafa M. Demir. 2019. "Chemically modified optical fibers in advanced technology: An overview." *Optics & Laser Technology* 115:404–432. https://doi.org/10.1016/j.optlastec.2019.02.025.

Singh, L., N. Agrawal, C. Saha, and B. K. Kaushik. 2022. "A plus shaped cavity in optical fiber based refractive index sensor." *IEEE Transactions on NanoBioscience* 21 (2):199–205. DOI: 10.1109/TNB.2021.3121779.

Singh, Lokendra, Niteshkumar Agrawal, Chinmoy Saha, Brij Mohan Singh, and Taresh Singh. 2022. "Highly sensitive plus shaped cavity in silicon fiber for RI detection of water samples." *Silicon*. DOI: 10.1007/s12633-021-01519-0.

Singh, Ragini, Santosh Kumar, Feng-Zhen Liu, Cheng Shuang, Bingyuan Zhang, Rajan Jha, and Brajesh Kumar Kaushik. 2020. "Etched multicore fiber sensor using copper oxide and gold nanoparticles decorated graphene oxide structure for cancer cells detection." *Biosensors and Bioelectronics* 168:112557. https://doi.org/10.1016/j.bios.2020.112557.

Smitha, S. L., K. M. Nissamudeen, Daizy Philip, and K. G. Gopchandran. 2008. "Studies on surface plasmon resonance and photoluminescence of silver nanoparticles." *Spectrochimica Acta Part A: Molecular and Biomolecular Spectroscopy* 71 (1):186–190. https://doi.org/10.1016/j.saa.2007.12.002.

Soler, Maria, Maria Carmen Estevez, Maria Cardenosa-Rubio, Alejandro Astua, and Laura M. Lechuga. 2020. "How nanophotonic label-free biosensors can contribute to rapid and massive diagnostics of respiratory virus infections: COVID-19 case." *ACS Sensors* 5 (9):2663–2678. DOI: 10.1021/acssensors.0c01180.

Song, Shiping, Hui Xu, and Chunhai Fan. 2006. "Potential diagnostic applications of biosensors: Current and future directions." *International Journal of Nanomedicine* 1 (4):433–440. DOI: 10.2147/nano.2006.1.4.433.

Srivastava, Swarnim, and Ekta Khare. 2021. "Biosensors based medical devices for disease monitoring therapy." *International Journal of Advanced Research in Science, Communication and Technology*:263–278. DOI: 10.48175/IJARSCT-988.

Stern, E. A., and R. A. Ferrell. 1960. "Surface plasma oscillations of a degenerate electron gas." *Physical Review* 120 (1):130–136. DOI: 10.1103/PhysRev.120.130.

Su, L., W. Jia, C. Hou, and Y. Lei. 2011. "Microbial biosensors: A review." *Biosens Bioelectron* 26 (5):1788–1799. DOI: 10.1016/j.bios.2010.09.005.

Sun, Qizhen, Deming Liu, Jian Wang, and Hairong Liu. 2008. "Distributed fiber-optic vibration sensor using a ring Mach-Zehnder interferometer." *Optics Communications* 281 (6):1538–1544. https://doi.org/10.1016/j.optcom.2007.11.055.

Szunerits, Sabine, and Rabah Boukherroub. 2018. "Graphene-based biosensors." *Interface Focus* 8 (3):20160132. DOI: 10.1098/rsfs.2016.0132.

Takeo, Takashi, and Hajime Hattori. 1982. "Optical fiber sensor for measuring refractive index." *Japanese Journal of Applied Physics* 21 (Part 1, No. 10):1509–1512. DOI: 10.1143/jjap.21.1509.

Tan, Alfred Jia Yee, Sing Ng, Paul Stoddart, and Hong Chua. 2020. "Trends and applications of U-shaped fiber optic sensors: A review." *IEEE Sensors Journal* 21:120–131. DOI: 10.1109/JSEN.2020.3014190.

Thakur, M. S., and K. V. Ragavan. 2013. "Biosensors in food processing." *Journal of Food Science and Technology* 50 (4):625–641. DOI: 10.1007/s13197-012-0783-z.

Tosi, Daniele. 2018. "Review of Chirped Fiber Bragg Grating (CFBG) fiber-optic sensors and their applications." *Sensors* 18 (7). DOI: 10.3390/s18072147.

Totsu, Kentaro, Yoichi Haga, and Masayoshi Esashi. 2004. "Ultra-miniature fiber-optic pressure sensor using white light interferometry." *Journal of Micromechanics and Microengineering* 15 (1):71–75. DOI: 10.1088/0960-1317/15/1/011.

Tran, Thuy, Olof Eskilson, Florian Mayer, Robert Gustavsson, Robert Selegård, Ingemar Lundström, Carl-Fredrik Mandenius, Erik Martinsson, and Daniel Aili. 2020. "Real-time nanoplasmonic sensor for IgG monitoring in bioproduction." *Processes* 8:1302. DOI: 10.3390/pr8101302.

Tric, Mircea, Mario Lederle, Lisa Neuner, Igor Dolgowjasow, Philipp Wiedemann, Stefan Wölfl, and Tobias Werner. 2017. "Optical biosensor optimized for continuous in-line glucose monitoring in animal cell culture." *Analytical and Bioanalytical Chemistry* 409 (24):5711–5721. DOI: 10.1007/s00216-017-0511-7.

Tyler, Scott W., John S. Selker, Mark B. Hausner, Christine E. Hatch, Thomas Torgersen, Carl E. Thodal, and S. Geoffrey Schladow. 2009. "Environmental temperature sensing using Raman spectra DTS fiber-optic methods." *Water Resources Research* 45 (4).

Unser, Sarah, Ian Bruzas, Jie He, and Laura Sagle. 2015. "Localized surface plasmon resonance biosensing: Current challenges and approaches." *Sensors (Basel, Switzerland)* 15 (7):15684–15716. DOI: 10.3390/s150715684.

Vasylieva, Natalia. 2012. "Implantable microelectrode biosensors for neurochemical monitoring of brain functioning." Agricultural sciences. INSA de Lyon; INSA de Lyon, 2012ISAL0078 [Thesis]. https://www.researchgate.net/publication/280899958_Implantable_microelectrode_biosensors_for_neurochemical_monitoring_of_brain_functioning#fullTextFileContent.

Vigneshvar, S., C. C. Sudhakumari, Balasubramanian Senthilkumaran, and Hridayesh Prakash. 2016. "Recent advances in biosensor technology for potential applications: An overview." *Frontiers in Bioengineering and Biotechnology* 4 (11). DOI: 10.3389/fbioe.2016.00011.

Wang, Y., G. Zhu, M. Li, R. Singh, C. Marques, R. Min, B. K. Kaushik, B. Zhang, R. Jha, and S. Kumar. 2021. "Water pollutants p-cresol detection based on Au-ZnO nanoparticles modified tapered optical fiber." *IEEE Transactions on NanoBioscience* 20 (3):377–384. DOI: 10.1109/TNB.2021.3082856.

Wiley, Benjamin, Yugang Sun, Brian Mayers, and Younan Xia. 2005. "Shape-controlled synthesis of metal nanostructures: The case of silver." *Chemistry: A European Journal* 11 (2):454–463. https://doi.org/10.1002/chem.200400927.

Willets, K. A., and R. P. Van Duyne. 2007. "Localized surface plasmon resonance spectroscopy and sensing." *Annual Review of Physical Chemistry* 58:267–297. DOI: 10.1146/annurev.physchem.58.032806.104607.

Wolfbeis, O. S., and B. M. Weidgans. 2006. "Fiber optic chemical sensors and biosensors: A view back. In *Optical Chemical Sensors*. NATO Science Series II: Mathematics, Physics and Chemistry, vol. 224, edited by F. Baldini, A. Chester, J. Homola, and S. Martellucci. Dordrecht: Springer. https://doi.org/10.1007/1-4020-4611-1_2.

Xavier, Jolly, Serge Vincent, Fabian Meder, and Frank Vollmer. 2018. "Advances in optoplasmonic sensors: Combining optical nano/microcavities and photonic crystals with plasmonic nanostructures and nanoparticles." *Nanophotonics* 7 (1):1–38. DOI: 10.1515/nanoph-2017-0064.

Xia, Younan, and Naomi J. Halas. 2005. "Shape-controlled synthesis and surface plasmonic properties of metallic nanostructures." *MRS Bulletin* 30 (5):338–348. DOI: 10.1557/mrs2005.96.

Yang, Tianxi, and Timothy V. Duncan. 2021. "Challenges and potential solutions for nanosensors intended for use with foods." *Nature Nanotechnology* 16 (3):251–265. DOI: 10.1038/s41565-021-00867-7.

Yoo, Eun-Hyung, and Soo-Youn Lee. 2010. "Glucose biosensors: An overview of use in clinical practice." *Sensors (Basel, Switzerland)* 10 (5):4558–4576. DOI: 10.3390/s100504558.

Yu, Huakang, Yusi Peng, Yong Yang, and Zhi-Yuan Li. 2019. "Plasmon-enhanced light: Matter interactions and applications." *npj Computational Materials* 5 (1):45. DOI: 10.1038/s41524-019-0184-1.

Zhang, X., E. M. Hicks, J. Zhao, G. C. Schatz, and R. P. Van Duyne. 2005. "Electrochemical tuning of silver nanoparticles fabricated by nanosphere lithography." *Nano Letters* 5 (7):1503–1507. DOI: 10.1021/nl050873x.

Zhang, Yuyan, and Srinivas Tadigadapa. 2004. "Calorimetric biosensors with integrated microfluidic channels." *Biosensors and Bioelectronics* 19 (12):1733–1743. https://doi.org/10.1016/j.bios.2004.01.009.

Zhou, Shuang, Yunfeng Zhao, Michael Mecklenburg, Dajin Yang, and Bin Xie. 2013. "A novel thermometric biosensor for fast surveillance of β-lactamase activity in milk." *Biosensors and Bioelectronics* 49:99–104. https://doi.org/10.1016/j.bios.2013.05.005.

Zhu, Chengzhou, Guohai Yang, He Li, Dan Du, and Yuehe Lin. 2015. "Electrochemical sensors and biosensors based on nanomaterials and nanostructures." *Analytical Chemistry* 87 (1):230–249. DOI: 10.1021/ac5039863.

Zhu, Guo, Niteshkumar Agrawal, Ragini Singh, Santosh Kumar, Bingyuan Zhang, Chinmoy Saha, and Chandrakanta Kumar. 2020. "A novel periodically tapered structure-based gold nanoparticles and graphene oxide: Immobilized optical fiber sensor to detect ascorbic acid." *Optics & Laser Technology* 127:106156. https://doi.org/10.1016/j.optlastec.2020.106156.

Zhu, Guo, Lokendra Singh, Yu Wang, Ragini Singh, Bingyuan Zhang, Fengzhen Liu, Brajesh Kumar Kaushik, and Santosh Kumar. 2020. "Tapered optical fiber-based LSPR biosensor for ascorbic acid detection." *Photonic Sensors*. DOI: 10.1007/s13320-020-0605-2.

2 Important Nanomaterials for Optical Fiber Plasmonic Biosensors

2.1 INTRODUCTION

Nanotechnology is a highly multidisciplinary study that combines knowledge from several fields of science and engineering, including physics, chemistry, biology, biochemistry, and material science (Tarafdar, Shikha, and Raliya 2013; Porter and Youtie 2009; Ossai and Raghavan 2018). With features like improved sensitivity, reliability, rapid response and recovery, reduced size, easy operation, and cost-effectiveness, nanotechnology-based sensing devices are in huge demand (Agrawal, Saha, Kumar, Singh, Zhang, and Kumar 2020). Nanomaterials (NMs) further contribute to enhancing these characteristics in biological and chemical sensors (Agrawal, Zhang, Saha, Kumar, Kaushik et al. 2020). NMs, owing to their remarkable physicochemical attributes like electrical conductivity, large surface area, melting points, wettability, scattering and absorption properties, catalytic activity, and optical sensitivity, have shown prominent advancements as compared to their equivalents (Kumar, Singh, Kaushik et al. 2019; Kumar et al. 2021). Nanosensors are indispensable for the detection of physicochemical alterations, assessing cell biochemistry, and quantifying industrial and environmental pollutants and their toxicity (Ma and Wu 2020). Because of their superior detection capabilities, noble metal nanoparticles (MNPs) based optical sensors with localized surface plasmon resonance (LSPR) have drawn considerable interest. With the advent of nanotechnology, significance of size and shape of materials correlating to their varying features was observed, and hence, NMs emerged to overpower their counterparts (Khan, Saeed, and Khan 2019) with key properties like a big proportion of surface atoms, high surface energy, decreased defects, and spatial confinement (Mathew, Joy, and George 2019). To increase the sensitivity and lower the limit of detection (*LoD*), NMs can be used to stabilize an increasing number of bioreceptor units, and even parts of the journey act themselves as transduction elements (Bolotsky et al. 2019). NMs such as MNPs, carbon nanotubes, graphene, polymer nanoparticles (NPs), semiconductor NMs, and quantum dots (QDs) have been intensively studied in the past decade (Lee, Mahendra, and Alvarez 2010; Zhu, Singh et al. 2020). Among these, MNPs have a wide scope in biosensing applications (Singh, Singh, Kumar et al. 2020), with properties such as improved reaction catalysis, large surface area, electron transfer, and better biocompatibility (Malekzad et al. 2017). Different kinds of sensing devices can be developed employing MNPs either alone or in combination with other nanostructures (NSs) (Guo et al. 2018). MNPs-based sensors exhibit improved signal amplification, sensitivity, and identification and quantification of different biomolecules (Islam et al. 2020; Yang, Zhu et al. 2020). Due to their superior sensitivity; nanoscale wires, carbon nanotubes, thin films, metal and metal oxide NPs, polymers, and biomaterials are some of the nanostructured materials used in nanosensors (Abu-Salah et al. 2010; Manikkoth et al. 2021). This chapter discusses the recent advances over NMs and based biomolecular sensors. Improvements in biosensor performance accounting for physical characteristics, structure, and shape; MNPs; and nano-hybrids are highlighted in this chapter. This chapter also presents an overview of different NMs used in chemical, biosensing, and other applications, along with the drawbacks and merits of diverse NSs. In further sections, special emphasis is given to synthesis and characterization of NMs, basics of NMs, properties, and growing applications; the necessity of NMs in biosensing applications; and their prospects.

DOI: 10.1201/9781003243199-2

NPs have garnered widespread interest due to their remarkable electrical, magnetic, thermal, and catalytic properties. Numerous biomedical industries have been credited with having a significant impact on the health of people worldwide. They are classified as metal-based NPs, metal oxide-based NPs, and carbon-based NPs. Noble MNPs have gained increased attention due to their optical and electrical properties. MNPs can be synthesized via several different techniques, including laser ablation, electrolysis, irradiation, chemical reduction, and photochemistry. They are favored as optical and electrochemical sensors. Colorimetric, fluorometric, and surface enhanced Raman scattering (SERS)-based MNPs-based optical sensors have been widely used to detect a wide variety of analytes, including anions, metal ions, dyes, and pesticides. MNPs are more sensitive than chromatographic, spectroscopic, or optical methods for detecting a wide variety of inorganic and organic contaminants in water when used as an electrochemical probe. This chapter emphasizes the importance of NMs in the development of plasmonic phenomenon-based optical fiber biosensors. The chapter also discusses recent advancements in preparation, electrochemical identification, and characterization procedures.

2.2 BASICS OF NANOMATERIAL AND ITS GROWING APPLICATIONS

Nanotechnology is a branch of science that is concerned with the discovery and development of novel nanoscale devices, systems, and functional materials (Singh et al. 2021). In particular, NMs with at least one critical dimension less than 100 nm are noteworthy (Singh et al. 2019). These NMs are employed in a range of areas such as nanoelectronics, nanosensors, food, and the pharmaceutical industry, as represented in Figure 2.1. They have unique features like large surface area, improved electrical and catalytic conductivity, and remarkable magnetic properties, which make them more significant and dynamic than their equivalents (Agrawal, Saha, Kumar, Singh, Zhang, Jha et al. 2020). With higher surface area, NMs emerge as very promising in biosensing applications, as this feature offers easy alteration of functional groups resulting in competent biomolecule immobilization (Agrawal, Zhang, Saha, Kumar, Pu et al. 2020). NMs have brought significant modulations in bioanalytical sciences in the last decades with a potential role in the development of this

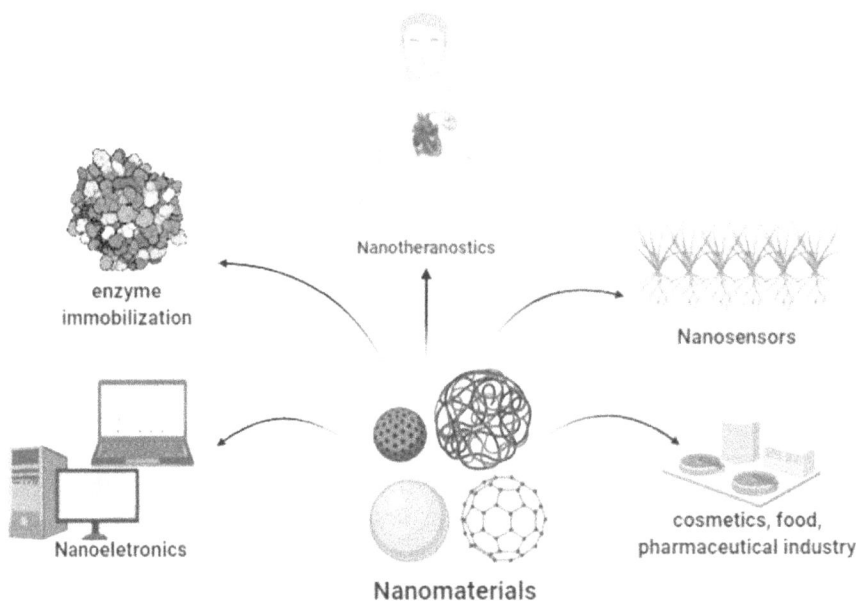

FIGURE 2.1   Several applications of nanomaterials (Cavalcante et al. 2021).

science in other scientific and industrial fields like electrochemistry, nano-catalysis, integrated analysis, waste management, biomedicine, food technology, bioengineering, etc. (Wang, Zhu, Li et al. 2021, Kumar, Guo et al. 2020). With exceptional electrocatalytic characteristics, NMs have become essential for a variety of biosensors, and they hold great promise for the creation of next-generation bioelectronic devices that combine biological recognition with electrical signal transduction, as well as play unique functions (Kumar and Singh 2021; Gan, Zhao, and Quan 2016).

The prime NMs, such as gold NPs (AuNPs) and silver NPs (AgNPs), find significant use in different biosensors (Wang, Zhu, Wang et al. 2021). Other noble NMs like copper (Cu), palladium (Pd), platinum (Pt), zinc (Zn), cobalt (Co), carbon nanotubes (CNTs), magnetic NPs, QDs, graphene oxide (GO) and its derivatives, and metal oxide NPs are extensively analyzed for their potential use in biosensing (Singh, Zhu et al. 2020). Different types of two-dimensional (2D) and three-dimensional (3D) NMs developed for *in-vitro* and *in-vivo* applications are displayed in Figure 2.2. Numerous types of NMs have been produced through nanotechnology; NPs are a broad category of materials that includes particle matter (Huang and Wang 2003). Classification of NMs is possible based on their shape, size, and unique characteristics (Singh, Kumar et al. 2020). Various classes include fullerenes, MNPs, ceramic NPs, and polymeric NPs, and they have unique physicochemical features due to their nanoscale size and higher surface area (Alcantara and Josephson 2012). Their optical properties, that exhibit a range of colors due to absorption in the visible region, have been shown to be influenced by their size, which has been demonstrated (Gohil and Choudhury 2019). Their size, structure, and shape also affect properties like reactivity and toughness (Tipper and Guillemois 2016); hence, accounting for such unique features, they are very useful in domestic and commercial sectors with applications in catalysis, imaging, medicine, and environmental applications (Njuguna et al. 2014). Numerous studies have been conducted on NMs based on 2D and 3D technology to expand the capabilities of various chemical and biological sensors (Yang, Zhang et al. 2020).

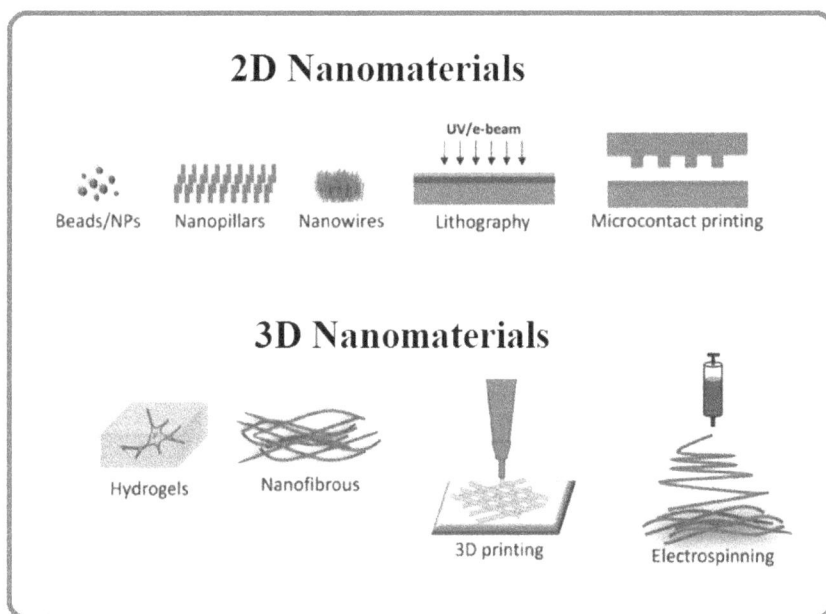

FIGURE 2.2   Types of topographical elements used in the development of 2D and 3D NMs for *in-vivo* and *in-vitro* applications.

Source: Reprinted with permission from *Journal of Drug Delivery Science and Technology*, Copyright 2021, Elsevier (Kumar, Aadil et al. 2020).

2.3   TYPES OF NANOMATERIAL

Nanomaterials are classified according to their size, structure, as well as chemical and physical properties (Jeevanandam et al. 2018). These NMs are optimized according to their plasmon properties, as shown in Figure 2.3. Broadly, these NMs are categorized as inorganic, organic, and carbon-based NMs, as shown in Figure 2.4. Inorganic NMs include metal NPs, magnetic NMs, alloys, up-conversion NPs, silica NPs, and QDs; and organic NMs include nanofibers, polymeric NPs, CNTs, graphene, liposomes, micelles, and dendrimers (Kyriakides et al. 2021). Due to their unique physicochemical properties, these NMs are used in a wide variety of biosensing applications (as illustrated in Figure 2.5). The graphical representation of various inorganic and organic NMs employed in biosensors is given in Figure 2.6 and Figure 2.7, respectively. These NMs are further categorized under (i) carbon-based NPs, (ii) ceramic NPs, (iii) MNPs, (iv) semiconductor NPs, (v) polymeric NPs, and (vi) lipid-based NPs (Pawar, Topcu Sendoğdular, and Gouma 2018), briefly discussed in the following subsections. Figure 2.8 shows the comparative study over zero-dimensional (0D), one-dimensional (1D), 2D, and 3D NMs.

2.3.1   METAL NANOPARTICLES

Metal nanoparticles are synthesized from their metal precursors and employ chemical, electrochemical, or photochemical methods for their synthesis (Iravani et al. 2014). Chemical methods use reducing agents for the reduction of metal-ion precursors in the solution for obtaining the MNPs. These possess higher surface energy and improved capacity to adsorb small molecules (Marinescu et al. 2020). Various MNPs such as Au, Ag, Pt, Pd, Cu, and Co NPs, including rare earth metals, have been used in fabricating the different biosensors (Zhu, Agrawal et al. 2020).

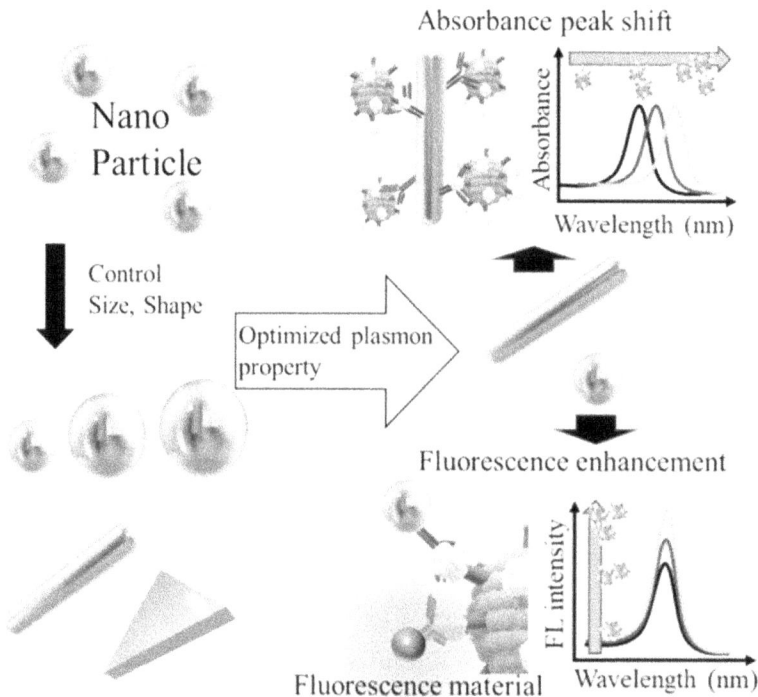

FIGURE 2.3 Optimization of nanomaterials: Controlling the dimensions of the nanoparticles results in the creation of optimal materials with the desired plasmonic properties (Takemura 2021).

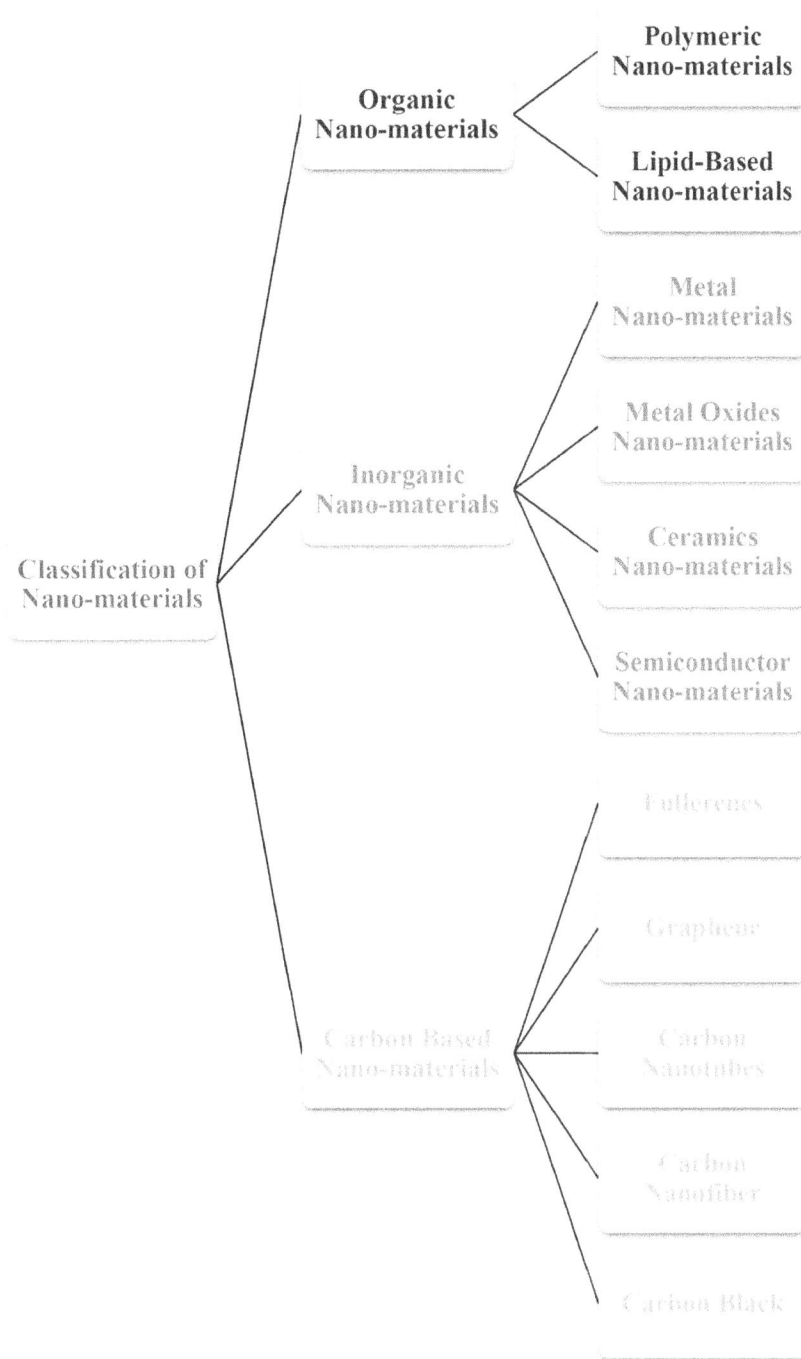

FIGURE 2.4 GENERAL CLASSIFICATION OF NANOMATERIALS.

Source: Reprinted with permission from *RSC Advances*, Copyright 2020, Royal Society of Chemistry (Foong et al. 2020).

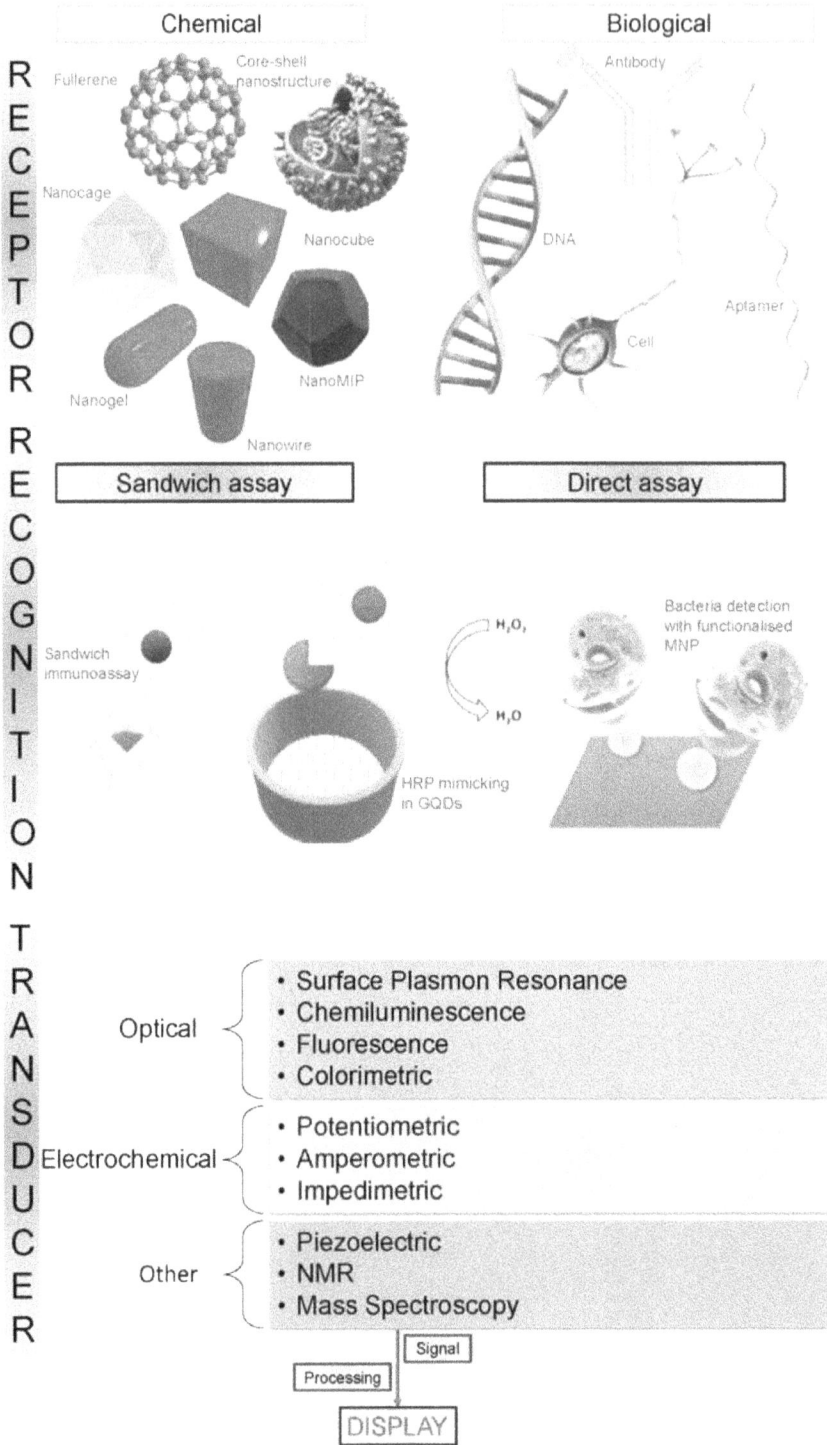

FIGURE 2.5   Roles of different nanomaterials in biosensing applications (Pirzada and Altintas 2019).

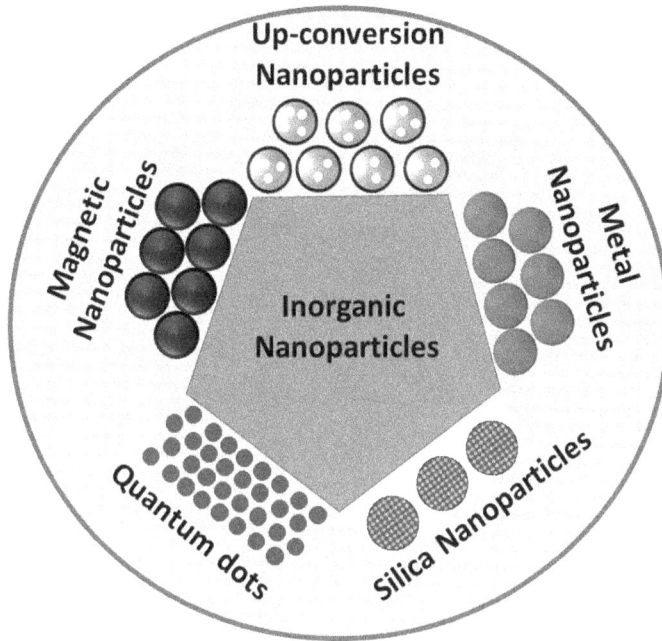

FIGURE 2.6 Types of inorganic nanomaterials.

Source: Reprinted with permission from *Journal of Drug Delivery Science and Technology*, Copyright 2021, Elsevier (Kumar, Aadil et al. 2020).

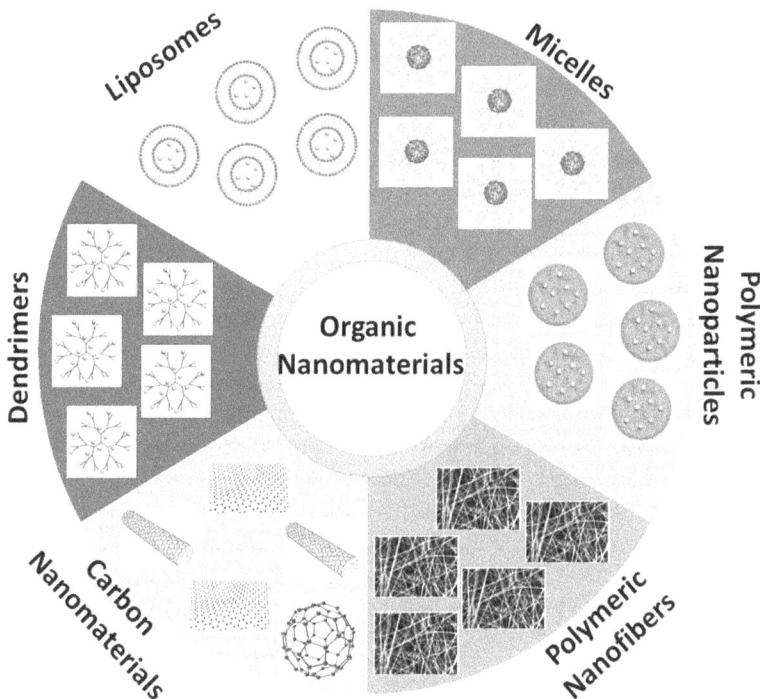

FIGURE 2.7 Types of organic nanomaterials.

Source: Reprinted with permission from *Journal of Drug Delivery Science and Technology*, Copyright 2021, Elsevier (Kumar, Aadil et al. 2020).

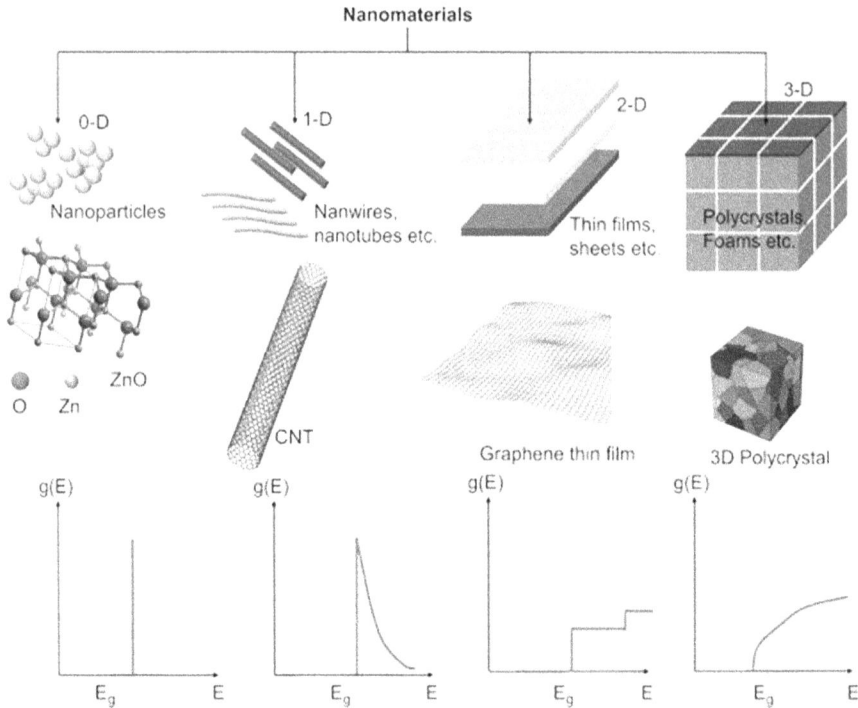

FIGURE 2.8 Zero-/one-/two-/three-dimensional nanomaterials and related density of electron versus density of states plots.

Source: Reprinted with permission from *Nanomaterials for Biosensors: Fundamentals and Applications.* Copyright 2020, Elsevier (Malhotra and Ali 2018).

Also, some of the alloys and dimers of MNPs like Ag@Au NPs are used in the detection of rhodamine B (RhB) and other biomolecules (Ha Pham, Dien, and Vu 2021, Lee et al. 2021).

The ability to immobilize biomolecules, catalyze electrochemical reactions, enhance electron transfer between electrode surfaces and proteins, and label biomolecules are all important functions of these materials (Kaushik et al. 2020; Cho, Kim, and Park 2020). MNPs have applicability both as analytical transducers in biosensing and as signal amplifiers (Singh, Singh, Zhang et al. 2020).

These NPs play a variety of functions in research, including biomolecule detection and imaging, as well as a variety of environmental and bioanalytical applications (Kalpana and Devi Rajeswari 2018). AuNPs, for example, are utilized to coat a sample before it is analyzed using scanning electron microscopy (SEM). This results in good quality SEM imaging as it enhances the electronic stream (Zhang et al. 2016). Metal nanoparticles-based sensors with improved sensitivity and selectivity exhibiting signal amplification have emerged as a potential class of biosensors (Wang, Wang et al. 2021). Because of their biocompatibility, distinctive optical and electrical characteristics, and ease of construction, AuNPs and AgNPs are the most often utilized noble MNPs in biosensing applications (Kumar, Singh, Zhu et al. 2019). Due to all these merits, these primary MNPs are synthesized, characterized, investigated, analyzed, and modified for different biosensing applications (Kumar, Singh, and Bedi 2018).

2.3.2 METAL NANORODS AND NANOTRIANGLES

Metal nanorods (MNRs), such as gold nanorods (AuNRs) and silver nanorods (AuNRs), are a fascinating family of nanoscale structures employed in a variety of medicinal and biotechnological applications, including sensing, imaging, and drug delivery. Their LSPR strongly depend on their shape and dimensions (size, aspect ratio). Especially in the case of AuNRs with higher aspect ratios (AR > 4), the longitudinal LSPR in the near-infrared (NIR) is 800–1300 nm, where absorption of biomatter is low, thus showing potential in a wide variety of biological applications (Loiseau et al. 2019; Tebbe et al. 2015). Also, surface modification of ultra-flat gold nanotriangles (AuNTs) with various shaped NPs is particularly important for SERS and plasmonic substrate photocatalytic activity (Koetz 2020). NRs and NTs-based biosensors with better sensitivity and selectivity and signal amplification have emerged as a promising biosensor class (Perez-Gonzalez et al. 2020).

2.3.3 SEMICONDUCTOR NANOPARTICLES

Semiconductor NPs have attributes of both nonmetals and metals and exhibit unique magnetic and optoelectronic properties (Ishtiaq et al. 2020). These NPs are very small (1–20 nm) with high surface area as well as quantum effect (Nair et al. 2018). They belong to the periodic table in groups II–VI, III–V, or IV–VI (Li et al. 2011). These particles with wide bandgaps display different features upon tuning. They are useful in many fields, including photocatalysis, electronics, photonics, and water splitting (Rani et al. 2018). GaN, GaP, InP, and InAs from groups III–V; ZnO, ZnS, CdS, CdSe, and CdTe from groups II–VI; and silicon and germanium from group IV are some examples of semiconductor NPs (Nikazar et al. 2020).

2.3.4 CARBON-BASED NANOPARTICLES

Carbon nanotubes and fullerenes are the two main components of carbon-based NPs. CNTs are graphene sheets coiled into tubes, while fullerenes are graphene sheets folded into tubes (Saito et al. 2014; Gao et al. 2021). These materials being highly stronger than steel are suitable for structural reinforcement (Saifuddin, Raziah, and Junizah 2013).

2.3.5 POLYMERIC NANOPARTICLES

Polymeric NPs are organic NPs that can take on a variety of shapes and forms depending on their preparation method, such as nano-capsular or nanospheres (Begines et al. 2020). The active chemicals and polymer are dispersed uniformly in a matrix-like structure in a nanosphere particle, while the nano-capsular particle exhibits a core-shell shape (Pal, Lee, and Cho 2020), and a polymer shell encloses the active compounds (Kumar, Kumar, and Paik 2013). Only a few of the advantages offered by polymeric NPs include controlled release, protection of the drug molecule, the ability to combine treatment with imaging, and selective targeting (Senapati et al. 2018). They are important in fields like medication delivery and diagnostics. The biocompatibility and biodegradability of medication delivery using polymeric NPs are excellent (Patra et al. 2018).

2.3.6 CERAMIC NANOPARTICLES

Ceramic NPs are inorganic solids made up of oxides, carbides, carbonates, and phosphates, among other elements. They exhibit exceptional thermal and chemical resistance (Krishna Prasad et al. 2020). They have a wide range of applications in the fields of photocatalysis, dye degradation, drug delivery, and imaging, among others (Gawande et al. 2016). They may prove to be viable drug delivery agents if certain characteristics such as size, surface area, porosity, and surface-to-volume ratio are carefully manipulated and optimized (Nikolova and Chavali 2020; Thomas et al. 2015). There is significant potential for these NPs to be used as drug delivery agents in a variety of diseases, including cancer, glaucoma, and a wide range of bacterial infections (Moreno-Vega et al. 2012; Noah 2020).

2.3.7 PEROVSKITE NANOPARTICLES

Perovskite structured NMs and their by-products have attained enormous interest in scientific research and potential technical applications because of their unique chemical and physical properties (Wang et al. 2017). These are synthesized to modify electrodes for the development of sensitive enzymatic electrochemical biosensor applications. Strontium titanate ($SrTiO_3$) NPs have a large surface area and offer a favorable microenvironment to keep the biological activity of the immobilized enzyme and promote fast direct electron transfer (DET) between glucose oxidase molecules and the electrode surface (Tian et al. 2018). Also, in a recent study, plasmon-based structures, such as the $SrPdO_3$ perovskite/AuNP-modified graphite electrode, demonstrated a low detection limit of 10 μM and high specificity toward glucose. These types of unique materials can be used for novel, nonenzymatic biochemical sensors (Atta et al. 2020).

2.3.8 MXENE-BASED NANOCOMPOSITES

MXenes are a 2D family of inorganic chemicals. These materials are made up of thin layers of transition metal carbides, nitrides, or carbonitrides that are only a few atoms thick. MXenes are unique because they are both hydrophilic and mostly synthesized from a top-down selective etching procedure (Shuck et al. 2020). MXenes have attracted much attention for their huge potential in biosensors for their high sensitivity and selectivity (Hasnan et al. 2022). Due to its outstanding features, including strong electrical conductivity and semiconductor capabilities, MXenes have been employed in a variety of disciplines, including catalyst creation, energy storage, and biosensors (Zhao et al. 2018). MXene-based fluorescent/optical biosensors and electrochemical biosensors are depicted in Figure 2.9.

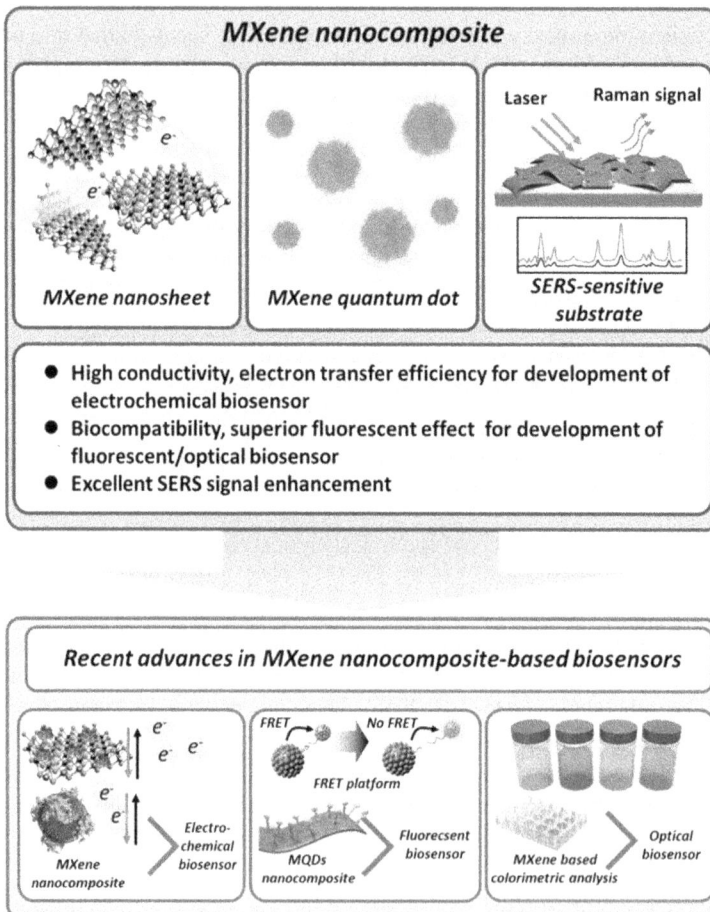

FIGURE 2.9 Recent advances in the development of advanced biosensors based on MXene nanocomposites (Yoon et al. 2020).

These show high biocompatibility and excellent SERS signal enhancement. A plasmonic-based MXene/AuNPs composite structure was used for sensitive and multiple detections of oncomiRs (cancer cells) for accurate cancer diagnostics (Mohammadniaei et al. 2020) and enzymatic glucose detection (Rakhi et al. 2016).

2.3.9 LIPID-BASED NANOPARTICLES

Lipid based NPs have a spherical shape and a diameter ranging from 10 to 100 nanometers. In addition to a solid lipid core, they also contain a matrix of lipophilic molecules that are water soluble (Mukherjee, Ray, and Thakur 2009). Emulsifiers and surfactants are used to stabilize the exterior core of these NPs. NPs have a great deal of potential in the biomedical field because of their roles as a drug delivery system and as a mechanism for the release of RNA in cancer therapy (Mitchell et al. 2021). As a result, the field of nanotechnology has enormous potential for advancement and is still far from being saturated in terms of innovation (Bayda et al. 2019). Hence, nanotechnology would show a similar exponential growth pattern as displayed by the other two fields in past decades (Chakravarty and Vora 2021).

2.4 SYNTHESIS OF NANOMATERIALS

Colloidal NPs, nano-powders, nanotubes, nanoclusters, thin films, nanowires, and other forms of NMs can be synthesized in a variety of ways. For the synthesis of NMs, physical, chemical, biological, and hybrid approaches have been established. MNPs are synthesized using chemical, electrochemical, and photochemical processes. Figure 2.10 depicts a flow chart of the many strategies that may be used to synthesize NMs. As discussed in previous sections, various NMs such as AuNPs, AgNPs, GO, Zn, Cu, and Pt are largely used in the development of biosensors. Key NMs such as AuNPs and AgNPs have major use in sensor development and are usually produced through

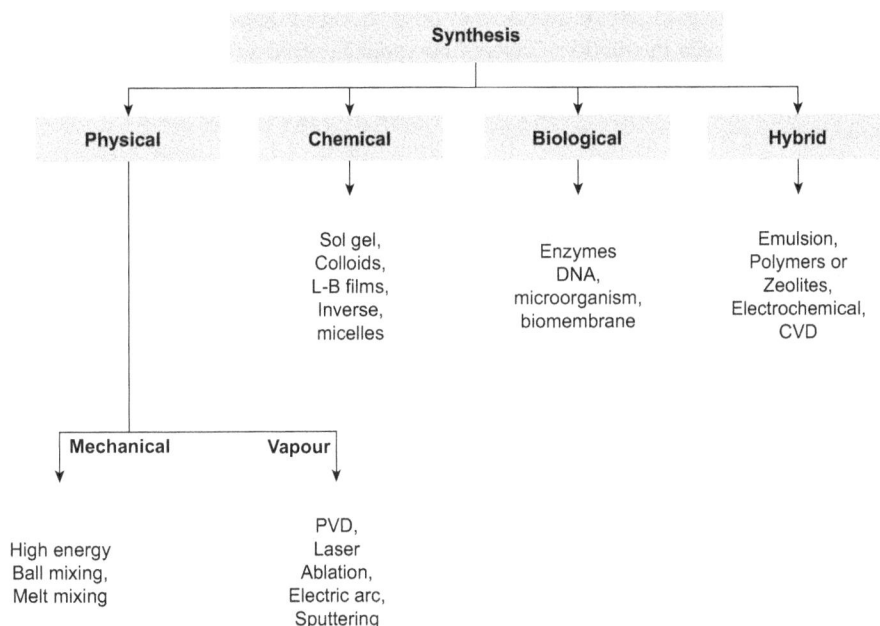

FIGURE 2.10 Techniques used for nanomaterials synthesis.

Source: Reprinted with permission from *Elsevier Book*, Copyright 2020, *Elsevier* (Malhotra and Ali 2018).

wet reduction methods. Further, the modified El-Sayed method is adopted to synthesize the gold nanorods. GO and its derivatives are synthesized using the Hummer method or modified Hummer method. Alkaline reduction method is employed for the synthesis of hybrid nanocomposites such as GO-magnetite NPs (RGO-Fe$_3$O$_4$ NPs).

2.4.1 WET CHEMICAL METHOD

The wet chemical method includes phase-transfer synthesis, colloidal chemistry, chemical methods, hydrothermal methods, and other precipitation (Nesheva 2001). This process may be used to make a variety of chemicals, including organic, inorganic, and certain metals (Tian et al. 2019). This method largely controls the size of a particle with great mono-dispersity (Majid and Bibi 2018). Turkevich et al. (1951) presented numerous wet chemical noteworthy procedures for the production of AuNPs using various reducing agents, such as citric acid and sodium borohydride (Dong et al. 2020). In the next stage of development, Brust et al. (1998) first reported the synthesis of AuNPs in a polar organic medium (Daniel and Astruc 2004).

2.4.2 PHYSICAL METHOD

The physical method is mostly used for the synthesis of MNPs and inorganic NMs and includes such techniques as mechanical alloying, grinding, and milling employing in this synthesis process. The most well-known physical methods are lithography, chemical vapor or vacuum deposition, and spray coating which are used in the development of carbon nanotubes.

2.4.3 EXFOLIATION METHOD

Mechanical exfoliation is one kind of top-down manufacturing process for emerging 2D materials. Exfoliation, commonly known as the scotch-tape method, is the genesis of effective 2D graphene since it creates the highest-quality thin layer with minimal imperfections due to the lack of chemical processing (Huang et al. 2020). Because of their strong intraplate chemical bonding but weak interplane van der Waals interactions, layered compounds serve as precursors for atomically thin 2D NMs. The efficient exfoliation of various 2D materials, such as boron nitride (BN), MXenes, molybdenum disulfide (MoS$_2$), and black phosphorous (BP) (Le et al. 2020).

2.5 CHARACTERIZATION OF NANOMATERIALS

Various methods have been used for the characterization of NMs to analyze their physicochemical properties. X-ray diffraction (XRD), polarized optical microscopy (POM), SEM, energy dispersive X-ray spectroscopy (EDX), X-ray photoelectron spectroscopy (XPn-S), IR, Brunauer-Emmett-Teller (BET), and transmission electron microscopy (TEM) are among the characterization methods utilized (Mourdikoudis, Pallares, and Thanh 2018; Manaia et al. 2017). The characterization results, such as absorbance spectrum, and TEM images of synthesized AuNPs, GO, and MoS$_2$-NPs, are indicated in Figures 2.11–2.13.

2.5.1 MORPHOLOGICAL CHARACTERIZATIONS

The morphological characteristics of NPs have long piqued the interest of researchers, as morphology has a significant impact on the majority of their physical and chemical properties. The morphology of NPs has a significant impact on their features, and hence morphological characterization is critical (Buzea, Pacheco, and Robbie 2007). Microscopic techniques, as discussed in the previous section, are the most widely employed techniques for morphological characterizations among other methods (Venkateshaiah et al. 2020).

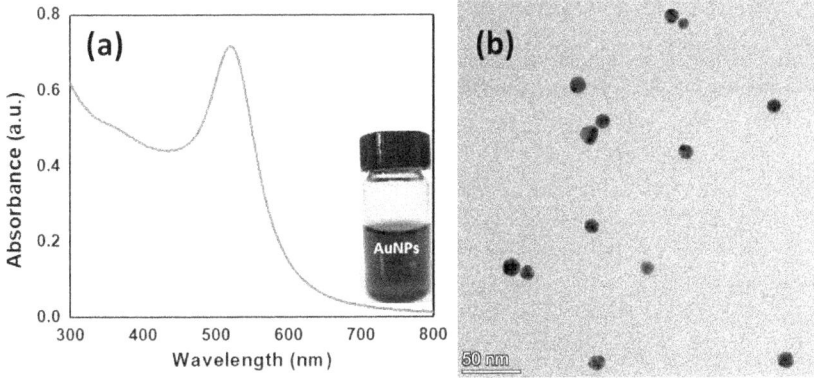

FIGURE 2.11 The characterization results of synthesized AuNPs: (a) pictorial view of AuNPs solution and its absorbance spectrum, and (b) HRTEM image.

Source: Reprinted with permission from *Optics Express.* Copyright, 2021, Optica (Li et al. 2021).

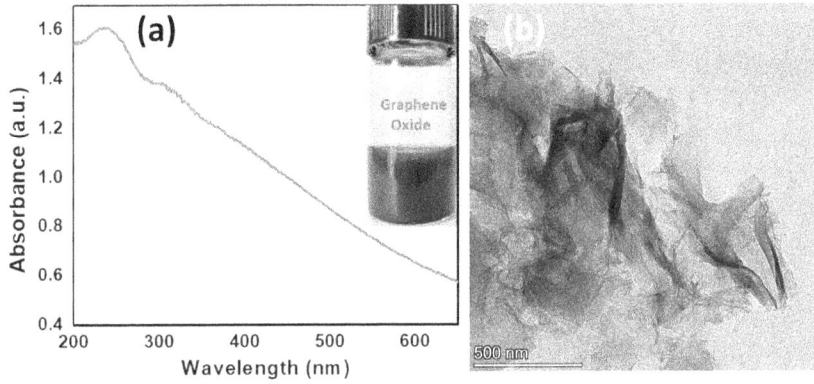

FIGURE 2.12 The characterization results of synthesized GO: (a) pictorial view of GO solution and its absorbance spectrum, and (b) HRTEM image.

Source: Reprinted with permission from *Optics Express.* Copyright, 2021, Optica (Li et al. 2021).

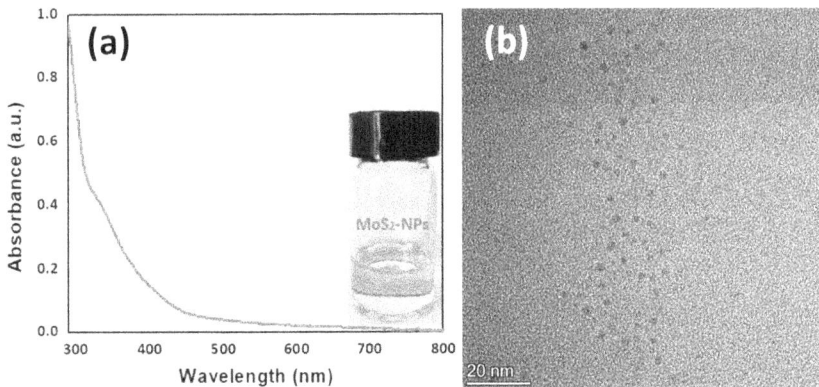

FIGURE 2.13 The characterization results of synthesized MoS_2-NPs: (a) pictorial view of MoS_2-NPs solution and its absorbance spectra, and (b) HRTEM image.

Source: Reprinted with permission from *Optics Express.* Copyright, 2021, Optica (Li et al. 2021).

2.5.2 Structural Characterizations

The structural characterization of bonding materials is essential when attempting to understand their composition and properties, as it provides critical information about the subject material's properties. To characterize the structural properties of NPs, various techniques, as discussed earlier, are frequently employed (Afolalu et al. 2019). Figure 2.14 shows the SEM images of (a) creatinine sensor probe and (b) GO-coated, (c) GO/AuNPs-coated, (d) GO/AuNPs/MoS2-NPs-immobilized sensor structures. Figure 2.15 indicates the typical EDX image for different NMs-coated probes such

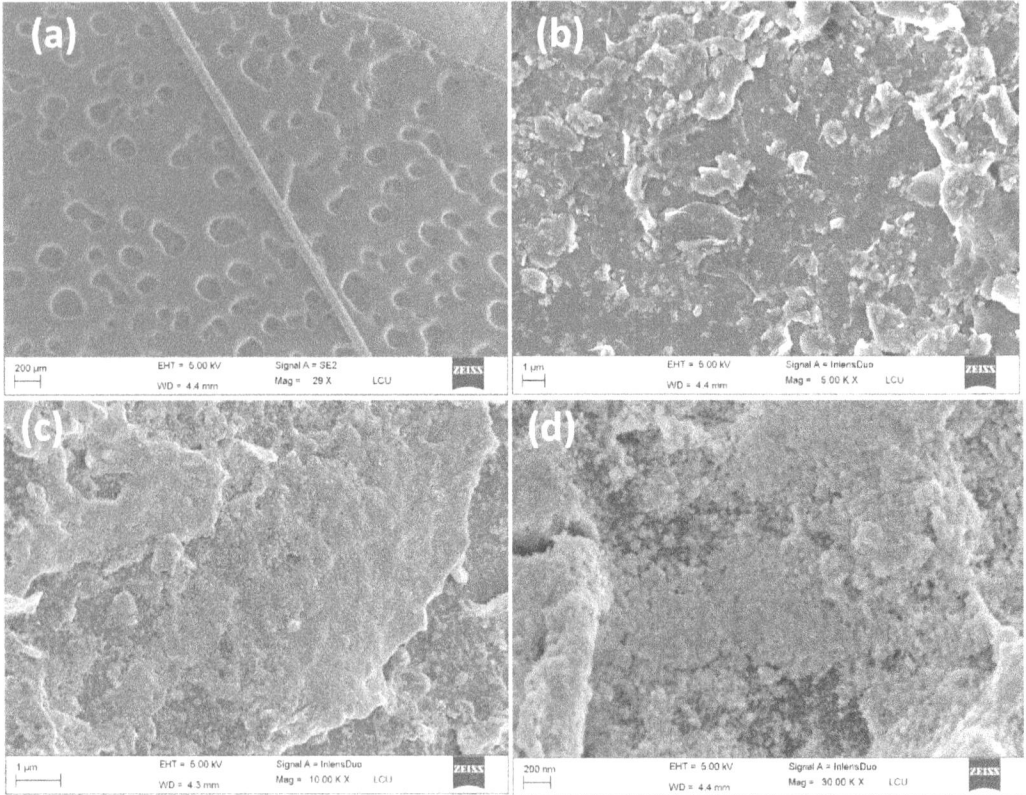

FIGURE 2.14 SEM images of (a) creatinine sensor probe and (b) GO-coated, (c) GO/AuNPs-coated, (d) GO/AuNPs/MoS$_2$-NPs-immobilized sensor structures.

Source: Reprinted with permission from *Optics Express.* Copyright, 2021, Optica (Li et al. 2021).

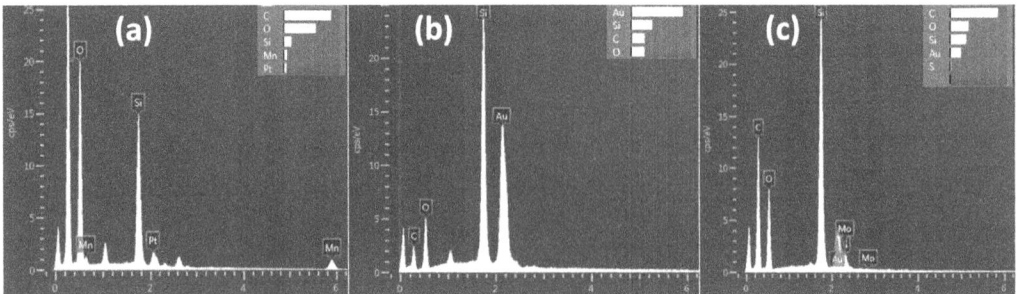

FIGURE 2.15 A typical EDX image for (a) GO-coated probe, (b) GO/AuNPs-coated probe, (c) GO/AuNPs/MoS$_2$-NPs-coated probe.

Source: Reprinted with permission from *Optics Express.* Copyright, 2021, Optica (Li et al. 2021).

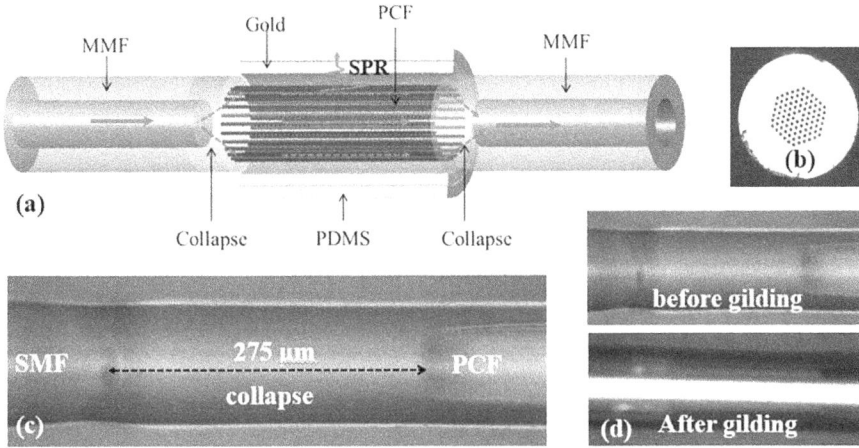

FIGURE. 2.16 (a) Multimode fiber-photonic crystal fiber–multimode fiber (MMF-PCF-MMF) structure. (b) Optical microscope image of a cross section of photonic crystal fiber. (c) Optical microscope image of the junction of photonic crystal and multimode fiber. (d) Optical microscope image of the sensing area before gilding and after gilding.

Source: Reprinted with permission from *Optics Express.* Copyright, 2019, Optica (Wang et al. 2019).

as GO, AuNPs, and MoS$_2$-NPs. This image indicates the presence of NMs over the nanocoated probe. There is also a different structure of specialty fiber configuration considered for the biosensing applications due to their high selectivity and sensitivity. A schematic of one such configuration is depicted in Figure 2.16, where the Au NMs are coated over the photonic crystal fiber (PCF) sensing region, where biomolecule sensing can be done using LSPR and propagating surface plasmon resonance (PSPR) phenomena.

2.5.3 Surface Area and Particle Size Characterization

The surface and size are again important attributes of NPs, and several methods are in use for their estimation. TEM, SEM, atomic force microscopy (AFM), XRD, and dynamic light scattering (DLS) are some of the methods used. The particle size may be better determined using characterization instruments. The zeta potential size analyzer/DLS is a very efficient tool for detecting the size of NPs at a very low level (Speranza et al. 2014). Figure 2.17 shows the SEM images of (a) tapered-in-taper sensor probe, (b) AuNPs-, (c) MoS$_2$-NPs/AuNPs-, (d) CeO$_2$-NPs/MoS$_2$-NPs/AuNPs-immobilized sensor probes.

2.5.4 Optical Characterizations

The optical characterization of NPs offers data on their absorption, reflectance, luminescence, and phosphorescence (Gao et al. 2015). The Beer-Lambert law and the fundamental concepts of lighting are the foundations for these definitions. In general, it is understood that NPs, particularly metallic and semiconductor NPs, exhibit a wide range of colors, making them particularly well suited for photo-related applications (Soto-Quintero et al. 2019). The values of absorption and reflectance of these materials must be estimated to fully comprehend the mechanistic aspects of each application (Khan, Saeed, and Khan 2017). For the optical characterization of NPs materials, several optical instruments, including photoluminescence, UV-Vis, and the null ellipsometer, are often utilized (Steinegger, Wolfbeis, and Borisov 2020).

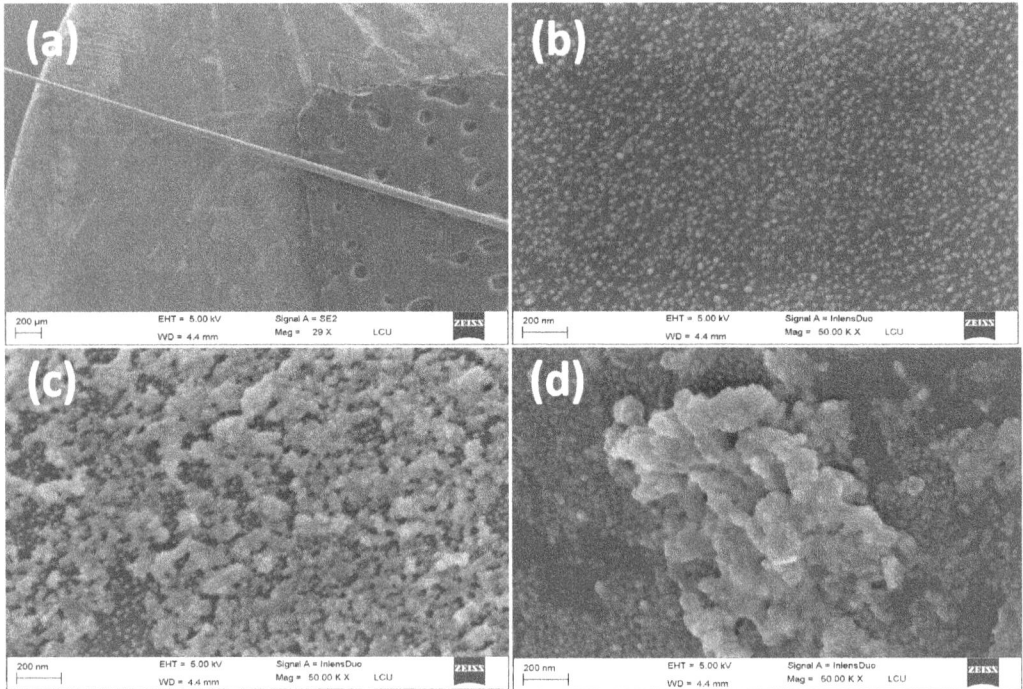

FIGURE 2.17   SEM images of (a) tapered-in-taper sensor probe, (b) AuNPs-, (c) MoS_2-NPs/AuNPs-, (d) CeO_2-NPs/MoS_2-NPs/AuNPs-immobilized sensor probe.

Source: Reprinted with permission from *Optics Express.* Copyright, 2021, Optica (Wang, Singh et al. 2021).

2.6   SUMMARY AND CONCLUSION

With the emergence of nanotechnology, new avenues are beginning for the development of biosensors. Aggregation of particles, photoemission, electrical and thermal conductivity, and catalytic activity are all important chemical and optical properties of NMs for the evolution of nano-bio-electronic devices. NMs enhance selectivity and sensitivity and provide stability to the biosensors. The NMs-based bioelectronics devices exhibit unique features of NMs; thus, these sensing devices continue to expand and demonstrate novel functionality. These NMs-based devices have significant implications in areas of environmental monitoring, food safety, security surveillance, and clinical diagnostics.

This chapter discusses NMs in detail, including their types, synthesis, characterization, physicochemical properties, and applications. The NMs possess exceptional physicochemical and plasmonic properties and hence have great relevance in several sensing applications. The unique properties of NMs, which include superior electrocatalytic capabilities, a high surface-to-volume ratio, and high stability, are critical for biomolecule detection. In recent times, various novel NMs such as MoS_2-NPs, and cerium oxide NPs (CeO_2-NPs) are used in the development of plasmonic-optical fiber sensors (P-OFSs). Wang et al. proposed a study for the detection of alanine aminotransferase (ALT), as indicated in Figure 2.18.

To further enhance and best utilize the unique properties of NMs, there is an increase in the synthesis of new NMs with different properties. An overview of the significance of the development of novel NMs with applications in biosensing is given in this chapter. The use of different functionalized carbon NMs, metal oxide NMs, metal NMs, polymeric NMs, QDs, graphene sheets, and other novel NMs in biosensor technology, and their innovations and advantages are discussed in this

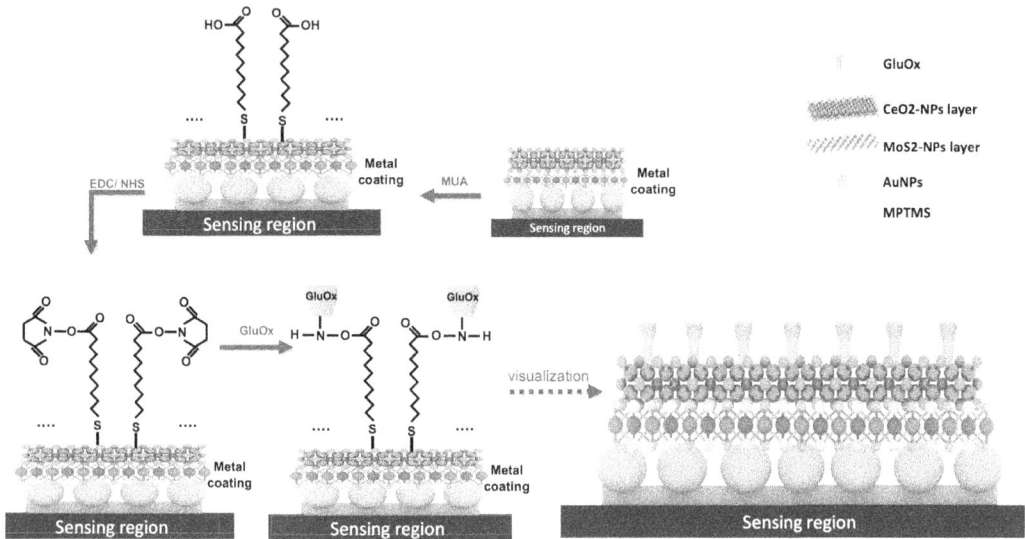

FIGURE 2.18 Alanine aminotransferase (ALT) sensor fabrication process using novel nanomaterials such as MoS$_2$-NPs and CeO$_2$-NPs.

Source: Reprinted with permission from *Optics Express.* Copyright, 2021, Optica (Wang, Singh et al. 2021).

chapter. Because of their unique properties, such as their large surface area, NPs have a promising future in a variety of applications. Moreover, the optical properties at nanoscale size make these relevant to photocatalytic applications. Synthetic techniques are also explored for their application in controlling different properties of NPs, like morphology, size, and magnetic properties. Despite their numerous applications, NPs can impose certain health risks as a result of their haphazard use and release into the natural environment, which should be taken into account when developing more convenient and environmentally friendly NPs. Another approach that is now gaining traction is the creation of biosensors by merging two or more new NMs. Strategies to combine different NMs, each with unique attributes, are in increasing demand for the enhancement of biosensors. Such hybrid NMs often show synergistic effects, facilitating the expansion of highly sensitive biosensors with wearable applications. There is a need for advanced research to achieve innovative technologies for the development of new NMs with improved sensitivity, selectivity, stability, and catalytic activity. NMs have become integral to bioanalytical devices owing to their increased sensitivity and detection capacity. The unique properties of such NMs also suggest the replacement of classic methods of transduction.

REFERENCES

Abu-Salah, Khalid M., Salman A. Alrokyan, Muhammad Naziruddin Khan, and Anees Ahmad Ansari. 2010. "Nanomaterials as analytical tools for genosensors." *Sensors (Basel, Switzerland)* 10 (1):963–993. DOI: 10.3390/s100100963.

Afolalu, S. A., S. B. Soetan, S. O. Ongbali, A. A. Abioye, and A. S. Oni. 2019. "Morphological characterization and physio-chemical properties of nanoparticle: Review." *IOP Conference Series: Materials Science and Engineering* 640:012065. DOI: 10.1088/1757-899x/640/1/012065.

Agrawal, N., C. Saha, C. Kumar, R. Singh, B. Zhang, R. Jha, and S. Kumar. 2020. "Detection of L-cysteine using silver nanoparticles and graphene oxide immobilized tapered SMS optical fiber structure." *IEEE Sensors Journal* 20 (19):11372–11379. DOI: 10.1109/JSEN.2020.2997690.

Agrawal, N., C. Saha, C. Kumar, R. Singh, B. Zhang, and S. Kumar. 2020. "Development of uric acid sensor using copper oxide and silver nanoparticles immobilized SMSMS fiber structure-based probe." *IEEE Transactions on Instrumentation and Measurement* 69 (11):9097–9104. DOI: 10.1109/TIM.2020.2998876.

Agrawal, N., B. Zhang, C. Saha, C. Kumar, B. K. Kaushik, and S. Kumar. 2020. "Development of dopamine sensor using silver nanoparticles and PEG-functionalized tapered optical fiber structure." *IEEE Transactions on Biomedical Engineering* 67 (6):1542–1547. DOI: 10.1109/TBME.2019.2939560.

Agrawal, N., B. Zhang, C. Saha, C. Kumar, X. Pu, and S. Kumar. 2020. "Ultra-sensitive cholesterol sensor using gold and zinc-oxide nanoparticles immobilized core mismatch MPM/SPS probe." *Journal of Lightwave Technology* 38 (8):2523–2529. DOI: 10.1109/JLT.2020.2974818.

Alcantara, David, and Lee Josephson. 2012. "Chapter 11: Magnetic nanoparticles for application in biomedical sensing." In *Frontiers of Nanoscience*, edited by Jesus M. de la Fuente and V. Grazu, 269–289. Amsterdam: Elsevier.

Atta, Nada, Ahmed Galal, Ekram El-Ads, and Aya Galal. 2020. "Efficient electrochemical sensor based on gold nanoclusters/carbon ionic liquid crystal for sensitive determination of neurotransmitters and anti-Parkinson drugs." *Advanced Pharmaceutical Bulletin* 10. DOI: 10.15171/apb.2020.006.

Bayda, Samer, Muhammad Adeel, Tiziano Tuccinardi, Marco Cordani, and Flavio Rizzolio. 2019. "The history of nanoscience and nanotechnology: From chemical-physical applications to nanomedicine." *Molecules (Basel, Switzerland)* 25 (1):112. DOI: 10.3390/molecules25010112.

Begines, Belén, Tamara Ortiz, María Pérez-Aranda, Guillermo Martínez, Manuel Merinero, Federico Argüelles-Arias, and Ana Alcudia. 2020. "Polymeric nanoparticles for drug delivery: Recent developments and future prospects." *Nanomaterials (Basel, Switzerland)* 10 (7):1403. DOI: 10.3390/nano10071403.

Bolotsky, Adam, Derrick Butler, Chengye Dong, Katy Gerace, Nicholas R. Glavin, Christopher Muratore, Joshua A. Robinson, and Aida Ebrahimi. 2019. "Two-dimensional materials in biosensing and healthcare: From in vitro diagnostics to optogenetics and beyond." *ACS Nano* 13 (9):9781–9810. DOI: 10.1021/acsnano.9b03632.

Brust, Mathias, Donald Bethell, Christopher J. Kiely, and David J. Schiffrin. 1998. "Self-assembled gold nanoparticle thin films with nonmetallic optical and electronic properties." *Langmuir* 14 (19):5425–5429. DOI: 10.1021/la980557g.

Buzea, C., Ivan I. Pacheco, and K. Robbie. 2007. "Nanomaterials and nanoparticles: Sources and toxicity." *Biointerphases* 2 (4): 17–71. DOI: 10.1116/1.2815690.

Cavalcante, Francisco T. T., Italo R. de A. Falcão, José E. da S. Souza, Thales G. Rocha, Isamayra G. de Sousa, Antônio L. G. Cavalcante, André L. B. de Oliveira, Maria C. M. de Sousa, and José C. S. dos Santos. 2021. "Designing of nanomaterials-based enzymatic biosensors: Synthesis, properties, and applications." *Electrochem* 2 (1). DOI: 10.3390/electrochem2010012.

Chakravarty, Malobika, and Amisha Vora. 2021. "Nanotechnology-based antiviral therapeutics." *Drug Delivery and Translational Research* 11 (3):748–787. DOI: 10.1007/s13346-020-00818-0.

Cho, Il-Hoon, Dong Hyung Kim, and Sangsoo Park. 2020. "Electrochemical biosensors: Perspective on functional nanomaterials for on-site analysis." *Biomaterials Research* 24 (1):6. DOI: 10.1186/s40824-019-0181-y.

Daniel, Marie-Christine, and Didier Astruc. 2004. "Gold nanoparticles: Assembly, supramolecular chemistry, quantum-size-related properties, and applications toward biology, catalysis, and nanotechnology." *Chemical Reviews* 104 (1):293–346. DOI: 10.1021/cr030698+.

Dong, Jiaqi, Paul L. Carpinone, Georgios Pyrgiotakis, Philip Demokritou, and Brij M. Moudgil. 2020. "Synthesis of precision gold nanoparticles using Turkevich method." *Kona: Powder Science and Technology in Japan* 37:224–232. DOI: 10.14356/kona.2020011.

Foong, Loke Kok, Mohammad Mehdi Foroughi, Armita Forutan Mirhosseini, Mohadeseh Safaei, Shohreh Jahani, Maryam Mostafavi, Nasser Ebrahimpoor, Maryam Sharifi, Rajender S. Varma, and Mehrdad Khatami. 2020. "Applications of nano-materials in diverse dentistry regimes." *RSC Advances* 10 (26):15430–15460. DOI: 10.1039/D0RA00762E.

Gan, Xiaorong, Huimin Zhao, and Xie Quan. 2016. "Two-dimensional MoS_2: A promising building block for biosensors." *Biosensors and Bioelectronics* 89. DOI: 10.1016/j.bios.2016.03.042.

Gao, Jingrong, Shan He, Anindya Nag, and Jonathan Woon Chung Wong. 2021. "A review of the use of carbon nanotubes and graphene-based sensors for the detection of aflatoxin M1 compounds in milk." *Sensors (Basel, Switzerland)* 21 (11):3602. DOI: 10.3390/s21113602.

Gao, Minmin, Liangliang Zhu, Wei Li Ong, Jing Wang, and Ghim Wei Ho. 2015. "Structural design of TiO_2-based photocatalyst for H_2 production and degradation applications." *Catalysis Science & Technology* 5 (10):4703–4726. DOI: 10.1039/C5CY00879D.

Gawande, Manoj B., Anandarup Goswami, François-Xavier Felpin, Tewodros Asefa, Xiaoxi Huang, Rafael Silva, Xiaoxin Zou, Radek Zboril, and Rajender S. Varma. 2016. "Cu and Cu-based nanoparticles: Synthesis and applications in catalysis." *Chemical Reviews* 116 (6):3722–3811. DOI: 10.1021/acs.chemrev.5b00482.

Gohil, Jaydevsinh M., and Rikarani R. Choudhury. 2019. "Chapter 2: Introduction to nanostructured and nano-enhanced polymeric membranes: Preparation, function, and application for water purification." In *Nanoscale Materials in Water Purification*, edited by Sabu Thomas, Daniel Pasquini, Shao-Yuan Leu, and Deepu A. Gopakumar, 25–57. Amsterdam: Elsevier.

Guo, Ting, Mei Lin, Junxing Huang, Chenglin Zhou, Weizhong Tian, Hong Yu, Xingmao Jiang, Jun Ye, Yujuan Shi, Yanhong Xiao, Xuefeng Bian, and Xiaoqian Feng. 2018. "The recent advances of magnetic nanoparticles in medicine." *Journal of Nanomaterials* 2018:7805147. DOI: 10.1155/2018/7805147.

Ha Pham, Thi Thu, Nguyen Dac Dien, and Xuan Hoa Vu. 2021. "Facile synthesis of silver/gold alloy nanoparticles for ultra-sensitive rhodamine B detection." *RSC Advances* 11 (35):21475–21488. DOI: 10.1039/D1RA02576G.

Hasnan, M., M. I. Megat, G. P. Lim, N. Nayan, C. F. Soon, A. A. Abd Halim, M. K. Ahmad, S. M. Said, M. S. Mohamed Ali, and I. M. Noor. 2022. "The investigation of chlorpyrifos (Cpy) detection of PEDOT:PSS-MXene(Ti_2CTX)-BSA-GO composite using P-ISFET reduction method." *Polymer Bulletin*. DOI: 10.1007/s00289-022-04105-5.

Huang, Y., Y. H. Pan, R. Yang, L. H. Bao, L. Meng, H. L. Luo, Y. Q. Cai, G. D. Liu, W. J. Zhao, Z. Zhou, L. M. Wu, Z. L. Zhu, M. Huang, L. W. Liu, L. Liu, P. Cheng, K. H. Wu, S. B. Tian, C. Z. Gu, Y. G. Shi, Y. F. Guo, Z. G. Cheng, J. P. Hu, L. Zhao, G. H. Yang, E. Sutter, P. Sutter, Y. L. Wang, W. Ji, X. J. Zhou, and H. J. Gao. 2020. "Universal mechanical exfoliation of large-area 2D crystals." *Nature Communications* 11 (1):2453. DOI: 10.1038/s41467-020-16266-w.

Huang, Y., and Z. L. Wang. 2003. "8.16: Mechanics of nanotubes." In *Comprehensive Structural Integrity*, edited by I. Milne, R. O. Ritchie, and B. Karihaloo, 551–579. Oxford: Pergamon.

Iravani, S., H. Korbekandi, S. V. Mirmohammadi, and B. Zolfaghari. 2014. "Synthesis of silver nanoparticles: Chemical, physical and biological methods." *Research in Pharmaceutical Sciences* 9 (6):385–406.

Ishtiaq, Marium, Mariya al-Rashida, Rima D. Alharthy, and Abdul Hameed. 2020. "Chapter 15: Ionic liquid-based colloidal nanoparticles: Applications in organic synthesis." In *Metal Nanoparticles for Drug Delivery and Diagnostic Applications*, edited by Muhammad Raza Shah, Muhammad Imran, and Shafi Ullah, 279–299. Amsterdam: Elsevier.

Islam, Tamanna, Md Mahedi Hasan, Abdul Awal, Md Nurunnabi, and A. J. Saleh Ahammad. 2020. "Metal nanoparticles for electrochemical sensing: Progress and challenges in the clinical transition of point-of-care testing." *Molecules (Basel, Switzerland)* 25 (24):5787. DOI: 10.3390/molecules25245787.

Jeevanandam, Jaison, Ahmed Barhoum, Yen S. Chan, Alain Dufresne, and Michael K. Danquah. 2018. "Review on nanoparticles and nanostructured materials: History, sources, toxicity, and regulations." *Beilstein Journal of Nanotechnology* 9:1050–1074. DOI: 10.3762/bjnano.9.98.

Kalpana, V. N., and V. Devi Rajeswari. 2018. "A review on green synthesis, biomedical applications, and toxicity studies of ZnO NPs." *Bioinorganic Chemistry and Applications* 2018:3569758. DOI: 10.1155/2018/3569758.

Kaushik, B. K., L. Singh, R. Singh, G. Zhu, B. Zhang, Q. Wang, and S. Kumar. 2020. "Detection of collagen-IV using highly reflective metal nanoparticles: Immobilized photosensitive optical fiber-based MZI structure." *IEEE Transactions on NanoBioscience* 19 (3):477–484. DOI: 10.1109/TNB.2020.2998520.

Khan, Ibrahim, Khalid Saeed, and Idrees Khan. 2017. "Nanoparticles: Properties, applications and toxicities." *Arabian Journal of Chemistry* 12 (7):908–931. DOI: 10.1016/j.arabjc.2017.05.011.

Khan, Ibrahim, Khalid Saeed, and Idrees Khan. 2019. "Nanoparticles: Properties, applications, and toxicities." *Arabian Journal of Chemistry* 12 (7):908–931. https://doi.org/10.1016/j.arabjc.2017.05.011.

Koetz, Joachim. 2020. "The effect of surface modification of gold nanotriangles for surface-enhanced Raman scattering performance." *Nanomaterials* 10 (11). DOI: 10.3390/nano10112187.

Krishna Prasad, N. V., K. Venkata Prasad, S. Ramesh, S. V. Phanidhar, K. Venkata Ratnam, S. Janardhan, H. Manjunatha, M. S. S. R. K. N. Sarma, and K. Srinivas. 2020. "Ceramic sensors: A mini-review of their applications." *Frontiers in Materials* 7 (368). DOI: 10.3389/fmats.2020.593342.

Kumar, K. Santhosh, Vijay Bhooshan Kumar, and Pradip Paik. 2013. "Recent advancement in functional core-shell nanoparticles of polymers: Synthesis, physical properties, and applications in medical biotechnology." *Journal of Nanoparticles* 2013:672059. DOI: 10.1155/2013/672059.

Kumar, Raj, Keshaw Ram Aadil, Shivendu Ranjan, and Vijay Bhooshan Kumar. 2020. "Advances in nanotechnology and nanomaterials based strategies for neural tissue engineering." *Journal of Drug Delivery Science and Technology* 57:101617. https://doi.org/10.1016/j.jddst.2020.101617.

Kumar, S., R. Singh, B. K. Kaushik, N. K. Chen, Q. S. Yang, and X. Zhang. 2019. "LSPR-based cholesterol biosensor using hollow core fiber structure." *IEEE Sensors Journal* 19 (17):7399–7406. DOI: 10.1109/JSEN.2019.2916818.

Kumar, S., R. Singh, Q. Yang, S. Cheng, B. Zhang, and B. K. Kaushik. 2021. "Highly sensitive, selective and portable sensor probe using germanium-doped photosensitive optical fiber for ascorbic acid detection." *IEEE Sensors Journal* 21 (1):62–70. DOI: 10.1109/JSEN.2020.2973579.

Kumar, Santosh, Zhu Guo, Ragini Singh, Qinglin Wang, Bingyuan Zhang, Shuang Cheng, Fengzhen Liu, Carlos Marques, Brajesh Kumar Kaushik, and Rajan Jha. 2020. "MoS$_2$ functionalized multicore fiber probes for selective detection of *Shigella* bacteria based on localized plasmon." *Journal of Lightwave Technology* pp. 1–1. DOI: 10.1109/JLT.2020.3036610.

Kumar, Santosh, Lokendra Singh, and Amna Bedi. 2018. "SPR based hybrid plasmonic waveguide sensor for detection of causes of anemia in Homosapiens." Proc. SPIE 10509, Plasmonics in Biology and Medicine XV, 105090G, 23 February. https://doi.org/10.1117/12.2285927.

Kumar, Santosh, and Ragini Singh. 2021. "Recent optical sensing technologies for the detection of various biomolecules: Review." *Optics & Laser Technology* 134:106620. DOI: 10.1016/j.optlastec.2020.106620.

Kumar, Santosh, Ragini Singh, Guo Zhu, Qingshan Yang, Xia Zhang, Shuang Cheng, Bingyuan Zhang, Brajesh Kumar Kaushik, and Fengzhen Liu. 2019. "Development of uric acid biosensor using gold nanoparticles and graphene oxide functionalized micro-ball fiber sensor probe." *IEEE Transactions on NanoBioscience* pp. 1–1. DOI: 10.1109/TNB.2019.2958891.

Kyriakides, Themis R., Arindam Raj, Tiffany H. Tseng, Hugh Xiao, Ryan Nguyen, Farrah S. Mohammed, Saiti Halder, Mengqing Xu, Michelle J. Wu, Shuozhen Bao, and Wendy C. Sheu. 2021. "Biocompatibility of nanomaterials and their immunological properties." *Biomedical Materials* 16 (4):042005. DOI: 10.1088/1748-605x/abe5fa.

Le, Thanh-Hai, Yuree Oh, Hyungwoo Kim, and Hyeonseok Yoon. 2020. "Exfoliation of 2D materials for energy and environmental applications." *Chemistry: A European Journal* 26 (29):6360–6401. https://doi.org/10.1002/chem.202000223.

Lee, Jaesang, Shaily Mahendra, and Pedro J. J. Alvarez. 2010. "Nanomaterials in the construction industry: A review of their applications and environmental health and safety considerations." *ACS Nano* 4 (7):3580–3590. DOI: 10.1021/nn100866w.

Lee, S., K. Sim, S. Y. Moon, J. Choi, Y. Jeon, J. M. Nam, and S. J. Park. 2021. "Controlled assembly of plasmonic nanoparticles: From static to dynamic nanostructures." *Adv Mater* 33 (46):e2007668. DOI: 10.1002/adma.202007668.

Li, Muyang, Ragini Singh, Carlos Marques, Bingyuan Zhang, and Santosh Kumar. 2021. "2D material assisted SMF-MCF-MMF-SMF based LSPR sensor for creatinine detection." *Optics Express* 29 (23):38150–38167. DOI: 10.1364/OE.445555.

Li, Xiangqian, Huizhong Xu, Zhe-Sheng Chen, and Guofang Chen. 2011. "Biosynthesis of nanoparticles by microorganisms and their applications." *Journal of Nanomaterials* 2011:270974. DOI: 10.1155/2011/270974.

Loiseau, Alexis, Victoire Asila, Gabriel Boitel-Aullen, Mylan Lam, Michèle Salmain, and Souhir Boujday. 2019. "Silver-based plasmonic nanoparticles for and their use in biosensing." *Biosensors* 9 (2). DOI: 10.3390/bios9020078.

Ma, Tengfei, and Hao Wu. 2020. "Industry development of derivative functionalized gold nanomaterials and their application in chemiluminescence bioanalysis: Based on the industrial practice of China's Central Yunnan urban agglomeration." *Journal of Chemistry* 2020:5474506. DOI: 10.1155/2020/5474506.

Majid, Abdul, and Maryam Bibi. 2018. "Wet chemical synthesis methods." In *Cadmium Based II-VI Semiconducting Nanomaterials: Synthesis Routes and Strategies*, edited by Abdul Majid and Maryam Bibi, 43–101. Cham: Springer International Publishing.

Malekzad, H., P. S. Zangabad, H. Mirshekari, M. Karimi, and M. R. Hamblin. 2017. "Noble metal nanoparticles in biosensors: Recent studies and applications." *Nanotechnology Reviews* 6 (3):301–329. DOI: 10.1515/ntrev-2016-0014.

Malhotra, Bansi Dhar, and Md Azahar Ali. 2018. "Chapter 1: Nanomaterials in biosensors: Fundamentals and applications." In *Nanomaterials for Biosensors*, edited by Bansi Dhar Malhotra and Md Azahar Ali, 1–74. Norwich, NY: William Andrew Publishing.

Manaia, Eloísa Berbel, Marina Paiva Abuçafy, Bruna Galdorfini Chiari-Andréo, Bruna Lallo Silva, João Augusto Oshiro Junior, and Leila Aparecida Chiavacci. 2017. "Physicochemical characterization of drug nanocarriers." *International Journal of Nanomedicine* 12:4991–5011. DOI: 10.2147/IJN.S133832.

Manikkoth, Sindhu Thalappan, Deepthi Panoth, Kunnambeth M. Thulasi, Fabeena Jahan, Anjali Paravannoor, and Baiju Kizhakkekilikoodayil Vijayan. 2021. "Chapter 7: Flexible smart nanosensors." In *Nanosensors for Smart Manufacturing*, edited by Sabu Thomas, Tuan Anh Nguyen, Mazaher Ahmadi, Ali Farmani, and Ghulam Yasin, 145–182. Amsterdam: Elsevier.

Marinescu, Liliana, Denisa Ficai, Ovidiu Oprea, Alexandru Marin, Anton Ficai, Ecaterina Andronescu, and Alina-Maria Holban. 2020. "Optimized synthesis approaches of metal nanoparticles with antimicrobial applications." *Journal of Nanomaterials* 2020:6651207. DOI: 10.1155/2020/6651207.

Mathew, Jinu, Josny Joy, and Soney C. George. 2019. "Potential applications of nanotechnology in transportation: A review." *Journal of King Saud University-Science* 31 (4):586–594. https://doi.org/10.1016/j.jksus.2018.03.015.

Mitchell, Michael J., Margaret M. Billingsley, Rebecca M. Haley, Marissa E. Wechsler, Nicholas A. Peppas, and Robert Langer. 2021. "Engineering precision nanoparticles for drug delivery." *Nature Reviews Drug Discovery* 20 (2):101–124. DOI: 10.1038/s41573-020-0090-8.

Mohammadniaei, M., A. Koyappayil, Y. Sun, J. Min, and M. H. Lee. 2020. "Gold nanoparticle/MXene for multiple and sensitive detection of oncomiRs based on synergetic signal amplification." *Biosens Bioelectron* 159:112208. DOI: 10.1016/j.bios.2020.112208.

Moreno-Vega, Aura-Ileana, Teresa Gómez-Quintero, Rosa-Elvira Nuñez-Anita, Laura-Susana Acosta-Torres, and Víctor Castaño. 2012. "Polymeric and ceramic nanoparticles in biomedical applications." *Journal of Nanotechnology* 2012:936041. DOI: 10.1155/2012/936041.

Mourdikoudis, Stefanos, Roger M. Pallares, and Nguyen T. K. Thanh. 2018. "Characterization techniques for nanoparticles: Comparison and complementarity upon studying nanoparticle properties." *Nanoscale* 10 (27):12871–12934. DOI: 10.1039/C8NR02278J.

Mukherjee, S., S. Ray, and R. S. Thakur. 2009. "Solid lipid nanoparticles: A modern formulation approach in drug delivery system." *Indian Journal of Pharmaceutical Sciences* 71 (4):349–358. DOI: 10.4103/0250-474X.57282.

Nair, Anju K., Anshida Mayeen, Leyana K. Shaji, Mooleparambil S. Kala, Sabu Thomas, and Nandakumar Kalarikkal. 2018. "Chapter 10: Optical characterization of nanomaterials." In *Characterization of Nanomaterials*, edited by Sneha Mohan Bhagyaraj, Oluwatobi Samuel Oluwafemi, Nandakumar Kalarikkal, and Sabu Thomas, 269–299. Sawston, Cambridge: Woodhead Publishing.

Nesheva, Diana. 2001. "Chapter 6: Nanocrystalline and amorphous thin film systems including low-dimensional chalcogenide materials." In *Handbook of Surfaces and Interfaces of Materials*, edited by Hari Singh Nalwa, 239–279. Burlington: Academic Press.

Nikazar, Sohrab, Vishnu Sankar Sivasankarapillai, Abbas Rahdar, Salim Gasmi, P. S. Anumol, and Muhammad Salman Shanavas. 2020. "Revisiting the cytotoxicity of quantum dots: An in-depth overview." *Biophysical Reviews* 12 (3):703–718. DOI: 10.1007/s12551-020-00653-0.

Nikolova, Maria P., and Murthy S. Chavali. 2020. "Metal oxide nanoparticles as biomedical materials." *Biomimetics (Basel, Switzerland)* 5 (2):27. DOI: 10.3390/biomimetics5020027.

Njuguna, J., F. Ansari, S. Sachse, H. Zhu, and V. M. Rodriguez. 2014. "1-nanomaterials, nanofillers, and nanocomposites: Types and properties." In *Health and Environmental Safety of Nanomaterials*, edited by James Njuguna, Krzysztof Pielichowski, and Huijun Zhu, 3–27. Sawston, Cambridge: Woodhead Publishing.

Noah, Naumih M. 2020. "Design and synthesis of nanostructured materials for sensor applications." *Journal of Nanomaterials* 2020:8855321. DOI: 10.1155/2020/8855321.

Ossai, Chinedu I., and Nagarajan Raghavan. 2018. "Nanostructure and nanomaterial characterization, growth mechanisms, and applications." *Nanotechnology Reviews* 7 (2):209–231. DOI: 10.1515/ntrev-2017-0156.

Pal, Nabanita, Jun-Hyeok Lee, and Eun-Bum Cho. 2020. "Recent trends in morphology-controlled synthesis and application of mesoporous silica nanoparticles." *Nanomaterials* 10 (11). DOI: 10.3390/nano10112122.

Patra, Jayanta Kumar, Gitishree Das, Leonardo Fernandes Fraceto, Estefania Vangelie Ramos Campos, Maria del Pilar Rodriguez-Torres, Laura Susana Acosta-Torres, Luis Armando Diaz-Torres, Renato Grillo, Mallappa Kumara Swamy, Shivesh Sharma, Solomon Habtemariam, and Han-Seung Shin. 2018. "Nano based drug delivery systems: Recent developments and future prospects." *Journal of Nanobiotechnology* 16 (1):71. DOI: 10.1186/s12951-018-0392-8.

Pawar, Milind, S. Topcu Sendoğdular, and Perena Gouma. 2018. "A brief overview of TiO_2 photocatalyst for organic dye remediation: Case study of reaction mechanisms involved in Ce-TiO_2 photocatalysts system." *Journal of Nanomaterials* 2018:5953609. DOI: 10.1155/2018/5953609.

Perez-Gonzalez, Victor, Jose Ortiz Castillo, Roberto Gallo-Villanueva, and Marc Madou. 2020. "Anisotropic gold nanoparticles: A survey of recent synthetic methodologies." *Coordination Chemistry Reviews* 425:213489. DOI: 10.1016/j.ccr.2020.213489.

Pirzada, Muqsit, and Zeynep Altintas. 2019. "Nanomaterials for healthcare biosensing applications." *Sensors* 19 (23). DOI: 10.3390/s19235311.

Porter, Alan L., and Jan Youtie. 2009. "How interdisciplinary is nanotechnology?" *Journal of Nanoparticle Research: An Interdisciplinary Forum for Nanoscale Science and Technology* 11 (5):1023–1041. DOI: 10.1007/s11051-009-9607-0.

Rakhi, R. B., Pranati Nayak, Chuan Xia, and Husam N. Alshareef. 2016. "Novel amperometric glucose biosensor based on MXene nanocomposite." *Scientific Reports* 6 (1):36422. DOI: 10.1038/srep36422.

Rani, Ankita, Rajesh Reddy, Uttkarshni Sharma, Priya Mukherjee, Priyanka Mishra, Aneek Kuila, Lan Ching Sim, and Pichiah Saravanan. 2018. "A review on the progress of nanostructure materials for energy harnessing and environmental remediation." *Journal of Nanostructure in Chemistry* 8 (3):255–291. DOI: 10.1007/s40097-018-0278-1.

Saifuddin, N., A. Z. Raziah, and A. R. Junizah. 2013. "Carbon nanotubes: A review on structure and their interaction with proteins." *Journal of Chemistry* 2013:676815. DOI: 10.1155/2013/676815.

Saito, Naoto, Hisao Haniu, Yuki Usui, Kaoru Aoki, Kazuo Hara, Seiji Takanashi, Masayuki Shimizu, Nobuyo Narita, Masanori Okamoto, Shinsuke Kobayashi, Hiroki Nomura, Hiroyuki Kato, Naoyuki Nishimura, Seiichi Taruta, and Morinobu Endo. 2014. "Safe clinical use of carbon nanotubes as innovative biomaterials." *Chemical Reviews* 114 (11):6040–6079. DOI: 10.1021/cr400341h.

Senapati, Sudipta, Arun Kumar Mahanta, Sunil Kumar, and Pralay Maiti. 2018. "Controlled drug delivery vehicles for cancer treatment and their performance." *Signal Transduction and Targeted Therapy* 3 (1):7. DOI: 10.1038/s41392-017-0004-3.

Shuck, Christopher E., Asia Sarycheva, Mark Anayee, Ariana Levitt, Yuanzhe Zhu, Simge Uzun, Vitaliy Balitskiy, Veronika Zahorodna, Oleksiy Gogotsi, and Yury Gogotsi. 2020. "Scalable synthesis of Ti$_3$C$_2$Tx MXene." *Advanced Engineering Materials* 22 (3):1901241. https://doi.org/10.1002/adem.201901241.

Singh, L., R. Singh, S. Kumar, B. Zhang, and B. K. Kaushik. 2020. "Development of collagen-IV sensor using optical fiber-based Mach-Zehnder interferometer structure." *IEEE Journal of Quantum Electronics* 56 (4):1–8. DOI: 10.1109/JQE.2020.3003022.

Singh, L., R. Singh, B. Zhang, B. K. Kaushik, and S. Kumar. 2020. "Localized surface plasmon resonance based hetero-core optical fiber sensor structure for the detection of L-cysteine." *IEEE Transactions on Nanotechnology* 19:201–208. DOI: 10.1109/TNANO.2020.2975297.

Singh, L., G. Zhu, R. Singh, B. Zhang, W. Wang, B. K. Kaushik, and S. Kumar. 2020. "Gold nanoparticles and uricase functionalized tapered fiber sensor for uric acid detection." *IEEE Sensors Journal* 20 (1):219–226. DOI: 10.1109/JSEN.2019.2942388.

Singh, Lokendra, Ragini Singh, Bingyuan Zhang, Shuang Chen, Brajesh Kumar Kaushik, and Santosh Kumar. 2019. "LSPR based uric acid sensor using graphene oxide and gold nanoparticles functionalized tapered fiber." *Optical Fiber Technology* 53:102043. DOI: 10.1016/j.yofte.2019.102043.

Singh, Lokendra, Guo Zhu, G. Kumar, D. Revathi, and Prakash Pareek. 2021. "Numerical simulation of all-optical logic functions at micrometer scale by using plasmonic metal-insulator-metal (MIM) waveguides." *Optics & Laser Technology* 135:106697. DOI: 10.1016/j.optlastec.2020.106697.

Singh, Ragini, Santosh Kumar, Feng-Zhen Liu, Cheng Shuang, Bingyuan Zhang, Rajan Jha, and Brajesh Kumar Kaushik. 2020. "Etched multicore fiber sensor using copper oxide and gold nanoparticles decorated graphene oxide structure for cancer cells detection." *Biosensors and Bioelectronics* 168:112557. https://doi.org/10.1016/j.bios.2020.112557.

Soto-Quintero, Albanelly, Nekane Guarrotxena, Olga García, and Isabel Quijada-Garrido. 2019. "Curcumin to promote the synthesis of silver NPs and their self-assembly with a thermoresponsive polymer in core-shell nanohybrids." *Scientific Reports* 9 (1):18187. DOI: 10.1038/s41598-019-54752-4.

Speranza, V., A. Sorrentino, F. De Santis, and R. Pantani. 2014. "Characterization of the polycaprolactone melt crystallization: Complementary optical microscopy, DSC, and AFM studies." *The Scientific World Journal* 2014:720157. DOI: 10.1155/2014/720157.

Steinegger, Andreas, Otto S. Wolfbeis, and Sergey M. Borisov. 2020. "Optical sensing and imaging of pH values: Spectroscopies, materials, and applications." *Chemical Reviews* 120 (22):12357–12489. DOI: 10.1021/acs.chemrev.0c00451.

Takemura, Kenshin. 2021. "Surface plasmon resonance (SPR)- and localized SPR (LSPR)-based virus sensing systems: Optical vibration of nano- and micro-metallic materials for the development of next-generation virus detection technology." *Biosensors* 11 (8):250.

Tarafdar, J., Sharma Shikha, and Ramesh Raliya. 2013. "Nanotechnology: Interdisciplinary science of applications." *African Journal of Biotechnology* 12:219–226. DOI: 10.5897/AJB12.2481.

Tebbe, Moritz, Christian Kuttner, Max Männel, Andreas Fery, and Munish Chanana. 2015. "Colloidally stable and surfactant-free protein-coated gold nanorods in biological media." *ACS Applied Materials & Interfaces* 7 (10):5984–5991. DOI: 10.1021/acsami.5b00335.

Thomas, S., C. Harshita, P. K. Mishra, and S. Talegaonkar. 2015. "Ceramic nanoparticles: Fabrication methods and applications in drug delivery." *Current Pharmaceutical Design* 21 (42):6165–6188. DOI: 10.21 74/1381612821666151027153246.

Tian, Minglei, Luwei Fang, Xuemin Yan, Wei Xiao, and Kyung Ho Row. 2019. "Determination of heavy metal ions and organic pollutants in water samples using ionic liquids and ionic liquid-modified sorbents." *Journal of Analytical Methods in Chemistry* 2019:1948965. DOI: 10.1155/2019/1948965.

Tian, P., L. Tang, K. S. Teng, and S. P. Lau. 2018. "Graphene quantum dots from chemistry to applications." *Materials Today Chemistry* 10:221–258. https://doi.org/10.1016/j.mtchem.2018.09.007.

Tipper, M., and E. Guillemois. 2016. "4-developments in the use of nanofibres in nonwovens." In *Advances in Technical Nonwovens*, edited by George Kellie, 115–132. Sawston, Cambridge: Woodhead Publishing.

Turkevich, John, Peter Cooper Stevenson, and James Hillier. 1951. "A study of the nucleation and growth processes in the synthesis of colloidal gold." *Discussions of the Faraday Society* 11 (0):55–75. DOI: 10.1039/DF9511100055.

Venkateshaiah, Abhilash, Vinod V. T. Padil, Malladi Nagalakshmaiah, Stanisław Waclawek, Miroslav Černík, and Rajender S. Varma. 2020. "Microscopic techniques for the analysis of micro and nanostructures of biopolymers and their derivatives." *Polymers* 12 (3):512. DOI: 10.3390/polym12030512.

Wang, Kuiyuan, Jinzhu Song, Xijian Duan, Jianshuai Mu, and Yan Wang. 2017. "Perovskite LaCoO$_3$ nanoparticles as enzyme mimetics: Their catalytic properties, mechanism, and application in dopamine biosensing." *New Journal of Chemistry* 41 (16):8554–8560. DOI: 10.1039/C7NJ01177F.

Wang, Meiling, Min Wang, Ganhong Zheng, Zhenxiang Dai, and Yongqing Ma. 2021. "Recent progress in sensing application of metal nanoarchitecture-enhanced fluorescence." *Nanoscale Advances* 3 (9):2448–2465. DOI: 10.1039/D0NA01050B.

Wang, Yong, Qing Huang, Wenjie Zhu, Minghong Yang, and Elfed Lewis. 2019. "Novel optical fiber SPR temperature sensor based on MMF-PCF-MMF structure and gold-PDMS film: Erratum." *Optics Express* 27 (8):10813–10813. DOI: 10.1364/OE.27.010813.

Wang, Yu, Guo Zhu, Muyang Li, Ragini Singh, Carlos Marques, Min Rui, Brajesh Kumar Kaushik, Bingyuan Zhang, Rajan Jha, and Santosh Kumar. 2021. "Water pollutants p-cresol detection based on Au-ZnO nanoparticles modified tapered optical fiber." *IEEE Transactions on NanoBioscience* 32. DOI: 10.1109/TNB.2021.3082856.

Wang, Zhi, Ragini Singh, Carlos Marques, Rajan Jha, Bingyuan Zhang, and Santosh Kumar. 2021. "Taper-in-taper fiber structure-based LSPR sensor for alanine aminotransferase detection." *Optics Express* 29 (26):43793–43810. DOI: 10.1364/OE.447202.

Wang, Zhi, Guo Zhu, Yu Wang, Muyang Li, Ragini Singh, Bingyuan Zhang, and Santosh Kumar. 2021. "Fabrication techniques and stability analysis of SMF-/MMF-based differently tapered optical fiber structures." *Applied Optics* 60 (7):2077–2082. DOI: 10.1364/AO.418875.

Yang, Qingshan, Xia Zhang, Santosh Kumar, Ragini Singh, Bingyuan Zhang, Cheng-Lin Bai, and Xipeng Pu. 2020. "Development of glucose sensor using gold nanoparticles and glucose-oxidase functionalized tapered fiber structure." *Plasmonics* 15. DOI: 10.1007/s11468-019-01104-7.

Yang, Qingshan, Guo Zhu, Lokendra Singh, Yu Wang, Ragini Singh, Bingyuan Zhang, Xia Zhang, and Santosh Kumar. 2020. "Highly sensitive and selective sensor probe using glucose oxidase/gold nanoparticles/graphene oxide functionalized tapered optical fiber structure for detection of glucose." *Optik* 208:164536. DOI: 10.1016/j.ijleo.2020.164536.

Yoon, Jinho, Minkyu Shin, Joungpyo Lim, Ji-Young Lee, and Jeong-Woo Choi. 2020. "Recent advances in MXene nanocomposite-based biosensors." *Biosensors* 10 (11). DOI: 10.3390/bios10110185.

Zhang, Xi-Feng, Zhi-Guo Liu, Wei Shen, and Sangiliyandi Gurunathan. 2016. "Silver nanoparticles: Synthesis, characterization, properties, applications, and therapeutic approaches." *International Journal of Molecular Sciences* 17 (9):1534. DOI: 10.3390/ijms17091534.

Zhao, Jinxiu, Lei Zhang, Xiao-Ying Xie, Xianghong Li, Yongjun Ma, Qian Liu, Wei-Hai Fang, Xifeng Shi, Ganglong Cui, and Xuping Sun. 2018. "Ti$_3$C$_2$Tx (T = F, OH) MXene nanosheets: Conductive 2D catalysts for ambient electrohydrogenation of N$_2$ to NH$_3$." *Journal of Materials Chemistry A* 6 (47):24031–24035. DOI: 10.1039/C8TA09840A.

Zhu, Guo, Niteshkumar Agrawal, Ragini Singh, Santosh Kumar, Bingyuan Zhang, Chinmoy Saha, and Chandrakanta Kumar. 2020. "A novel periodically tapered structure-based gold nanoparticles and graphene oxide: Immobilized optical fiber sensor to detect ascorbic acid." *Optics & Laser Technology* 127:106156. https://doi.org/10.1016/j.optlastec.2020.106156.

Zhu, Guo, Lokendra Singh, Yu Wang, Ragini Singh, Bingyuan Zhang, Fengzhen Liu, Brajesh Kumar Kaushik, and Santosh Kumar. 2020. "Tapered optical fiber-based LSPR biosensor for ascorbic acid detection." *Photonic Sensors*. DOI: 10.1007/s13320-020-0605-2.

3 Design Methodology

3.1 INTRODUCTION

The contribution of optical fiber-based plasmonic sensors is profound and versatile in different kinds of biosensing applications. Because of their wide range of applications, such as clinical diagnostics, biomolecule detection, gas sensing, temperature and pressure monitoring, medicine, security, food safety, chemical sensing, and point-of-care, these sensors have piqued the interest of the research community. In recent years, the research has also been extended to include the detection of pathogenic microorganisms (bacteria, viruses, mycobacteria, fungi, and protozoa) using plasmonic biosensors. This chapter presents the recent developments in surface plasmon resonance (SPR)/localized surface plasmon resonance (LSPR) sensing, detection schemes, their realization at the surface of s nanostructure, configuration, components employed, and application of the sensors in the field of biosensing technologies. Herein, mainly challenging and oriented developments in fiber-optic-based plasmonic biosensor-centric literature are discussed and summarized, indicating potentially valuable future research avenues. Because of its popularity and versatility, there is no specific definition and description of the working concept of the nano-biosensor. In terms of in vivo health assessment and diagnosis, this bright new star shines in many application fields, such as those used to monitor the presence of contaminants, toxins, humidity, environmental pollutants, heavy metal toxicity, and even carcinogens.

The development of accurate and cheap biosensors increases the potential for commercial application and its increased use in the healthcare sector (Neethirajan et al. 2018). All sorts of biosensing technical studies, for instance, electrochemical (Akolpoglu et al. 2019), thermometric (Vasuki et al. 2019), luminescent (Roda et al. 2016), amperometric (Pan et al. 2017), potentiometric (Ding and Qin 2020), and optical methods (Huertas et al. 2019) have been reported. The research community is increasingly attracted by biosensors, especially optical methods-based sensors that are being used in diagnostic and bioanalytical applications (Andryukov et al. 2020). Pregnancy testing and glucose testing are two such examples of the successful application of biosensing devices (Malhotra and Ali 2018). In this study, we restricted our discussion to fiber-optic plasmonic biosensors, which are categorized under optical method-based biosensors. The application of the fiber-optic technique in sensor-based devices provides various advantages such as anti-electromagnetic interference, multiplex machine, extreme condition capability (chemical etching, high temperatures, and radial zoon), dielectric sensor design, application of distributed fiber sensor, and mechanical advantages due to the low-profile cylindrical geometry (Simon and Denis 2019; Habel 2019). Remarkably, the concept of plasmonic sensing within the context of optical fiber sensors (OFSs) was proposed for the first time in the 1980s (Allsop and Neal 20p[19]). Many physicists, chemists, biologists, and material scientists were attracted to this new type of sensor, and as a result, it made a strong entry into the world of sensors due to its numerous applications in the area of biosensing (Petryayeva and Krull 2011; Prabowo, Purwidyantri, and Liu 2018). Fiber-optic-based plasmonic sensors with the ability to measure variations from single or multiple light beams are used in several research and commercial applications (Allsop and Neal 2019). Optical sensing technology, in particular, SPR/LSPR shows a range of advantages such as remote sensing, portability, lightweight, label-free detection, ease of fabrication, anti-electromagnetic interference, small-scale size, multiplexing function, biocompatibility, high data accuracy, real-time monitoring, and small detection time (Sharma, Jha, and Gupta 2007; Masson 2020). The SPR phenomenon-based sensor was widely investigated and tested for gas detection for the first time in 1982, demonstrating the variation in optical parameters of the film caused by the gas exposer (Nylander, Liedberg, and Lind 1982).

This chapter is divided into five sections to elucidate the design methodology of plasmonic OFSs (P-OFSs). Section 3.2 describes developments in sensor structural design, including commonly used tapered and hetero-core sensor designs. This section also extensively covers previous studies based

DOI: 10.1201/9781003243199-3

on structural designs of various sensors. Sections 3.3 is dedicated to the developments in nano-coating process and characterization of nanomaterials and immobilized probes. This section also emphasizes recent advances and approaches for nanocoating of probes that are reported to improve the sensitivity of plasmonic sensors. Section 3.4 broadly deals with sensor developments and a wide range of applications. Section 3.5 indicates a summary, major findings, and observations of the present chapter as well as the limitations of available sensor designs and the possibilities of advances in structural design for the performance boosting of optic-plasmonic sensors.

3.2 STRUCTURAL DEVELOPMENTS

Many structural developments and advancements are discussed in this section to help the reader understand how P-OFSs work. Discussion includes the tapering technique (Semwal and Gupta 2018; Mustapha Kamil et al. 2018; Velázquez-González et al. 2017), chemical etching method (Srivastava, Verma, and Gupta 2012), bending of fiber (Srivastava et al. 2012; Wang and Liu 2018), fiber Bragg grating (Zhou et al. 2021), hetero-core-structure (Wang and Liu 2018), addition of a highly sensitive dielectric layer (Tabassum and Gupta 2017), the micro-ball structure (Kumar, Singh, Zhu et al. 2019), and so on. Chemical etching and bending techniques, for example, have drawbacks such as increased surface roughness, improbability of results, and uncontrolled fabrication (Singh, Raghuwanshi, and Prakash 2019). Furthermore, the tapering technique and hetero-core structure demonstrate promising performance and aid in sensor sensing sensitivity (Yang, Zhang et al. 2019). These structures are created using a variety of normal fibers, including single-mode fiber (SMF), photosensitive fiber (PSF), multimode fiber (MMF), multicore fiber (MCF), photonic-crystal fiber (PCF), hollow-core fiber (HCF), and others (Zhou et al. 2019). The basic optical fiber structures, as indicated in Figure 3.1, are designed by varying the parameters like core diameter, alignment,

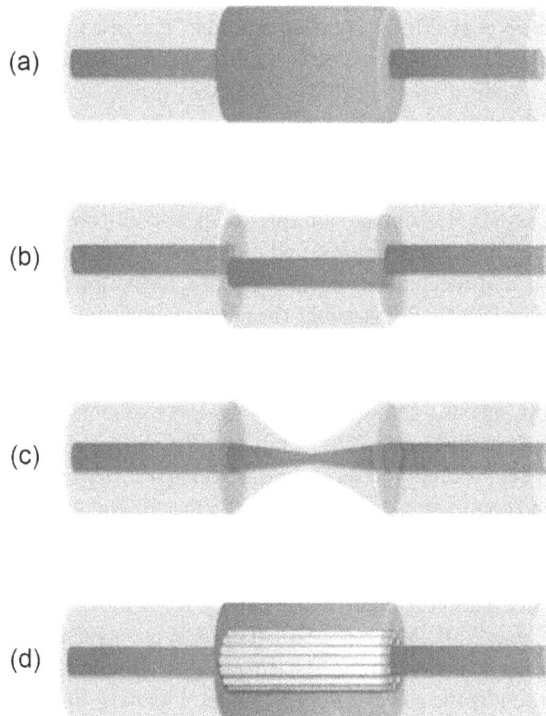

FIGURE 3.1 Optical fiber structures development designed by varying (a) the core diameter, (b) the alignment, (c) the shape, and (d) the type of the fibers (Socorro-Leránoz et al. 2019).

shape, and type of fiber (Lopez-Torres, Elosua, and Arregui 2020). Various advanced machines are available to develop such structures, including a combiner manufacturing system (CMS), fusion splicer, among others (Kaushik et al. 2020). Fabrication of some vital and effective structures is covered in the following subsections.

3.2.1 Tapered Structure

With the rapid progress in micro-/nanotechnology, spatial miniaturization has been one of the current trends of OFSs. It is obvious that reducing the size of a sensing structure is usually an essential step to impart the sensor with faster response, higher sensitivity, low power consumption, and better spatial resolution. Hence, a tapered fiber is one of the best candidates for this purpose. Tapered fibers offer a number of efficient optical and mechanical properties, including the following:

- Large evanescent fields: A considerable fraction of the propagating light can get transmitted as the evanescent field beyond the tapered fiber physical boundary, and this can be exploited for sensors and high-Q resonators.
- Great configurability: Tapered fibers preserve the original optical fiber dimensions at their pigtails, allowing for low-loss interconnection to fiberized components and detectors. Due to the large refractive index (RI) contrast between silica and air, bend radii of the order of a few micrometers can be readily achieved with low induced bend loss, allowing for highly compact devices with complex geometries (e.g., two-dimensional [2D] and three-dimensional [3D] resonators.
- Low-loss connection: Since tapered fibers are manufactured by adiabatically stretching optical fibers, they maintain the original fiber size at their input and output ends, which allows for easy splicing to standard fibers and other fiberized components. One can easily fabricate tapered fibers having insertion loss smaller than 0.1 dB.
- Strong confinement: A tapered fiber can confine light within the diffraction limit for lengths that are only limited by the loss. This allows the ready observation of nonlinear interactions, such as supercontinuum generation, at relatively modest power levels.

Additionally, tapered fiber-based sensors exhibit all the beneficial characteristic of OFSs, including greater sensitivity, reduced size, reduced weight, immunity to electromagnetic interference, reduced cost, lightweight, large bandwidth, ease in implementing multiplexed or distributed sensors, and compatibility with optical communication technology. All these advantages make the tapered fiber a novel miniaturized platform for optical sensing.

Based on different tapered fiber-based structures, a variety of physical, chemical, and biological sensors have been demonstrated so far. Some of the most popular microfiber-based structures are:

  I. Single tapered fiber
 II. Cascaded tapered fiber
III. Tapered fiber gratings
 IV. Tapered fiber resonators
  V. Functionally activated tapered fiber

For fabricating a tapered fiber, the most favored processes are based on the top-down physical drawing method that reduces large-volume materials (often from glass fibers) to thin fibers by means of microfiber drawing. The tapered fibers fabricated from these top-down processes have excellent geometric uniformity and surface smoothness, which are essential for achieving low optical loss and high signal-to-noise ratio.

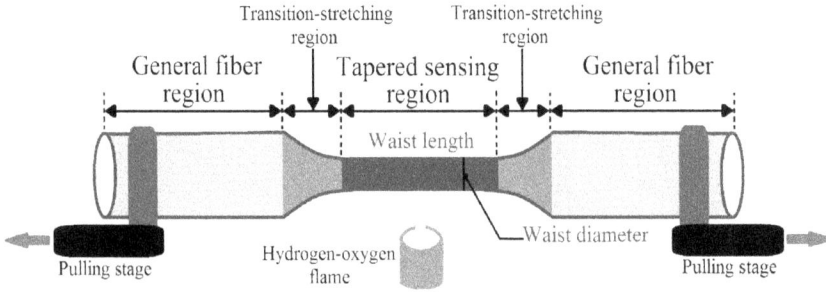

FIGURE 3.2 Flame and brush for tapered fiber drawing technique.

Source: Reprinted with permission from *Biomedical Optics Express.* Copyright, 2019, Optica (Kumar, Kaushik et al. 2019).

In 1970, the first use of tapered fiber was reported for increasing the light-receiving area of an avalanche photodiode (Nishida et al. 1970). Flame-brush techniques have been popularly used for fabricating tapered fiber. This is the most widely used tapered fiber drawing technique. Bilodeau et al. reported this technique for the first time for manufacturing tapered fiber and couplers in 1988 (Bilodeau et al. 1988). The schematic of a typical flame-brushing technique is shown in Figure 3.2. In this technique, an SMF is heated above a gas burner flame and then stretched by means of axial pulling force applied at the two sides. The pulling reduces the diameter at the hot zone of the flame (where the temperature is above the softening temperature of the fiber material), and as a result, microfiber gets fabricated. By controlling the flame movement and the fiber pulling rate, one can define the microfiber shape to an extremely high degree of accuracy. Generally, a low-carbon fuel such as hydrogen is used in the burner to minimize the contamination of fiber with incompletely burned carbon particles. Occasionally, oxygen is also supplied to the burner to control the temperature and size of the flame (Tong and Sumetsky 2010).

Apart from being very simple and cost-effective, an advantage of this technique is that it provides access to both pigtailed ends of the tapered fiber which is very important for practical applications, such as telecommunication and sensing, where connectivity and system integration are highly essential. Optical fiber tapering is a unique and effective technique used to raise the penetration depth and allow the evanescent waves (EWs) to interrelate with the external environment (Korposh et al. 2019). The guided wave, while leaking from the fiber core, decays exponentially to the external surface of cladding section at the taper waist region. The evanescent fields are generated in the cladding and decay exponentially in the normal fiber (Mustapha et al. 2015; Roy and Knight 2017). Figure 3.3(a) illustrates the schematic of a single-tapered optic-fiber structure, while the process of wave propagation along the fiber structure is described in Figure 3.3(b). The tapered transition section is dichotomized as (i) adiabatic transition and (ii) nonadiabatic transition (Agrawal, Saha, Kumar, Singh, Zhang, Jha et al. 2020). In an adiabatic transition, maximum efficiency has been revealed from the fundamental mode, and additional modes are not so important, whereas in nonadiabatic conditions, most of the optical signals transmitted in the tapered fiber leak into the external environment as EWs (Song 2016). (Zhu et al. 2020). As shown in Figure 3.3(a), the tapered fiber structure consists of three major sections: left transition, uniform waist, and right transition. This technique is highly effective, and no mode squeezing phenomena are possible in the tapered fiber sensor structure (Zhang, Zhuang et al. 2019). The tapered structure probe fabricated by the conventional flame-brush technique is hardly reproducible in such geometry. Tapered structural reproducibility is very high due to the use of various advanced machinery, including the CMS multipurpose machine and advanced fusion splicer machine. The currently available fiber taper sensors have high sensitivity and good reproducibility in both geometry and sensor performance, which takes a solid step toward practical applications. As a result, in the last few years, various noted biosensing studies

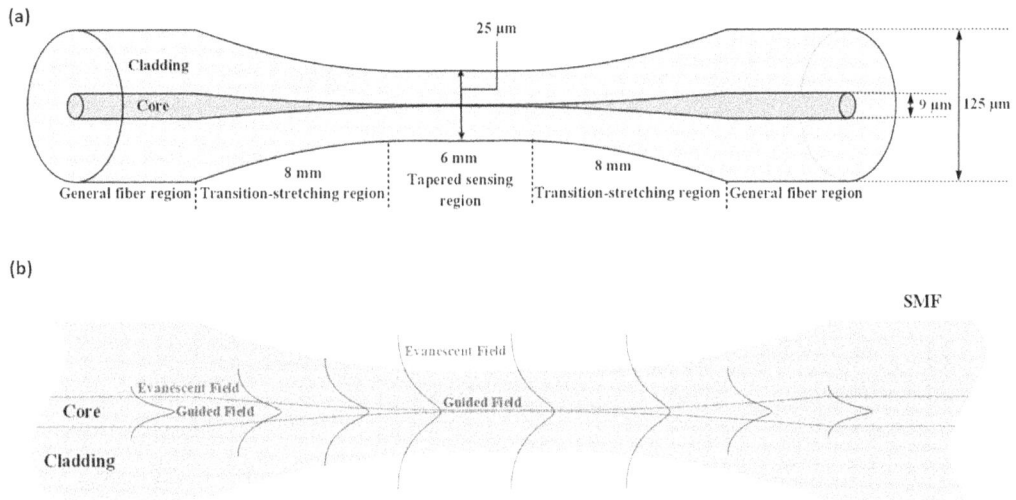

FIGURE 3.3 (a) Single tapered fiber probe and (b) wave propagation through tapered fiber structure.

Source: Reprinted with permission from Optik, Copyright 2020, Elsevier (Yang, Zhu et al. 2020).

(in vivo and in vitro detection) based on tapered fiber structure are presented for dopamine sensor (Agrawal, Zhang, Saha, Kumar, Kaushik et al. 2020), cholesterol sensor (Zhang, Qi, et al. 2019), glucose sensor (Li et al. 2018), uric acid sensor (Singh, Zhu et al. 2020), ascorbic acid sensor, and cancer cell detection (Li et al. 2014).

3.2.2 HETERO-CORE STRUCTURE

The hetero-core optic-fiber structures are obtained by the splicing of two or more dissimilar core fibers structures. Dissimilar optical fibers are connected in a hetero-core structure, resulting in mode field mismatch loss and transition loss. A transformation has to be carried out for effective mode matching. Various hetero-core fiber structures are reported for the development of fiber-optic-based plasmonic biosensors, such as SMF-MMF-SMF (SMS) hetero-core optic-fiber probe (Wang, Farrell, and Yan 2008; Singh, Singh, Zhang et al. 2020), MMF-PSF-MMF (MPM) probe, SMF-PSF-SMF (SPS) fiber probe (Agrawal, Zhang, Saha, Kumar, Pu et al. 2020), SMF-MMF-SMF-MMF-SMF (SMSMS) hetero-core fiber probe (Agrawal, Saha, Kumar, Singh, Zhang, and Kumar 2020), MMF-SMF-MMF (MSM) fiber probe (Singh, Singh, Kumar et al. 2020), and SMF-MMF-PSF-MMF-SMF (SMPMS) optic-fiber probe (Kaushik et al. 2020).

3.2.3 OTHER STRUCTURES

Similarly, for the development of plasmonic biosensors, there are few reports related to other novel fiber structures, such as tapered SMF-MMF-SMF (TSMS) fiber probe (Agrawal, Saha, Kumar, Singh, Zhang, Jha et al. 2020) and micro-ball structure (Kumar et al. 2020). The optical fiber's sensor structure, such as the U-bent, has also been reported. In one study, this type of structure was used for DNA detection (Yang, Yu et al. 2019b). Figure 3.4 shows the schematic of the fabrication process for a fiber structure composed of an SMF-MCF (1.5 cm)-MMF (2 cm)-SMF-based hetero-core sensor structure. Figure 3.5(a–c) shows the tapered-in-taper optical fiber structure and its probe fabrication process.

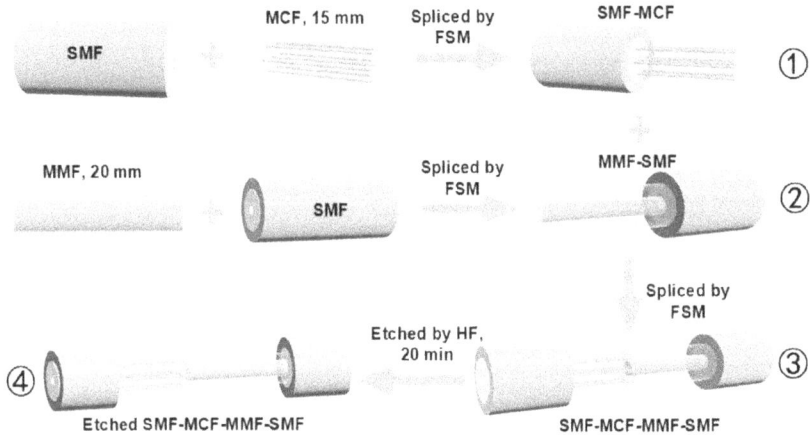

FIGURE 3.4 The fabrication process for a fiber structure composed of SMF-MCF (1.5 cm)-MMF (2 cm)-SMF-based hetero-core sensor structure.

Source: Reprinted with permission from Optics Express. Copyright, 2021, Optica (Li et al. 2021).

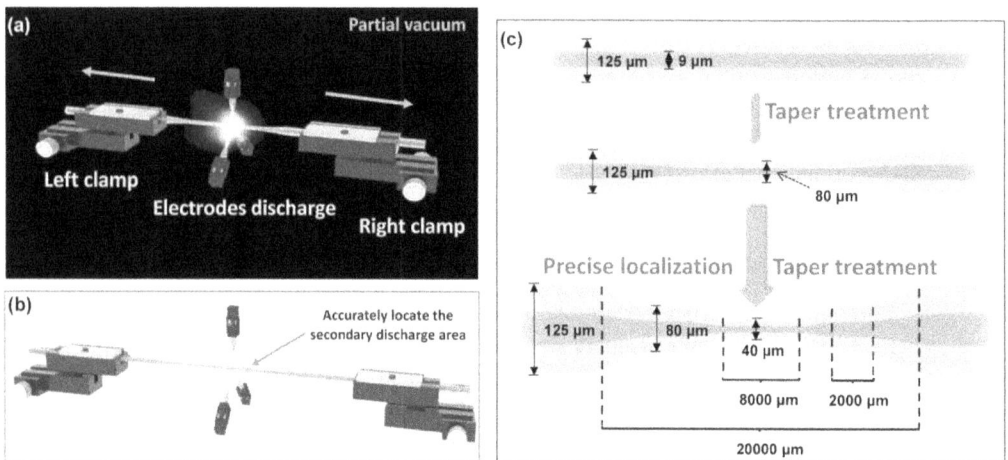

FIGURE 3.5 (A–C) Tapered-in-taper optical fiber structure and probe fabrication process.

Source: Reprinted with permission from *Optics Express.* Copyright, 2021, Optica (Wang et al. 2021).

3.3   NANOCOATING PROCESS AND CHARACTERIZATION

In this section, the nanocoating process and characterization of tapered fiber are discussed. Advances in science and nanotechnology have made it easier to come up with new ways to make nanoparticles (NPs), nanosheets, and new nanomaterials (NMs) (Jeevanandam et al. 2018). NMs such as gold NPs (AuNPs) (Lee et al. 2018), silver NPs (AgNPs) (Loiseau et al. 2019), zinc-oxide NPs (ZnO-NPs) (Tomaev et al. 2019), copper-oxide NPs (CuO-NPs) (Gupta, Pathak, and Semwal 2019), selenium NPs (Amjadi, Hallaj, and Salari 2018), graphene oxide (GO) and its derivatives (Omar et al. 2019), bimetallic NPs (BNPs) (Sytwu, Vadai, and Dionne 2019), and novel NPs (NNPs) (Erdem et al. 2018) are largely reported for the development of plasmonic sensors. These NMs are very efficient at scattering and absorbing light (El-Shafai et al. 2019). It is possible to tune the optical

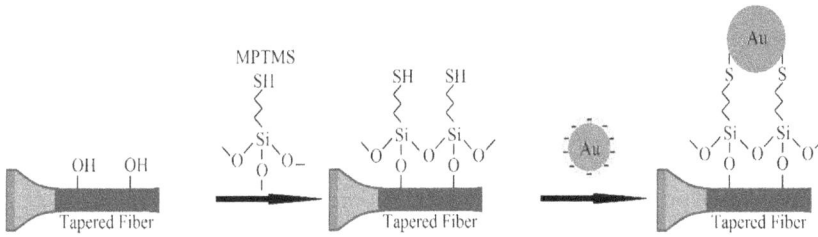

FIGURE 3.6 Gold nanoparticles nanocoating over taper fiber structure.

Source: Reprinted with permission from *Biomedical Optics Express.* Copyright, 2019, Optica (Kumar, Kaushik et al. 2019).

response from the ultraviolet to the near-infrared (NIR) by varying the shape, composition, and size of NMs (Bhatia, Verma, and Sinha 2019). The various processes are involved in the development of P-OFSs, including bare fiber structure fabrication, cleaning, salinization, nanocoating, and functionalization (Lee and Jun 2019). The brief process involved in the nanocoating of a sensor probe is revealed in Figure 3.6.

These nanostructures (NSs) are emerging to have promising uses in photochemical reactions, especially in improving the catalytic properties of metal NPs. Some metal NPs support an SPR and LSPR phenomenon that converts incident light into a strong electromagnetic field, heat conduction, or thermal conductivity and enhances chemical reactions (Sytwu, Vadai, and Dionne 2019; Jeong et al. 2019). During the development process, various advanced instruments are used for the characterization of NSs and NM-coated probes. The ultraviolet-visible (UV-Vis) spectrophotometer is employed to check the absorbance spectrum. Atomic force microscopy (AFM) and high-resolution transmission electron microscopy (HRTEM) are applied to the morphology exploration of the chemosynthetic NMs. The uniformity of NMs coatings over the immobilized sensor probe is examined using scanning electron microscopy (SEM) and energy-dispersive X-ray spectroscopy (EDX) in the following step of characterization (Devasahayam 2019).

3.4 SENSOR DEVELOPMENT AND APPLICATIONS

3.4.1 BIOMEDICAL AND DIAGNOSTIC APPLICATIONS

The development of biosensors can be traced to the biological monitoring of carcinogens, serum antigens, as well as pathogens of many metabolic diseases. The researchers then used biosensors based on serum analysis to monitor and evaluate diseases such as diabetes, cancer, allergic reactions, and many others in a broader diagnostic application. Nano-biosensors have become a research hot spot and have many clinical applications, including glucose detection in patients with diabetes, urinary tract bacterial infection detection, HIV-AIDS detection, and even cancer diagnosis. It is worth noting that all these efforts have far-reaching implications for human health and that the detection and diagnosis of these diseases were difficult, time-consuming, and expensive before biosensors were widely used. Therefore, the emergence of biosensors for the diagnosis of these diseases and related faults undoubtedly proves beneficial. With the development of nanotechnology, people can incorporate nanoscale intervention in the detection of biosensors to improve the sensing performance. At the same time, using NMs to fix the detection system, the high-priced enzyme can be recovered and reused to further improve the economy. In addition, the implementation of these nanoscale-technological innovations like micro- and nano-electromechanical systems, combining chips based on smart sensing materials at the nanoscale with microarray-based detection technologies, has made it possible to detect more than one disease. Under controlled conditions, magnetic NPs can be synthesized to improve the selectivity of biochemical reactions and to separate heavy metals with similar properties to iron from biological serum. The possibility of blood-related diseases is well proved by the presence of ferritin and hemoglobin in the serum sample. Because this process uses optimized magnetic coupling of antigens in the body, a diagnosis based on this principle can be called diagnostic magnetic resonance. In addition, more complex responses have been studied experimentally using nano-biosensors, and these responses have been incorporated into various sensing mechanisms for various clinical tests. The plasmonic phenomenon-based OFSs are broadly divided based on their detecting compounds as presented in the following sections.

3.4.1.1 Glucose Detection

Diabetes or metabolic disorder is a major public health problem. According to a report by the World Health Organization, the number of patients with diabetes is expected to reach 300 million by 2025 (Tabish 2007). High blood glucose levels can cause health problems such as diabetic retinopathy and kidney failure (Chawla, Chawla, and Jaggi 2016). As a result, rapid and accurate detection are critical for diabetes. Various biosensors based on plasmonic phenomena have been reported for glucose detection, as shown in Table 3.1. It can be concluded that various NMs, such as AuNPs, AgNPs, and so on, are used to increase the sensitivity of sensors. Glucose sensors are categorized under enzymatic sensors (Hwang et al. 2018), such as glucose oxidase (GOx) for improving the selectivity, and nonenzymatic (Huang et al. 2016) sensors. The mechanism used for glucose detection using the LSPR phenomenon is shown in Figure 3.7. The plasmonic phenomenon-based glucose sensors as summarized in Table 3.1 have a wide range of features like robustness, tiny size, low cost, antielectromagnetic interference, and real-time monitoring (Yang, Zhang et al. 2020; Gupta and Kant 2018).

3.4.1.2 Cholesterol Detection

Cholesterol is one of the prime sterols in the human body system, and its unusual concentration is acknowledged as a warning sign for diabetes, stroke, hypertension, and cardiovascular and heart diseases (Agrawal, Zhang, Saha, Kumar, Pu et al. 2020). Different plasmonic phenomenon-based biosensors are reported for cholesterol detection as indicated in Table 3.2. To allow the EWs to interact with surrounding analytes, various structural modifications are proposed based on tapered and hetero-core structures (Correia et al. 2018), which predominantly include SMF-HCF, MPM (MMF-PSF-MMF), and SPS (SMF-PSF-SMF) structures. The study presented in Table 3.2

TABLE 3.1

Summary of Different SPR/LSPR Phenomenon-Based Glucose Biosensors

Material used	Mechanism	Structure used	Linearity range	Limit of detection	Sensitivity	Ref.
AuNPs	LSPR	Tapered SMF	0–10 mM	322 μM	0.9261 nm/mM	Yang, Zhang et al. 2020
GO/AuNPs/GOx	LSPR	Tapered SMF	0–11 mM	2.26 mM	1.06 nm/mM	Yang, Zhu et al. 2020
Silver (Ag) film	SPR	Tilted fiber Bragg grating (TFBG) SMF	3–8 mM	N.R.	0.5 dB/mM	Zhang et al. 2018
AuNPs	SPR	Optical fiber (core diameter = 400 μm)	0.01–30 mM	80 nM	N.R.	Yuan et al. 2018
AuNPs/GOx	SPR	U-shaped fiber	N.R.	N.R.	2.899 nm dB/%	Chen et al. 2018
AuNPs	SPR	TFBG (SMF)	1 μM–500 μM	N.R.	2.61 dB/μM	Wang et al. 2018
AuNPs	SPR	Tapered SMF	N.R.	N.R.	~2180 nm/RIU	Li et al. 2018

Note: AuNP, gold nanoparticle; GO, graphene oxide; GOx, glucose oxidase; LSPR, localized surface plasmon resonance; N.R., not reported; RIU, refractive index unit; SMF, single-mode fiber; SPR, surface plasmon resonance.

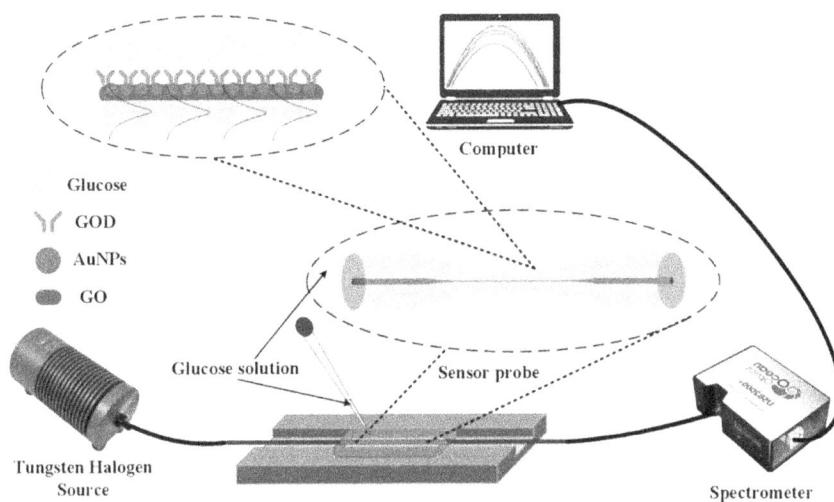

FIGURE 3.7 Experimental setup for the detection of glucose.

Source: Reprinted with permission from Optik, Copyright 2020, Elsevier (Yang, Zhu et al. 2020).

TABLE 3.2
Summary of Different SPR/LSPR Phenomenon-Based Cholesterol Biosensors

Material used	Mechanism	Structure used	Linear ranges	Detection limit	Sensitivity	Ref.
AuNPs	LSPR	Simple SMF	10 nM–1 µM	53.1 nM	0.125%/mM	Kumar, Kaushik et al. 2019
AgNPs/GO	LSPR	Plastic clad silica SMF	0.0–10 mM	1.131 mM	5.14 nm/mM	Semwal and Gupta 2018
AuNPs	LSPR	SMF-HCF	50 nM–1 µM	25.5 nM	16.149 nm/µM	Kumar, Singh, Kaushik et al. 2019
AuNPs and ZnO-NPs	LSPR	AuNPs (10 nm)/ ZnO-NPs/ MPM fiber structure	0.1–10 mM	0.6161 mM	0.6898 nm/mM	Agrawal, Zhang, Saha, Kumar, Pu et al. 2020
		AuNPs (30 nm)/ZnO-NPs/ MPM fiber structure	0.1–10 mM	1.2777 mM	0.3319 nm/mM	
		AuNPs (10 nm)/ ZnO-NPs/ SPS fiber structure	1–10 mM	2.1748 mM	0.1976 nm/mM	
Cyclodextrin capped AuNPs	LSPR	Tapered structure	IE-18– IE-6	N.R.	N.R.	Zhang, Qi et al. 2019

Note: AgNP, silver nanoparticle; AuNP, gold nanoparticle; GO, graphene oxide; HCF, hollow-core fiber; LSPR, localized surface plasmon resonance; MMF, multimode fiber; MPM, MMF-PSF-MMF; N.R., not reported; PSF, photosensitive fiber; SMF, single-mode fiber; SPR, surface plasmon resonance; SPS, SMF-PSF-SMF; ZnO-NP, zinc oxide nanoparticle.

also illustrates the therapeutic potential of smaller AuNPs in improving sensor sensitivity (Xie et al. 2018). The mechanism used for the detection of cholesterol using LSPR-OFSs is shown in Figure 3.8. The study based on SPR/LSPR sensors reveals the highest biocompatibility with extremely promising results.

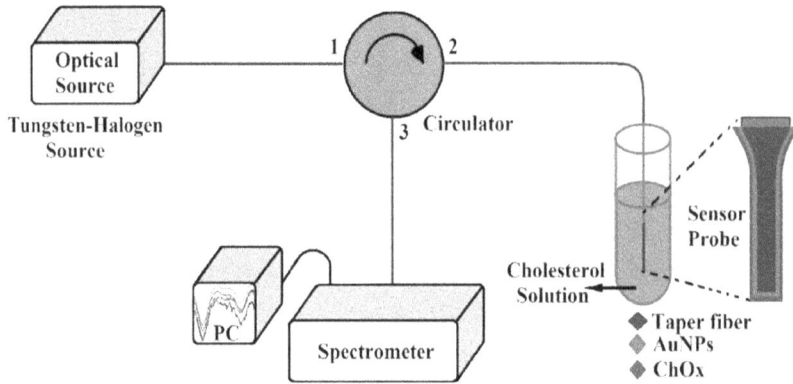

FIGURE 3.8   An experimental setup for cholesterol detections.

Source: Reprinted with permission from *Biomedical Optics Express.* Copyright, 2019, Optica (Kumar, Singh, Kaushik et al. 2019).

3.4.1.3   Bacteria Detection

Several modern techniques for bacterial diagnosis and detection have been developed, including electrochemical sensors, chemiluminescence, fiber-optic biosensors, impedimetric immune sensors, microfluidic devices, and conductometric methods (Farré and Barceló 2020). These methods require specialists and characterization of pathogenic microorganisms at high concentrations (Alahi and Mukhopadhyay 2017). They also take a long time to diagnose, are quite expensive, and include complicated systems that do not always produce good sense, making them inconsistent for the centers that lack infrastructure and basic care (Rajapaksha et al. 2019).

Recently, many scientists have turned their attention toward plasmonic NPs based on SPR/LSPR biosensors to detect or clinically diagnose bacteria because of its higher sensitivity, less complexity, reliability, reproducibility, reusability, rapid testing, less cost, and selective recognition of bacteria (Liu et al. 2020; Mauriz, Dey, and Lechuga 2019). Figure 3.9 depicts an experimental apparatus for detecting *Escherichia coli* bacteria using SPR immune sensors. This sensing platform (plasmonic sensor) is promising and shows a broad range of applications in diverse clinical, bacterial, and microbial diagnoses and monitoring, as well as quality monitoring of food and water for different pathogenic microorganisms (Leonard et al. 2003; Yoo and Lee 2015). Different plasmonic phenomenon-based biosensors are reported for bacteria detection as indicated in Table 3.3.

3.4.1.4   Virus Detection

The health risks of people due to several viral diseases have increased over the past few years with these diseases causing many health problems worldwide, and they may lead to various chronic diseases (Lindahl and Grace 2015; Saylan et al. 2019). This necessitates the accurate and rapid detection of viruses in real-world samples. To check these real-world samples, various methods are used, and a large number of biosensors have been reported for this purpose. Plasmonic sensors for virus detection have piqued the interest of researchers in recent years. Various SPR/LSPR phenomenon-based P-OFSs have been reported for rapid detection of viruses such as dengue and avian influenza, as shown in Table 3.4. A schematic of the experimental setup for avian-influenza-virus-subtype-H6 detection using fiber-optic SPR sensors is presented in Figure 3.10.

3.4.1.5   Cell Detection

Detection of cells and their structures is vital for understanding the progression of chronic diseases such as cancer (Gonzalez, Hagerling, and Werb 2018). Early cell detection is crucial for major

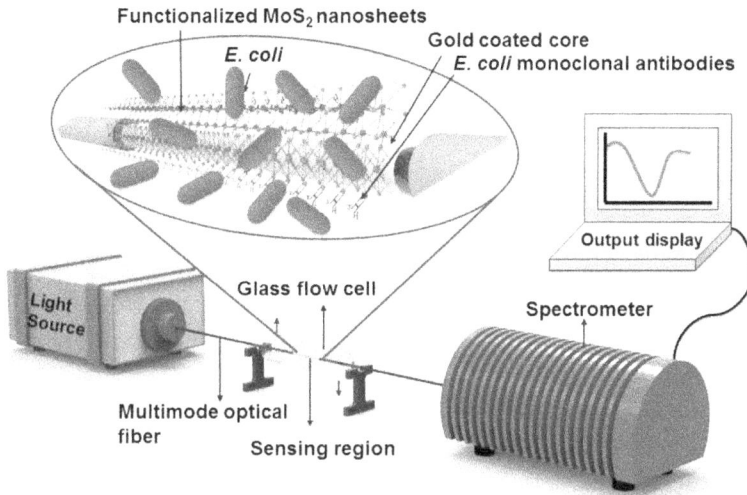

FIGURE 3.9 Experimental setup for *Escherichia coli* detection.

Source: Reprinted with permission from Biosensors and Bioelectronics, Copyright 2020, Elsevier (Kaushik et al. 2019).

TABLE 3.3
Summary of Different SPR/LSPR Biosensors for the Diverse Types of Bacteria Detections

Material used	Mechanism	Detection	Structure used	Linear range	Detection limit	Sensitivity	Ref.
MoS$_2$	SPR	*Escherichia coli*	Step index MMF	1000–8000 CFU/mL	94 CFU/mL	2.9nm/1000 CFU mL^{-1}	Kaushik et al. 2019
AuNPs	LSPR	Anti-biotin	Plastic-clad silica MMF	52.4 nM and 349 nM	29.5 nM	N.R.	Wu et al. 2016
AgNPs and GO	SPR	*E. coli*	Simple SMF	1.0×10^3 to 5.0×10^7 CFU/mL	5.0×10^2 CFU/mL	5489 nm/RIU	Zhou et al. 2018

Note: AgNP, silver nanoparticle; AuNP, gold nanoparticle; CFU, colony-forming unit; GO, graphene oxide; LSPR, localized surface plasmon resonance; MMF, multimode fiber; N.R., not reported; RIU, refractive index unit; SMF, single-mode fiber; SPR, surface plasmon resonance.

TABLE 3.4
Summary of Different SPR/LSPR Biosensors for the Detection of Diverse Types of Viruses

Material used	Mechanism	Detection	Structure used	Linear range	Detection limit	Sensitivity	Ref.
Gold film	SPR	Avian influenza virus subtype H6	Standard MMF	N.R.	5.14×105 EID$_{50}$/0.1 mL	N.R.	Zhao et al. 2016
AuNPs	LSPR	Dengue	Standard MMF	N.R.	1.54 nM	43 nm/ (ng/mm^2)	Camara et al. 2013
Gold film	SPR	Dengue	Standard fiber	0.0001–0.01 nM	N.R.	39.96° nM^{-1}	Omar et al. 2018

Note: AuNP, gold nanoparticle; LSPR, localized surface plasmon resonance; MMF, multimode fiber; N.R., not reported; SPR, surface plasmon resonance.

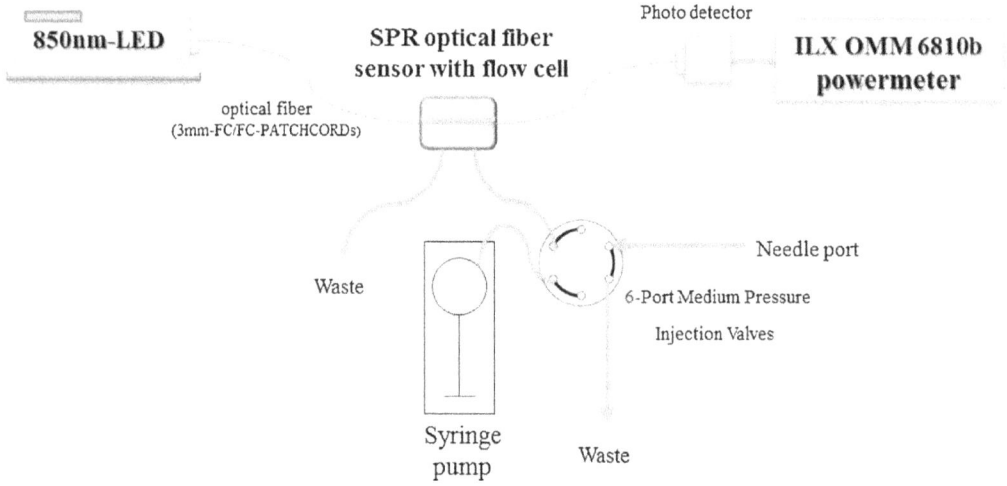

FIGURE 3.10 Experimental setup avian influenza virus subtype H6 detection.

Source: Reprinted with permission from Journal of Virological Methods, Copyright 2020, Elsevier (Zhao et al. 2016).

TABLE 3.5

Summary of Different SPR/LSPR Biosensors for the Detection of Cells

Material used	Mechanism	Detection	Structure used	Linear range	Detection limit	Sensitivity	Ref.
AuNPs	LSPR	N-glycan and cancer cells	U-shaped fiber	1×10^2–1×10^6 cells/mL	30 cells/mL	N.R.	Luo et al. 2019
			Straight fiber	5×10^3–1×10^6 cells/mL	879 cells/mL	N.R.	
AuNPs	LSPR	Thyroglobulin (T_g) detection	Silica core, glass-clad MMF	1 pg/mL – 10 ng/mL)	0.19 pg/mL	13.07 RIU^{-1}	Kim et al. 2019
Gold	SPR	Cytokeratin	Tilted fiber Bragg gratings	N.R.	1 pM	N.R.	Ribaut et al. 2017
CuO and AuNPs	LSPR	Cancer cells	Multicore fiber structure	1×10^2–1×10^6 cells/mL	3, 2, 2, 2, 4,10 cells/mL	N.R.	Singh, Kumar; et al. 2020

Note: AuNP, gold nanoparticle; CuO, copper oxide; LSPR, localized surface plasmon resonance; MMF, multimode fiber; N.R., not reported; RIU, refractive index unit; SPR, surface plasmon resonance.

chronic diseases, such as the thyroglobulin test, which is indicated as a tumor marker test and is used in thyroid cancer treatment (Kim et al. 2019). As shown in Table 3.5, various optical fiber structures such as simple fiber structure, U-shaped structure, tilted fiber Bragg grating (FBG), and so on were reported for the detections of various types of cells. Among these structures, the U-shaped structure-based LSPR sensor has overcome the limitation of lower sensitivity cell detection (Luo et al. 2019). The setup used for the detection of N-glycan and cancer cells using U-shaped optic-fiber structure LSPR sensors is shown in Figure 3.11.

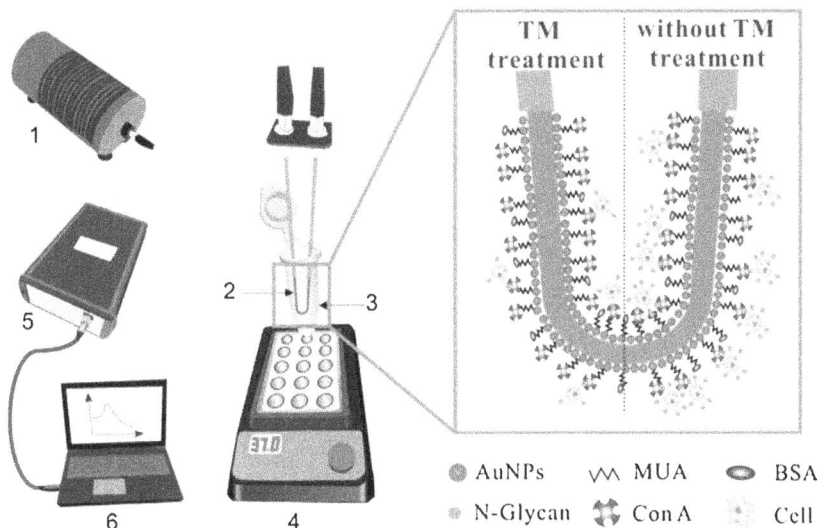

FIGURE 3.11 Experimental setup for the detection of cancer cells.

Source: Reprinted with permission from Biosensors and Bioelectronics, Copyright 2020, Elsevier (Luo et al. 2019).

3.4.1.6 DNA Biomolecules Detection

A label-free microfluidic biosensor platform based on SPR/LSPR phenomenon DNA biomolecules detection and real-time polymerase reaction is discussed here. DNA polymerization is an important reaction in the replication of DNA in all types of cells and organisms. To detect the specificity of DNA targets based on RI changes of NM immobilized probes, a prominent notice must be given. Nonspecific DNA binding to the NMs is avoided by functionalization with 6-mercaptohexanol (MCH) (Roether et al. 2019). The experimental setup for DNA biomolecule detection using U-bent-annealing fiber structure LSPR sensors is shown in Figure 3.12. Several SPR/LSPR phenomenon-based OFSs are used for quick detection of DNA hybridization and biomolecules, and these are shown in Table 3.6. The methodologies presented herein for detecting DNA biomolecules and other targets aid in the development of next-generation DNA biosensors and also indicate the possibility of integrating with microfluidic and point-of-care biosensing devices (Soares et al. 2014; Fu, Lu, and Lai 2019). Various companies, such as Biacore Life Science, MediSense, and Texas Instruments, deal with commercial biosensors at the outset; other SPR/LSPR-based sensor technology is yet to be applied extensively for biosensing applications (Shukla and Suneetha 2017).

3.4.2 Environmental Applications

Because there is so much uncertainty in the experimental environment at all times, this is a broad and complex area of application. Therefore, a detailed and comprehensive assessment of the target levels (such as heavy metals, temperature, and air humidity) in various environments is required for detecting environmental disturbances. In recent years, the use of nanomaterial sensors in detection and monitoring has drawn increasing attention due to their strong flexibility and accuracy. Nanomaterial-based sensing tools like cantilever electronic probes can be used to accurately monitor the presence of specific classes of substances in the environment. According to one study, fluorescent probes or kits based on Chinese hamster ovary cells can be used to measure various toxicants substances in extraordinary complex and diverse water body samples. The basic idea behind this function is that highly complex exogenous compounds, such as environmental endocrine disruptors,

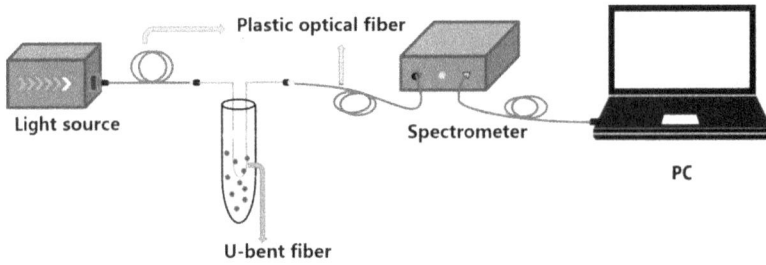

FIGURE 3.12 Experimental setup for the detection of DNA biomolecule using U-bent-annealing fiber structure LSPR sensors (Yang, Yu et al. 2019a).

TABLE 3.6

Summary of Different SPR/LSPR Biosensors for the Detection of DNA and RNA

Material used	Mechanism	Detection	Structure used	Linear range	Detection limit	Sensitivity	Ref.
GoldNanodisk	LSPR	DNA hybridization	Simple SMF	N.R.	10 fM	227 nm/RIU	Kaye et al. 2017
Graphene/ ITO Nanorod	LSPR	DNA biomolecule	U-bent-annealing fiber	0.1 to 100 nM	0.1 nM	690.7 nm/RIU	Yang, Yu et al. 2019a

Note: LSPR, localized surface plasmon resonance; N.R., not reported; RIU, refractive index unit; SMF, single-mode fiber.

can cause the dysfunction of an intact hormonal system and thus separate carcinogens and other harmful intermediates from sample. Similarly, Purohit et al. used biosensors to interact with abiotic environments to optimize biological-recovery applications and bioremediation. In this case, bioremediation technology is primarily used to purify harmful pollutants and improve environmental quality. Also, when engineers design experiments with specific nanomaterials, it will be thought that more practical and positive value can be found. Nanomaterials can be used to make a single sensor that can detect many different types of contaminants simultaneously. Many biosensors have been developed for the quantitative detection of inorganic phosphate, nitrate and biological oxygen demand, and other parameters, at the same time. They have been proved to have the function of environmental remediation. This is all facilitated by nanomaterials and substrate-specific detection mechanisms. An assumption was made that we can try to integrate many kinds of nanomaterials, and through this inspiration, nano-biosensors can adapt and detect its rich and complex environment, while also has advantages like energy, economic, and time savings.

3.4.3 MISCELLANEOUS APPLICATIONS

Nano-biosensors can still be instrumental in other detection methods. The main role of the nano-biosensor is to control the entry of a mixture of matrix and nutrient media into the bioreactor in a practical industrial operation. On the industrial scale, these sensors can enhance loads of commercial preparations and separations. As an example, the separation of impurities from ores is a key step in the metallurgical process. The complex combination of impurities in ores can be selectively separated through different configurations of nano-biosensors.

3.5 SUMMARY AND CONCLUSION

To recognize bio-elements, various techniques have been adopted, such as colorimetric, fluorescence, optical methods, and surface-enhanced Raman scattering (Aloisi et al. 2019). Different optical plasmonic-based techniques such as SPR and LSPR are also largely employed in biosensing applications. These are very useful for their large contribution to label-free detection, which has attracted many researchers in recent years (Rubab et al. 2018). Various configurations such as simple fiber structure, tapered structure, bend structure, FBG, tilted FBG, micro-ball fiber structure, etc., are broadly investigated. It has been found that optical fiber-based biosensors are mainly developed by changing (i) core diameter, (ii) alignment, (iii) shape, and (iv) type of fibers (Socorro-Leránoz et al. 2019). It has also been found that the parameters that mainly indicate the performance of plasmonic-OFSs (sensitivity, selectivity, detection limit, linearity, and accuracy) are greatly improved due to the structural modifications such as tapered structure and hetero-core structure (Caucheteur, Guo, and Albert 2015; Arghir et al. 2016). In the case of glucose sensors, the lowest limit of detection (80 nM) and a higher range of linearity (0.01–30 mM) were detected with AuNPs-immobilized SPR sensors (Yuan et al. 2018). As shown in Table 3.1, the sensing performance of an optic-fiber sensor structure with a larger core diameter (400 m) improves significantly. During cholesterol detection, enhancement in the performance parameters such as limit of detection (25.5 nM), sensitivity (16.15 nm/μM), and linear range (50 nM—1 μM) was observed with LSPR phenomenon-based AuNPs-immobilized-SMF-HCF sensing probe (shown in Table 3.2) (Kumar, Singh, Kaushik et al. 2019). Furthermore, for the diagnosis and detection of bacteria, various SPR/LSPR phenomenon-based biosensors have been reported in the past, as mentioned in Table 3.3. As indicated in Table 3.3, the SPR-AuNPs-GO-SMF *E. coli* sensor probe reveals the great sensing parameters such as limit of detection (5×10^2 CFU/mL), sensitivity, and linear range. Similarly, highly sensitive viruses, cells, and RNA/DNA plasmonic biosensors have been reported in the past as indicated in Tables 3.4, 3.5, and 3.6, respectively.

Many front-runner companies are working on developing highly efficient biosensors and plasmonic-based biosensors (Shukla and Suneetha 2017). The recent development and innovations in SPR/LSPR-based OFSs show their acceptance in label-free detection. There are still many opportunities for the development and successful construction of biosensor platforms that address the health hazards in environmental issues requiring increased understanding, information, commonality, and commercialization (Bhalla et al. 2016).

The plasmonic sensing area has been widely explored in recent years and is considered to be among the top emerging technologies. As mentioned earlier, SPR/LSPR phenomenon-based OFSs offer many potential applications in key areas, including prospective health monitoring and diagnostics, medicine, biotechnology, drug treatment, and nutrition monitoring. This in-depth review describes the potential applications and challenges for the enhancement of the sensitivity of plasmonic-OFSs. OFSs related to plasmonic NSs have been used to monitor analytes in environmental survey, health diagnostics, environmental food safety, and security.

More than 500 companies around the globe are working on research and development of biosensors, especially for point-of-care and other medical diagnosis applications. Plasmonic-based sensing has tremendously stimulated growth in the development of rapid and accurate biosensors (Shukla and Suneetha 2017). P-OFSs have the potential to provide the platform for multiplexed analysis and specificity toward detection, which is crucial for medical diagnostics.

REFERENCES

Agrawal, N., C. Saha, C. Kumar, R. Singh, B. Zhang, R. Jha, and S. Kumar. 2020. "Detection of L-cysteine using silver nanoparticles and graphene oxide immobilized tapered SMS optical fiber structure." *IEEE Sensors Journal*:1–1. DOI: 10.1109/JSEN.2020.2997690.

Agrawal, N., C. Saha, C. Kumar, R. Singh, B. Zhang, and S. Kumar. 2020. "Development of uric acid sensor using copper oxide and silver nanoparticles immobilized SMSMS fiber structure-based probe." *IEEE Transactions on Instrumentation and Measurement* 69 (11):9097–9104.

Agrawal, N., B. Zhang, C. Saha, C. Kumar, B. K. Kaushik, and S. Kumar. 2020. "Development of dopamine sensor using silver nanoparticles and PEG-functionalized tapered optical fiber structure." *IEEE Transactions on Biomedical Engineering* 67 (6):1542–1547. DOI: 10.1109/TBME.2019.2939560.

Agrawal, N., B. Zhang, C. Saha, C. Kumar, X. Pu, and S. Kumar. 2020. "Ultra-sensitive cholesterol sensor using gold and zinc-oxide nanoparticles immobilized core mismatch MPM/SPS probe." *Journal of Lightwave Technology* 38 (8):2523–2529.

Akolpoglu, M. Birgul, Ugur Bozuyuk, Pelin Erkoc, and Seda Kizilel. 2019. "Chapter 9: Biosensing-drug delivery systems for in vivo applications." In *Advanced Biosensors for Health Care Applications*, edited by Inamuddin, Raju Khan, Ali Mohammad and Abdullah M. Asiri, 249–262. Amsterdam: Elsevier.

Alahi, Md Eshrat E., and Subhas Chandra Mukhopadhyay. 2017. "Detection methodologies for pathogen and toxins: A review." *Sensors (Basel, Switzerland)* 17 (8):1885. DOI: 10.3390/s17081885.

Allsop, Thomas, and Ron Neal. 2019. "A review: Evolution and diversity of optical fibre plasmonic sensors." *Sensors (Basel, Switzerland)* 19 (22):4874. DOI: 10.3390/s19224874.

Aloisi, Alessandra, Antonio Della Torre, Angelantonio De Benedetto, and Rosaria Rinaldi. 2019. "Biorecognition in spectroscopy-based biosensors for heavy metals-water and waterborne contamination analysis." *Biosensors* 9 (3):96. DOI: 10.3390/bios9030096.

Amjadi, Mohammad, Tooba Hallaj, and Rana Salari. 2018. "A highly sensitive plasmonic sensor for detection of selenium based on the shape transformation of silver nanoprisms." *Sensors and Actuators B: Chemical* 273:1307–1312. https://doi.org/10.1016/j.snb.2018.07.027.

Andryukov, Boris G., Natalya N. Besednova, Roman V. Romashko, Tatyana S. Zaporozhets, and Timofey A. Efimov. 2020. "Label-free biosensors for laboratory-based diagnostics of infections: Current achievements and new trends." *Biosensors* 10 (2). DOI: 10.3390/bios10020011.

Arghir, Iulia, Koen Schouteden, Peter Goos, Filip Delport, Dragana Spasic, and Jeroen Lammertyn. 2016. "Thermal annealing of gold coated fiber optic surfaces for improved plasmonic biosensing." *Sensors and Actuators B Chemical* 229:678–685. DOI: 10.1016/j.snb.2016.02.034.

Bhalla, Nikhil, Pawan Jolly, Nello Formisano, and Pedro Estrela. 2016. "Introduction to biosensors." *Essays in Biochemistry* 60 (1):1–8. DOI: 10.1042/EBC20150001.

Bhatia, Pradeep, S. S. Verma, and M. M. Sinha. 2019. "Optical properties simulation of magneto-plasmonic alloys nanostructures." *Plasmonics* 14 (3):611–622. DOI: 10.1007/s11468-018-0839-7.

Bilodeau, F., K. O. Hill, S. Faucher, and D. C. Johnson. 1988. "Low-loss highly overcoupled fused couplers: Fabrication and sensitivity to external pressure." *Journal of Lightwave Technology* 6 (10):1476–1482. DOI: 10.1109/50.7904.

Camara, Alexandre R., Paula M. P. Gouvêa, Ana Carolina M. S. Dias, Arthur M. B. Braga, Rosa F. Dutra, Renato E. de Araujo, and Isabel C. S. Carvalho. 2013. "Dengue immunoassay with an LSPR fiber optic sensor." *Optics Express* 21 (22):27023–27031. DOI: 10.1364/OE.21.027023.

Caucheteur, Christophe, Tuan Guo, and Jacques Albert. 2015. "Review of plasmonic fiber optic biochemical sensors: Improving the limit of detection." *Analytical and Bioanalytical Chemistry* 407 (14):3883–3897. DOI: 10.1007/s00216-014-8411-6.

Chawla, Aastha, Rajeev Chawla, and Shalini Jaggi. 2016. "Microvasular and macrovascular complications in diabetes mellitus: Distinct or continuum?" *Indian Journal of Endocrinology and Metabolism* 20 (4):546–551. DOI: 10.4103/2230-8210.183480.

Chen, Kuan-Chieh, Yu-Le Li, Chao-Wei Wu, and Chia-Chin Chiang. 2018. "Glucose sensor using U-shaped optical fiber probe with gold nanoparticles and glucose oxidase." *Sensors (Basel, Switzerland)* 18 (4):1217. DOI: 10.3390/s18041217.

Correia, R., S. James, S. W. Lee, S. P. Morgan, and S. Korposh. 2018. "Biomedical application of optical fibre sensors." *Journal of Optics* 20 (7):073003. DOI: 10.1088/2040-8986/aac68d.

Devasahayam, Sheila. 2019. "Chapter 17: Nanotechnology and nanomedicine in market: A global perspective on regulatory issues." In *Characterization and Biology of Nanomaterials for Drug Delivery*, edited by Shyam S. Mohapatra, Shivendu Ranjan, Nandita Dasgupta, Raghvendra Kumar Mishra and Sabu Thomas, 477–522. Amsterdam: Elsevier.

Ding, Jiawang, and Wei Qin. 2020. "Recent advances in potentiometric biosensors." *TrAC Trends in Analytical Chemistry* 124:115803. https://doi.org/10.1016/j.trac.2019.115803.

El-Shafai, Nagi, Mohamed E. El-Khouly, Maged El-Kemary, Mohamed Ramadan, Ibrahim Eldesoukey, and Mamdouh Masoud. 2019. "Graphene oxide decorated with zinc oxide nanoflower, silver and titanium dioxide nanoparticles: Fabrication, characterization, DNA interaction, and antibacterial activity." *RSC Advances* 9 (7):3704–3714. DOI: 10.1039/C8RA09788G.

Erdem, Özgecan, Yeseren Saylan, Nilüfer Cihangir, and Adil Denizli. 2018. "Molecularly imprinted nanoparticles based plasmonic sensors for real-time enterococcus faecalis detection." *Biosensors and Bioelectronics* 126. DOI: 10.1016/j.bios.2018.11.030.

Farré, Marinella, and Damià Barceló. 2020. "6-Microfluidic devices: Biosensors." In *Chemical Analysis of Food*. 2nd ed., edited by Yolanda Pico, 287–351. Cambridge, MA: Academic Press.

Fu, Zirui, Yi-Cheng Lu, and James J. Lai. 2019. "Recent advances in biosensors for nucleic acid and exosome detection." *Chonnam Medical Journal* 55 (2):86–98. DOI: 10.4068/cmj.2019.55.2.86.

Gonzalez, Hugo, Catharina Hagerling, and Zena Werb. 2018. "Roles of the immune system in cancer: From tumor initiation to metastatic progression." *Genes & Development* 32 (19–20):1267–1284. DOI: 10.1101/gad.314617.118.

Gupta, Banshi D., and Ravi Kant. 2018. "Recent advances in surface plasmon resonance based fiber optic chemical and biosensors utilizing bulk and nanostructures." *Optics & Laser Technology* 101:144–161. DOI: 10.1016/j.optlastec.2017.11.015.

Gupta, Banshi D., Anisha Pathak, and Vivek Semwal. 2019. "Carbon-based nanomaterials for plasmonic sensors: A review." *Sensors (Basel, Switzerland)* 19 (16):3536. DOI: 10.3390/s19163536.

Habel, Wolfgang R. 2019. "Optical fiber methods in nondestructive evaluation." In *Handbook of Advanced Nondestructive Evaluation*, edited by Nathan Ida and Norbert Meyendorf, 595–642. Cham: Springer International Publishing.

Huang, Jun, Mengshi Li, Peipei Zhang, Pengfei Zhang, and Liyun Ding. 2016. "Temperature controlling fiber optic glucose sensor based on hydrogel-immobilized GOD complex." *Sensors and Actuators B: Chemical* 237:24–29. https://doi.org/10.1016/j.snb.2016.06.062.

Huertas, Cesar S., Olalla Calvo-Lozano, Arnan Mitchell, and Laura M. Lechuga. 2019. "Advanced evanescent-wave optical biosensors for the detection of nucleic acids: An analytic perspective." *Frontiers in Chemistry* 7 (724). DOI: 10.3389/fchem.2019.00724.

Hwang, Dae-Woong, Saram Lee, Minjee Seo, and Taek Dong Chung. 2018. "Recent advances in electrochemical non-enzymatic glucose sensors: A review." *Analytica Chimica Acta* 1033:1–34. https://doi.org/10.1016/j.aca.2018.05.051.

Jeevanandam, Jaison, Ahmed Barhoum, Yen S. Chan, Alain Dufresne, and Michael K. Danquah. 2018. "Review on nanoparticles and nanostructured materials: History, sources, toxicity and regulations." *Beilstein Journal of Nanotechnology* 9:1050–1074. DOI: 10.3762/bjnano.9.98.

Jeong, Hyeon-Ho, Eunjin Choi, Elizabeth Ellis, and Tung-Chun Lee. 2019. "Recent advances in gold nanoparticles for biomedical applications: From hybrid structures to multi-functionality." *Journal of Materials Chemistry B* 7 (22):3480–3496. DOI: 10.1039/C9TB00557A.

Kaushik, B. K., L. Singh, R. Singh, G. Zhu, B. Zhang, Q. Wang, and S. Kumar. 2020. "Detection of collagen-IV using highly reflective metal nanoparticles: Immobilized photosensitive optical fiber-based MZI structure." *IEEE Transactions on NanoBioscience* 19 (3):477–484. DOI: 10.1109/TNB.2020.2998520.

Kaushik, Siddharth, Umesh K. Tiwari, Sudipta S. Pal, and Ravindra K. Sinha. 2019. "Rapid detection of *Escherichia coli* using fiber optic surface plasmon resonance immunosensor based on biofunctionalized molybdenum disulfide (MoS_2) nanosheets." *Biosensors and Bioelectronics* 126:501–509. https://doi.org/10.1016/j.bios.2018.11.006.

Kaye, Savannah, Zheng Zeng, Mollye Sanders, Krishnan Chittur, Paula M. Koelle, Robert Lindquist, Upender Manne, Yongbin Lin, and Jianjun Wei. 2017. "Label-free detection of DNA hybridization with a compact LSPR-based fiber-optic sensor." *The Analyst* 142 (11):1974–1981. DOI: 10.1039/c7an00249a.

Kim, Hyeong-Min, Dae Hong Jeong, Ho-Young Lee, Jae-Hyoung Park, and Seung-Ki Lee. 2019. "Improved stability of gold nanoparticles on the optical fiber and their application to refractive index sensor based on localized surface plasmon resonance." *Optics & Laser Technology* 114:171–178. https://doi.org/10.1016/j.optlastec.2019.02.002.

Korposh, Sergiy, Stephen W. James, Seung-Woo Lee, and Ralph P. Tatam. 2019. "Tapered optical fibre sensors: Current trends and future perspectives." *Sensors (Basel, Switzerland)* 19 (10):2294. DOI: 10.3390/s19102294.

Kumar, S., R. Singh, B. K. Kaushik, N. Chen, Q. S. Yang, and X. Zhang. 2019. "LSPR-based cholesterol biosensor using hollow core fiber structure." *IEEE Sensors Journal* 19 (17):7399–7406.

Kumar, S., R. Singh, G. Zhu, Q. Yang, X. Zhang, S. Cheng, B. Zhang, B. K. Kaushik, and F. Liu. 2019. "Development of uric acid biosensor biosensor using gold nanoparticles and graphene oxide functionalized micro-ball fiber sensor probe." *IEEE Transactions on NanoBioscience*:1–1. DOI: 10.1109/TNB.2019.2958891.

Kumar, S., R. Singh, G. Zhu, Q. Yang, X. Zhang, S. Cheng, B. Zhang, B. K. Kaushik, and F. Liu. 2020. "Development of uric acid biosensor using gold nanoparticles and graphene oxide functionalized microball fiber sensor probe." *IEEE Transactions on NanoBioscience* 19 (2):173–182.

Kumar, Santosh, Brajesh Kumar Kaushik, Ragini Singh, Nan-Kuang Chen, Qing Shan Yang, Xia Zhang, Wenjun Wang, and Bingyuan Zhang. 2019. "LSPR-based cholesterol biosensor using a tapered optical fiber structure." *Biomedical Optics Express* 10 (5):2150–2160. DOI: 10.1364/BOE.10.002150.

Lee, Jin-Ho, Hyeon-Yeol Cho, Hye Kyu Choi, Ji-Young Lee, and Jeong-Woo Choi. 2018. "Application of gold nanoparticle to plasmonic biosensors." *International Journal of Molecular Sciences* 19 (7):2021. DOI: 10.3390/ijms19072021.

Lee, Sang Hun, and Bong-Hyun Jun. 2019. "Silver nanoparticles: Synthesis and application for nanomedicine." *International Journal of Molecular Sciences* 20 (4):865. DOI: 10.3390/ijms20040865.

Leonard, Paul, Stephen Hearty, Joanne Brennan, Lynsey Dunne, John Quinn, Trinad Chakraborty, and Richard O'Kennedy. 2003. "Advances in biosensors for detection of pathogens in food and water." *Enzyme and Microbial Technology* 32:3–13. DOI: 10.1016/S0141-0229(02)00232-6.

Li, Kaiwei, Guigen Liu, Yihui Wu, Peng Hao, Wenchao Zhou, and Zhiqiang Zhang. 2014. "Gold nanoparticle amplified optical microfiber evanescent wave absorption biosensor for cancer biomarker detection in serum." *Talanta* 120:419–424. https://doi.org/10.1016/j.talanta.2013.11.085.

Li, Muyang, Ragini Singh, Carlos Marques, Bingyuan Zhang, and Santosh Kumar. 2021. "2D material assisted SMF-MCF-MMF-SMF based LSPR sensor for creatinine detection." *Optics Express* 29 (23):38150–38167. DOI: 10.1364/OE.445555.

Li, Yanpeng, Hui Ma, Lin Gan, Qi Liu, Zhijun Yan, Deming Liu, and Qizhen Sun. 2018. "Immobilized optical fiber microprobe for selective and high sensitive glucose detection." *Sensors and Actuators B: Chemical* 255:3004–3010. https://doi.org/10.1016/j.snb.2017.09.123.

Lindahl, Johanna F., and Delia Grace. 2015. "The consequences of human actions on risks for infectious diseases: A review." *Infection Ecology & Epidemiology* 5:30048–30048. DOI: 10.3402/iee.v5.30048.

Liu, Juanjuan, Mahsa Jalali, Sara Mahshid, and Sebastian Wachsmann-Hogiu. 2020. "Are plasmonic optical biosensors ready for use in point-of-need applications?" *Analyst* 145 (2):364–384. DOI: 10.1039/C9AN02149C.

Loiseau, Alexis, Victoire Asila, Gabriel Boitel-Aullen, Mylan Lam, Michèle Salmain, and Souhir Boujday. 2019. "Silver-based plasmonic nanoparticles for and their use in biosensing." *Biosensors* 9 (2):78. DOI: 10.3390/bios9020078.

Lopez-Torres, Diego, Cesar Elosua, and Francisco J. Arregui. 2020. "Optical fiber sensors based on microstructured optical fibers to detect gases and volatile organic compounds: A review." *Sensors* 20 (9). DOI: 10.3390/s20092555.

Luo, Zewei, Yimin Wang, Ya Xu, Xu Wang, Zhijun Huang, Junman Chen, Yongxin Li, and Yixiang Duan. 2019. "Ultrasensitive U-shaped fiber optic LSPR cytosensing for label-free and in situ evaluation of cell surface N-glycan expression." *Sensors and Actuators B: Chemical* 284:582–588. https://doi.org/10.1016/j.snb.2019.01.015.

Malhotra, Bansi Dhar, and Md Azahar Ali. 2018. "Chapter 7: Nanostructured biomaterials for in vivo biosensors." In *Nanomaterials for Biosensors*, edited by Bansi Dhar Malhotra and Md Azahar Ali, 183–219. Norwich, NY: William Andrew Publishing.

Masson, Jean-Francois. 2020. "Portable and field-deployed surface plasmon resonance and plasmonic sensors." *Analyst* 145 (11):3776–3800. DOI: 10.1039/D0AN00316F.

Mauriz, Elba, Priyanka Dey, and Laura M. Lechuga. 2019. "Advances in nanoplasmonic biosensors for clinical applications." *Analyst* 144 (24):7105–7129. DOI: 10.1039/C9AN00701F.

Mustapha Kamil, Y., M. H. Abu Bakar, M. A. Mustapa, M. H. Yaacob, N. H. Z. Abidin, A. Syahir, H. J. Lee, and M. A. Mahdi. 2018. "Label-free dengue E protein detection using a functionalized tapered optical fiber sensor." *Sensors and Actuators B: Chemical* 257:820–828. https://doi.org/10.1016/j.snb.2017.11.005.

Mustapha, Yasmin, M. Mustapa, Muhammad Hafiz Abu Bakar, Baktiar Musa, Amir Syahir, Mohd Yaacob, and Mohd Adzir Mahdi. 2015. "Refractive index sensor with asymmetrical tapered fiber based on evanescent field sensing." 2015 IEEE International Broadband and Photonics Conference (IBP), Bali, Indonesia, 23–25 April. DOI: 10.1109/IBP.2015.7230762.

Neethirajan, Suresh, Vasanth Ragavan, Xuan Weng, and Rohit Chand. 2018. "Biosensors for sustainable food engineering: Challenges and perspectives." *Biosensors* 8 (1). DOI: 10.3390/bios8010023.

Nishida, K., Y. Nannichi, T. Uchida, and I. Kitano. 1970. "An avalanche photodiode with a tapered light-focusing fiber guide." *Proceedings of the IEEE* 58 (5):790–791. DOI: 10.1109/PROC.1970.7734.

Nylander, Claes, Bo Liedberg, and Tommy Lind. 1982. "Gas detection by means of surface plasmon resonance." *Sensors and Actuators* 3:79–88. https://doi.org/10.1016/0250-6874(82)80008-5.

Omar, Nur Alia Sheh, Yap Wing Fen, Jaafar Abdullah, Che Engku Noramalina Che Engku Chik, and Mohd Adzir Mahdi. 2018. "Development of an optical sensor based on surface plasmon resonance phenomenon for diagnosis of dengue virus E-protein." *Sensing and Bio-Sensing Research* 20:16–21. https://doi.org/10.1016/j.sbsr.2018.06.001.

Omar, Nur Alia Sheh, Yap Wing Fen, Silvan Saleviter, Wan Mohd Ebtisyam Mustaqim Mohd Daniyal, Nur Ain Asyiqin Anas, Nur Syahira Md Ramdzan, and Mohammad Danial Aizad Roshidi. 2019. "Development of a graphene-based surface plasmon resonance optical sensor chip for potential biomedical application." *Materials (Basel, Switzerland)* 12 (12):1928. DOI: 10.3390/ma12121928.

Pan, H. M., S. Gonuguntla, S. Li, and D. Trau. 2017. "3.33 conjugated polymers for biosensor devices." In *Comprehensive Biomaterials II*, edited by Paul Ducheyne, 716–754. Oxford: Elsevier.

Petryayeva, Eleonora, and Ulrich J. Krull. 2011. "Localized surface plasmon resonance: Nanostructures, bioassays and biosensing: A review." *Analytica Chimica Acta* 706 (1):8–24. https://doi.org/10.1016/j.aca.2011.08.020.

Prabowo, Briliant Adhi, Agnes Purwidyantri, and Kou-Chen Liu. 2018. "Surface plasmon resonance optical sensor: A review on light source technology." *Biosensors* 8 (3):80. DOI: 10.3390/bios8030080.

Rajapaksha, P., A. Elbourne, S. Gangadoo, R. Brown, D. Cozzolino, and J. Chapman. 2019. "A review of methods for the detection of pathogenic microorganisms." *Analyst* 144 (2):396–411. DOI: 10.1039/C8AN01488D.

Ribaut, Clotilde, Médéric Loyez, Jean-Charles Larrieu, Samia Chevineau, Pierre Lambert, Myriam Remmelink, Ruddy Wattiez, and Christophe Caucheteur. 2017. "Cancer biomarker sensing using packaged plasmonic optical fiber gratings: Towards in vivo diagnosis." *Biosensors and Bioelectronics* 92:449–456. https://doi.org/10.1016/j.bios.2016.10.081.

Roda, Aldo, Mara Mirasoli, Elisa Michelini, Massimo Di Fusco, Martina Zangheri, Luca Cevenini, Barbara Roda, and Patrizia Simoni. 2016. "Progress in chemical luminescence-based biosensors: A critical review." *Biosensors and Bioelectronics* 76:164–179. https://doi.org/10.1016/j.bios.2015.06.017.

Roether, Johanna, Kang-Yu Chu, Norbert Willenbacher, Amy Q. Shen, and Nikhil Bhalla. 2019. "Real-time monitoring of DNA immobilization and detection of DNA polymerase activity by a microfluidic nanoplasmonic platform." *Biosensors and Bioelectronics* 142:111528. https://doi.org/10.1016/j.bios.2019.111528.

Roy, Debdulal, and Alex E. Knight. 2017. "Scanning near-field optical microscopy and related techniques." In *Encyclopedia of Spectroscopy and Spectrometry.* 3rd ed., edited by John C. Lindon, George E. Tranter, and David W. Koppenaal, 1–6. Oxford: Academic Press.

Rubab, Momna, Hafiz Muhammad Shahbaz, Amin N. Olaimat, and Deog-Hwan Oh. 2018. "Biosensors for rapid and sensitive detection of *Staphylococcus aureus* in food." *Biosensors and Bioelectronics* 105:49–57. https://doi.org/10.1016/j.bios.2018.01.023.

Saylan, Yeşeren, Özgecan Erdem, Serhat Ünal, and Adil Denizli. 2019. "An alternative medical diagnosis method: Biosensors for virus detection." *Biosensors* 9 (2):65. DOI: 10.3390/bios9020065.

Semwal, V., and B. D. Gupta. 2018. "LSPR- and SPR-based fiber-optic cholesterol sensor using immobilization of cholesterol oxidase over silver nanoparticles coated graphene oxide nanosheets." *IEEE Sensors Journal* 18 (3):1039–1046.

Sharma, A. K., R. Jha, and B. D. Gupta. 2007. "Fiber-optic sensors based on surface plasmon resonance: A comprehensive review." *IEEE Sensors Journal* 7 (8):1118–1129. DOI: 10.1109/JSEN.2007.897946.

Shukla, Ira, and V. Suneetha. 2017. "Biosensors: Growth and market scenario." *Research Journal of Pharmacy and Technology* 10:3573–3579. DOI: 10.5958/0974-360X.2017.00647.3.

Simon, Pevec, and Donlagić Denis. 2019. "Multiparameter fiber-optic sensors: A review." *Optical Engineering* 58 (7):1–26. DOI: 10.1117/1.OE.58.7.072009.

Singh, M., S. K. Raghuwanshi, and O. Prakash. 2019. "Ultra-sensitive fiber optic gas sensor using graphene oxide coated long period gratings." *IEEE Photonics Technology Letters* 31 (17):1473–1476. DOI: 10.1109/LPT.2019.2932764.

Singh, L., R. Singh, S. Kumar, B. Zhang, and B. K. Kaushik. 2020. "Development of collagen-IV sensor using optical fiber-based Mach-Zehnder interferometer structure." *IEEE Journal of Quantum Electronics* 56 (4):1–8. DOI: 10.1109/JQE.2020.3003022.

Singh, L., R. Singh, B. Zhang, B. K. Kaushik, and S. Kumar. 2020. "Localized surface plasmon resonance based hetero-core optical fiber sensor structure for the detection of L-cysteine." *IEEE Transactions on Nanotechnology* 19:201–208.

Singh, L., G. Zhu, R. Singh, B. Zhang, W. Wang, B. K. Kaushik, and S. Kumar. 2020. "Gold nanoparticles and uricase functionalized tapered fiber sensor for uric acid detection." *IEEE Sensors Journal* 20 (1):219–226.

Singh, Ragini, Santosh Kumar, Feng-Zhen Liu, Cheng Shuang, Bingyuan Zhang, Rajan Jha, and Brajesh Kumar Kaushik. 2020. "Etched multicore fiber sensor using copper oxide and gold nanoparticles decorated graphene oxide structure for cancer cells detection." *Biosensors and Bioelectronics* 168:112557. https://doi.org/10.1016/j.bios.2020.112557.

Soares, Leonor, Andrea Csáki, Jacqueline Jatschka, Wolfgang Fritzsche, Orfeu Flores, Ricardo Franco, and Eulália Pereira. 2014. "Localized Surface Plasmon Resonance (LSPR) biosensing using gold nano-triangles: Detection of DNA hybridization events at room temperature." *Analyst* 139 (19):4964–4973. DOI: 10.1039/C4AN00810C.

Socorro-Leránoz, A. B., D. Santano, I. Del Villar, and I. R. Matias. 2019. "Trends in the design of wavelength-based optical fibre biosensors (2008–2018)." *Biosensors and Bioelectronics: X* 1:100015. https://doi.org/10.1016/j.biosx.2019.100015.

Song, Y. W. 2016. "3: Carbon nanotube and graphene photonic devices [This chapter was first published as Chapter 3 "Carbon nanotube and graphene photonic devices: Nonlinearity enhancement and novel preparation approaches" by Y.-W. Song in *Carbon Nanotubes and Graphene for Photonic Applications*, ed. S. Yamashita, Y. Saito and J. H. Choi, Woodhead Publishing Limited, 2013, ISBN: 978-0-85709-417-9.] In *Photodetectors*, edited by Bahram Nabet, 47–85. Sawston, Cambridge: Woodhead Publishing.

Srivastava, Sachin K., Vikas Arora, Sameer Sapra, and Banshi D. Gupta. 2012. "Localized surface plasmon resonance-based fiber optic U-shaped biosensor for the detection of blood glucose." *Plasmonics* 7 (2):261–268. DOI: 10.1007/s11468-011-9302-8.

Srivastava, Sachin K., Roli Verma, and Banshi Gupta. 2012. "Surface plasmon resonance based fiber optic glucose biosensor." *Proceedings of SPIE* 8351:69. DOI: 10.1117/12.915978.

Sytwu, Katherine, Michal Vadai, and Jennifer A. Dionne. 2019. "Bimetallic nanostructures: Combining plasmonic and catalytic metals for photocatalysis." *Advances in Physics: X* 4 (1):1619480. DOI: 10.1080/23746149.2019.1619480.

Tabassum, R., and B. D. Gupta. 2017. "Influence of oxide overlayer on the performance of a fiber optic SPR sensor with Al/Cu layers." *IEEE Journal of Selected Topics in Quantum Electronics* 23 (2):81–88. DOI: 10.1109/JSTQE.2016.2553442.

Tabish, Syed Amin. 2007. "Is diabetes becoming the biggest epidemic of the twenty-first century?" *International Journal of Health Sciences* 1 (2):V–VIII.

Tomaev, Vladimir, Vladimir Polischuk, T. Vartanyan, and E. Vasil'ev. 2019. "Surface plasmon resonance in zinc nanoparticles." *Glass Physics and Chemistry* 45:238–241.

Tong, Limin, and Michael Sumetsky. 2010. "Subwavelength and nanometer diameter optical fibers." Advanced Topics in Science and Technology in China (ATSTC), Springer Berlin, Heidelberg. DOI: https://doi.org/10.1007/978-3-642-03362-9.

Vasuki, S., V. Varsha, R. Mithra, S. Dharshni, R. Abinaya, N. Dharshini, and N. Sivarajasekar. 2019. "Thermal biosensors and their applications." *American International Journal of Research in Science, Technology, Engineering & Mathematics* 262–264.

Velázquez-González, J. S., D. Monzón-Hernández, F. Martínez-Piñón, D. A. May-Arrioja, and I. Hernández-Romano. 2017. "Surface plasmon resonance-based optical fiber embedded in PDMS for temperature sensing." *IEEE Journal of Selected Topics in Quantum Electronics* 23 (2):126–131. DOI: 10.1109/JSTQE.2016.2628022.

Wang, Fang, Yang Zhang, Zexu Liu, Huizhen Yuan, Zhenlin Wu, Dapeng Zhou, Zhenguo Jing, and Wei Peng. 2018. "Highly sensitive glucose detection using Au nanoparticles based fiber optic SPR sensor." 26th International Conference on Optical Fiber Sensors, Lausanne, 24 Sep.

Wang, Q., G. Farrell, and W. Yan. 2008. "Investigation on single-mode: Multimode-single-mode fiber structure." *Journal of Lightwave Technology* 26 (5):512–519.

Wang, Qi, and Yu Liu. 2018. "Review of optical fiber bending/curvature sensor." *Measurement* 130:161–176. https://doi.org/10.1016/j.measurement.2018.07.068.

Wang, Zhi, Ragini Singh, Carlos Marques, Rajan Jha, Bingyuan Zhang, and Santosh Kumar. 2021. "Taper-in-taper fiber structure-based LSPR sensor for alanine aminotransferase detection." *Optics Express* 29 (26):43793–43810. DOI: 10.1364/OE.447202.

Wu, Chin-Wei, Chang-Yue Chiang, Chien-Hsing Chen, Chung-Sheng Chiang, Chih-To Wang, and Lai-Kwan Chau. 2016. "Self-referencing fiber optic particle plasmon resonance sensing system for real-time biological monitoring." *Talanta* 146:291–298. https://doi.org/10.1016/j.talanta.2015.08.047.

Xie, Zhenzhen, Mandapati V. Ramakrishnam Raju, Andrew C. Stewart, Michael H. Nantz, and Xiao-An Fu. 2018. "Imparting sensitivity and selectivity to a gold nanoparticle chemiresistor through thiol monolayer functionalization for sensing acetone." *RSC Advances* 8 (62):35618–35624. DOI: 10.1039/C8RA06137H.

Yang, Qingshan, Xia Zhang, Santosh Kumar, Ragini Singh, Bingyuan Zhang, Chenglin Bai, and Xipeng Pu. 2020. "Development of glucose sensor using gold nanoparticles and glucose-oxidase functionalized tapered fiber structure." *Plasmonics* 15 (3):841–848. DOI: 10.1007/s11468-019-01104-7.

Yang, Qingshan, Guo Zhu, Lokendra Singh, Yu Wang, Ragini Singh, Bingyuan Zhang, Xia Zhang, and Santosh Kumar. 2020. "Highly sensitive and selective sensor probe using glucose oxidase/gold nanoparticles/graphene oxide functionalized tapered optical fiber structure for detection of glucose." *Optik* 208:164536. https://doi.org/10.1016/j.ijleo.2020.164536.

Yang, Wen, Jing Yu, Xiangtai Xi, Yang Sun, Yiming Shen, Weiwei Yue, Chao Zhang, and Shouzhen Jiang. 2019a. "Preparation of graphene/ITO nanorod metamaterial/U-bent-annealing fiber sensor and DNA biomolecule detection." *Nanomaterials (Basel, Switzerland)* 9 (8):1154. DOI: 10.3390/nano9081154.

Yang, Wen, Jing Yu, Xiangtai Xi, Yang Sun, Yiming Shen, Weiwei Yue, Chao Zhang, and Shouzhen Jiang. 2019b. "Preparation of graphene/ITO nanorod metamaterial/U-bent-annealing fiber sensor and DNA biomolecule detection." *Nanomaterials* 9 (8). DOI: 10.3390/nano9081154.

Yang, Wenlei, Shuo Zhang, Tao Geng, Le Li, Guoan Li, Yijia Gong, Kai Zhang, Chengguo Tong, Chunlian Lu, Weimin Sun, and Libo Yuan. 2019. "High sensitivity refractometer based on a tapered-single mode-no core-single mode fiber structure." *Sensors (Basel, Switzerland)* 19 (7):1722. DOI: 10.3390/s19071722.

Yoo, Seung, and Sang Yup Lee. 2015. "Optical biosensors for the detection of pathogenic microorganisms." *Trends in Biotechnology* 34. DOI: 10.1016/j.tibtech.2015.09.012.

Yuan, Huizhen, Wei Ji, Shuwen Chu, Siyu Qian, Fang Wang, Jean-Francois Masson, Xiuyou Han, and Wei Peng. 2018. "Fiber-optic surface plasmon resonance glucose sensor enhanced with phenylboronic acid modified Au nanoparticles." *Biosensors and Bioelectronics* 117:637–643. https://doi.org/10.1016/j.bios.2018.06.042.

Zhang, Nancy Meng Ying, Miao Qi, Zhixun Wang, Zhe Wang, Mengxiao Chen, Kaiwei Li, Ping Shum, and Lei Wei. 2019. "One-step synthesis of cyclodextrin-capped gold nanoparticles for ultra-sensitive and highly-integrated plasmonic biosensors." *Sensors and Actuators B: Chemical* 286:429–436. https://doi.org/10.1016/j.snb.2019.01.166.

Zhang, W., W. Zhuang, M. Dong, L. Zhu, and F. Meng. 2019. "Dual-parameter optical fiber sensor for temperature and pressure discrimination featuring cascaded tapered-FBG and ball-EFPI." *IEEE Sensors Journal* 19 (14):5645–5652. DOI: 10.1109/JSEN.2019.2905635.

Zhang, Xuejun, Ze Wu, Fu Liu, Qiangqiang Fu, Xiaoyong Chen, Jian Xu, Zhaochuan Zhang, Yunyun Huang, Yong Tang, Tuan Guo, and Jacques Albert. 2018. "Hydrogen peroxide and glucose concentration measurement using optical fiber grating sensors with corrodible plasmonic nanocoatings." *Biomedical Optics Express* 9 (4):1735–1744. DOI: 10.1364/BOE.9.001735.

Zhao, Xihong, Yu-Chia Tsao, Fu-Jung Lee, Woo-Hu Tsai, Ching-Ho Wang, Tsung-Liang Chuang, Mu-Shiang Wu, and Chii-Wann Lin. 2016. "Optical fiber sensor based on surface plasmon resonance for rapid detection of avian influenza virus subtype H6: Initial studies." *Journal of Virological Methods* 233:15–22. https://doi.org/10.1016/j.jviromet.2016.03.007.

Zhou, Chen, Haimin Zou, Ming Li, Chengjun Sun, Dongxia Ren, and Yong-Xin Li. 2018. "Fiber optic surface plasmon resonance sensor for detection of *E. coli* O157:H7 based on antimicrobial peptides and AgNPs-rGO." *Biosensors and Bioelectronics* 117. DOI: 10.1016/j.bios.2018.06.005.

Zhou, H., G. Ma, M. Zhang, H. Zhang, and C. Li. 2019. "A high sensitivity optical fiber interferometer sensor for acoustic emission detection of partial discharge in power transformer." *IEEE Sensors Journal*:1–1. DOI: 10.1109/JSEN.2019.2951613.

Zhou, H. Y., G. M. Ma, M. Zhang, H. C. Zhang, and C. R. Li. 2021. "A high sensitivity optical fiber interferometer sensor for acoustic emission detection of partial discharge in power transformer." *IEEE Sensors Journal* 21 (1):24–32. DOI: 10.1109/JSEN.2019.2951613.

Zhu, Guo, Niteshkumar Agrawal, Ragini Singh, Santosh Kumar, Bingyuan Zhang, Chinmoy Saha, and Chandrakanta Kumar. 2020. "A novel periodically tapered structure-based gold nanoparticles and graphene oxide: Immobilized optical fiber sensor to detect ascorbic acid." *Optics & Laser Technology* 127:106156. https://doi.org/10.1016/j.optlastec.2020.106156.

4 Gold Nanoparticles Assisted Optical Fiber-Based Plasmonic Biosensors

4.1 INTRODUCTION

In recent years, plasmonic phenomenon-based sensors have attracted unprecedented attention in various areas such as military application, drug testing, environmental pollution, food health, and biosensing applications due to their excellent current-illumination characteristics (Tong, Xia, and Peng 2019). A brief discussion about the prominent role of gold nanoparticles (AuNPs) in the development of biosensors based on different plasmonic optical fiber sensors (P-OFSs) is discussed and reported in this chapter. In the detection of various biomarkers, AuNPs show excellent biocompatibility, are convenient to synthesize, easily interact with various molecules (like polypeptides, antibodies, carboxyl groups, RNA, DNA, polyethylene glycol [PEG], etc.) (Zhu, Agrawal et al. 2020). In addition, excellent chemical properties, stability, and easy adjustment for geometric size and shape make AuNPs a superior choice over other inorganic nanoparticles (NPs) (Agrawal et al. 2021). The AuNPs have been integrated with various special fiber structures, such as tapered, grating structure, side polished fiber, U-shaped structures, partially uncoated fiber, and D-shaped fiber structures to enhance the plasmonic characteristics of the sensor (Chack, Agrawal, and Raghuwanshi 2014; Agrawal, Saha, Kumar, Singh, Zhang, and Kumar 2020).

The AuNPs allow excitation of collective oscillation of conduction electrons with sub-wavelength features (Agrawal, Zhang, Saha, Kumar, Kaushik et al. 2020). The general setup of the AuNPs-based fiber-optic plasmonic sensor is shown in Figure 4.1. When reflectance intensity (RI) of the medium changes, the coupling condition of evanescent waves (EWs) and surface plasmon waves (SPWs) changes (Singh, Agrawal, Saha, and Kaushik 2022; Agrawal, Saha, Kumar, Singh, Zhang, Jha et al. 2020). Thus, as a potential application of optical technology, plasmonics sensors modified by noble metallic material like AuNPs can play a game-changing role in the detection of RI change (Singh, Singh, Umar et al. 2020). This absorbance depends on the absorptivity, which increases for a higher RI, concentration of AuNPs coated on the fiber, and fiber length (Singh, Agrawal, Saha, Singh et al. 2022). The development of surface plasmon resonance (SPR) technology can be summarized from the study of intrinsic optical properties of metal films to various other extensible applications. Typical of those sensing tools are lab biosensor chip and color-based biosensors.

4.2 SYNTHESIS, CHARACTERIZATION, PROPERTIES, AND APPLICATIONS OF GOLD NANOPARTICLES

In general, AuNPs in the range of 5–100 nm are synthesized and reported for the development of plasmonic phenomenon-based sensors that are used for biomedical to environmental parameter detection. In general, AuNPs are synthesized via the citrate reduction method, like the well-known Turkevich method. Through the formation of monodisperse AuNPs by a series of redox and disproportionation reactions, and simple changes in temperature and dosage, the size of the resulting nanoparticles can be adjusted directly (Young et al. 2011). Throughout the redox reaction, citrate anions act as a reductant and play an important reductant role in the formation of stable colloidal AuNPs. It is worth noting that the diameter of spherical AuNPs is closely related to their corresponding SPR peak wavelength, and the typical particle size and the corresponding

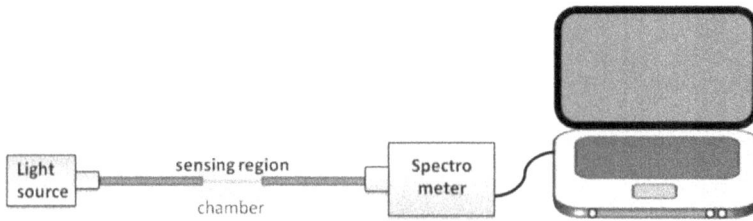

FIGURE 4.1 The setup of the gold nanoparticle-based fiber-optic sensor (Houngkamhang et al. 2018).

TABLE 4.1
Size-Dependent Change in Peak SPR Wavelength of Spherical AuNPs

Size of gold nanoparticle	Peak SPR wavelength
5 nm	515–520 nm
10 nm	515–520 nm
20 nm	524 nm
30 nm	526 nm
40 nm	530 nm
50 nm	535 nm
60 nm	540 nm
80 nm	553 nm
100 nm	572 nm

Source: Sigma-Aldrich (Shah et al. 2014).

Note: AuNP, gold nanoparticle; SPR, surface plasmon resonance.

plasmon wavelength are summarized in Table 4.1. It is clear from the table that simply tuning the AuNP's size allows the wavelength in visible region to be tuned. Transmission electron microscopy (TEM) images of AuNPs and Au nanorods as a function of increasing dimensions are presented in Figure 4.2. In this figure, the size of Au spheres (a–e) is limited to 4–40 nm, while the aspect ratio of Au nanorods (f–k) is confined from 1.3 to 5. Further, optical absorption spectra of Au nanorods are reported in Figure 4.3. Unstable AuNPs tend to aggregate, changing the color of the solution from wine red to blue/purple, and resulting in black clumps within transparent color solution. The localized surface plasmon resonance (LSPR) effect of AuNPs is caused by the absorption of the energy of incident light; thus, the potential detection ability of the LSPR sensor can be evaluated by measuring the reflected light intensity. Further, Figure 4.4 shows the green synthesis of AuNPs from a variety of biological sources. The different processes are introduced for the synthesis of AuNPs as indicated in Table 4.1.

4.2.1 TURKEVICH METHOD

The typical process is demonstrated in this section to synthesize the AuNPs using the Turkevich method, with size of 10.5 ± 0.5 nm. First, 150 mL of HAuCl4 (100 mM) solution is mixed with 14.85 mL deionized (DI) water and heated to boiling. Then, carefully add the 1.8 mL trisodium citrate (38.8 mM) of DI water solution while stirring at a constant speed. Stop stirring after 10 minutes and keep boiling for 5 minutes. During this process, the solution transits from black color to a clear

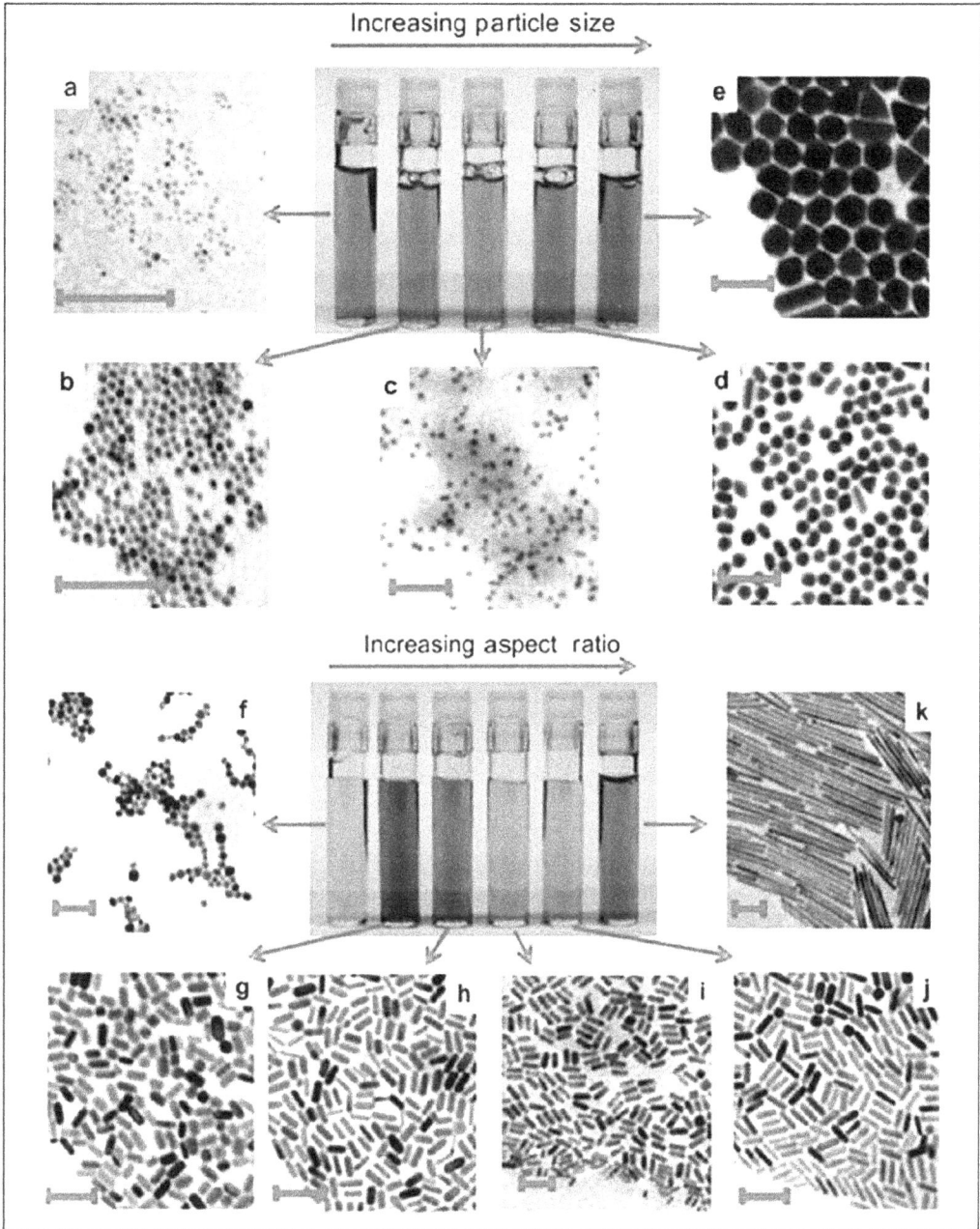

FIGURE 4.2 TEM images of gold nanospheres (upper panels) and gold nanorods (lower panels) as a function of increasing dimensions. The size of the Au spheres (a–e) is limited to 4–40 nm, while the aspect ratio of Au nanorods (f–k) is confined from 1.3 to 5 (Mody et al. 2010).

wine-red color. The inset of Figure 4.5(a) illustrates the final synthesized AuNPs. A high-resolution transmission electron microscopy (HRTEM) image about the distribution of AuNPs in aqueous is shown in Figure 4.5(b). Using ImageJ 10.0 software for the analysis in Figure 4.5(c), an HRTEM image of AuNPs can be obtained indicating formation of stable AuNPs with a particle size of 10.5 ± 0.5 nm. After observing, the synthesized AuNPs solution can be kept at room temperature for up to

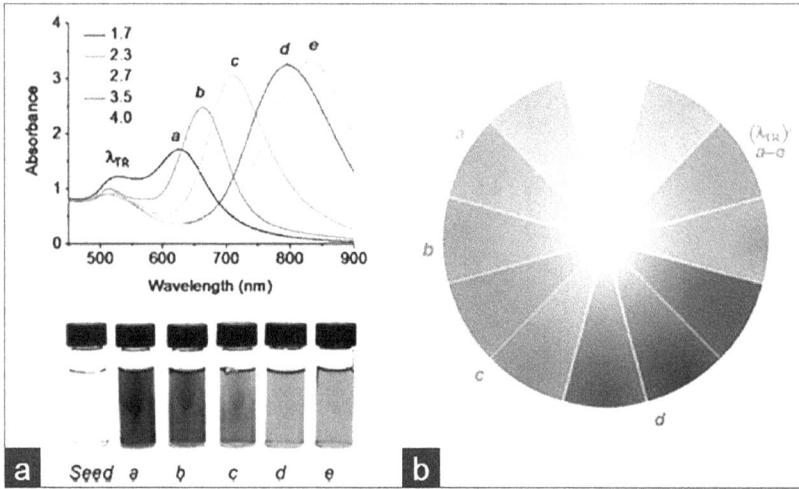

FIGURE 4.3 (a) Optical absorption spectra of gold nanorods with different aspect ratios (a–e). (b) Color wheel, concerning gold nanorods labeled (a–e). TR, transverse resonance (Mody et al. 2010).

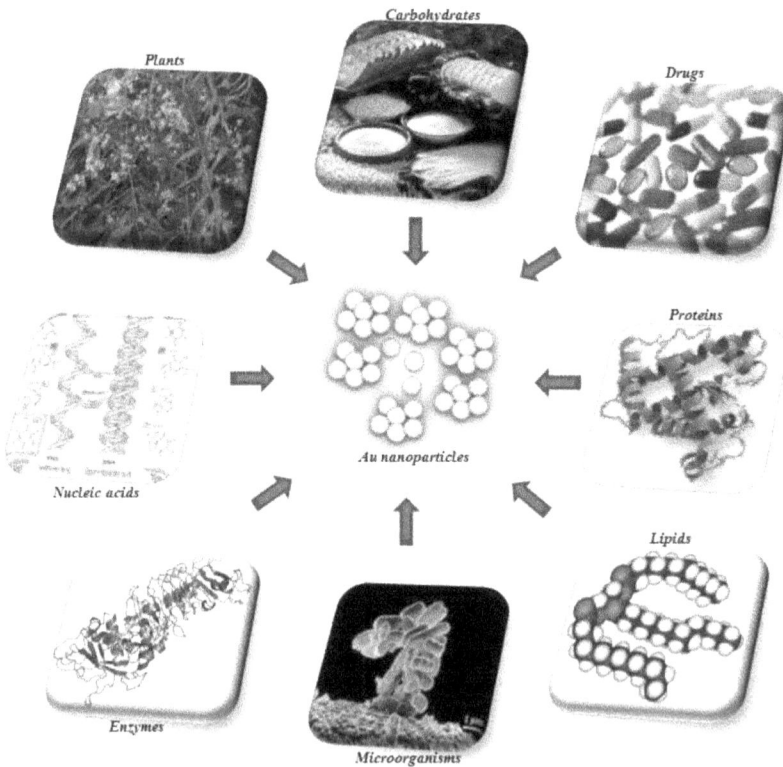

FIGURE 4.4 Different biological sources ranging from biomolecules (carbohydrates, lipids, enzymes, nucleic acids, and proteins), drugs, plants, and microorganisms, which are used in green synthesis of gold nanoparticles due to the combined reducing and capping property of different biocomponents present in them. (Image credit: wikipedia.org) (Shah et al. 2014).

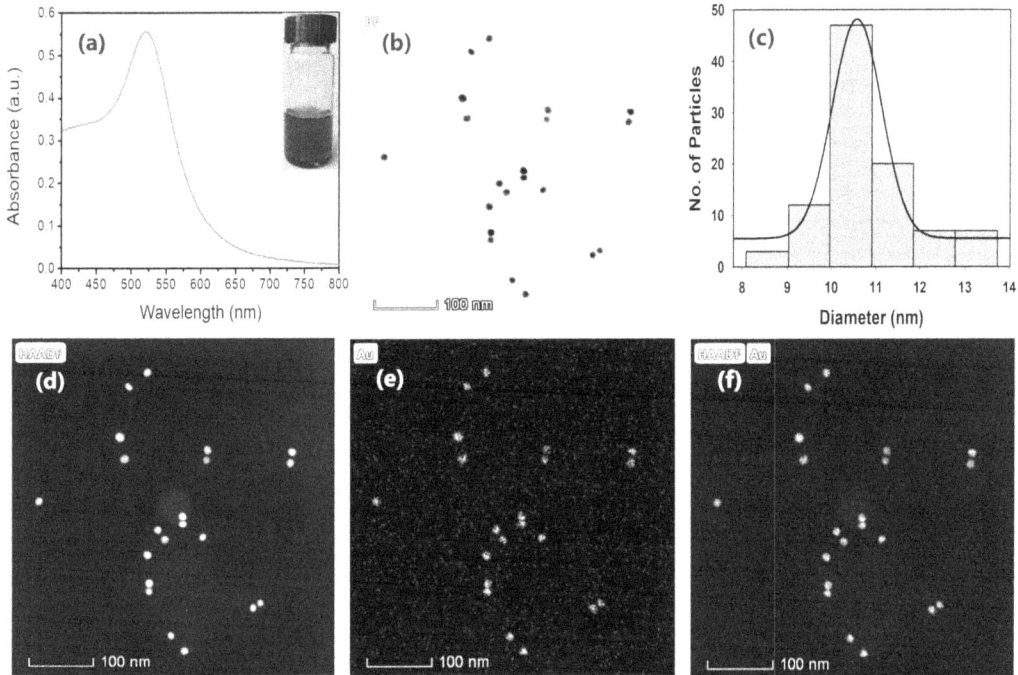

FIGURE 4.5 Synthesized gold nanoparticle using Turkevich method and characterization results: (a) synthesized solution and absorbance spectrum, (b) HRTEM image of AuNP, (c) nanoparticle analysis (histogram) of TEM image shows that mean diameter of AuNPs is 10.5 ± 0.5 nm, and (d–f) EDX analysis of AuNPs shows the presence of Au as synthesized particles (Kumar, Kaushik et al. 2019).

3 months without agglomeration. Figure 4.5(d–f) describe the energy dispersive X-ray spectroscopy (EDX) of AuNPs to bear out synthesized spherical particles as Au.

4.2.2 Brust Method

The well-known Brust method, first proposed in 1994 and related to Faraday's concept of two-phase system, is mainly used to synthesize small AuNPs with particle sizes below 10 nm. In Figure 4.6, the process can be simply described as the transfer of gold salts from an aqueous solution to toluene (as organic solvent), through vigorous agitation and tetraoctylammonium bromide (TOAB, a kind of phase transfer agent). Sodium borohydride was added, then, to reduce the gold. In the presence of alkanethiol, AuNPs can be stabilized without agglomeration formation. By regulating the ratio of thiol to Au, the reaction solution transit from orange color to brown color, that means the particle size around 1.5–5.2 nm of the AuNPs has been synthesized successfully (Calandra et al. 2010).

4.2.3 Seeded Growth Method

Seeded mediated growth is the preferred technique for synthesizing AuNPs with special shapes like tubes, cubes, and rods. The key step of this technique, in brief, is to first add sodium borohydride (a strong reductant) in the salt of the gold sample to produce small particles of Au called seed particles. These seeds are then added in metal salt solution for reaction. While the un-nucleated Au seeds, with the help of structural-directing agent and weak reductant ascorbic acid (work as strong reductants), grow rapidly to form special shapes. The shape of fresh synthesized AuNPs can change

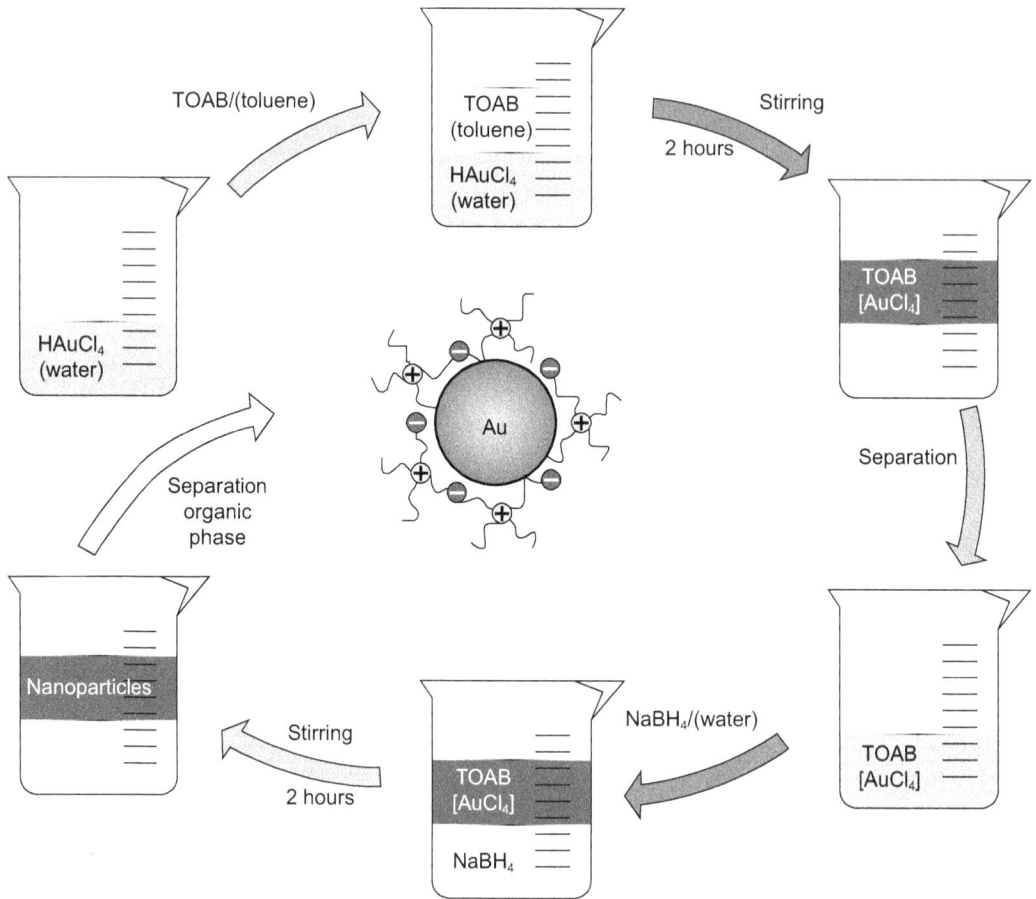

FIGURE 4.6 Steps involved in the synthesis of AuNPs using the Brust method (Calandra et al. 2010).

the anisotropic growth state of seed particles by changing the concentration of basis seed, reducing agent, and structure-directing agent (Jana, Gearheart, and Murphy 2001).

4.2.4 ELECTROCHEMICAL METHOD

Reetz et al. first proposed the method of preparing AuNPs by the electrochemical method using a simple two-electrode battery (Reetz and Helbig 1994). In this method, the glassy carbon electrodes are modified with multiwalled carbon nanotubes (MWCNTs), and the size of transition metal particles can be adjusted by adjusting the tetra-alkylammonium salt (the stabilizer of metal clusters in nonaqueous media) (Herizchi et al. 2016).

4.2.5 MISCELLANEOUS METHODS

Digestive ripening based on the mechanism of digestion and maturation, is a widely approved method for preparing monodisperse AuNPs with uniform size due to the advantage of simple operation and excellent repeatability. The size of NPs can be adjusted by controlling the temperature and time of heat treatment and digesting the kinds of curing agents. Furthermore, other unique methods for synthesized AuNPs are as follows: microwave, electrochemistry, solvothermal method, laser ablation, photochemical reduction, and ultrasonic waves (Shah et al. 2014).

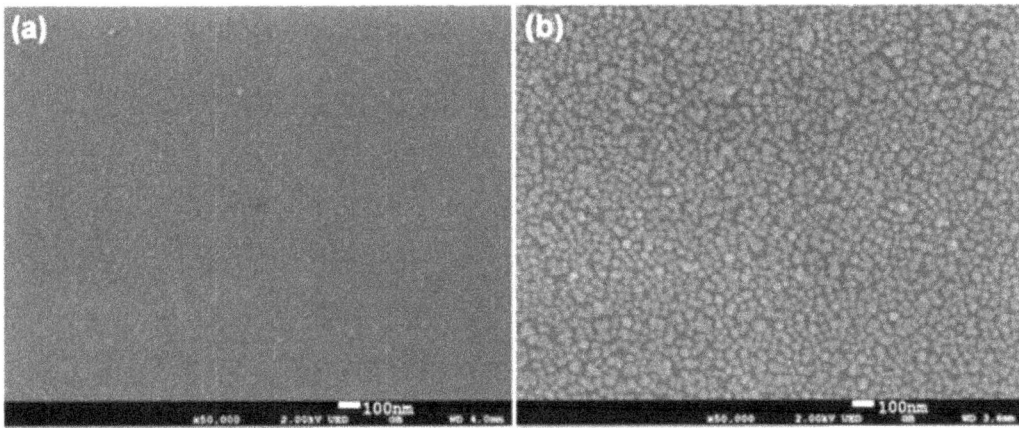

FIGURE 4.7 Topographical FESEM image showing the elemental information of the optical fiber (a) before and (b) after it is coated with gold nanoparticles (Houngkamhang et al. 2018).

The synthesized AuNP properties vary on account of their micro-morphometric parameters, like shape, distribution, size, and environment. To investigate these related parameters, some characterization machines, such as dynamic light scattering (DLS), ultraviolet-visible (UV-Vis), atomic force microscopy (AFM), and high-resolution transmission electron microscope (HRTEM) are employed to ensure the optical properties of AuNPs. In 2007, Haiss et al. reported a method to calculate the size of NPs (Haiss et al. 2007b). The process involves the micromorphological distribution of synthesized spheroidal AuNPs in aqueous sample with the help of UV-Vis spectra (Haiss et al. 2007a). The instruments such as scanning electron microscopy (SEM), energy-dispersive X-ray spectroscopy (EDS or XEDS), and field emission scanning electron microscopy (FESEM) are used to check the morphology of nanomaterials (NMs) and NMs over the sensing region. The sample HRTEM image of synthesized AuNPs is shown in Figure 4.5(b). This will help us to check the size and shape of synthesized NMs. The sample EDS images of synthesized AuNPs present in Figure 4.5(d–f) indicate the presence of proposed NMs over the surface of the sensor probe. The morphology distribution on the fiber surface before and after the AuNPs coating process is compared with FESEM images in Figure 4.7(a and b), separately. FESEM is an advanced technology used to capture the microstructure image of the materials. A FESEM is used to visualize very small topographic details on the surface or entire or fractioned objects. Researchers in biology, chemistry, and physics apply this technique to observe structures that may be as small as 1 nm.

4.3 SOME BIOSENSOR DESIGN BASED ON AuNPs

The fabrication process for the development of AuNPs assisted optical fiber-based plasmonic biosensors is briefly covered in this section. The schematic of the AuNPs coated optical fiber is indicated in Figure 4.8, as used in the development of P-OFSs. This kind of fiber-optic sensor has the characteristics of a simple but cost-effective manufacturing process and thus exhibits huge potential to be adapted to in situ applications in the future.

A detailed description of the sensor development steps for an AuNPs assisted tapered fiber structure is presented here by Santosh et. al (Kumar, Kaushik et al. 2019). The tapered fiber probe is fabricated using oxygen butane flame or hydrogen-oxygen through flame and brush technology. In this technique, an SMF is heated above a gas burner flame and then stretched by means of axial pulling force applied at the two sides. The pulling reduces the diameter at the hot zone of the flame (where the temperature is above the softening temperature of the fiber material) and, as a result, the tapered fiber gets fabricated as illustrated in Figure 4.9. By controlling the flame movement and

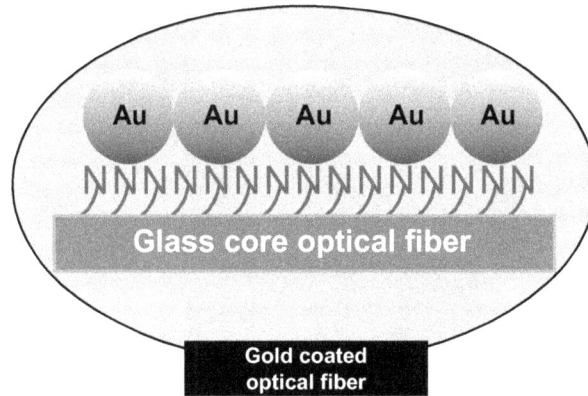

FIGURE 4.8   Gold nanoparticles coated optical fiber (Houngkamhang et al. 2018).

the fiber pulling rate, one can define the microfiber shape to an extremely high degree of accuracy. Generally, a low-carbon fuel such as hydrogen is used in the burner to minimize the contamination of fiber with incompletely burned carbon particles. Occasionally, oxygen is also supplied to the burner to control the temperature and size of the flame. In addition, there is a constant and suitable heating temperature, which helps to avoid a broken fiber or an uneven shape during the stretching process. Therefore, it is indispensable for the good-enough parameters of the computer program to ensure the stability and reproducibility of the experiment. To exhibit the lowest stress and strain of fabricated probes, several key parameters like waist diameter, stretch dimension, and flow power are optimized as ~4 µm, 15,000 µm, and 40 µm, respectively.

In the next step, synthesized AuNPs are immobilized over the sensor surface. For this, tapered fiber used for immobilization is cleaned by a three-step process. The fiber needs careful handling during various processes to prevent it from breaking since the waist diameter of taper fiber is very low (~4 µm). The whole process can be summed up as three-step cleaning and two-step soaking; however, it is worth noting that the whole process is to prevent the fragile fiber probe. Therefore, it is necessary to describe the manufacturing process in detail as follows. First, the sensing regions of the same-batch optical fibers are aligned and immersed in acetone solution for 20 minutes. This step can make the probes surface smooth. The dried fibers are then placed in piranha solution for 30 minutes. Piranha solution (seven parts of H_2SO_4 in three parts of H_2O_2) can effectively hydrolyze the organic substance on the surface of the probe and form a homogeneous layer of hydroxyl groups. The probes are then carefully removed, the residual materials are cleaned with DI water and dried at 70°C under vacuum conditions. The fibers are then meticulously encapsulated in an ethanol solution of (3-mercaptopropyl) trimethoxysilane (MPTMS, 250 µL of MPTMS in 25 mL of ethanol). After 12 hours of reaction, here, MPTMS as coupling agent can form homogeneously mercapto monolayers on the probe surface, which is beneficial to the adhesion of AuNPs. As for the next step, the unbound MPTMS is then cleaned with alcohol, and the dry probes are encapsulated with care in a freshly prepared AuNPs solution for 48 hours. Over time, AuNPs became attached to the SH group with MPTMS. The entire reaction process is visualized in Figure 4.10. The final clean step is to carefully remove the unbonded monomers on the surface of the probes using ethanol. At this point, a batch of AuNPs-modified sensor probes is obtained. To ensure the quality of the AuNPs coating technique, a carefully placed AuNPs sensing area is observed using SEM on a 3 × 3 mm silicon wafer. From Figure 4.11(a), a partial sensing region and transition-stretching region in excellent shape can be observed clearly. Figure 4.11(b) shows a uniform distribution of AuNPs on the surface of sensing region.

In the next step, the enzymatic functionalization of the sensor probe using cholesterol oxidase (ChOx) can be described in detail as follows. The clean probe is first encapsulated in an aqueous

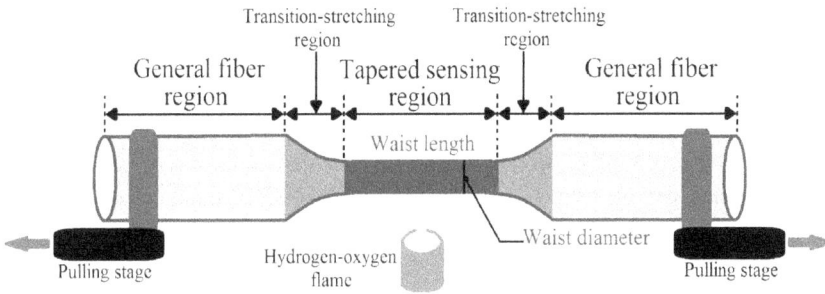

FIGURE 4.9 Typical schematic view of the fiber tapering process using hydrogen-oxygen flame-brushing technique (Kumar, Kaushik et al. 2019).

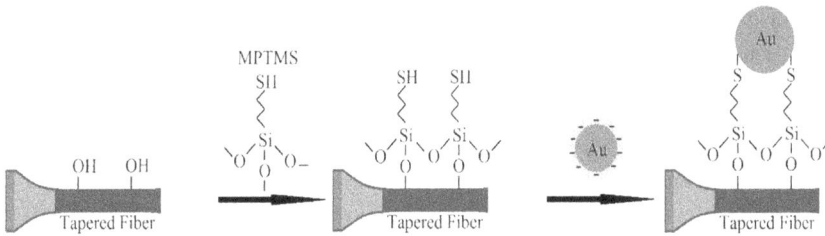

FIGURE 4.10 Immobilization of AuNPs over tapered optical fiber surface (Kumar, Kaushik et al. 2019).

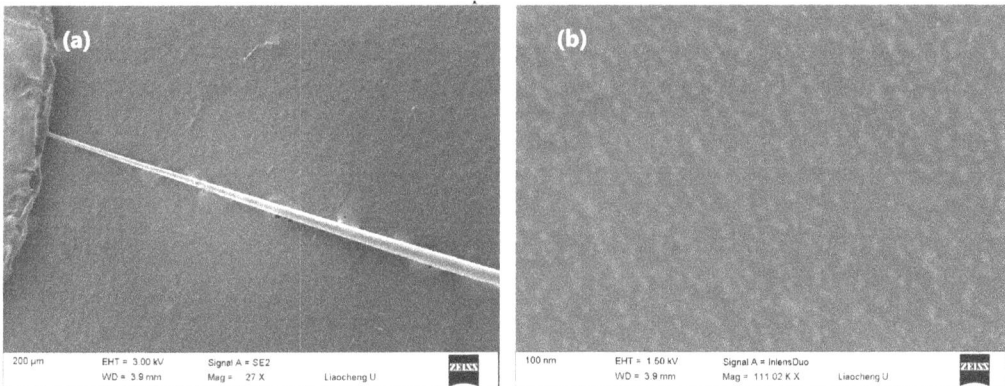

FIGURE 4.11 Scanning electron micrographs of AuNPs-immobilized taper fiber (a) at lower magnification to check the shape of the sensor probe, and (b) at higher magnification to check the morphology of AuNPs over the sensing surface of the sensor probe (Kumar, Kaushik et al. 2019).

solution of the MUA. After 5 hours of reaction, a uniform film of carboxyl group is formed on the surface of the probe. The probe is then removed and carefully soaked in the EDC/NHS (N-ethyl-N′-(3-(dimethylamino)propyl)carbodiimide/N-hydroxysuccinimide) mixture for 10 minutes. During this time, EDC acts as a coupling agent that effectively activates the surface carboxyl groups, while NHS makes enzyme immobilization more reliable. Finally, the treated probe is carefully encapsulated in a fresh ChOx solution (pH 7.4, 0.32 mg of ChOx in 0.5 mL of phosphate-buffered saline (PBS) solution) for 12 hours. After this process, the ChOx-functionalized sensor probes are obtained and stored carefully in a refrigerator at 4°C. Before the measurement purpose, dipping in cold PBS solution for 15 minutes is necessary for the sensor probes.

4.4   RECENT DEVELOPMENT OF GOLD NANOPARTICLES ASSISTED PLASMONIC BIOSENSORS

A label-free biosensing device, AuNPs modified P-OFSs is demonstrated in this section. These sensors are subdivided into different categories based on their application in the biosensing field. The in-depth study over AuNPs-assisted biosensors for the detection of (i) glucose, (ii) cholesterol, (iii) other biomolecules, (iv) bacteria and viruses, and (v) DNA/RNA and cells are presented in the following subsections.

4.4.1   GOLD NANOPARTICLES ASSISTED GLUCOSE SENSOR

Diabetes mellitus has always been a serious topic for human health. In middle-aged and older adults, the incidence of glycuresis is high, and there is no effective cure. Therefore, early monitoring and treatment of blood sugar are particularly vital. As an important blood glucose index, it is of significance to develop a glucose biosensor with high sensitivity and selectivity. In addition, glucose biosensors are not only limited to the diagnosis of glycuresis but have a pivotal position in many fields like biotechnology applications and food industry. In recent years, optical fiber-based glucose biosensors have become popular due to their miniaturization, high portability, multiplexing capabilities, remote access, and cost-benefit (Yang, Zhang et al. 2020). The Au-coated plasmonic fibers optic biosensor with different structure and sensing mechanisms are analyzed in this section. The range of studies for the detection of glucose using plasmonic-based technique are represented in Table 4.2.

4.4.2   GOLD NANOPARTICLES ASSISTED CHOLESTEROL SENSOR

Cholesterol is an indispensable element in human blood, cells, and tissues. Moreover, the detection of cholesterol is significant in clinical diagnosis. A high level of cholesterol is associated with many serious diseases like myxedema, hyperthyroidism, anemia, coronary artery disease, cardiovascular disease, and high blood pressure. The traditional detection method is to use an electrochemical

---

TABLE 4.2

Summary of Different Gold Nanoparticles Assisted Plasmonic Biosensors for Glucose Detection

Material used	Mechanism	Structure used	Linearity range	Limit of detection	Sensitivity	Ref.
AuNPs	LSPR	Tapered SMF	0–10 mM	322 µM	0.9261 nm/mM	Yang, Zhang et al. 2020
GO/AuNPs/GOx	LSPR	Tapered SMF	0–11 mM	2.26 mM	1.06 nm/mM	Yang, Zhu et al. 2020
AuNPs	SPR	Optical fiber (core diameter= 400 µm)	0.01–30 mM	80 nM	N.R.	Yuan et al. 2018
AuNPs/GOx	SPR	U-shaped fiber	N.R.	N.R.	2.899 nm dB/%	Chen et al. 2018
AuNPs	SPR	TFBG (SMF)	1–500 µM	N.R.	2.61 dB/µM	Wang et al. 2018
AuNPs	SPR	Tapered SMF	N.R.	N.R.	~2180 nm/RIU	Li et al. 2018
Silver (Ag) film	SPR	TFBG SMF	3–8 mM	N.R.	0.5 dB/mM	Zhang et al. 2018

Note: AuNP, gold nanoparticle; GO, graphene oxide; GOx, glucose oxidase; LSPR, localized surface plasmon resonance; N.R., not reported; RIU, refractive index unit; SMF, single-mode fiber; SPR, surface plasmon resonance; TFBG, tilted fiber Bragg grating.

sensor to detect the cholesterol level in the sample. However, the sensitivity of this method is not high, which affects the accuracy of the result. In recent years, biosensors based on plasma phenomena have attracted much attention due to their great advantages such as high portability, high sensitivity, and simple operation. Different studies with AuNPs assisted plasmonic biosensors were conducted for the detection of bacterias and viruses. A few of the notable studies are mentioned next.

Here, an optical fiber-based sensor probe with good shape of a tapered structure is fabricated and fixed with AuNPs (10.5 ± 0.5 nm of particle size) and cholesterol oxidase (ChOx) on the sensing region in proper order to improve selectivity and sensitivity. The typical experimental setup for cholesterol detection using a AuNPs-immobilized LSPR phenomenon-based sensor is presented in Figure 4.12. The proposed sensor probe exhibits excellent performance in cholesterol quantity detection, that the detection limit is 53.1 nm in the linear range of 0–10 mM as well as in the range of 10 nM–10 mM; the sensitivity, liner R2, and resolution are 0.125%/mM, 0.9952, and 0.12, respectively. Compared to the existing sensors, this fabrication technique and workability of the developed sensor probe reveal more versatility and better performance over the various sensing performance parameters such as stability, reproducibility, linearity, selectivity, and reusability (Kumar, Kaushik et al. 2019). The measurement results such as LSPR spectra, linearity plot, and selectivity plot are shown in Figures 4.13 and 4.14. The range of studies for the detection of cholesterol using plasmonic based technique are represented with Table 4.3.

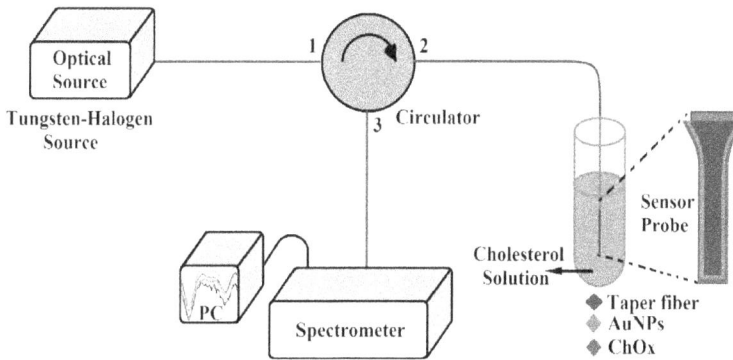

FIGURE 4.12 Typical experimental setup for cholesterol detection using AuNPs-immobilized LSPR phenomenon-based sensor (Kumar, Kaushik et al. 2019).

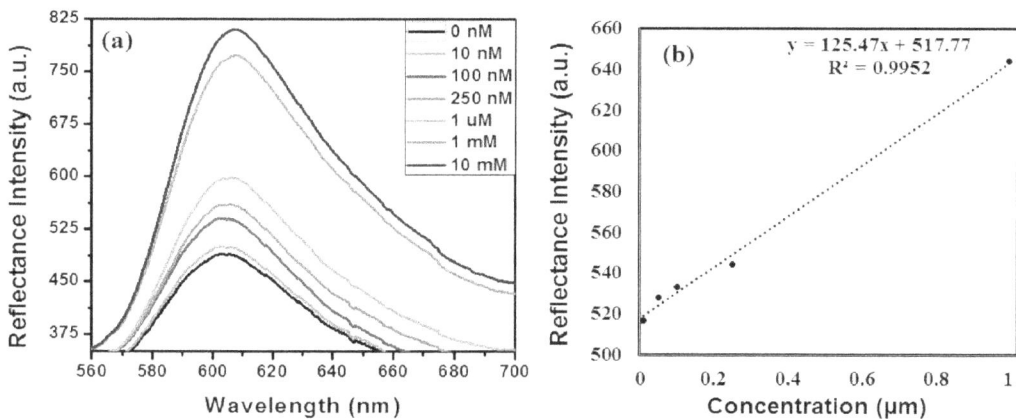

FIGURE 4.13 Measurement results of cholesterol sensor: (a) LSPR spectra and (b) linearity plot (Kumar, Kaushik et al. 2019).

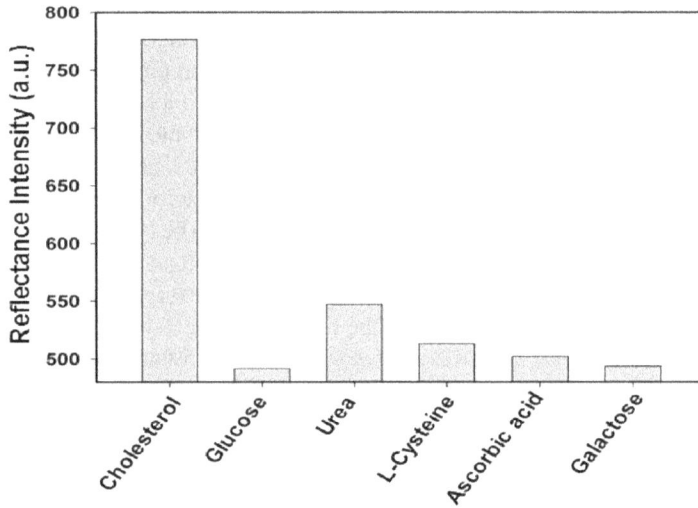

FIGURE 4.14   Selectivity test of AuNPs-immobilized LSPR phenomenon-based cholesterol sensor (Kumar, Kaushik et al. 2019).

TABLE 4.3

Summary of Different Gold Nanoparticles Assisted Plasmonic Biosensors for Cholesterol Detection

Material used	Mechanism	Structure used	Linear range	Detection limit	Sensitivity	Ref.
AuNPs	LSPR	Simple SMF	10 nM—1 µM	53.1 nM	0.125%/mM	Kumar, Kaushik et al. 2019
AgNPs/GO	LSPR	Plastic-clad silica SMF	0–10 mM	1.131 mM	5.14 nm/mM	Semwal and Gupta 2018
AuNPs	LSPR	SMF-HCF	50 nM—1 µM	25.5 nM	16.149 nm/µM	Kumar, Singh, Kaushik et al. 2019
AuNPs and ZnO-NPs	LSPR	AuNPs (10 nm)/ZnO-NPs/ MPM fiber structure	0.1–10 mM	0.6161 mM	0.6898 nm/mM	Agrawal, Zhang, Saha, Kumar, Pu et al. 2020
		AuNPs (30 nm)/ZnO-NPs/ MPM fiber structure	0.1–10 mM	1.2777 mM	0.3319 nm/mM	
		AuNPs (10 nm)/ ZnO-NPs/ SPS fiber structure	1–10 mM	2.1748 mM	0.1976 nm/mM	
Cyclodextrin capped AuNPs	LSPR	Tapered structure	IE-18–IE-6	N.R.	N.R.	(Song et al. 2019)

Note: AuNP, gold nanoparticle; GO, graphene oxide; HCF, hollow-core fiber; LSPR, localized surface plasmon resonance; MMF, multimode fiber; MPM, MMF-PSF-MMF; N.R., not reported; PSF, photosensitive fiber; SMF, single-mode fiber; SPS, SMF-PSF-SMF; ZnO-NP, zinc-oxide nanoparticle.

4.4.3   Gold Nanoparticles Assisted Other Important Biosensors

A large range of biomolecules can be detected using plasmonic based technique and represented in tabular form in Table 4.4. The biomolecules such as uric acid (UA), L-cysteine (L-Cys), alanine aminotransferase (ALT), creatinine, and ascorbic acid (AA) are presented in proposed table. The

TABLE 4.4

Summary of Different Gold Nanoparticles Assisted Plasmonic Biosensors for Other Biomolecules Detection

Detection	Material used	Linear range	Detection limit	Sensitivity	Ref.
Ascorbic acid	AuNPs and ZnO-NPs	1–200 μM	12.56 μM	6 nm/mM	Zhu, Singh et al. 2020
		10–200 μM	25.78 μM	5.7 nm/mM	
Uric acid	AuNPs (10 nm)	10–800 μM	175.89 μM	0.0073 nm/μM	Singh, Zhu et al. 2020
	AuNPs (30 nm)	10–800 μM	280.07 μM	0.0131 nm/μM	
Uric acid	AuNPs	50 μM–1 mM	N.R.	0.005%/mM	Kumar, Singh, Zhu et al. 2019
	AuNPs/GO	10 μM–1 mM	65.60 μM	2.1%/mM	
Uric acid	GO/AuNPs	10–800 μM	206 μM	0.0082 nm/μM	Kumar, Kaushik et al. 2019
L-Cysteine	AuNPs/GO	0 μM–1 mM	152.5 μM	0.0012 nm/μM	Singh, Singh, Zhang et al. 2020
Alanine aminotransferase	AuNPs/MoS$_2$-NPs/ CeO$_2$-NPs	10–1000 U/L	10.61 U/L	4.1 pm/(U/L)	Wang et al. 2021
Creatinine	AuNPs, GO, molybdenum disulfide nanoparticles (MoS$_2$-NPs)	0–2000 μM	128.4 μM	0.0025 nm/μM	Li et al. 2021

Note: AuNP, gold nanoparticle; CeO$_2$-NP, cerium oxide nanoparticle; GO, graphene oxide; MoS$_2$-NP, molybdenum disulfide nanoparticle; N.R., not reported; ZnO-NP, zinc-oxide nanoparticle.

different studies with AuNPs assisted plasmonic biosensors are presented for the detection of various biomolecules. A few of the notable studies are indicated later.

ALT can be detected in a variety of organs and tissues, including the liver, adipose tissue, and intestine and is recognized as a barometer of liver health. In this study, a kind of optical fiber with tapered-in-tapered (TIT) structure has been developed initially. In addition, besides the AuNPs, other special nanomaterials like molybdenum disulfide nanoparticles (MoS$_2$-NPs) and Ceria nanoparticles (CeO$_2$-NPs) are innovatively used to modify the sensing region to enhance the subsequent adhesion of functionalized enzymes. After detection, the probe shows a good linear relationship with the quantitative test samples. The experimental setup of detection of LSPR-based ALT sensor is demonstrated in Figure 4.15.

Due to the presence of many interfering substances in the serum samples, the traditional, widely used electrochemical methods cannot effectively distinguish the target analysis with low signal resolution. Although some sensors have a better linear fitting ratio, the result of the linearity range is too small to cover the normal range of human enzyme activity. In this work, a novel LSPR-based biosensor associated with TIT structure based SMF was developed. The novel nanomaterial-based LSPR sensor has great potential and undisputed research value, and it outshines the traditional ALT enzyme detection method. The measurement results of the alanine aminotransferase sensor, such as LSPR spectra, linearity plot, and selectivity test, are presented in Figures 4.16 and 4.17.

4.4.4 Gold Nanoparticles Assisted Biosensors for Bacteria and Virus Detection

Traditional methods, such as the virus detection systems (non-polymerase chain reaction) on the market, have complete easy-operational processes and concurrent analysis of multiple samples. However, due to the limitation of sensitivity, it seems hard to analyze the signals of samples at very low concentrations, which leads to false-negative results. In recent years, a new kind of detection method was developed, based on well-known SPR and LSPR, that can capture specific viral

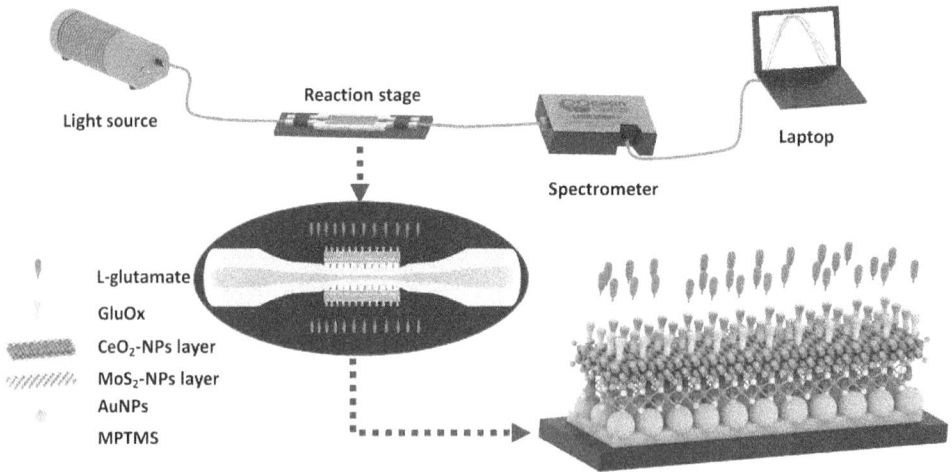

FIGURE 4.15 Experimental setup for ALT detection using the LSPR sensor (Wang et al. 2021).

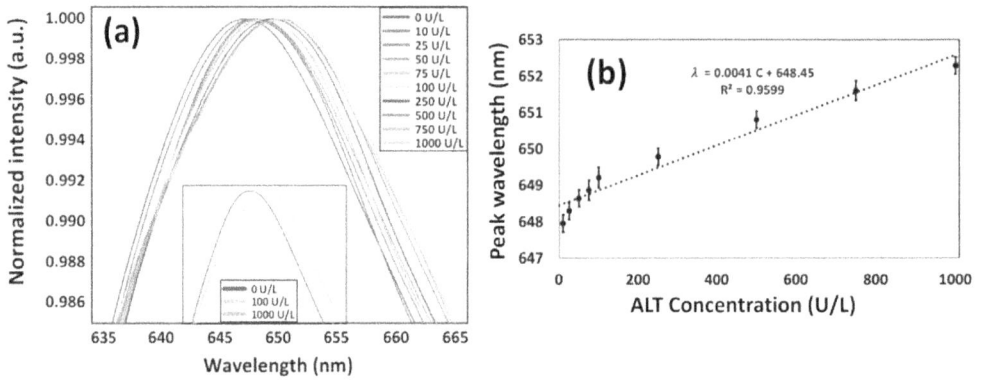

FIGURE 4.16 Measurement results of alanine aminotransferase sensor: (a) LSPR spectra and (b) linearity plot (Wang et al. 2021).

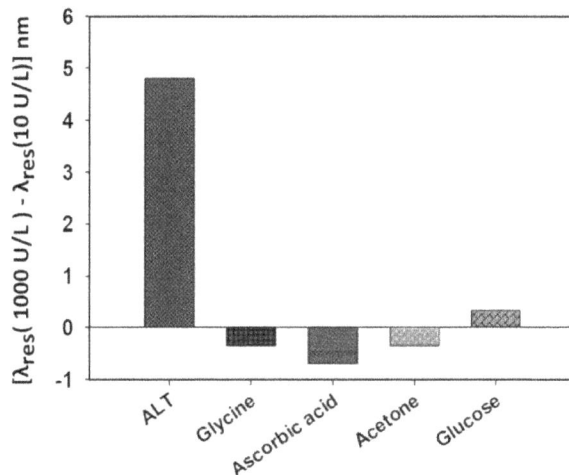

FIGURE 4.17 Selectivity test of AuNPs-immobilized LSPR phenomenon based alanine aminotransferase sensor (Wang et al. 2021).

analytes through receptors on the sensing region. This method is simple but highly sensitive and can amplify the signal of the sample at very low concentration to complete the response analysis. In addition, through experimental analysis, it is found that the size and shape of plasma particles can be adjusted as well as the structure of metal film can be designed to further improve the sensitivity of the sensor. At the same time, the system based on SPR builds a system in reusability and miniaturization. Compared with the SPR sensor system, the LSPR-sensing system is more advantageous to miniaturization. It has made greater progress in the research on effective observation of light response. There is no doubt that SPR and LSPR systems have a bright future, but there is still a long way to go. Overall, research on the SPR- and LSPR-based virus detection has demonstrated great potential to challenge existing traditional detection methods. The prospects for the next generation of virus detection technology are to ensure basic requirements like high sensitivity and anti-interference ability but also to design it to be as simple as possible to operate, convenient, faster, and more universal. As a guideline, an integrated biosensor system could be developed for simultaneous analysis of multiple analytes in one test step. To realize this idea, the choice of auxiliary material and aptamer and the corresponding optimization modification method must be determined. In the future, once this new concept of SPR or LSPR virus detection sensors becomes popular, people will be able to quickly detect virus anytime and anywhere through mobile phones, wearable devices, etc. This will profoundly change future measures to prevent and control viral epidemics. A few of the notable, past studies with AuNPs assisted biosensors used in the work of virus and bacteria quantity detection are mentioned in the following section.

4.4.5 GOLD NANOPARTICLE-BASED SENSOR FOR DENGUE IMMUNOASSAY

The theoretical assumption for early detection of dengue virus based on the SPR system is that one fixing ligand can bind to four different dengue serotypes, and their visualizations are shown in Figures 4.18 and 4.19 (Jahanshahi et al. 2014). Dengue fever is an acute, insect-borne disease that mainly affects adults. Due to the complexity and high cost of specific dengue detection, which causes a considerable impact on human health and the local economy, the research community is committed to explore detection technology that has low cost, is simple to operate, and is fast and reliable to replace the traditional detection methods. In this section, a novel LSPR-based all-fiber (62.5 μm/125 μm) sensor using the principle of specular reflection from AuNPs coating layer is proposed for the diagnosis of acute-stage dengue. The biosensor is simply made by immobilizing an anti-dengue NS1 antibody over AuNPs layer on the end-face of the probe. The developed sensing probe is well used for quantity detection of NS1 antigen with the limit of quantification as 0.074 μg/mL = 1.54 nM, and excellent linear correlation among wavelength shifts to NS1 antigen concentration. From the results, the sensor can detect dengue NS1 antigen in symptomatic patient samples as expected, as well as it

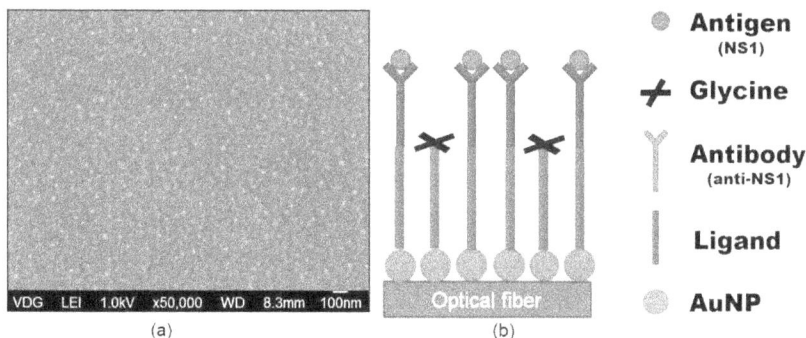

FIGURE 4.18 SEM image of AuNPs on the end-face of an optical fiber. (b) Fiber end-face with AuNPs, ligand, anti-NS1 antibody, glycine, and adsorbed dengue NS1 antigen (Camara et al. 2013).

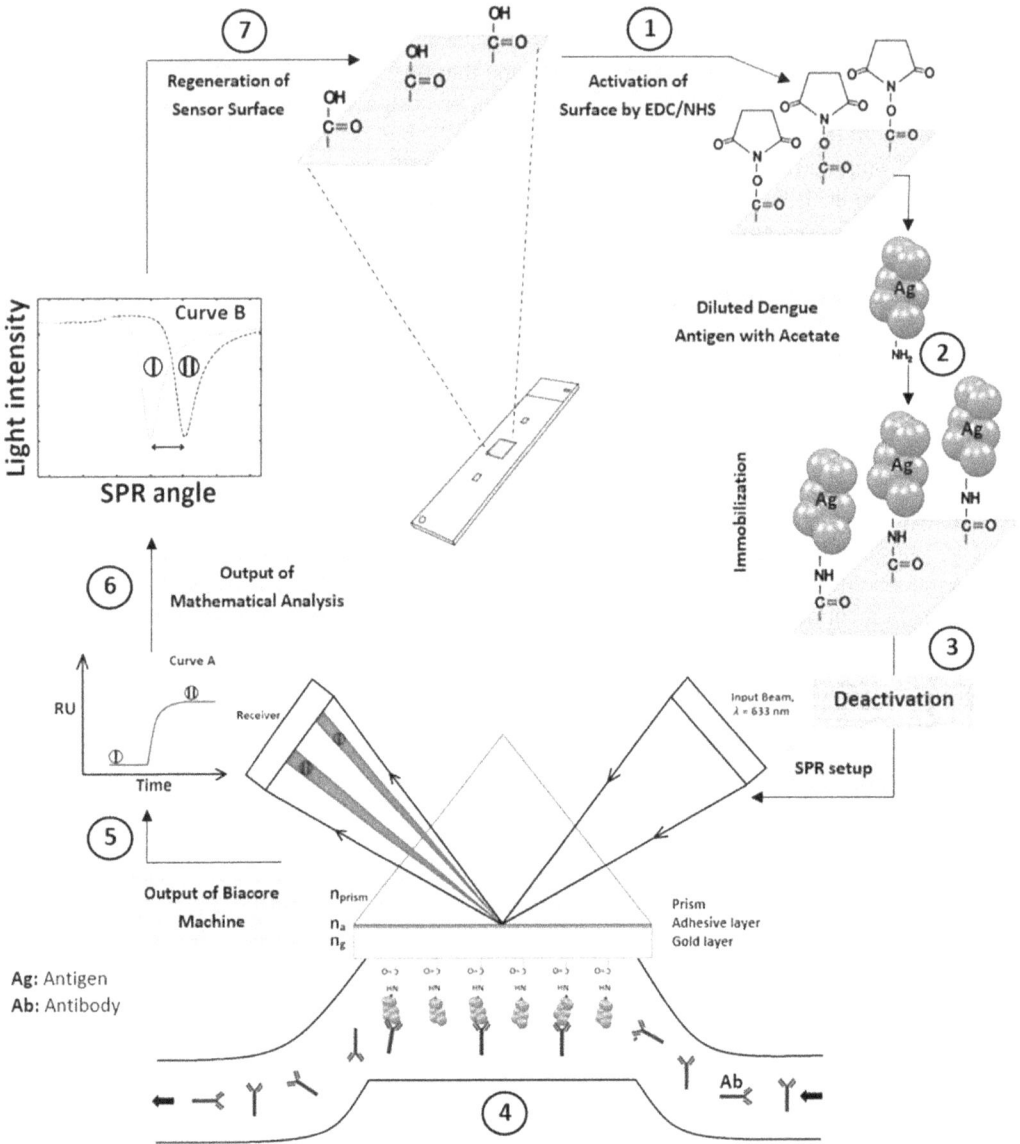

FIGURE 4.19 Dengue virus diagnosis SPR phenomenon (Jahanshahi et al. 2014).

shows potential for use for acute-infectious dengue diagnosis (Camara et al. 2013). Studies for the detection of bacteria and virus using plasmonic-based technique is presented in Table 4.5.

4.4.6 GOLD NANOPARTICLES ASSISTED BIOSENSORS FOR DNA/RNA AND CELLS DETECTION

The plasmonic phenomenon-based DNA/RNA and cells detection is explored at a higher level as the AuNPs-coating technique used in SPR-based platforms shows high antioxidant properties and a straightforward procedure. Therefore, in the detection process, the uniform DNA/RNA-specific molecules modified on the end-face of SPR culture-medium can successfully capture DNA/RNA molecules in samples, thus achieving high sensitivity detection to cells and DNA/RNA. A few AuNPs assisted selected plasmonic-based studies for the detection of cells and DNA/RNA are as follows.

TABLE 4.5

Summary of Different Gold Nanoparticles Assisted Plasmonic Biosensors for Bacteria and Virus Detection

Detection	Material used	Linear range	Detection limit	Sensitivity	Ref.
IgG	Gold film	N.R.	37 ng/mL	3915 nm/RIU	Zhou et al. 2018
Cytokeratin cells	Gold film	N.R.	1 pM	N.R.	Ribaut et al. 2017
Dengue	Gold film	0.0001–0.01 nM	N.R.	$39.96°$ nM^{-1}	Omar et al. 2018
Avian influenza virus subtype H6	Gold film	N.R.	5.14×105 EID$_{50}$/ 0.1 mL	N.R.	Zhao et al. 2016
Anti-biotin	AuNPs	52.4–349 nM	29.5 nM	N.R.	Wu et al. 2016
Dengue	AuNPs	N.R.	1.54 nM	43 nm/(ng/mm^2)	Camara et al. 2013
Malaria	Gold film	N.R.	0.007	14285.71 nm/RIU (Ring phase)	Chaudhary, Kumar, and Kumar 2021
			0.019	10000 nm/RIU (Trophozoite phase)	
			0.029	8206.09 nm/RIU (Schizont phase)	

Note: AuNP, gold nanoparticle; IgG, immunoglobulin G; N.R., not reported; RIU, refractive index unit.

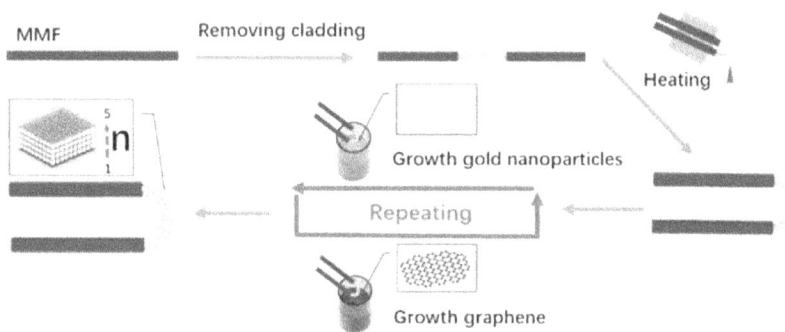

FIGURE 4.20 Preparation procedure of n*(Au/G)@U-MMF sensor probe to measure time- and concentration-dependent DNA hybridization kinetics (Li et al. 2020).

In this section, the fabrication technology of U-type optical fiber is introduced in detail, and the characteristics of the U-shape optical fiber are studied. Thanks to the ease of fabrication and excellent sensitivity, the structure exhibits strong potential for sensing. As shown in Figure 4.20, a U-shaped multimode fiber-based LSPR biosensor has been fabricated using AuNPs and multilayer graphene as 3D modification material. AuNPs and graphene films are prepared by reducing chloroauric acid and liquid/chemical methods, respectively. The obtained 3D U-shaped probes are applied to investigate the time–concentration relationship of DNA hybridization kinetics. The sensitivity of the sensor is 1251.44 nM/RIU in the detection range of 0.1–100 nM, and the detection limit is 0.1 nM. In addition, the probe exhibits high stability and repeatability in the test process. This shows that the technology has excellent performance and can be further studied in single nucleotide analysis, disease biomarkers, transcriptional profiling, and gene screening (Li et al. 2020). Figure 4.21 presents a basic diagram of the polymer-templated AuNPs immobilized optical fiber-based LSPR sensor for quantity measurement of IgG. The range of studies for the detection of DNA/RNA and cells using plasmonic-based technique are represented in Table 4.6.

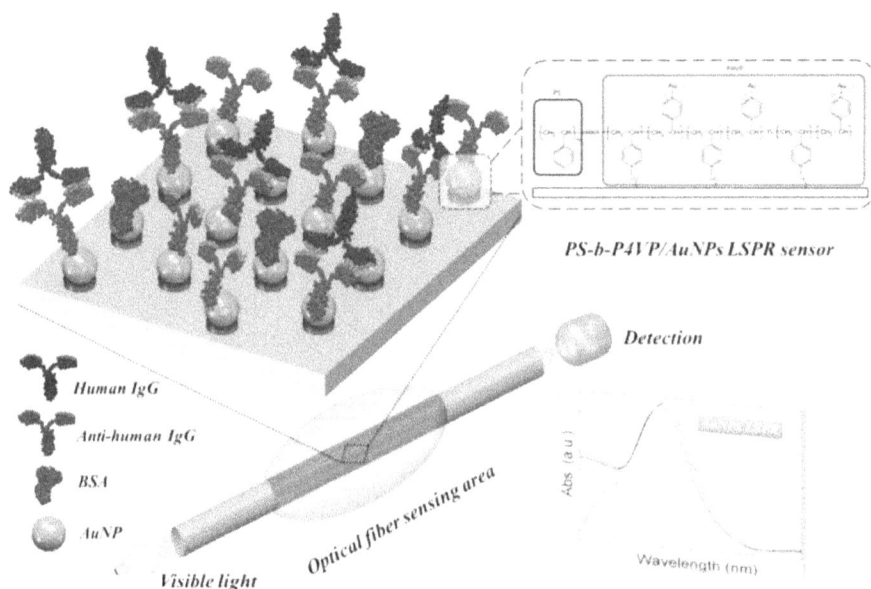

FIGURE 4.21 Polymer-templated gold nanoparticles immobilized optical fiber-based LSPR sensor for the measurement of IgG.

Source: Reprinted with permission from *ACS Sensors*, Copyright 2022, American Chemical Society (Lu et al. 2019).

TABLE 4.6

Different Gold Nanoparticles Assisted Plasmonic Biosensors for DNA/RNA and Cells Detection

Detection	Material used	Linear range	Detection limit	Sensitivity	Ref.
Cancer cells	AuNPs/CuO	$1 \times 10^2 - 1 \times 10^6$ cells/mL	3, 2, 2, 2, 4,10 cells/mL	N.R.	Singh, Kumar et al. 2020
Thyroglobulin (Tg) detection	AuNPs	1 pg/mL–10 ng/mL	0.19 pg/mL	13.07 RIU^{-1}	Kim et al. 2019
N-glycan and cancer cells	AuNPs (U-shaped fiber)	$1 \times 10^2 - 1 \times 10^6$ cells/mL	30 cells/mL	N.R.	Luo et al. 2019
	AuNPs (Straight fiber)	$5 \times 10^3 - 1 \times 10^6$ cells/mL	879 cells/mL	N.R.	
Thrombin	AuNPs	1–35 nM	1 nM	3.21×10^7 dB/M	Lao et al. 2019
Collagen-IV	AuNPs/ZnO-NPs	N.R.	314.04 ng/mL	0.0031 nm/ng/mL	Kaushik et al. 2020
DNA hybridization	Gold nanodisks	N.R.	10 fM	227 nm/RIU	Kaye et al. 2017
DNA hybridization	3D composite structure of AuNPs and multilayer graphene films	N.R.	0.1 nM	1251.44 nm/RIU	Li et al. 2020
Cytokeratin	Gold film	N.R.	1 pM	N.R.	Ribaut et al. 2017
Human IgG	Polymer-templated AuNPs	N.R.	1.2 nM	570%/RIU	Lu et al. 2019

Note: AuNP, gold nanoparticle; CuO, copper oxide; N.R., not reported; RIU, refractive index unit; ZnO-NP, zinc-oxide nanoparticle.

4.5 SUMMARY AND CONCLUSION

In this chapter, a AuNPs-based plasmonic sensor is presented and demonstrated for different types of biosensing applications. The comparative study over a large range of AuNPs assisted P-OFSs are reported in this chapter. The AuNPs with different sizes ranging from 5 to 100 nm are synthesized and used in the development of P-OFSs. In the design of plasmonic biosensors, there are various ways to improve the sensing performance and sensitivity, including (i) synthesizing NP arrays of different sizes and shapes and (ii) adjusting and controlling the local electric field intensity near the substrate of the plasma sensor to improve the sensing performance and sensitivity. In addition, the particle spacing of a NPs array is also a key factor affecting the sensing performance, which can be adjusted by special polymer additive (methotrexate and testosterone). The in-depth study of the properties of AuNPs plays an important role in the development of plasma sensors for various scenarios in areas like gene transcriptional profiling, disease biomarkers, gene screening, and single nucleotides. In comparison with other conventional sensors for biosensing applications, plasmonic-based sensors exhibit cost-efficiency, sensitivity, label-free detection, better antioxidation, and biological compatibility.

The classical synthetic routes of AuNPs are introduced in this chapter, as well as the sensing system based on nanoscale LSPR or micro-scale SPR, which are considered as a new generation of optical fiber detection technology. Finally, the mechanisms of AuNPs to antibacterial agents are investigated and discussed. In addition to this, major areas of improvements are (i) miniaturization of P-OFSs based on portable and economical biosensing for detection of different biomolecules and (ii) development of eco-friendly (green) synthesis methods to synthesis AuNPs efficiently, which can be scaled up and will be sustainable.

REFERENCES

Agrawal, N., C. Saha, C. Kumar, R. Singh, B. Zhang, R. Jha, and S. Kumar. 2020. "Detection of L-cysteine using silver nanoparticles and graphene oxide immobilized tapered SMS optical fiber structure." *IEEE Sensors Journal* 20 (19):11372–11379. DOI: 10.1109/JSEN.2020.2997690.

Agrawal, N., C. Saha, C. Kumar, R. Singh, B. Zhang, and S. Kumar. 2020. "Development of uric acid sensor using copper oxide and silver nanoparticles immobilized SMSMS fiber structure-based probe." *IEEE Transactions on Instrumentation and Measurement* 69 (11):9097–9104. DOI: 10.1109/TIM.2020.2998876.

Agrawal, N., B. Zhang, C. Saha, C. Kumar, B. K. Kaushik, and S. Kumar. 2020. "Development of dopamine sensor using silver nanoparticles and PEG-functionalized tapered optical fiber structure." *IEEE Transactions on Biomedical Engineering* 67 (6):1542–1547. DOI: 10.1109/TBME.2019.2939560.

Agrawal, N., B. Zhang, C. Saha, C. Kumar, X. Pu, and S. Kumar. 2020. "Ultra-sensitive cholesterol sensor using gold and zinc-oxide nanoparticles immobilized core mismatch MPM/SPS probe." *Journal of Lightwave Technology* 38 (8):2523–2529.

Agrawal, Niteshkumar, Reshu Saxena, Lokendra Singh, Chinmoy Saha, and Santosh Kumar. 2021. "Recent advancements in plasmonic optical biosensors: A review." *ISSS Journal of Micro and Smart Systems*. DOI: 10.1007/s41683-021-00079-0.

Calandra, Pietro, Giuseppe Calogero, Alessandro Sinopoli, and Pietro Giuseppe Gucciardi. 2010. "Metal nanoparticles and carbon-based nanostructures as advanced materials for cathode application in dye-sensitized solar cells." *International Journal of Photoenergy* 2010:109495. DOI: 10.1155/2010/109495.

Camara, Alexandre R., Paula M. P. Gouvêa, Ana Carolina M. S. Dias, Arthur M. B. Braga, Rosa F. Dutra, Renato E. de Araujo, and Isabel C. S. Carvalho. 2013. "Dengue immunoassay with an LSPR fiber optic sensor." *Optics Express* 21 (22):27023–27031. DOI: 10.1364/OE.21.027023.

Chack, Devendra, Niteshkumar Agrawal, and S. K. Raghuwanshi. 2014. "To analyse the performance of tapered and MMI assisted splitter on the basis of geographical parameters." *Optik* 125 (11):2568–2571. https://doi.org/10.1016/j.ijleo.2013.11.019.

Chaudhary, V. S., D. Kumar, and S. Kumar. 2021. "Gold-immobilized photonic crystal fiber-based SPR biosensor for detection of malaria disease in human body." *IEEE Sensors Journal* 21 (16):17800–17807. DOI: 10.1109/JSEN.2021.3085829.

Chen, Kuan-Chieh, Yu-Le Li, Chao-Wei Wu, and Chia-Chin Chiang. 2018. "Glucose sensor using U-shaped optical fiber probe with gold nanoparticles and glucose oxidase." *Sensors (Basel, Switzerland)* 18 (4):1217. DOI: 10.3390/s18041217.

Haiss, W., N. T. Thanh, J. Aveyard, and D. G. Fernig. 2007a. "Determination of size and concentration of gold nanoparticles from UV-vis spectra." *Analytical Chemistry* 79 (11):4215–4221. DOI: 10.1021/ac0702084.

Haiss, Wolfgang, Nguyen T. K. Thanh, Jenny Aveyard, and David G. Fernig. 2007b. "Determination of size and concentration of gold nanoparticles from UV-vis spectra." *Analytical Chemistry* 79 (11):4215–4221. DOI: 10.1021/ac0702084.

Herizchi, Roya, Elham Abbasi, Morteza Milani, and Abolfazl Akbarzadeh. 2016. "Current methods for synthesis of gold nanoparticles." *Artificial Cells, Nanomedicine, and Biotechnology* 44 (2):596–602. DOI: 10.3109/21691401.2014.971807.

Houngkamhang, Nongluck, Sittan Charoensuwan, O. Sonthipakdee, Kawin Nawattanapaiboon, Armote Somboonkaew, and R. Amarit. 2018. "Gold-nanoparticle-based fiber optic sensor for sensing the refractive index of environmental solutions." *Chiang Mai Journal of Science* 45:2168–2177.

Jahanshahi, Peyman, Erfan Zalnezhad, Shamala Devi Sekaran, and Faisal Rafiq Mahamd Adikan. 2014. "Rapid immunoglobulin M-based dengue diagnostic test using surface plasmon resonance biosensor." *Scientific Reports* 4 (1):3851. DOI: 10.1038/srep03851.

Jana, N. R., L. Gearheart, and C. J. Murphy. 2001. "Seed-mediated growth approach for shape-controlled synthesis of spheroidal and rod-like gold nanoparticles using a surfactant template." *Advanced Materials* 13 (18):1389–1393. https://doi.org/10.1002/1521-4095(200109)13:18<1389::AID-ADMA1389>3.0.CO;2-F.

Kaushik, B. K., L. Singh, R. Singh, G. Zhu, B. Zhang, Q. Wang, and S. Kumar. 2020. "Detection of collagen-IV using highly reflective metal nanoparticles: Immobilized photosensitive optical fiber-based MZI structure." *IEEE Transactions on NanoBioscience* 19 (3):477–484. DOI: 10.1109/TNB.2020.2998520.

Kaye, Savannah, Zheng Zeng, Mollye Sanders, Krishnan Chittur, Paula M. Koelle, Robert Lindquist, Upender Manne, Yongbin Lin, and Jianjun Wei. 2017. "Label-free detection of DNA hybridization with a compact LSPR-based fiber-optic sensor." *The Analyst* 142 (11):1974–1981. DOI: 10.1039/c7an00249a.

Kim, Hyeong-Min, Dae Hong Jeong, Ho-Young Lee, Jae-Hyoung Park, and Seung-Ki Lee. 2019. "Improved stability of gold nanoparticles on the optical fiber and their application to refractive index sensor based on localized surface plasmon resonance." *Optics & Laser Technology* 114:171–178. https://doi.org/10.1016/j.optlastec.2019.02.002.

Kumar, S., R. Singh, B. K. Kaushik, N. Chen, Q. S. Yang, and X. Zhang. 2019. "LSPR-based cholesterol biosensor using hollow core fiber structure." *IEEE Sensors Journal* 19 (17):7399–7406.

Kumar, S., R. Singh, G. Zhu, Q. Yang, X. Zhang, S. Cheng, B. Zhang, B. K. Kaushik, and F. Liu. 2019. "Development of uric acid biosensor biosensor using gold nanoparticles and graphene oxide functionalized micro-ball fiber sensor probe." *IEEE Transactions on NanoBioscience*:1–1. DOI: 10.1109/TNB.2019.2958891.

Kumar, Santosh, Brajesh Kumar Kaushik, Ragini Singh, Nan-Kuang Chen, Qing Shan Yang, Xia Zhang, Wenjun Wang, and Bingyuan Zhang. 2019. "LSPR-based cholesterol biosensor using a tapered optical fiber structure." *Biomedical Optics Express* 10 (5):2150–2160. DOI: 10.1364/BOE.10.002150.

Lao, J., L. Han, Z. Wu, X. Zhang, Y. Huang, Y. Tang, and T. Guo. 2019. "Gold nanoparticle-functionalized surface plasmon resonance optical fiber biosensor: In situ detection of thrombin with 1 n·M detection limit." *Journal of Lightwave Technology* 37 (11):2748–2755. DOI: 10.1109/JLT.2018.2822827.

Li, Can, Zhen Li, Shuanglu Li, Yanan Zhang, Baoping Sun, Yuehao Yu, Haiyang Ren, Shouzhen Jiang, and Weiwei Yue. 2020. "LSPR optical fiber biosensor based on a 3D composite structure of gold nanoparticles and multilayer graphene films." *Optics Express* 28 (5):6071–6083. DOI: 10.1364/OE.385128.

Li, Muyang, Ragini Singh, Carlos Marques, Bingyuan Zhang, and Santosh Kumar. 2021. "2D material assisted SMF-MCF-MMF-SMF based LSPR sensor for creatinine detection." *Optics Express* 29 (23):38150–38167. DOI: 10.1364/OE.445555.

Li, Yanpeng, Hui Ma, Lin Gan, Qi Liu, Zhijun Yan, Deming Liu, and Qizhen Sun. 2018. "Immobilized optical fiber microprobe for selective and high sensitive glucose detection." *Sensors and Actuators B: Chemical* 255:3004–3010. https://doi.org/10.1016/j.snb.2017.09.123.

Lu, Mengdi, Hu Zhu, C. Geraldine Bazuin, Wei Peng, and Jean-Francois Masson. 2019. "Polymer-templated gold nanoparticles on optical fibers for enhanced-sensitivity localized surface plasmon resonance biosensors." *ACS Sensors* 4 (3):613–622. DOI: 10.1021/acssensors.8b01372.

Luo, Zewei, Yimin Wang, Ya Xu, Xu Wang, Zhijun Huang, Junman Chen, Yongxin Li, and Yixiang Duan. 2019. "Ultrasensitive U-shaped fiber optic LSPR cytosensing for label-free and in situ evaluation of cell surface N-glycan expression." *Sensors and Actuators B: Chemical* 284:582–588. https://doi.org/10.1016/j.snb.2019.01.015.

Mody, Vicky V., Rodney Siwale, Ajay Singh, and Hardik R. Mody. 2010. "Introduction to metallic nanoparticles." *Journal of Pharmacy & Bioallied Sciences* 2 (4):282–289. DOI: 10.4103/0975-7406.72127.

Omar, Nur Alia Sheh, Yap Wing Fen, Jaafar Abdullah, Che Engku Noramalina Che Engku Chik, and Mohd Adzir Mahdi. 2018. "Development of an optical sensor based on surface plasmon resonance phenomenon for diagnosis of dengue virus E-protein." *Sensing and Bio-Sensing Research* 20:16–21. https://doi.org/10.1016/j.sbsr.2018.06.001.

Reetz, Manfred T., and Wolfgang Helbig. 1994. "Size-selective synthesis of nanostructured transition metal clusters." *Journal of the American Chemical Society* 116 (16):7401–7402. DOI: 10.1021/ja00095a051.

Ribaut, Clotilde, Médéric Loyez, Jean-Charles Larrieu, Samia Chevineau, Pierre Lambert, Myriam Remmelink, Ruddy Wattiez, and Christophe Caucheteur. 2017. "Cancer biomarker sensing using packaged plasmonic optical fiber gratings: Towards in vivo diagnosis." *Biosensors and Bioelectronics* 92:449–456. https://doi.org/10.1016/j.bios.2016.10.081.

Semwal, V., and B. D. Gupta. 2018. "LSPR- and SPR-based fiber-optic cholesterol sensor using immobilization of cholesterol oxidase over silver nanoparticles coated graphene oxide nanosheets." *IEEE Sensors Journal* 18 (3):1039–1046.

Shah, M., V. Badwaik, Y. Kherde, H. K. Waghwani, T. Modi, Z. P. Aguilar, H. Rodgers, W. Hamilton, T. Marutharaj, C. Webb, M. B. Lawrenz, and R. Dakshinamurthy. 2014. "Gold nanoparticles: Various methods of synthesis and antibacterial applications." *Frontiers in Bioscience (Landmark Ed)* 19:1320–1344. DOI: 10.2741/4284.

Singh, L., N. Agrawal, C. Saha, and B. K. Kaushik. 2022. "A plus shaped cavity in optical fiber based refractive index sensor." *IEEE Transactions on NanoBioscience* 21 (2):199–205. DOI: 10.1109/TNB.2021.3121779.

Singh, L., R. Singh, B. Zhang, B. K. Kaushik, and S. Kumar. 2020. "Localized surface plasmon resonance based hetero-core optical fiber sensor structure for the detection of L-cysteine." *IEEE Transactions on Nanotechnology* 19:201–208. DOI: 10.1109/TNANO.2020.2975297.

Singh, L., G. Zhu, R. Singh, B. Zhang, W. Wang, B. K. Kaushik, and S. Kumar. 2020. "Gold nanoparticles and uricase functionalized tapered fiber sensor for uric acid detection." *IEEE Sensors Journal* 20 (1):219–226.

Singh, Lokendra, Niteshkumar Agrawal, Chinmoy Saha, Brij Mohan Singh, and Taresh Singh. 2022. "Highly sensitive plus shaped cavity in silicon fiber for RI detection of water samples." *Silicon*. DOI: 10.1007/s12633-021-01519-0.

Singh, Ragini, Santosh Kumar, Feng-Zhen Liu, Cheng Shuang, Bingyuan Zhang, Rajan Jha, and Brajesh Kumar Kaushik. 2020. "Etched multicore fiber sensor using copper oxide and gold nanoparticles decorated graphene oxide structure for cancer cells detection." *Biosensors and Bioelectronics* 168:112557. https://doi.org/10.1016/j.bios.2020.112557.

Singh, Sachin, Dr Singh, Ahmad Umar, Pooja Lohia, Hasan Albargi, L. Castañeda, and D. K. Dwivedi. 2020. "2D nanomaterial-based surface plasmon resonance sensors for biosensing applications." *Micromachines* 11:779. DOI: 10.3390/mi11080779.

Song, Hang, Hongxin Zhang, Zhuo Sun, Ziyang Ren, Xiaoyu Yang, and Qi Wang. 2019. "Triangular silver nanoparticle U-bent fiber sensor based on localized surface plasmon resonance." *AIP Advances* 9 (8):085307. DOI: 10.1063/1.5111820.

Tong, Rui-jie, Feng Xia, and Yun Peng. 2019. "Current status of optical fiber biosensor based on surface plasmon resonance." *Biosensors and Bioelectronics* 142:111505. DOI: 10.1016/j.bios.2019.111505.

Wang, Fang, Yang Zhang, Zexu Liu, Huizhen Yuan, Zhenlin Wu, Dapeng Zhou, Zhenguo Jing, and Wei Peng. 2018. "Highly sensitive glucose detection using Au Nanoparticles based fiber optic SPR sensor." 26th International Conference on Optical Fiber Sensors, Lausanne, 24 Sep.

Wang, Zhi, Ragini Singh, Carlos Marques, Rajan Jha, Bingyuan Zhang, and Santosh Kumar. 2021. "Taper-in-taper fiber structure-based LSPR sensor for alanine aminotransferase detection." *Optics Express* 29 (26):43793–43810. DOI: 10.1364/OE.447202.

Wu, Chin-Wei, Chang-Yue Chiang, Chien-Hsing Chen, Chung-Sheng Chiang, Chih-To Wang, and Lai-Kwan Chau. 2016. "Self-referencing fiber optic particle plasmon resonance sensing system for real-time biological monitoring." *Talanta* 146:291–298. https://doi.org/10.1016/j.talanta.2015.08.047.

Yang, Qingshan, Xia Zhang, Santosh Kumar, Ragini Singh, Bingyuan Zhang, Chenglin Bai, and Xipeng Pu. 2020. "Development of glucose sensor using gold nanoparticles and glucose-oxidase functionalized tapered fiber structure." *Plasmonics* 15 (3):841–848. DOI: 10.1007/s11468-019-01104-7.

Yang, Qingshan, Guo Zhu, Lokendra Singh, Yu Wang, Ragini Singh, Bingyuan Zhang, Xia Zhang, and Santosh Kumar. 2020. "Highly sensitive and selective sensor probe using glucose oxidase/gold nanoparticles/graphene oxide functionalized tapered optical fiber structure for detection of glucose." *Optik* 208:164536. https://doi.org/10.1016/j.ijleo.2020.164536.

Young, Joseph K., Nastassja A. Lewinski, Robert J. Langsner, Laura C. Kennedy, Arthi Satyanarayan, Vengadesan Nammalvar, Adam Y. Lin, and Rebekah A. Drezek. 2011. "Size-controlled synthesis of monodispersed gold nanoparticles via carbon monoxide gas reduction." *Nanoscale Research Letters* 6 (1):428–428. DOI: 10.1186/1556-276X-6-428.

Yuan, Huizhen, Wei Ji, Shuwen Chu, Siyu Qian, Fang Wang, Jean-Francois Masson, Xiuyou Han, and Wei Peng. 2018. "Fiber-optic surface plasmon resonance glucose sensor enhanced with phenylboronic acid modified Au nanoparticles." *Biosensors and Bioelectronics* 117:637–643. https://doi.org/10.1016/j.bios.2018.06.042.

Zhang, Xuejun, Ze Wu, Fu Liu, Qiangqiang Fu, Xiaoyong Chen, Jian Xu, Zhaochuan Zhang, Yunyun Huang, Yong Tang, Tuan Guo, and Jacques Albert. 2018. "Hydrogen peroxide and glucose concentration measurement using optical fiber grating sensors with corrodible plasmonic nanocoatings." *Biomedical Optics Express* 9 (4):1735–1744. DOI: 10.1364/BOE.9.001735.

Zhao, Xihong, Yu-Chia Tsao, Fu-Jung Lee, Woo-Hu Tsai, Ching-Ho Wang, Tsung-Liang Chuang, Mu-Shiang Wu, and Chii-Wann Lin. 2016. "Optical fiber sensor based on surface plasmon resonance for rapid detection of avian influenza virus subtype H6: Initial studies." *Journal of Virological Methods* 233:15–22. https://doi.org/10.1016/j.jviromet.2016.03.007.

Zhou, Zhan, Zhuosen Wang, Yiping Tang, Jinwei Gao, Cheng Cheng Zhang, and Qianming Wang. 2018. "Multimodal tracking dopamine using a hybrid inorganic-organic silver nanoparticle and its cellular imaging performance." *Journal of Luminescence* 204:394–400. https://doi.org/10.1016/j.jlumin.2018.08.045.

Zhu, Guo, Niteshkumar Agrawal, Ragini Singh, Santosh Kumar, Bingyuan Zhang, Chinmoy Saha, and Chandrakanta Kumar. 2020. "A novel periodically tapered structure-based gold nanoparticles and graphene oxide: Immobilized optical fiber sensor to detect ascorbic acid." *Optics & Laser Technology* 127:106156. https://doi.org/10.1016/j.optlastec.2020.106156.

Zhu, Guo, Lokendra Singh, Yu Wang, Ragini Singh, Bingyuan Zhang, Fengzhen Liu, Brajesh Kumar Kaushik, and Santosh Kumar. 2020. "Tapered optical fiber-based LSPR biosensor for ascorbic acid detection." *Photonic Sensors*. DOI: 10.1007/s13320-020-0605-2.

5 Silver Nanoparticles Assisted Optical Fiber-Based Plasmonic Biosensors

5.1 INTRODUCTION

The ancient Greek and Roman empires are the first to use silver (Ag) as an antibacterial and antiseptic (Spear 2010). The healing and preservation powers of Ag were mostly used to protect blood vessels from bacterial infections and to make water and other fluids potable (Alexander 2009). On a worldwide scale, Ag has been found to be an effective weapon against disease factors. Silver's antibacterial effect is caused by interactions between Ag ions and the mercaptan groups of enzymes and proteins required by bacteria, resulting in cell death (Dakal et al. 2016). Silver has been designed as nanoparticles (NPs) for decades (less than 100 nm in size) (Agrawal et al. 2021). Thanks to their small size and new material characteristics, Ag nanoparticles (AgNPs) have attracted a lot of interest in the last decade. Their nanometer-scale size allowed them to be deployed in a plethora of novel applications with a variety of bulk material features, including high ultraviolet-visible (UV-Vis) absorption signals that might be used as a nonlabeling sensing approach for biomolecular interactions (Singh, Agrawal, and Saha 2021; Konop et al. 2016; Klasen 2000). AgNPs have a variety of optical properties that have led to new ways of sensing applications, based on many techniques such as colorimetric, scattering, surface-enhanced Raman spectroscopy (SERS), surface plasmonic resonance (SPR), localized SPR (LSPR), and metal enhanced fluorescence (MEF) techniques, all with extremely low limits of detection (LoDs) (Singh et al. 2022, Calderón-Jiménez et al. 2017). AgNPs may be incorporated directly as labels, or they may be necessary for the application's design to fulfill other duties (such as administration of medication) and simply give this extremely effective additional advantage (Xu et al. 2020). Although plasmonic sensing has a lot of potentials, the detection thresholds for most practical applications need to be enhanced (Agrawal, Zhang, Saha, Kumar, Pu et al. 2020). A significant amount of current research is focused on improving the adjustable characteristics of AgNPs in order to increase their responsiveness in plasmonic sensors (Dawadi et al. 2021). In this chapter, a novel optical biosensor assembled with an AgNPs surface has been preliminarily constructed for the detection of different biomolecules, bacteria, viruses, cells, protein, and DNA/RNA (Akter et al. 2018). Focus on Ag-based NPs, thanks to their unique characteristics, has undoubtedly played the most essential role in the realization of the most recent plasmonic applications. This chapter begins with the techniques for making AgNPs with regulated size, homogeneity, and shape (Loiseau et al. 2019). In plasma resonance of precious metals, the Ag LSPR excitation effect is the best; the wavelength range is larger. In addition, Ag has a thinner LSPR band, less dissipation, and a higher refractive index (RI) for plasmon applications than Au. The size and form of the nanostructure (NSs), as well as the surrounding dielectric, may effectively control these plasmon characteristics. Nanorods, nanowires, nanoprisms, and nanoflowers are examples of AgNPs structures of various forms that are frequently employed. For asymmetrically formed AgNPs (e.g., nanowires and nanorods), two plasmon absorbance bands, with SPR peaks between 300 and 800 nm, corresponding to the longitudinal and transverse modes detectable by UV-Vis spectrometer, exist. A coating or shell is used to protect the morphology and surface structure of silver nanorods against halide ions, mercaptan, UV light, heat, and acid. This determines the plasmon band of the Ag nanorods. For example, with greater polymer concentrations, the LSPR band of poly 10 (N-isopropylacrylamide) (PNIPAM) modified Ag nanocolumnar is slightly red-shifted from 514 nm

DOI: 10.1201/9781003243199-5

to 516–522 nm, with an increase in absorbance over the whole spectrum range (Haider and Kang 2015). At the same time, hot areas at the tip of the complete particle surface and the junction of NPs drew a lot of attention, causing SERS to behave abnormally (Zhu et al. 2020). This flower-like structure features a spiky surface and a high number of nanogaps, allowing for wideband plasma scattering spectra in the visible range of 350–750 nm (Zhang et al. 2017).

In addition to their excellent optical properties, AgNPs have excellent electrical conductivity. Thus, according to Ali et al. (Ali et al. 2016), integrating AgNPs into polyacrylonitrile fibers to generate carbon nanofibers (CNFs) boosted the conductive performance of the CNFs. The electrical properties of CNFs have been found to be affected by AgNPs in a concentration-dependent manner. In another study, Huang et al. studied the electrochemical response of AgNPs implanted in composite graphite for the development of electrochemical biosensors (Huang et al. 2014). Graphite–epoxy composite (GEC) dispersion, AgNPs/GEC, and AgNPs/GEC mixed with polyaniline (AgNPs/PANI/GEC) are the three types of composite electrodes employed (Ibrahim et al. 2021). Both composite electrodes treated with AgNPs exhibited a linear increase in redox peak currents, showing that the current sensitivity of the AgNPs-modified composite electrodes has improved. Following that, AgNPs might act as a redox biomolecule capable of oxidation and reduction (Krajczewski and Kudelski 2019). The dissolution of AgNPs, which are employed to build a cholesterol-detecting biosensor, enabled for analyte detection using this redox characteristic. Cholesterol oxidase (ChOx) is used to convert cholesterol to cholest-4-en-3-one and H_2O_2, with H_2O_2 converting AgNPs to Ag+ ions, resulting in a color change from yellow to pinkish/colorless, depending on the quantity of H_2O_2 produced (Ibrahim et al. 2021).

AgNPs are being used because of their unique optoelectronic features, such as their adjustable plasmonic capabilities and excellent electrochemical qualities. A very low LoD toward DNA/RNA, antibody/antigens, and enzymes has shown AgNPs' good electrical conductivity and great sensitivity. In addition, as compared to other metals, Ag has a strong resistance to oxidation and chemical inertness. A general overview on synthesis, characterization, properties, and applications of AgNPs is presented in Section 5.2. A historical perspective of AgNPs and based biosensors and generalized overview are covered in Section 5.3. Moreover, discussion on important features, limitations, and advantages for AgNPs-based biosensor is also thoroughly discussed in this section. The recent developments over AgNPs-based plasmonic biosensors for different applications are well covered. This application covers from biomolecule detection to virus/bacteria/DNA/RNA detection. Figure 5.1

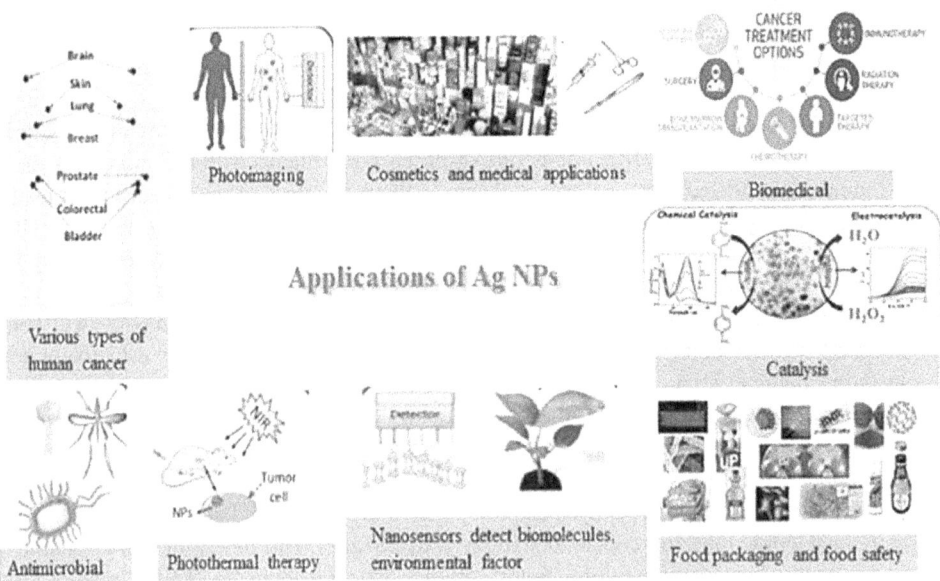

FIGURE 5.1   Various applications of silver nanoparticles (Hawa et al. 2021).

shows the various applications of AgNPs. This information might aid researchers in making judg-ments and considering the design and development of innovative biosensors with high efficiency. The summary, future considerations, and suggestions for a robust and effective biosensing detection approach employing AgNPs-based sensing devices are included in Section 5.4.

5.2 SYNTHESIS, CHARACTERIZATION, PROPERTIES, AND APPLICATIONS OF SILVER NANOPARTICLES

Metal NPs are presently being extensively researched in various fields, covering renewable energy, cos-metics, medicine, environmental concerns, sensor systems, optoelectronic devices, mechanics, and SERS, to name a few. Alkali metal detection in drinking water, adsorbent materials, and water filtration are only a few of the uses for NPs in the environment. The use of functionalized NPs for molecular selective biosens-ing has emerged as popular multidisciplinary research avenue in biology, chemistry, and materials science. Noble metals, particularly AgNPs, have unique and adjustable plasmonic characteristics, and altering the size and form of these metal nanostructures (NSs) enables modifying their reaction to the surrounding environment. Figure 5.2 shows the schematic of the various forms of metal NPs (MNPs).

5.2.1 SYNTHESIS METHODS FOR SILVER NANOPARTICLES AND COMPOSITES

Silver NPs unique opto-electronic capabilities, along with their tiny surface area, have allowed them to be used in sensing applications. With very low detection limits, AgNPs are widely employed for identifying a variety of health and environmental contaminants such as heavy metal ions and other toxic organic compounds (Agrawal, Saha, Kumar, Singh, Zhang, and Kumar 2020). The toxicity of AgNPs has been lowered considerably in recent years utilizing green production techniques (Agrawal, Zhang, Saha, Kumar, Kaushik et al. 2020). The transmission electron microscopy (TEM) image presenting AgNPs with different geometry and shapes such as quasi-spherical, hollow spher-ical, cubic, and Au-Ag nanostars is available in Figure 5.3.

5.2.1.1 Spherical Silver Nanoparticles

To synthesize the spherical AgNPs, various methods are reported by different researchers. An elec-trochemical method is widely used for the preparation of spherical AgNPs. In 2009, Cao et al. described an electrochemical method for the preparation of spherical AgNPs, mostly chemical reduction phenomenon is used in this method (Cao et al. 2009). Similarly, Zhang et al. described the electrochemical method for the synthesis of spherical AgNPs (Zhang et al. 2011):

Electrochemical method: To put it simply, the compound solution 24.55 mL, pure water 24 mL, silver nitrate aqueous solution (0.05 mol/L, 0.05 mL), sodium citrate (0.075 mol/L, 0.5 mL), sodium citrate (0.075 mol/L, 0.5 mL) are prepared at room temperature and then spined in the air. After stirring for a few minutes, 0.25 mL (0.1 mol/L) sodium borohydride is added to the mixture. The color of the AgNPs mixed solution is changed from colorless to dark yellow, suggesting that spherical AgNPs have been successfully produced.

Chemical reduction method: Chemical reduction is used to synthesize Ag-NPs. PVP (a reducing agent and particle stabilizer) and AgNO$_3$ are utilized as starting ingredients. PVP is dissolved in 43 g in 30 mL distilled water, while AgNO$_3$ is dissolved in 0.03 g in 30 mL distilled water. These two solutions are mixed together to make a white solution with a 6:1 PVP to AgNO$_3$ ratio. In a beaker, stir the mixture at 1300 rpm using a magnetic stirrer. Drop by drop, aqueous ammonia is added to the PVP and AgNO$_3$ mixed solution until the milky solution became clear. The production of tiny Ag ion particles occurs as a consequence of this process. After that, the solution is baked for around 40 hours at 160°C in an oven. Small particles evolve into bigger particles at this temperature. The cre-ation of Ag-NPs is indicated by the development of a yellowish clear solution. The Ag-NPs solution is kept in the refrigerator at 4°C before use. The synthesis of Ag-NPs is validated using techniques such as high-resolution transmission electron microscopy (HRTEM) and UV-Vis spectroscopy. The synthesis result of polyvinyl alcohol (PVA)-coated AgNPs using chemical reduction method is shown in Figure 5.4.

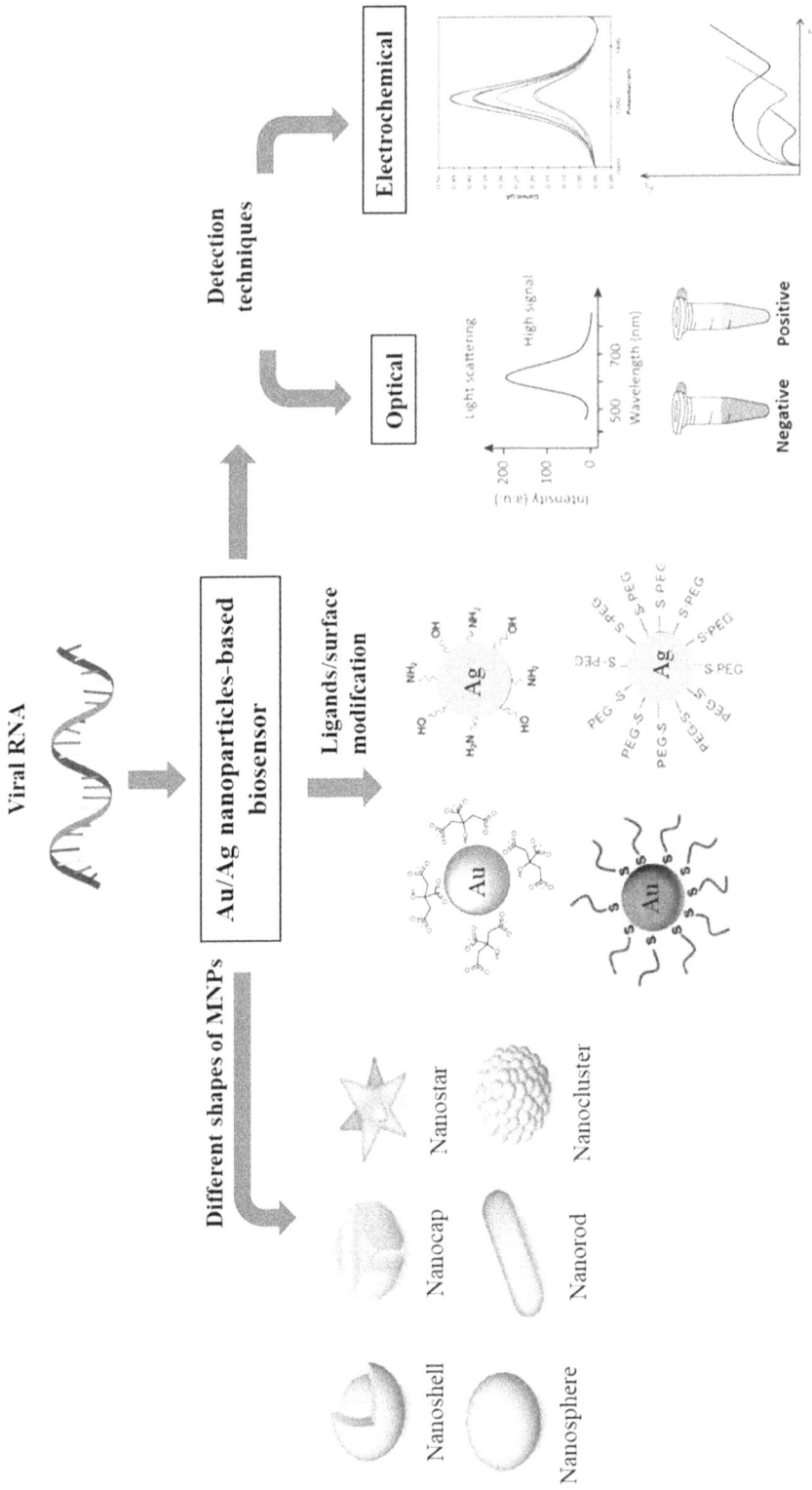

FIGURE 5.2 The various forms of metal nanoparticles (MNPs) like AgNPs, as well as the usage of ligands to stabilize the MNPs. Optical and electrochemical sensing methods are used to confirm the MNPs' optical and electrochemical characteristics (Ibrahim et al. 2021).

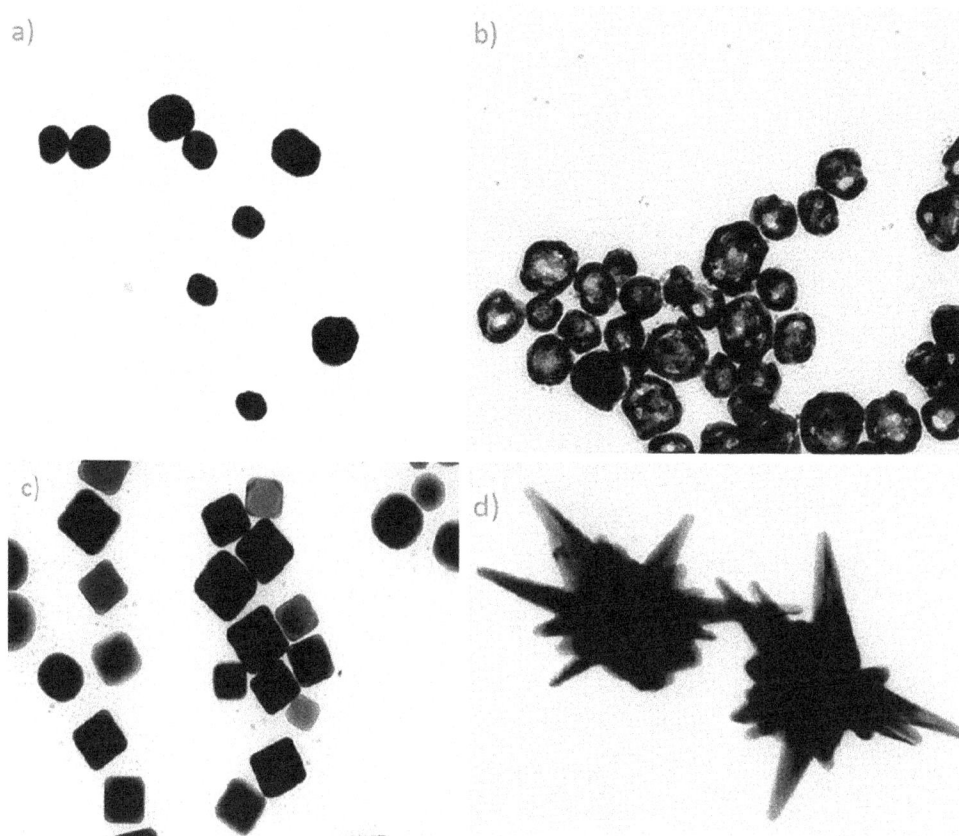

FIGURE 5.3 TEM micrographs of AgNPs with various geometries and shapes: (a) quasi-spherical AgNPs, (b) hollow spherical AgNPs, (c) cubic AgNPs, (d) Au-Ag nanostars (Krajczewski, Kołątaj, and Kudelski 2017).

TABLE 5.1

Summary of Basic Methodologies for Synthesizing AgNPs and Matching Form and Size and Their Applications

Shapes	Sizes (nm)	Synthesis methods	Applications
Spheres	10–100	Chemical reduction	Plasmonic and sensing; catalysis; antimicrobial
Triangles	Width: 100 Height: 50	Chemical reduction; NSL	Plasmonic and sensing; analytical devices (SERS); photovoltaics; molecular detection (Alzheimer disease)
Nanocubes	20–45	Polyol process	Cysteine sensing by plasmons of silver nanocubes; analytical devices (SERS)
Nanowires	Length: 60	Polyol process	Plasmonic and molecule sensing; provide conductive coatings (transparent conductors and flexible electronics)
Nanorods	Length: 250–300	Photochemical; thermal; ORG	Plasmonic and sensing; analytical devices (SERS)
Nanobars	Length: 100	Polyol process	Plasmonic and sensing; analytical devices (SERS)
Pyramides	Edge length: 50–200	Chemical reduction	Plasmonic and sensing; analytical devices (SERS)
Flower-like	200–300	Wet-chemical method	Analytical devices (SERS); catalysis

Source: See Loiseau et al. 2019.

Note: NSL, nanosphere lithography; ORG, oxidation reduction growth; SERS, surface-enhanced Raman scattering.

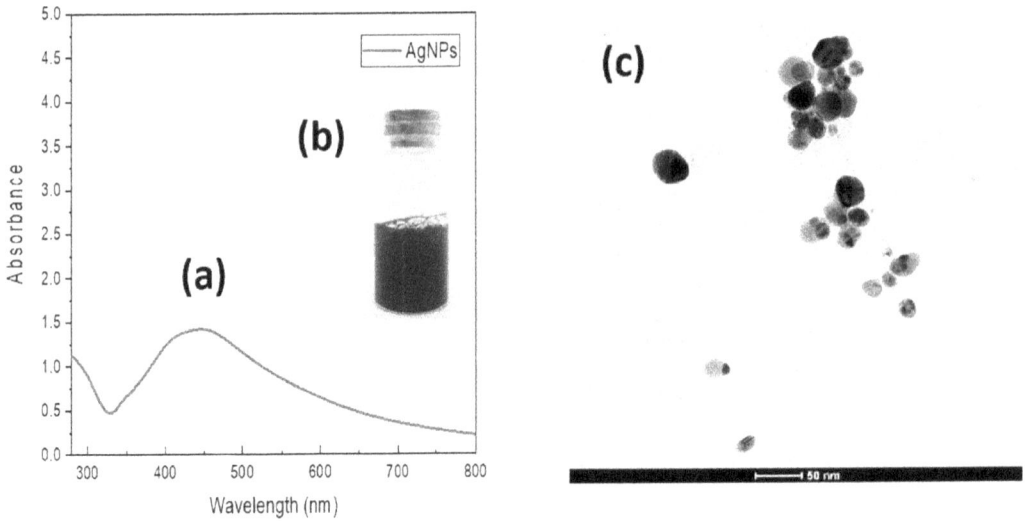

FIGURE 5.4 Synthesis result of PVA-coated AgNPs using chemical reduction method: (a) absorbance spectrum, (b) dark brown colloidal solution of PVA-coated AgNPs solution, and (c) TEM image (Yuniarni et al. 2020).

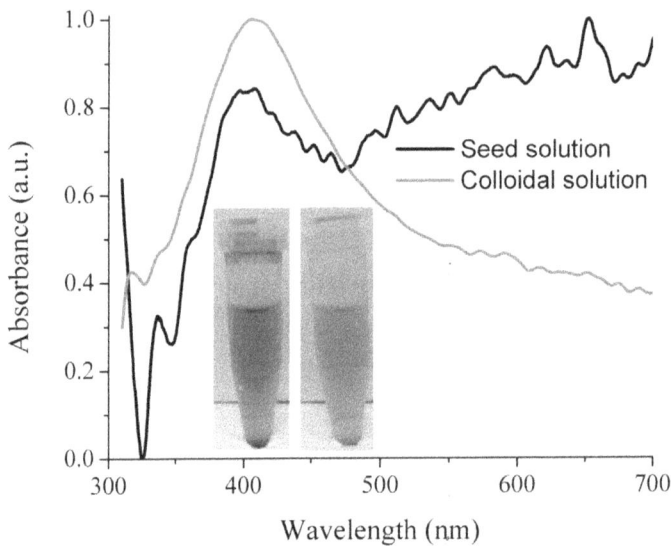

FIGURE 5.5 Absorbance spectra of seed and colloidal solution of AgNP synthesis in the range of 6–28 nm (Ortega-Mendoza et al. 2014).

The spherical AgNPs are widely used in the development of plasmonic sensor. For this purpose, AgNPs is synthesized in the range of 5–100 nm, as reported in previous studies. The absorbance spectra for Au colloidal solution with size particles between 6 and 28 nm are shown in Figure 5.5. The absorbance spectra of AgNPs colloidal solution with nanoparticle size of around 60 nm are reported as shown in Figure 5.6. In this case, the absorption peak is absorbed at 436 nm.

5.2.1.2 Triangular Silver Nanoparticles

The triangular AgNPs were also reported and utilized in various applications including the development of biosensors. The following are the general procedures for making triangular AgNPs: The previously mentioned spherical AgNPs are treated with 30% hydrogen peroxide (H_2O_2), which is continually swirled and combined during the operation. The color of the solution varies in a variety of ways throughout the addition process, as shown in Figure 5.7. The drop of hydrogen peroxide is discontinued when the solution became blue, and a triangle of AgNPs is formed. Figure 5.8 shows a scanning electron microscope (SEM) image of synthesized triangular AgNPs. The direct chemical reduction approach is used to make the Ag triangular plate NPs in this research. The formation of silver triangle plate NPs begins with the formation of a stable nanosheet core, followed by crystal growth of silver triangle plate NPs. Due to differences in the stirring of various sections throughout the re-synthesis process, the size of the generated triangular plate NPs is not consistent (Song et al. 2019).

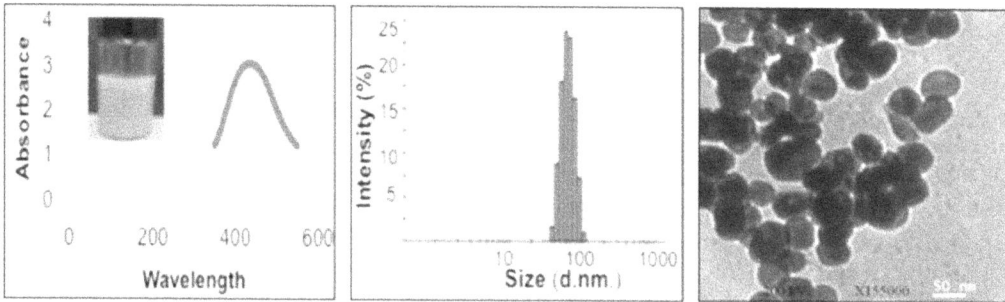

FIGURE 5.6   Absorbance spectra of AgNPs colloidal solution with nanoparticle size of around 60 nm; absorption peak is absorbed at 436 nm (Bhardwaj and McGoron 2013).

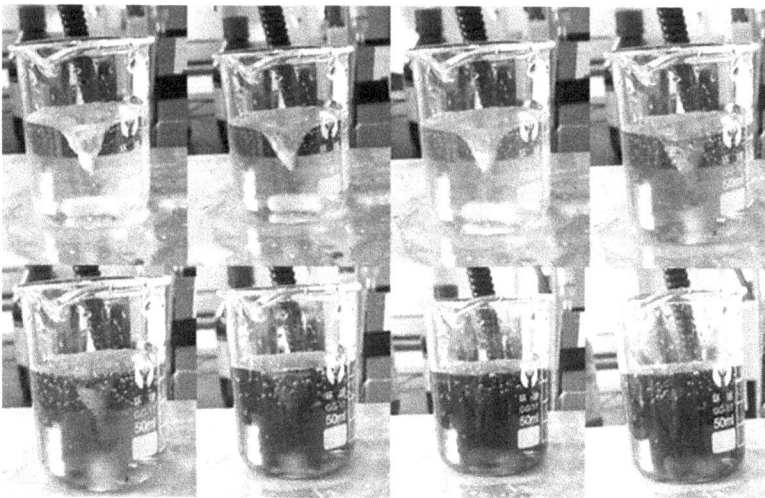

FIGURE 5.7   Color change of solution in the process of synthesizing silver triangle plate nanoparticles (Song et al. 2019).

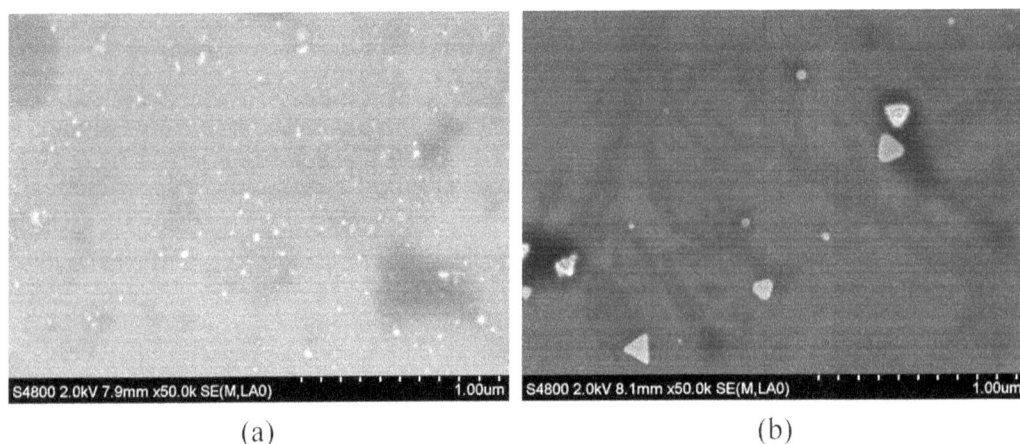

(a)   (b)

FIGURE 5.8   SEM images of AgNPs: (a) spherical AgNPs and (b) triangular silver nanoparticles (Song et al. 2019).

5.2.1.3   Synthesis of PVA-AgNPs Composites

AgNPs are immediately produced in the PVA matrix in a few stages, thanks to the PVA's reducibility to $AgNO_3$. To begin, in order to produce a colorless transparent PVA solution, 0.5 g of PVA is dissolved in 25 mL of hot deionized (DI) water with magnetic stirring. The $AgNO_3$ solution (4 mM, 125 mL) is then added to the aqueous PVA solution, and the solution is magnetically heated gently at 60°C–70°C for 2 hours. The color of the solution gradually deepens from an achromatic color to a faint yellowish equilibrium color, and the PVA-AgNPs composites are cooled at 20°C–24°C. The absorption spectra of colloidal AgNPs and PVA-AgNPs synthesized and inserted synthesized AgNPs solution is presented in Figure 5.9. Further, Figure 5.10 includes a TEM picture of colloidal AgNPs with and without PVA stabilizers. The PVA-AgNPs create a wide absorption band and sharpen the absorption spectra curve, indicating a lower particle size. The morphology (crystallites) of AgNPs has roughly spherical geometry with dispersive particle dispersion, according to TEM images.

5.2.1.4   Green Synthesis of Ag Nanoparticles

To make AgNPs, physical and chemical techniques such as microwave synthesis, thermal breakdown, sonochemical synthesis, microemulsion synthesis, solvothermal synthesis, co-precipitation, and photoreduction are utilized. While most chemical and physical procedures create AgNPs with high purity and the correct form and size, they also have drawbacks, such as the requirement for costly equipment, high energy consumption, hazardous organic solvents, significant amounts of toxic waste, and trouble purifying nanoparticles. Furthermore, hazardous chemicals may be deposited on the surfaces of AgNPs generated by chemical techniques, rendering them unsuitable and improper for medical and biological use. The need for environmentally friendly, energy-saving, cost-effective, and low-harm new synthetic processes is growing. As a result, in the recent decade, the green synthesis of AgNPs utilizing safe reaction media and nontoxic solvents has gotten a lot of interest. The biosynthetic method is used to make AgNPs, using reductants sourced from bacteria, fungi, algae, and plants. Amino acids, enzymes, carbohydrates, and other bioorganic substances have also been used to make AgNPs. Plants are being intensively investigated for the manufacture of AgNPs because of various benefits, such as the lack of a complicated microbe culture management procedure, quicker reaction times, and ease of scaling up for large-scale synthesis. The green synthesis of AgNPs utilizing plant-based reductants, as well as a few additional bioreductants, is covered in the following subsections.

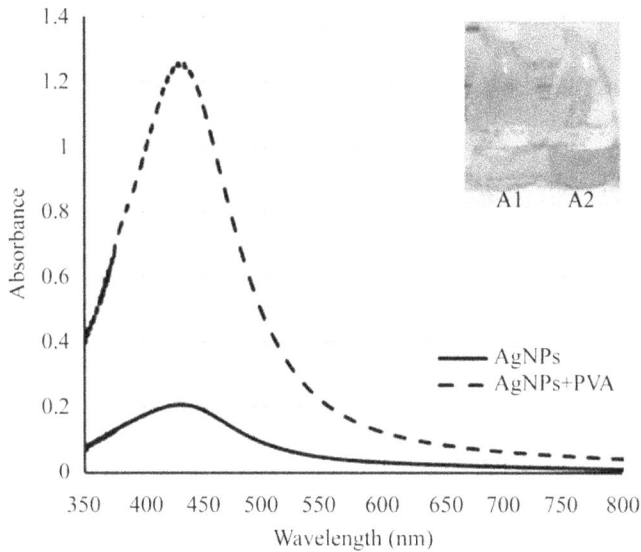

FIGURE 5.9 Absorption spectra of colloidal AgNPs synthesized and inserted synthesized AgNPs solution (Mahmudin et al. 2015).

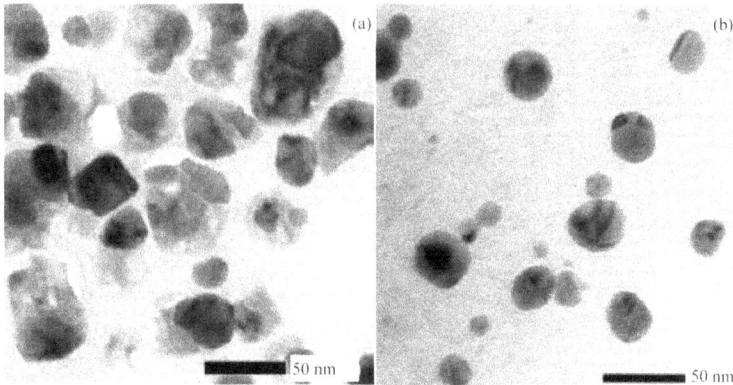

FIGURE 5.10 TEM image of colloidal AgNPs (a) without stabilizer polyvinyl alcohol (PVA) and (b) with the stabilizer of PVA (Mahmudin et al. 2015).

5.2.1.5 Synthesis of AgNPs Using Green Route Method

As illustrated in Figure 5.11, AgNPs are synthesized using a simple one-pot green method (Chaloeipote et al. 2021). *Pistia stratiotes* leaves (30 g) are chopped into tiny pieces and rinsed with deionized water. They are cooked for 30 minutes at 95°C in 500 mL DI water before being cooled to room temperature. Whatman Grade 1 filter paper is used to filter the reducing solution. The decreasing *P. stratiotes* solution is then filled with 0.04 g AgNO$_3$) in 20 mL DI water. The combination solutions are exposed to blue-light irradiation in a dark environment at room temperature for 1 hour to decrease Ag ion into AgNPs. The color shift from yellow to brown, indicating successful AgNPs production, may be seen with the naked eye. The various factors affecting the synthesis of AgNPs ae present in Figure 5.12.

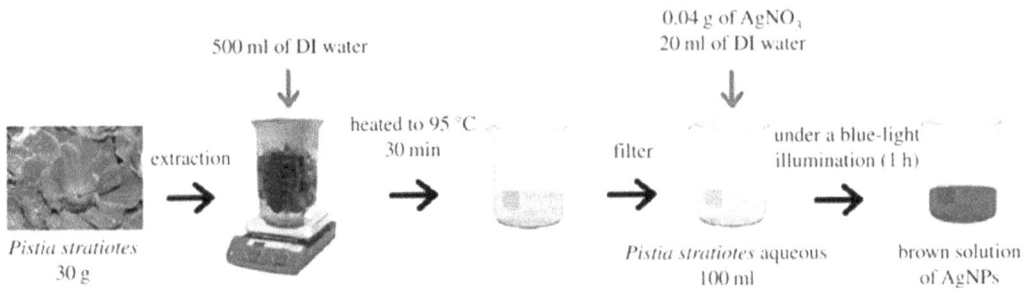

FIGURE 5.11 Synthesis of AgNPs using green route method (Chaloeipote et al.).

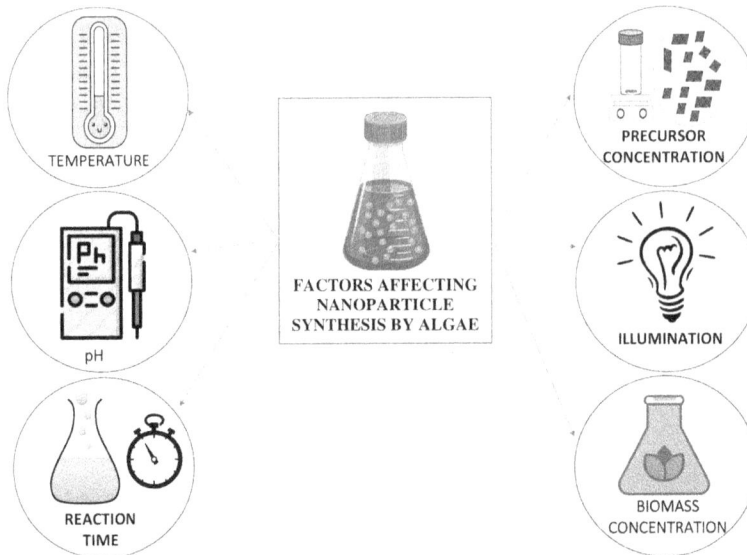

FIGURE 5.12 Factors affecting the synthesis of silver nanoparticles (Chugh, Viswamalya, and Das 2021).

5.3   DIVERSE USAGE OF SILVER NANOPARTICLES

Silver NPs are one of the most extensively used NPs due to their potential catalytic, electrical, magnetic, chemical, optical, and electrochemical properties. Chemical and biological techniques depend on the use of suitable reducing agents to reduce Ag+ to Ag. Chemical reducing reagents are often hazardous and nonbiocompatible substances. Biological reducing agents have been researched as biodegradable and benign compounds for the production of AgNPs as discussed earlier. Plants, fungi, and bacteria may all be employed to make AgNPs. However, additional capping agents, such as polymers, may be required to increase the stability of AgNPs. As a result, they have been widely used in industrial, biomedical, and environmental settings. For industrial applications, AgNPs built on multiwalled carbon nanotubes (MWCNTs) are employed as heterogeneous catalysts to change bicarbonate to format. This technology is employed in the storage of energy and the production of synthetic fuels. AgNPs-GO nanoparticle binding in bismuth-doped manganese oxide nanoparticles is also employed in oxygen reduction processes and might be utilized in sustainable energy technologies. Tannic acid blocking AgNPs are employed to immobilize galactosidase for food processing. In terms of catalysis and photonics, AgNPs stabilized on alumina also exhibit essential optical features. AgNPs have received a lot of interest in the biological field. They have been used to treat malignancies including pancreatic, prostate, breast, ovarian, and blood cancers as well as other sorts of cancers. They have also been looked at as antibacterial, antifungal, insecticidal, and antioxidant agents. Their role in environmental pollution reduction has also been investigated. AgNPs derived from metal organic framework (MOF) precursors, for example, have a high affinity and adsorption capability for hazardous bromine ions. It has also been established that they can remove pollutants such as total nitrogen, ammonium nitrogen, and total phosphate. They also showed promise in degrading the dyes reactive black, methyl orange, Congo red, and methylene blue. Orooji et al. released a review on current advancements in the degradation and removal of contaminants from the environment using AgNPs. The detection of environmental contaminants, particularly organic pollutants, utilizing AgNPs-based electrochemical sensors is investigated. The plasmonic properties of AgNPs have attracted considerable interest from various researchers. Due to their unique physical, chemical, electrical, and size-related optical properties, AgNPs are now used for catalytic activity, wastewater treatment, biosensing, targeted drug delivery, antibacterial activity, and other applications. An example of an AgNP-modified probe and a schematic of an AgNP-coated probe surface are presented in Figures 5.13 and 5.14, respectively.

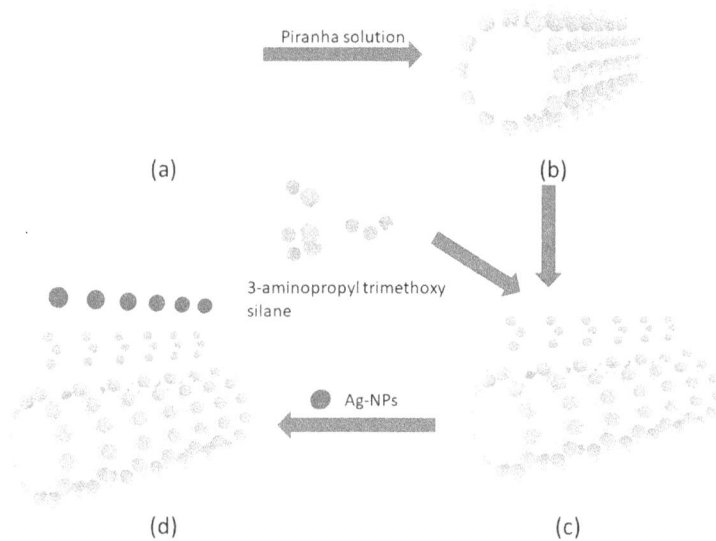

FIGURE 5.13 An example of a silver nanoparticle detecting probe: (a) the exposed core without the cladding; (b) hydroxylated fiber surface; (c) 3-aminopropyl trimethoxy silane bonded to the fiber surface; and (d) silver nanoparticles attached to the fiber surface (Song et al. 2019).

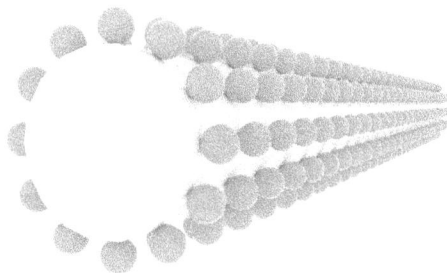

FIGURE 5.14 Surface of an optical fiber coated with AgNPs (Song et al. 2019).

Nanotechnology has allowed the development of low-dimensional material characteristics in the last 10 years, allowing them to be used in a variety of sectors including as sensors, optics, energy, catalysis, and biology. Noble metal nanomaterials (NMs), for example, are created via a bottom-up technique with a variety of morphologies, including spheres, cubes, stars, flowers, and wires, and display important chemical-physical characteristics that allow for novel interactions with the environment. The ability to generate AgNPs with precise shape and surface functionalization, resulting in unique characteristics, astounds researchers. Furthermore, sophisticated characterization techniques enable researchers to investigate how well they react to variations in pH, redox potentials, temperature, light, and magnetic fields.

5.3.1 Silver Nanoparticles Assisted Biosensors for Biomolecules Detection

The different studies over AgNPs assisted plasmonic biosensors were presented for the detection of glucose/cholesterol/other biomolecules. A few of the notable biochemical detection studies are reported next.

This section demonstrates a label-free approach for detecting triacylglycerides using LSPR phenomenon-based optical fiber sensors (OFSs). In order to determine the sensor's sensitivity, the wavelength shift as a function of concentration is used to determine the peak absorption wavelength. A triacylglycerides solution with a concentration range of 0–7 mM is used to test the sensor. With a response time of 40 seconds, the sensor demonstrates the greatest sensitivity at 37°C and pH 7.4 of the triacylglycerides emulsion. In the whole spectrum of triacylglycerides, a sensitivity of 28.5 nm/mM of triacylglycerides solution is achieved with a LoD of 0.016 mM. As a result, this biosensor is well suited for real-time live monitoring and remote sensing applications because of its excellent selectivity, stability, and reproducibility. Figures 5.15 and 5.16 show the functionalization of an enzyme (lipase) and a schematic design of the experimental setup for characterizing an LSPR-based fiber-optic biosensor for the detection of triacylglycerides. As illustrated in Figure 5.17, there are hypothesized mechanisms of AgNPs-induced cytotoxicity in cancer cell lines. AgNPs are currently applied in a number of advanced applications.

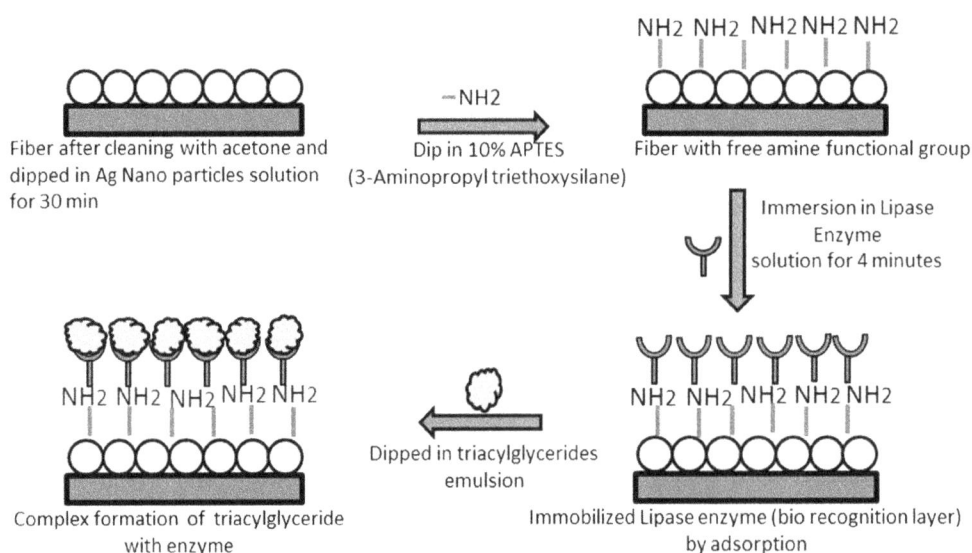

FIGURE 5.15 Enzyme (lipase) functionalization of triacylglycerides sensor (Anjli et al. 2017).

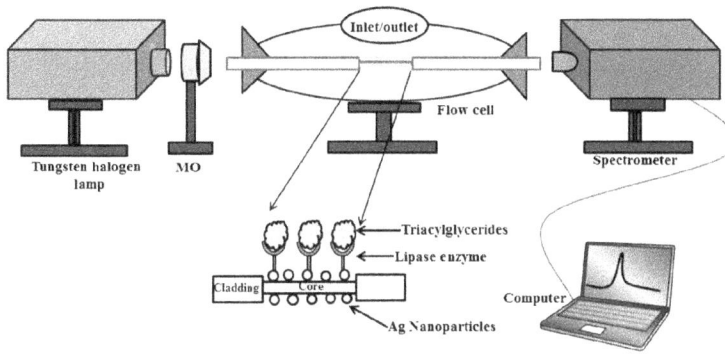

FIGURE 5.16 Experimental setup for characterizing the LSPR-based fiber-optic biosensor for the detection of triacylglycerides (Anjli et al. 2017).

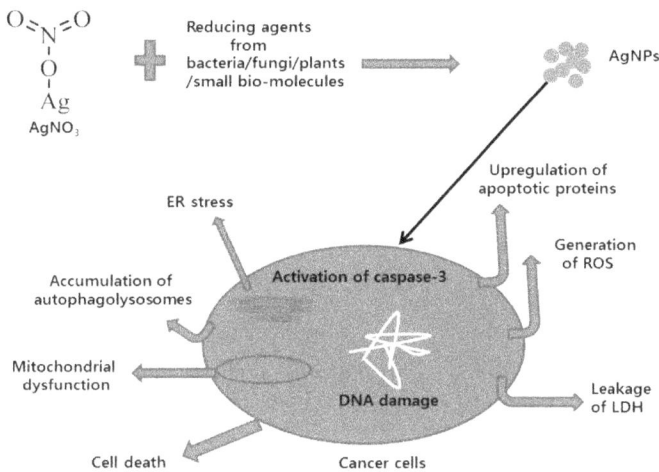

FIGURE 5.17 The possible mechanisms of AgNP-induced cytotoxicity in cancer cell lines: endoplasmic reticulum (ER) stress, lactate dehydrogenase (LDH), and reactive oxygen species (ROS) (Zhang et al. 2016).

TABLE 5.2
Summary of Silver Nanoparticles Assisted Plasmonics Optical Fiber Sensor Studies Available in Open Source

Material used	Mechanism	Detection	Linear range	LOD	Sensitivity	Ref.
PVA, graphene, and AgNPs	LSPR	Glucose	N.R.	N.R.	700.3 nm/RIU	Jiang et al. 2017
AgNPs/GO	LSPR	Cholesterol	0.0–10 mM	1.131 mM	5.14 nm/mM	Semwal and Gupta 2018
Ag film	SPR	Glucose	3–8 mM	N.R.	0.5 dB/mM	Zhang et al. 2018
AgNPs	LSPR	Dopamine	10 nM–1 μM	0.0058 μM	9.7 nm/ μM	Agrawal et al. 2019
PVAAgNPs/GO	LSPR	L-Cysteine	0 μM–1 mM	126.6 μM	0.0009 nm/μM	Singh et al. 2020
AgNPs/GO	LSPR	L-Cysteine	10 nM–1 mM	63.25 μM	7.0 nm/ mM	Agrawal, Saha, Kumar, Singh, Zhang, Jha et al. 2020
AgNPs	LSPR	Triacylglycerides	N.R.	0.016 mM	28.5 nm/mM	Anjli et al. 2017
Ag film	SPR	Triacylglycerides	N.R.	0.1 mM	3.17 nm/mM	Baliyan et al. 2013

Note: AgNP, silver nanoparticle; GO, graphene oxide; LSPR, localized surface plasmon resonance; PVA, polyvinyl alcohol; N.R., not reported; RIU, refractive index unit; SPR, surface plasmon resonance.

5.4 SUMMARY AND CONCLUSION

In this chapter, studies based on different sizes and shapes of AgNPs are elaborately reported. Also covered are the comparative performances based on these AgNPs. However, when comparing the triangular AgNP sensor to the spherical AgNPs sensor, the triangular AgNPs sensor exhibits a bigger red shift of the wavelength as the RI range shrinks. The experimental findings published by Song et al. show that triangular AgNPs may significantly increase the plasmonic sensor's sensitivity (Song et al. 2019). In summary, future applications of AgNPs include multiplexing detection, large-scale parallel biological detection for high-throughput drug screening, diagnostic level detection for clinical detection, study of molecular-level biological interactions, and plasma-scale measurement of molecular distances of tens of nanometers. All of these require more research. AgNPs are being evaluated as possible nanoprobes for biosensing applications. As a result, this biosensor is well suited for real-time live monitoring and remote sensing applications because of its excellent selectivity, stability, and reproducibility. They have attracted a lot of attention as optical probes for detecting several biomolecules, bacteria, cells, virus, and DNA/RNA. Pesticides, organic dyes, pharmaceuticals, microorganisms, nitro-aromatics, biomolecules, and mycotoxins have all been detected using AgNPs-based optical sensors.

Scientists use a variety of research strategies to generate metal NPs, including physical and chemical methods. However, these methods are expensive for a variety of synthesized substances. They may result in the existence of NPs of dangerous chemical organisms on the surface, which might be damaging in a variety of biological and medicinal applications. The urge to find environmentally acceptable technology for "green synthesis" of NPs is rising. In terms of the "green" approach, the AgNPs is one of the most investigated NMs and the most favored target. Plant extract-based NPs are becoming more common in research and development. Plant structures may be exploited to make diverse MNPs both intracellularly and extracellularly. Metal-rich soils and high-metal-medium seed plants provide good examples of intracellular systems for processing NPs. Extracellular processing NPs are made from extract leaves, which are made by boiling or mounding leaves in water or ethanol. *Medicago sativa* is a plant that uses its biomolecule to synthesize Ag and Au-NPs. It is the first plant to be employed for extracellular NPs manufacturing. Plants have gotten a lot of interest as a medium for NPs manufacturing since then. AgNPs has been found to have applications in the treatment of wounds and burns, as well as in the production of NMs for bone implants and dental materials, antibacterial, antiviral, antifungal, anti-arthropod, antigenic, antilarvicidal and anticancer agents. Until the development of AgNPs, $AgNO_3$ was a widely utilized antibacterial agent in clinical practice. In recent years, the usage of nanostructured materials in nanotechnology has increased dramatically. It has interesting biological implications for detecting and preventing various disorders. AgNPs are utilized for dental titanium implants because they may be readily coated with titanium or titanium alloys. AgNPs have a broad range of applications in medicine, cosmetics, biosensors, therapies, and other fields.

Several efforts have been made in recent years to create novel green synthesis processes. Green synthesis is based on the utilization of microorganisms or plants, making it an environmentally responsible and long-term method for NP synthesis. The vast range of applications for AgNPs and their various production methods are highlighted in this chapter. Because of their cost-effective technique of manufacturing and extraction, algal synthesis of AgNPs is the most popular among all living microorganisms. Cell extract, cell-free extract, and live cells may all be used in algae-mediated synthesis. The majority of these approaches include the use of biomolecules as synthesis capping agents. Despite its many benefits, algae-based AgNPs manufacturing is currently restricted due to a lack of knowledge regarding the actual process of synthesis. To build large-scale bioreactors for commercial-level production, further research is needed to tackle difficulties with kinetics, yield, and cell survival. Furthermore, substantial study is needed to identify and assess the involvement of various biomolecules as reducing and capping agents.

However, if the method is combined with the use of external capping agents, the NP's stability may be manually controlled. This will most likely allow for the production of more efficient NPs. As new technologies are developed, it is possible to produce algae-mediated NPs with better control and quality, enhancing the characteristics and functionality of these NPs to be used in industrial applications. AgNPs should be used to fight germs because of this. Additionally, there is a pressing need for intensive research and development in the use of diverse AgNPs and the evaluation of their impacts on human health and the environment. Second, new technologies must be created to avoid systemic negative effects. AgNPs have been demonstrated to slow down antiviral activity in several investigations; however, the specific mechanism remains a mystery, and further research is required. Traditional physical and chemical synthesis techniques may one day be replaced by environmentally friendly and technologically sophisticated AgNPs production methods.

Fluorescence, absorption-based SPR, LSPR, reflectance, and colorimetry are some of the optical biosensor's detection approaches. Analytes may be identified using optical detection of reflectivity, colorimetry, SPR, and fluorescent biosensors thanks to the optical characteristics of AgNPs, which have a local surface plasma with a visible resonant wavelength and can exhibit distinct color according to certain wavelengths. Sensors that create light signals directly from biological receptors and biomarkers (e.g., colorimetric, absorption, reflection, chemiluminescence, or fluorescence) are referred to as optical biosensors. Both label-based and label-free techniques may be used to detect signals from optical biosensors. Biometric events are quantified using optical tags, such as fluorescent dyes or enzymes, which are used in label-based systems. A colorimetric, reflecting, fluorescent, or luminescent sensor is then used to create the light signal. A transducer in label-free mode produces the measured optical signal as soon as the material interacts with it, as opposed to labeled mode. This technology does not need the use of tags or chemical coupling steps to monitor biometric events.

REFERENCES

Agrawal, N., C. Saha, C. Kumar, R. Singh, B. Zhang, R. Jha, and S. Kumar. 2020. "Detection of L-cysteine using silver nanoparticles and graphene oxide immobilized tapered SMS optical fiber structure." *IEEE Sensors Journal* 20 (19):11372–11379. DOI: 10.1109/JSEN.2020.2997690.

Agrawal, N., C. Saha, C. Kumar, R. Singh, B. Zhang, and S. Kumar. 2020. "Development of uric acid sensor using copper oxide and silver nanoparticles immobilized SMSMS fiber structure-based probe." *IEEE Transactions on Instrumentation and Measurement* 69 (11):9097–9104. DOI: 10.1109/TIM.2020.2998876.

Agrawal, N., B. Zhang, C. Saha, C. Kumar, B. K. Kaushik, and S. Kumar. 2019. "Development of dopamine sensor using silver nanoparticles and PEG-functionalized tapered optical fiber structure." *IEEE Transactions on Biomedical Engineering* 67 (6):1542–1547. DOI: 10.1109/TBME.2019.2939560.

Agrawal, N., B. Zhang, C. Saha, C. Kumar, B. K. Kaushik, and S. Kumar. 2020. "Development of dopamine sensor using silver nanoparticles and PEG-functionalized tapered optical fiber structure." *IEEE Transactions on Biomedical Engineering* 67 (6):1542–1547. DOI: 10.1109/TBME.2019.2939560.

Agrawal, Niteshkumar, Lokendra Singh, Chinmoy Saha, and Santosh Kumar. 2022. "Recent advancements in plasmonic optical biosensors: A review." *ISSS Journal of Micro and Smart Systems* 11:31–42. DOI: 10.1007/s41683-021-00079-0.

Agrawal, Niteshkumar, Bingyuan Zhang, Chinmoy Saha, Chandrakanta Kumar, Xipeng Pu, and Santosh Kumar. 2020. "Ultra-sensitive cholesterol sensor using gold and zinc-oxide nanoparticles immobilized core mismatch MPM/SPS probe." *Journal of Lightwave Technology* 38 (8):2523–2529.

Akter, Mahmuda, Md Tajuddin Sikder, Md Mostafizur Rahman, A. K. M. Atique Ullah, Kaniz Fatima Binte Hossain, Subrata Banik, Toshiyuki Hosokawa, Takeshi Saito, and Masaaki Kurasaki. 2018. "A systematic review on silver nanoparticles-induced cytotoxicity: Physicochemical properties and perspectives." *Journal of Advanced Research* 9:1–16. https://doi.org/10.1016/j.jare.2017.10.008.

Alexander, J. W. 2009. "History of the medical use of silver." *Surgical Infections (Larchmt)* 10 (3):289–292. DOI: 10.1089/sur.2008.9941.

Ali, Zainal Abidin, Rosiyah Yahya, Shamala Devi Sekaran, and R. Puteh. 2016. "Green synthesis of silver nanoparticles using apple extract and its antibacterial properties." *Advances in Materials Science and Engineering* 2016:4102196. DOI: 10.1155/2016/4102196.

Anjli, Baliyan, Usha Sruthi Prasood, D. Gupta Banshi, Gupta Rani, and Sharma Enakshi Khular. 2017. "Localized surface plasmon resonance-based fiber-optic sensor for the detection of triacylglycerides using silver nanoparticles." *Journal of Biomedical Optics* 22 (10):1–10. DOI: 10.1117/1.JBO.22.10.107001.

Baliyan, Anjli, Priya Bhatia, Banshi D. Gupta, Enakshi K. Sharma, Arti Kumari, and Rani Gupta. 2013. "Surface plasmon resonance based fiber optic sensor for the detection of triacylglycerides using gel entrapment technique." *Sensors and Actuators B: Chemical* 188:917–922. https://doi.org/10.1016/j.snb.2013.07.090.

Bhardwaj, Vinay, and Anthony McGoron. 2013. "AgNPs-based label-free colloidal SERS nanosensor for the rapid and sensitive detection of stress-proteins expressed in response to environmental-toxins." *Journal of Biosensors and Bioelectronics* S12. DOI: 10.4172/2155-6210.S12-005.

Calderón-Jiménez, Bryan, Monique E. Johnson, Antonio R. Montoro Bustos, Karen E. Murphy, Michael R. Winchester, and José R. Vega Baudrit. 2017. "Silver nanoparticles: Technological advances, societal impacts, and metrological challenges." *Frontiers in Chemistry* 5. DOI: 10.3389/fchem.2017.00006.

Cao, Z., Zeng Meng-Xue, Zhang Ling, Huang Xi-Xi, Wang Ming-Xing, Gong Fu-Chun, and Tan Shu-Zhen. 2009. "Novel optical nanobiosensor assembled with silver nanoparticles on gold surface." 2009 4th IEEE International Conference on Nano/Micro Engineered and Molecular Systems, 5–8 Jan.

Chaloeipote, Gun, Jaruwan Samarnwong, Pranlekha Traiwatcharanon, Teerakiat Kerdcharoen, and Chatchawal Wongchoosuk. 2021. "High-performance resistive humidity sensor based on Ag nanoparticles decorated with graphene quantum dots." *Royal Society Open Science* 8 (7):210407. DOI: 10.1098/rsos.210407.

Chugh, Deeksha, V. S. Viswamalya, and Bannhi Das. 2021. "Green synthesis of silver nanoparticles with algae and the importance of capping agents in the process." *Journal of Genetic Engineering and Biotechnology* 19 (1):126. DOI: 10.1186/s43141-021-00228-w.

Dakal, Tikam Chand, Anu Kumar, Rita S. Majumdar, and Vinod Yadav. 2016. "Mechanistic basis of anti-microbial actions of silver nanoparticles." *Frontiers in Microbiology* 7:1831–1831. DOI: 10.3389/fmicb.2016.01831.

Dawadi, Sonika, Saurav Katuwal, Aakash Gupta, Uttam Lamichhane, Ranjita Thapa, Shankar Jaisi, Ganesh Lamichhane, Deval Prasad Bhattarai, and Niranjan Parajuli. 2021. "Current research on silver nanoparticles: Synthesis, characterization, and applications." *Journal of Nanomaterials* 2021:6687290. DOI: 10.1155/2021/6687290.

Haider, Adnan, and Inn-Kyu Kang. 2015. "Preparation of silver nanoparticles and their industrial and biomedical applications: A comprehensive review." *Advances in Materials Science and Engineering* 2015:165257. DOI: 10.1155/2015/165257.

Hawa, Ainil, Azirah Ali, Sagadevan Suresh, and Zaharah Wahid. 2021. "Silver nanoparticles in various new applications." IntechOpen Press, London. DOI: 10.5772/intechopen.96105.

Huang, Ke-Jing, Yu-Jie Liu, Hai-Bo Wang, and Ya-Ya Wang. 2014. "A sensitive electrochemical DNA biosensor based on silver nanoparticles-polydopamine@graphene composite." *Electrochimica Acta* 118:130–137. DOI: 10.1016/j.electacta.2013.12.019.

Ibrahim, Nadiah, Nur D. Jamaluddin, Ling L. Tan, and Nurul Y. Mohd Yusof. 2021. "A review on the development of gold and silver nanoparticles-based biosensor as a detection strategy of emerging and pathogenic RNA virus." *Sensors* 21 (15). DOI: 10.3390/s21155114.

Jiang, Shouzhen, Zhe Li, Chao Zhang, Saisai Gao, Zhen Li, Hengwei Qiu, Chonghui Li, Cheng Yang, Mei Liu, and Yanjun Liu. 2017. "A novel U-bent plastic optical fibre local surface plasmon resonance sensor based on a graphene and silver nanoparticle hybrid structure." *Journal of Physics D: Applied Physics* 50 (16):165105. DOI: 10.1088/1361-6463/aa628c.

Klasen, H. 2000. "A historical review of the use of silver in the treatment of burns. Part I: Early uses." *Burns: Journal of the International Society for Burn Injuries* 26:117–130. DOI: 10.1016/S0305-4179(99)00108-4.

Konop, Marek, Tatsiana Damps, Aleksandra Misicka, and Lidia Rudnicka. 2016. "Certain aspects of silver and silver nanoparticles in wound care: A mini-review." *Journal of Nanomaterials* 2016:7614753. DOI: 10.1155/2016/7614753.

Krajczewski, Jan, Karol Kołątaj, and Andrzej Kudelski. 2017. "Plasmonic nanoparticles in chemical analysis." *RSC Advances* 7 (28):17559–17576. DOI: 10.1039/C7RA01034F.

Krajczewski, Jan, and Andrzej Kudelski. 2019. "Shell-isolated nanoparticle-enhanced Raman spectroscopy." *Frontiers in Chemistry* 7:410–410. DOI: 10.3389/fchem.2019.00410.

Loiseau, Alexis, Victoire Asila, Gabriel Boitel-Aullen, Mylan Lam, Michèle Salmain, and Souhir Boujday. 2019. "Silver-based plasmonic nanoparticles for and their use in biosensing." *Biosensors* 9 (2). DOI: 10.3390/bios9020078.

Mahmudin, Lufsyi, Edi Suharyadi, Agung Utomo, and Kamsul Abraha. 2015. "Optical properties of silver nanoparticles for surface plasmon resonance (SPR)-based biosensor applications." *Journal of Modern Physics* 6:1071–1076. DOI: 10.4236/jmp.2015.68111.

Ortega-Mendoza, J. Gabriel, Alfonso Padilla-Vivanco, Carina Toxqui-Quitl, Placido Zaca-Morán, David Villegas-Hernández, and Fernando Chávez. 2014. "Optical fiber sensor based on localized surface plasmon resonance using silver nanoparticles photodeposited on the optical fiber end." *Sensors (Basel, Switzerland)* 14 (10):18701–18710. DOI: 10.3390/s141018701.

Semwal, V., and B. D. Gupta. 2018. "LSPR- and SPR-based fiber-optic cholesterol sensor using immobilization of cholesterol oxidase over silver nanoparticles coated graphene oxide nanosheets." *IEEE Sensors Journal* 18 (3):1039–1046.

Singh, L., N. Agrawal, and C. Saha. 2021. "Investigation of glucose sensor by using plasmonic MIM waveguide based M." 2021 IEEE MTT-S International Microwave and RF Conference (IMARC), 17–19 Dec.

Singh, L., R. Singh, B. Zhang, B. K. Kaushik, and S. Kumar. 2020. "Localized surface plasmon resonance based hetero-core optical fiber sensor structure for the detection of L-cysteine." *IEEE Transactions on Nanotechnology* 19:201–208. DOI: 10.1109/TNANO.2020.2975297.

Singh, Lokendra, Niteshkumar Agrawal, Chinmoy Saha, Brij Mohan Singh, and Taresh Singh. 2022. "Highly sensitive plus shaped cavity in silicon fiber for RI detection of water samples." *Silicon*. DOI: 10.1007/s12633-021-01519-0.

Song, Hang, Hongxin Zhang, Zhuo Sun, Ziyang Ren, Xiaoyu Yang, and Qi Wang. 2019. "Triangular silver nanoparticle U-bent fiber sensor based on localized surface plasmon resonance." *AIP Advances* 9 (8):085307. DOI: 10.1063/1.5111820.

Spear, M. 2010. "Silver: An age-old treatment modality in modern times." *Plastic Surgical Nursing* 30 (2):90–3. DOI: 10.1097/PSN.0b013e3181deea2e.

Xu, Li, Yi-Yi Wang, Jie Huang, Chun-Yuan Chen, Zhen-Xing Wang, and Hui Xie. 2020. "Silver nanoparticles: Synthesis, medical applications and biosafety." *Theranostics* 10 (20):8996–9031. DOI: 10.7150/thno.45413.

Yuniarni, Diah, Nur Intan Pratiwi, Aminah Umar, and Cuk Imawan. 2020. "Synthesis of silver nanoparticles (AgNPs) using sodium chloride (NaCl) for iron (III) ions detection based on colorimetric and optical changes." *Journal of Physics: Conference Series* 1528:012062. DOI: 10.1088/1742-6596/1528/1/012062.

Zhang, Heng, Zhenyi Chen, Taihao Li, Na Chen, Wenjie Xu, and Shupeng Liu. 2017. "Surface-enhanced Raman scattering spectra revealing the inter-cultivar differences for Chinese ornamental *Flos Chrysanthemum*: A new promising method for plant taxonomy." *Plant Methods* 13 (1):92. DOI: 10.1186/s13007-017-0242-y.

Zhang, Qiao, Na Li, James Goebl, Zhenda Lu, and Yadong Yin. 2011. "A systematic study of the synthesis of silver nanoplates: Is citrate a 'magic' reagent?" *Journal of the American Chemical Society* 133 (46):18931–18939. DOI: 10.1021/ja2080345.

Zhang, Xi-Feng, Zhi-guo Liu, Wei Shen, and Sangiliyandi Gurunathan. 2016. "Silver nanoparticles: Synthesis, characterization, properties, applications, and therapeutic approaches." *International Journal of Molecular Sciences* 17.

Zhang, Xuejun, Ze Wu, Fu Liu, Qiangqiang Fu, Xiaoyong Chen, Jian Xu, Zhaochuan Zhang, Yunyun Huang, Yong Tang, Tuan Guo, and Jacques Albert. 2018. "Hydrogen peroxide and glucose concentration measurement using optical fiber grating sensors with corrodible plasmonic nanocoatings." *Biomedical Optics Express* 9 (4):1735–1744. DOI: 10.1364/BOE.9.001735.

Zhu, Guo, Niteshkumar Agrawal, Ragini Singh, Santosh Kumar, Bingyuan Zhang, Chinmoy Saha, and Chandrakanta Kumar. 2020. "A novel periodically tapered structure-based gold nanoparticles and graphene oxide: Immobilized optical fiber sensor to detect ascorbic acid." *Optics & Laser Technology* 127:106156. https://doi.org/10.1016/j.optlastec.2020.106156.

6 Graphene Oxide Coated Gold Nanoparticles-Based Fiber-Optic LSPR Sensor

6.1 INTRODUCTION

As mentioned earlier, the absorption-based fiber-optic sensor using a localized surface plasmon resonance (LSPR) sensor using gold nanoparticles is popular due to its advantages, including low cost, simple to develop, disposable (Luo et al. 2013; Nayak, Parhi, and Jha 2015; Bharadwaj and Mukherji 2014; Nayak, Parhi, and Jha 2016), and helps in identifying biological and chemical substances (Yonzon et al. 2004). This type of biosensor has some more advantages like quick response time, linear response, the capability of simultaneous sensing, and need for smaller pixel size (Malinsky et al. 2001). In this regard, gold nanoparticles (AuNPs) are very popular due to their significant electronic (Brust et al. 1998), thermo-optical (Richardson et al. 2006), electrochemical (Guo and Wang 2007), and optical (Huang et al. 2007) properties as well as properties of catalytic behavior. Due to this, there are wide and significant applications in the fields of chemistry, physics, biology (Sperling et al. 2008), and medicine (Huang et al. 2007). AuNPs have also been gaining interest because of their many advanced properties such as size and shape-dependent optical properties and wide use in biosensing applications (Henglein 1993).

The unique advantages such as size and shape-dependent optical property (strong absorption band in the visible region) and wide usefulness of AuNPs in sensing technology make it impactful technology (Mock et al. 2002; Smitha et al. 2008). Due to compact size and higher surface activity, these biosensors are selective and used commonly in chemical and biochemical sensing (Haes and Van Duyne 2002; Ortega-Mendoza et al. 2014; Luo et al. 2013; Urrutia, Goicoechea, and Arregui 2015; Tagad et al. 2013). Therefore, AuNPs are suitable candidates for the design of optical fiber-based LSPR sensors. However, these NPs are in solution form and tend to aggregate with time. So, to address the problem of aggregation, the encapsulation of NPs is required.

The optical properties (especially its bandgap) of graphene can be enhanced by the controlled absorption of oxygen for different sensing applications. After encapsulating the AuNPs with graphene oxide (GO), its colloidal stability increases, and it also controls the distance between the core particles. These things help to avoid the aggregation of NPs. Due to this, the chemical stability of gold increases and helps in the development of plasmonic sensors for biosensing applications. GO is a kind of special inorganic material that has a high affinity to bind proteins and helps in biosensing (Guo and Wang 2007). This helps GO in localization, immobilization of biotinylated biomolecules, and in vitro detection. Bovine serum albumin (BSA) is commonly used during the study of the proteins due to its structural similarity with human serum albumin (HSA). BSA also plays an important role in disease and drug-related peptides and proteins (Onaş et al. 2020). However, direct immobilization of protein molecules such as BSA on the surface of the gold is not possible as the bonding energy is low (Chen et al. 2007). These types of BSA proteins can be attached to GO through covalent bonding (Chiu and Huang 2014). In this case, the amine group (-NH$_2$) of BSA binds with the carboxylic acid group (–COOH) available on the GO surface and forms a strong covalent bond.

The graphene and its derivatives such as graphene oxide (GO) and reduced graphene oxide (rGO) are widely employed these days in the fabrication of plasmonic and other optical sensors. These sensors are applied in a range of applications such as chemical, gas, biomolecules, physical parameters

DOI: 10.1201/9781003243199-6

sensing, and environmental parameter/health monitoring applications. Graphene has been widely utilized in biosensing applications because of its numerous advantages that include a high electron transfer rate, large surface area, its ability to immobilize molecules, and increased electrical conductivity. The graphene enhances the performance of the plasmonic sensor via effective charge transfer, which increases vertical charge-density oscillations. It has been previously reported that the performance of optic-plasmonic sensors can be controlled by the properties of the capping material, surface charge, and interparticle interaction, which are more effective than the size of the particle. Accordingly, it is important to investigate the capping material, the surface charge, and the interparticle interaction of the plasmonic optical fiber sensors (P-OFSs). Previously, much effort was spent to boost the development of P-OFSs. In 2014, by depositing GO over a monolayer of gold nanoparticles (AuNPs), chemically attached to a functionalized fused silica substrate, Michela Cittadini et al. prepared a localized surface plasmon resonance (LSPR) phenomenon based gas sensor for selective detection of multiple gases (Cittadini et al. 2014). In 2017, based on a GO and silver nanoparticle (AgNPs) hybrid structure, Jiang et al. proposed a novel U-bend P-OFSs, which has the capability to detect glucose and ethanol (Jiang et al. 2017). In 2019, using a graphene/indium-tin-oxide (ITO) nanorod metamaterial hybrid structure, Yang et al. developed a U-bent P-OFSs that enables biomolecule detection (Yang et al. 2019). In 2019, to detect a DNA-polymerase reaction, Johanna Roether et al. presented the application of nanoplasmonic technology that is coupled with microfluidics (Roether et al. 2019). In 2019, Hang Song et al. developed a triangular AgNP U-bent fiber sensor with a sensitivity of 1116.8 nm/RIU (Song et al. 2019).

Further, fiber-based LSPR sensors can work in reflection as well as in transmission modes. Fiber-tip sensor (in reflection mode) probes are well suited in situ as point probes, which is not feasible with conventional fiber-based SPR systems used in transmission mode (Jian et al. 2014; Bekmurzayeva et al. 2021).

In this chapter, a fiber-based sensor with GO encapsulated gold nanoparticles has been studied in both reflection and transmission modes. The probe fabrication and results are discussed in Sections 6.2.3 and 6.3, respectively. Further, a study on gold nanoparticles and GO-assisted optical fiber-based fiber-optic biosensors has been discussed for the detection of several biomolecules.

6.2   EXPERIMENTAL SECTION

6.2.1   SYNTHESIS OF AuNPs AND GO

AuNPs are synthesized using a well-established Turkevich protocol (Turkevich, Stevenson, and Hillier 1951). First, a stock solution of aqueous gold chloride solution (50 mM) is prepared. Thereafter, a small amount (0.2 mL, 50 mM) of gold chloride solution is mixed with 39.15 mL of deionized (DI) water. The solution is heated and stirred until it is boiled. Thereafter, sodium citrate trihydrate (0.647 mL of 5 mg/mL) is mixed. The solution is stirred and heated until it becomes red wine in color.

Following that, GO can be synthesized via a modified Hummer's method (Hummers and Offeman 1958). To begin, graphite flakes (1 g) are mixed with NaCl (20 g). Following that, 150 mL of DI water is added to the mixture, and the graphite powder is filtered and dried. Following that, graphite powder is combined with sulfuric acid and stirred in an ice bath, followed by the addition of sodium nitrate (1 g) to the solution. Following that, $KMnO_4$ is slowly added to the mixture to avoid raising the temperature of the solution. At room temperature, this solution is stirred for 24 hours. The solution was then brought to a temperature of 30°C, and 40 mL of DI water was added. Following that, add the H_2O_2 and 100 mL of DI water once more. Filtration and collection of the by-product in a conical flask take place. Further, 250 mL of DI water needs to be added. The solution is centrifuged at 6000 rpm for 10 minutes and then the supernatant is centrifuged again at 15,000 rpm for 60 minutes, giving us the final GO particles. Here, Figure 6.1 illustrates the schematic of the formation graphite layer into GO. In this process, mainly an allotrope of carbon,

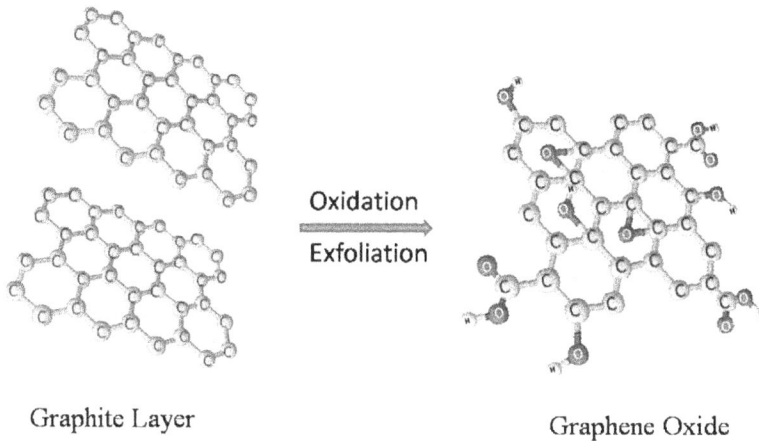

FIGURE 6.1 Conversion of graphite layer into graphene oxide.

Source: Reprinted with permission from Journal of Physics D: Applied Physics. Copyright, 2016, IOP (Nayak, Parhi, and Jha 2016).

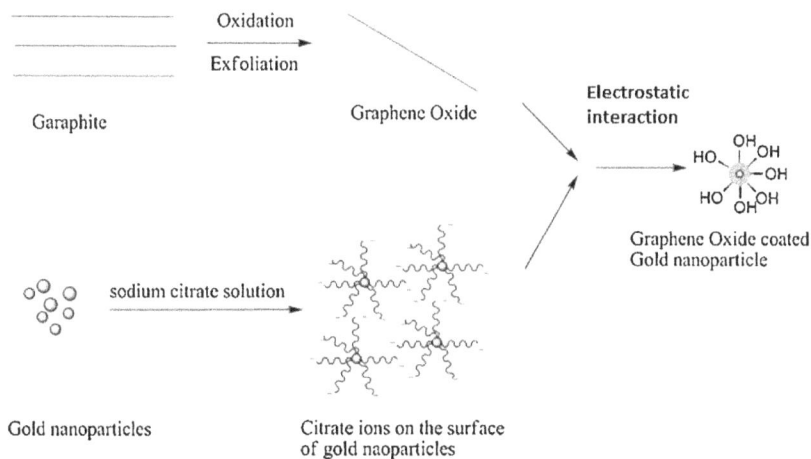

FIGURE 6.2 Encapsulation process of AuNPs with GO.

Source: Reprinted with permission from *Journal of Physics D: Applied Physics.* Copyright, 2016, IOP (Nayak, Parhi, and Jha 2015).

graphite layers are oxidized using $KMnO_4$ and $NaNO_3$ in the vicinity of a sulfuric acid environment. Selective oxidation of unsaturated aliphatic double bonds in this process is mainly carried out by Mn_2O_7. Thereafter, the graphite layer exfoliate in this process is obtained in the form of GO.

6.2.2 PREPARATION OF GO ENCAPSULATED AuNPs

In this process, the synthesis process of GO encapsulated AuNPs (GOE-AuNPs) has been discussed. In this process, 5 mL of prepared AuNPs solution and 30 mL of GO need to be mixed, and the mixture needs to be stirred for 1 hour. Thereafter, the need to centrifuge the mixture at high speed to form the GOE-AuNPs. This process is well illustrated in Figure 6.2. Here, encapsulation of AuNPs with GO is mainly performed due to electrostatic interaction between AuNPs with citrate ions and GO. The functional group COOH and OH also plays an important role during encapsulation.

6.2.3   PREPARATION OF FIBER PROBE

This process is crucial where the fiber of the 200-µm core diameter with NA = 0.37 is frequently used for biosensor development. The end faces need to be polished with a different polishing film of roughness such as 15 µm, 5 µm, 3 µm, and 1 µm to get a smooth end surface for better light coupling. Then, 1 cm cladding is removed from one end of plastic-cladded silica (PCS) fiber using methanol and KOH solution to fabricate the tip-based sensor probe. If we can remove the cladding from the middle of the fiber, then this type of probe will work in a transmission mode. After fabrication, the fiber probe needs to be functionalized using a silane reagent (Sai, Kundu, and Mukherji 2009). This process starts with the addition of a fiber probe in sulfochromic solution (10 mL of concentrated H_2SO_4 added to 1 mg of $K_2Cr_2O_7$ in 1 mL of DI water) for 8–10 minutes, and thereafter washed the probe in DI water, thrice. Here, the sulfochromic solution helps in developing additional Si-OH on the fiber surface to get the covalent bonding of amino-silane molecules. The probe is kept in the oven at 115°C for 4 hours. This needs to be dipped in the silane solution in the presence of nitrogen gas for 3 minutes duration. Acetic acid also plays a critical role in this process, preventing the aggregation of GOE-AuNPs on the fiber surface and preventing the formation of a multilayer of silane. For the monolayer of silane, there will be a single layer of GOE-AuNPs. If acetic acid will not be there, then multilayers of silane will be there; as a result, there will be a chance of aggregation of GOE-AuNPs on the sensing area of the fiber. Thereafter, the predesign needs to be washed thrice and kept in the dry nitrogen environment and is further heated at 110°C for 2 hours. The schematic of this process is well illustrated in Figure 6.3.

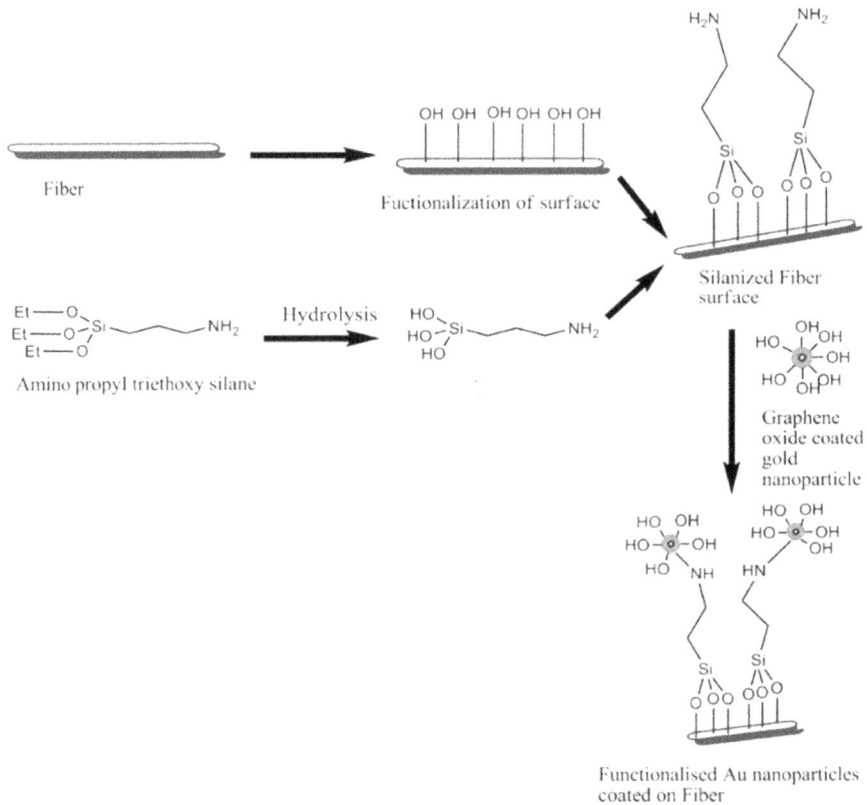

FIGURE 6.3   Process of attachment of GO encapsulated AuNPs on the fiber surface.

Source: Reprinted with permission from *Journal of Physics D: Applied Physics.* Copyright, 2016, IOP (Nayak, Parhi, and Jha 2015).

6.3 RESULTS AND DISCUSSION

The synthesized GO has been characterized by using X-ray diffraction and is found in Figure 6.4. A strong diffraction peak is seen at 2θ = 10.8°, corresponding to the (0 0 2) plane of GO, and another small diffraction peak is observed at 2θ = 26.7°, by the literature (Zangmeister 2010).

Further, to confirm the formation of GO, the inset of Figure 6.4 shows the Raman spectra of GO. In this case, two strong peaks are observed. The first peak (i.e., D-peak found at 1356 cm⁻¹) shows the breathing mode of aromatic rings with dangling bonds in-plane terminations and the second peak (i.e., G-peak found at 1610 cm⁻¹) shows the bond stretching of sp^2 carbon pairs in both rings and chains. Both peaks have comparable intensities, in this case, indicating the presence of functional groups on the planar carbon backbones (Zangmeister 2010; Kundu et al. 2010). Before immobilizing AuNPs on the optical fiber tip, Au-NPs in solution, GO dispersed in water, and GOE-AuNPs were characterized using a UV-Vis spectrometer, as illustrated in Figure 6.5. The line with

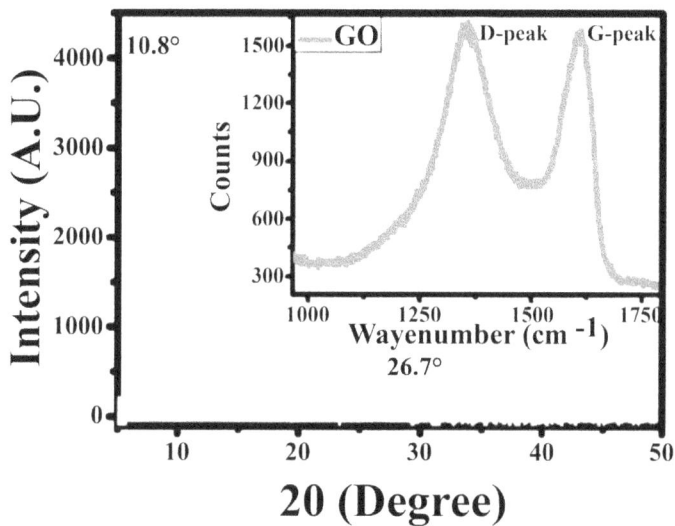

FIGURE 6.4 X-ray diffraction pattern of GO, and the inset shows Raman spectra of GO.

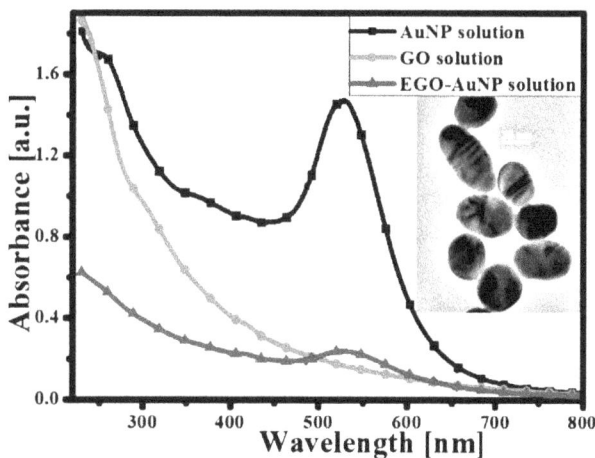

FIGURE 6.5 UV-Vis spectra of AuNPs, GO, and GOE. TEM image of AuNPs is shown in inset.

square represents the change of peak absorbance wavelength for AuNPs dispersed in water, with peak absorbance occurring at $\lambda = 528$ nm due to LSPR. The line with circle represents the variation of absorbance for GO at different values of incident wavelength. Similarly, the line with up triangles shows the UV-Vis spectra for GOE-AuNPs in solution form. The inset of Figure 6.5 represents the transmission electron microscopy (TEM) image of the synthesized Au-NPs. To calculate the average particle diameter, Figure 6.6 shows the plot to determine the size distribution of AuNPs. The average size of AuNPs has been found to be around 28 nm; however, a maximum number of particles have size around 25 nm. Figure 6.7 illustrates the experimental setup for the proposed tip-based optical fiber sensor.

A tungsten-halogen light source was used to initiate the light at the first end of the bifurcated cable, and a sensor probe was spliced to the second end of the bifurcated cable in the experimental setup. The GOE-AuNPs functionalized probe is dipped into the bio-sample, where light interacts. Following that, reflected light is collected and sent to the spectrometer via the third end of the bifurcated cable, as illustrated in Figure 6.7.

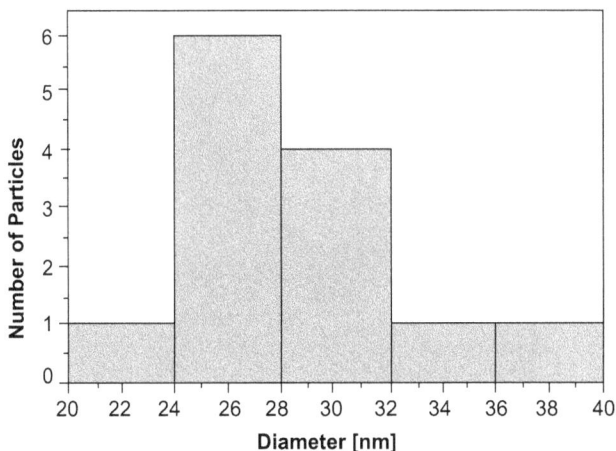

FIGURE 6.6   Histogram of AuNPs size distribution

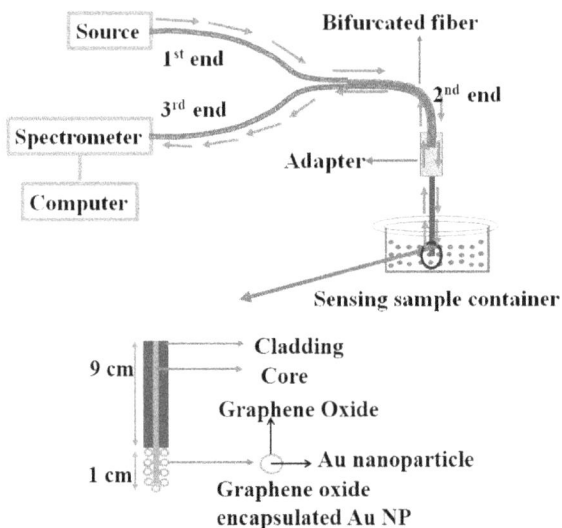

FIGURE 6.7   Experimental setup for BSA detection.

During the experiment, the functionalized tip of the fiber is dipped into the gold nanoparticle solution. AuNPs is very sensitive, if it aggregates before coating on a fiber surface, then the performance of the sensor can decrease. Due to this reason, in this case, GO has been used to encapsulate the AuNPs and enhance the stability of the sensor probe. Thus, the proposed structure is GOE-AuNPs-based structure and used for further sensing purpose. It is interesting to know that thickness of GO over AuNPs is approximately 1.7 nm, which is confirmed through TEM image as shown in Figure 6.8.

The absorbance variation of the probe dipped in GOE-AuNPs solution over a range of dip times is shown in Figure 6.9. The absorbance peaks at approximately 517 nm and increases with dipping

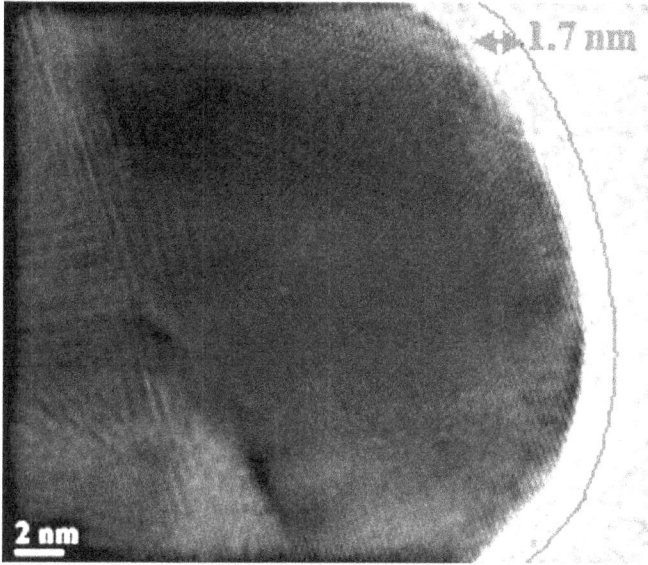

FIGURE 6.8 TEM image of GOE-AuNPs particle.

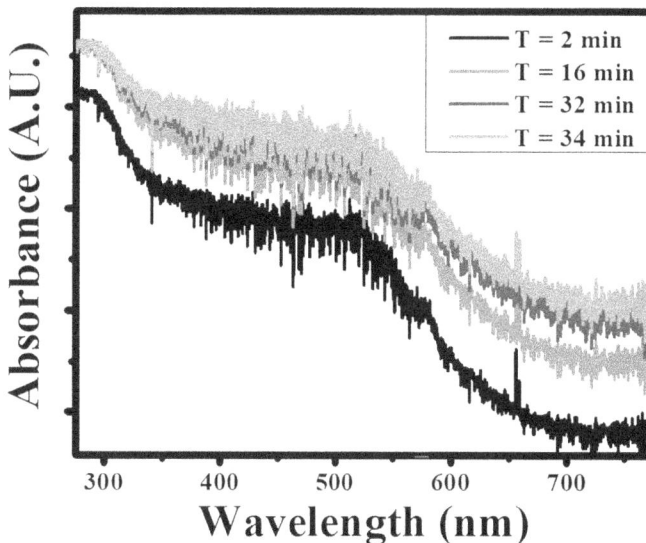

FIGURE 6.9 Absorbance variation with different dip time of the probe in GOE-AuNPs solution.

time. This increase in peak absorbance indicates that the GOE-AuNPs are getting attached to the silanized probe with time. As the time of dip increases, the number of GOE-AuNPs getting attached increases. So from Figure 6.9, it is clear that the maximum number of GOE-AuNPs are getting attached after around 34 minutes of dipping time. Similarly, the immobilization of GOE-AuNPs has been confirmed through field emission scanning electron microscopy (FESEM).

Figure 6.10(a–d) shows the FESEM images of the fiber probe immobilized with GOE-AuNPs with different magnifications. From Figure 6.10(d), it is clearly visible that the very small particles have been immobilized on the core of the fiber probe. Thereafter, sensor performance checked through absorbance measurement in the presence of different RI of analyte as shown in Figure 6.11.

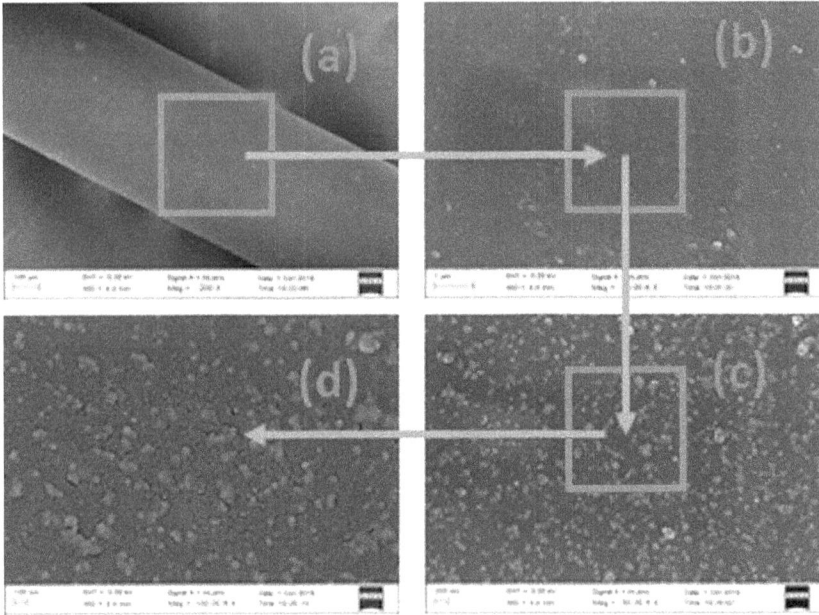

FIGURE 6.10   FESEM image of a fiber probe immobilized with GOE-AuNPs.

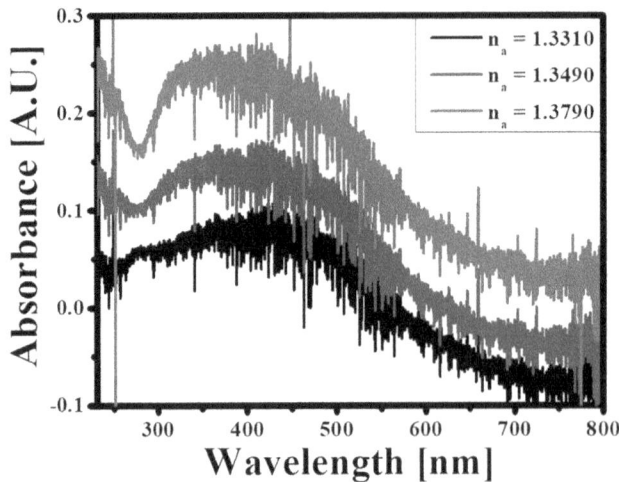

FIGURE 6.11   Absorbance measurement in the presence of different analyte RI through proposed, GOE-AuNPs-based sensor probe.

As can be seen from Figure 6.9 and Figure 6.11, the absorbance spectra are very noisy and broad; therefore, it is quite difficult to track the variation in peak absorbance with change in analyte refractive index. This may primarily be due to the fact that light interacting with the whole system twice in reflection makes the system noisy. This can be addressed by system operation in transmission mode as explained next.

Before performing the experiment, the UV-Vis spectrometer has been used to characterize the synthesized AuNPs solution. As per Figure 6.12, it can be determined that the peak absorbance wavelength of synthesized AuNPs is 524 nm. This can also be verified in normalized transmittance that is calculated and compared theoretically using Mie theory (Bohren and Huffman 2008). The absorbances by the NPs are calculated by Eq. (6.1):

$$A_{NPs} = \frac{\pi R^2 Q_{ext} dN_d}{2.303}$$ (6.1)

Here, d is the path length due to the spectrometer, and N_d shows the density of particles. Using Eq. (6.1), the absorption spectra have been calculated for AuNPs.

To verify the absorbance spectrum, AuNPs is diluted in DI water, and its absorbance is measured. It has been found that the absorbance spectrum matched the experimental results. The detailed derivation of the Eq. (6.1) has been discussed in Appendix E. Further, the absorption spectra can be calculated for the proposed sensor using Eq. (6.2) (Ruddy, MacCraith, and Murphy 1990):

$$A_{fiber} = k\left[\sqrt{2}\left(4\lambda\right)/3\left(2\pi rNA\right)\right]Q_{ext}cL$$ (6.2)

where r is the optical fiber radius for coupling of light, λ is the wavelength of the incident light, NA is the numerical aperture, c is the concentration of the absorbent molecules, Q_{ext} is the extinction coefficient of absorbing medium (here, GOE-AuNPs), k is the correction factor, and L is the length of the sensing layer.

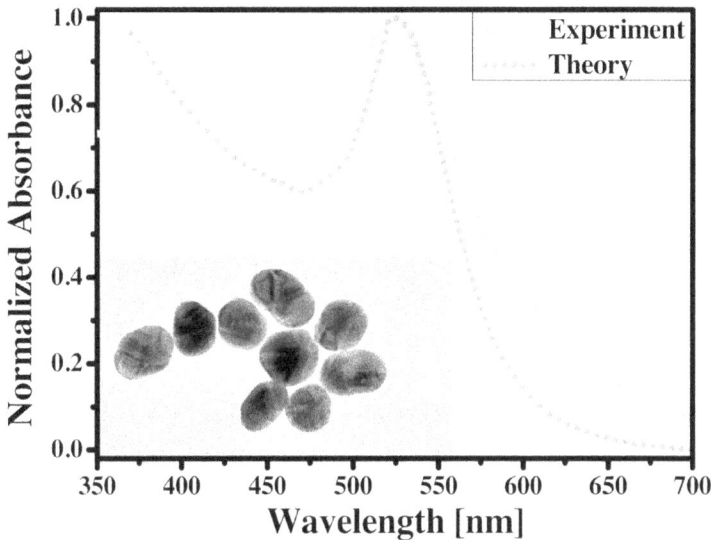

FIGURE 6.12 Absorbance measurement of AuNPs solution and image of AuNPs in inset.

Source: Reprinted with permission from *Sensors and Actuators B: Chemical.* Copyright, 2016, Elsevier (Nayak, Parhi, and Jha 2015).

In Figure 6.12, the theoretical absorbance curve is shown by a dotted line in which peak absorbance is found at 521 nm wavelength for 30 nm of AuNPs. The percentage error in theoretical and experimental results is less than 0.1% due to the assumption that AuNPs is spherical in shape during computation. Also, the concentration differences of AuNPs during theory and experiment may be the reason for deviation of the absorbance spectrum. In this work, AuNPs' diameter is considered as 30 nm, and its concentration (in the form of number density of the particles per unit volume) is $10^{17}/m^3$. The width difference arises during experiment and theoretical study that is due to the nonuniform distribution of AuNPs during the experiment. The shape of all the NPs is considered to be spherical in theory, but in the experiment, the shape is not exactly spherical as appears from the TEM result. To determine the average size of AuNPs, a TEM image of freshly synthesized AuNPs was taken, as illustrated in the inset of Figure 6.12. The particle diameter has been calculated by averaging the diameter of 15 AuNPs measured from the TEM image. The average diameter of synthesized AuNPs is 30 nm with 0.1%. The stability of synthesized AuNPs is around 2 months, and after that its color may fade away due to AuNPs agglomeration. This can also be analyzed through absorbance measurement of freshly prepared AuNPs and 2-month-old AuNPs as shown in Figure 6.13. Additionally, the absorbance spectrum of agglomerated AuNPs (width of 155 nm) is wider than the absorbance spectrum of freshly prepared AuNPs (width of 115 nm).

Thus, discussion of AuNPs agglomeration in the development of biosensors is quite important. This problem can be avoided by AuNPs encapsulation scheme that can be possible using GO as discussed in this chapter. The characterization results of freshly prepared GO are discussed in Figure 6.2. Figure 6.14 shows a high-resolution transmission electron microscopy (HRTEM) image for GOE-AuNPs at different magnifications. It can be observed that 2-nm-thick GO is coated over the AuNPs that helps to avoid the aggregation of AuNPs (i.e., formation of bigger NPs). This helps to get the narrow absorbance spectrum and avoid multiple resonance peaks.

The experimental setup for sensing with the developed sensor probe is shown in Figure 6.15. This type of setup consists of tungsten-halogen light source, spectrometer, adaptors, SubMiniature version A (SMA) connectors, and SMA fiber patch cords. In this case, one end of the sensor probe is connected through the source, and the other end is connected through the spectrometer. First, the

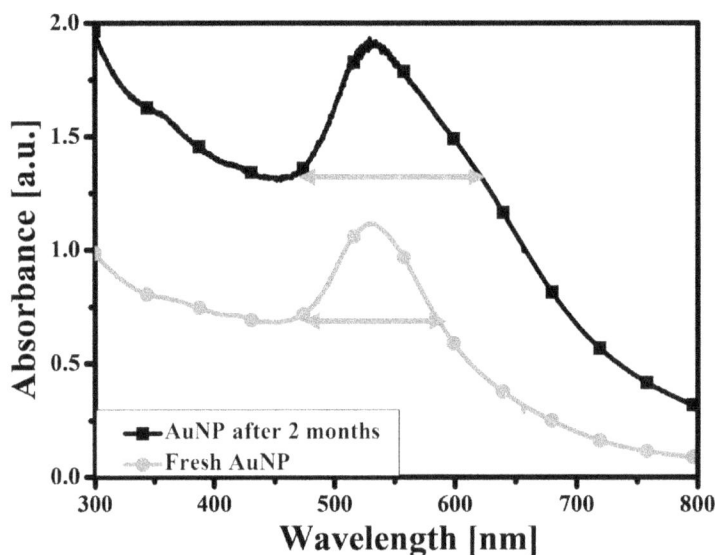

FIGURE 6.13 Absorbance spectrum of freshly prepared AuNPs and AuNPs after 2 months.

Source: Reprinted with permission from *Sensors and Actuators B: Chemical.* Copyright, 2016, Elsevier (Nayak, Parhi, and Jha 2015).

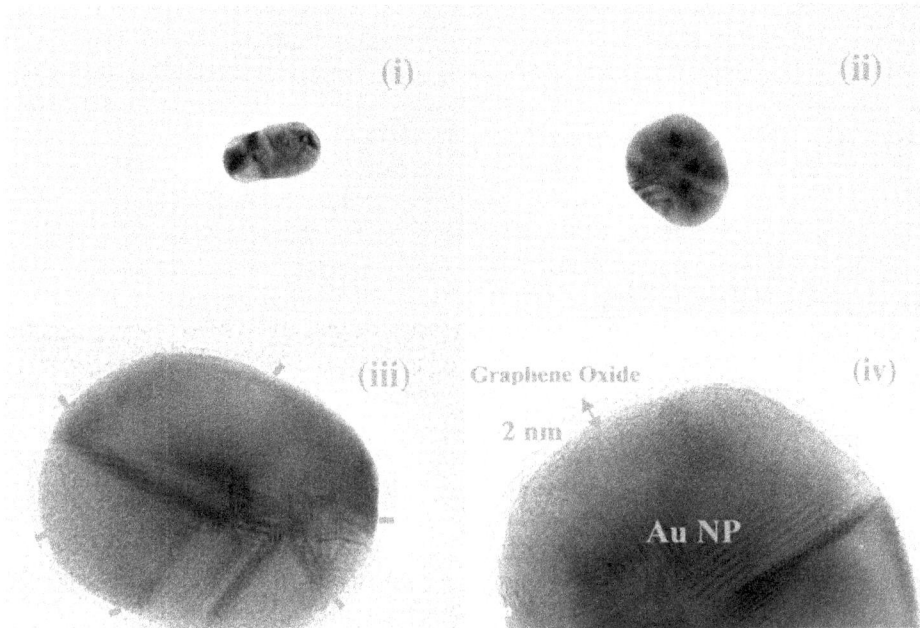

FIGURE 6.14 HRTEM image of GO-encapsulated AuNP.

Source: Reprinted with permission from *Sensors and Actuators B: Chemical.* Copyright, 2016, Elsevier (Nayak, Parhi, and Jha 2015).

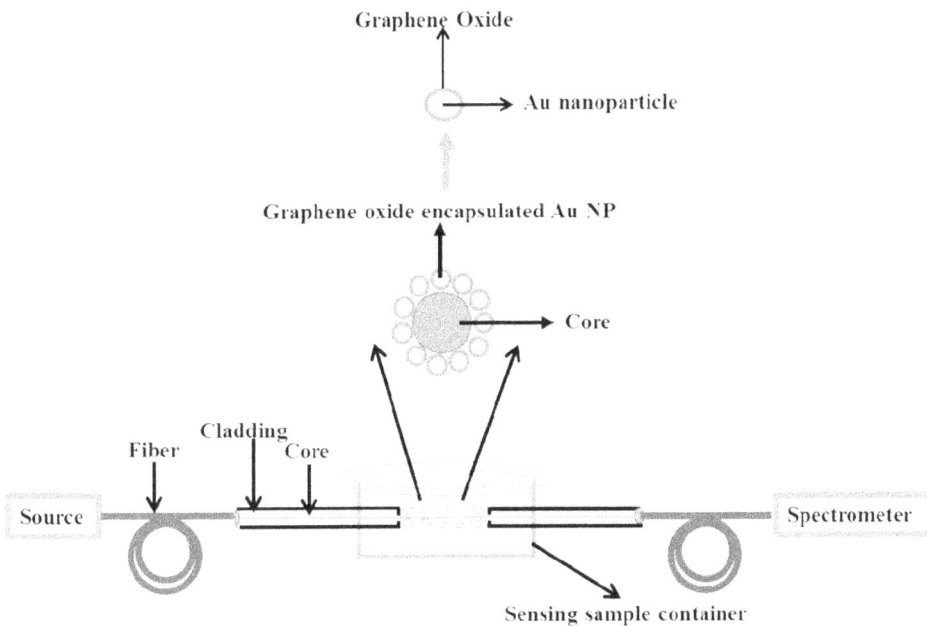

FIGURE 6.15 Experimental setup for transmission measurement through GOE-AuNPs.

Source: Reprinted with permission from *Sensors and Actuators B: Chemical.* Copyright, 2016, Elsevier (Nayak, Parhi, and Jha 2015).

spectrum of the reference signal and the spectrum of the dark signal need to be saved. In most of the cases, the absorbance mode needs to be activated with averaging the 100 spectra. The sensing area needs to be dipped in the analytes until a stable signal is received. Thereafter, analyte needs to be removed and the sensing area washed using DI water and then sensor probe dried. In this way, absorbance spectra can be recorded for the different RIs of analytes. In this case, a sensor probe is washed with DI water four to five times before the measurement of new sucrose solution. In Figure 6.16, the absorbance spectra of AuNPs, GO, and GOE-AuNPs are shown clearly.

In this case, the peak absorbance wavelength of AuNPs is 524 nm, and its absorbance value is 0.570. In this spectrum, a small peak arises between 250 nm and 300 nm that is due to the small amount of unreacted gold precursor (chloroauric acid) found in synthesized AuNPs. This peak is due to charge transfer from the ligand to metal band of the $AuCl_4^-$ ion (Gangopadhayay and Chakravorty 1961).

In the GO spectrum, two characteristic peaks occur at 230 nm and 301 nm that are also called $\pi \rightarrow \pi^*$ transition of C-C and $n \rightarrow \pi^*$ transition of the carbonyl groups, respectively, as shown in Figure 6.16. The absorbance value of GOE-AuNPs solution is 0.40, and it lies between GO and AuNPs in the visible region. Here, the reason for a decrease in peak absorbance of GOE-AuNPs is the damping effect. The imaginary part of the system's effective RI is greater than it is without encapsulated AuNPs.

Further, to know the performance study of the proposed sensor, the absorbance spectrum is measured using a developed sensor probe in the presence of different RI of sucrose solutions. Here, it has been observed that sucrose solutions are taken in the range of RIs value 1.3395 to 1.3790.

In this case, changes are found in the value of absorbance value but there are not any shift in peak absorbance wavelength, it is constant at 537.5 nm in the case of change in the concentration of sucrose solution. Absorbance variation with respect to time is shown in the inset of Figure 6.17. Initially for 10 minutes duration, its absorbance value increases sharply, it means, maximum particles of GOE-AuNPs are bounded with salinized probe. Thereafter, for the next 40 minutes, absorbance increases gradually, and it is saturated in the next 20–30 minutes.

In this case, further sensitivity of the sensor is calculated by plotting the absorbance plot with respect to different RIs of solution. Figure 6.18 shows the variation of peak absorbance at 537.5 nm wavelength with respect to the different concentrations of sucrose solution in the range of

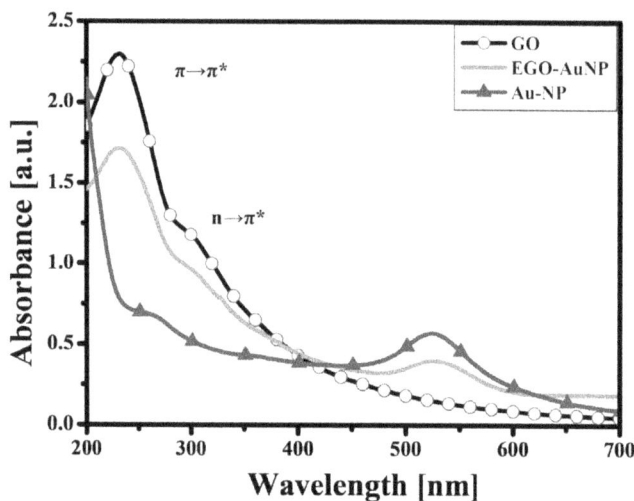

FIGURE 6.16 Absorbance variation in the case of AuNPs, GO, and GOE-AuNPs solution.

Source: Reprinted with permission from *Sensors and Actuators B: Chemical.* Copyright, 2016, Elsevier (Nayak, Parhi, and Jha 2015).

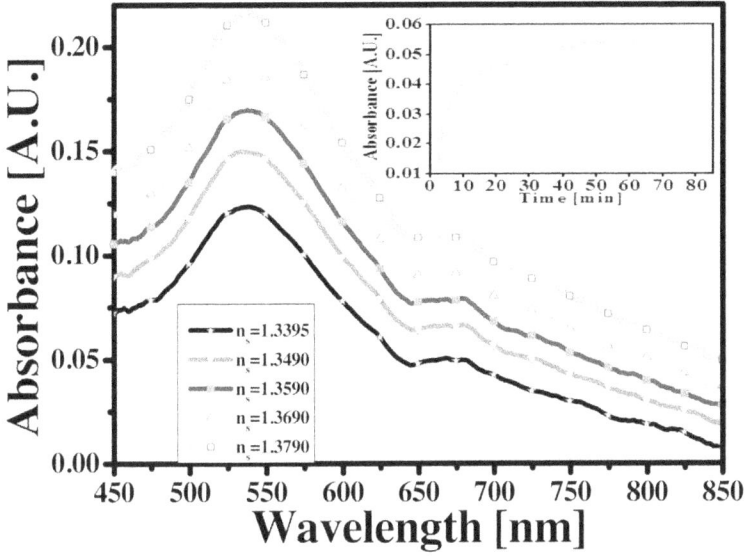

FIGURE 6.17 Absorbance variation for different RI of sensing layer. Absorbance variation with time is shown in the inset.

Source: Reprinted with permission from *Sensors and Actuators B: Chemical.* Copyright, 2016, Elsevier (Nayak, Parhi, and Jha 2015).

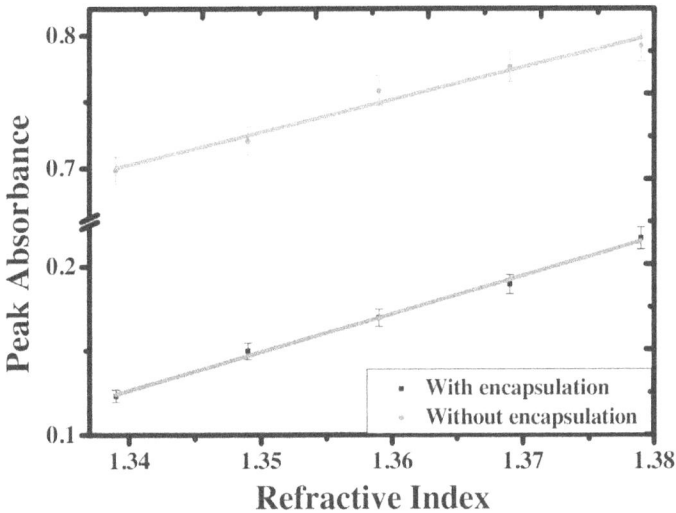

FIGURE 6.18 Absorbance variation in the presence of different RIs of sensing layer with and without encapsulation.

Source: Reprinted with permission from *Sensors and Actuators B: Chemical.* Copyright, 2016, Elsevier (Nayak, Parhi, and Jha 2015).

1.3395–1.3790 for the case of with and without GO encapsulation over AuNPs. In this case, the slope of the linear fitted curve shows the sensitivity of the sensor and unit of sensitivity is ΔA/RIU (change in absorbance per refractive index unit). Thus, in this case, sensitivity of GOE-AuNPs is calculated as 2.288 ΔA/RIU.

The line represents the linear fit in the case of GOE-AuNPs with intercept equal to −2.939 and $R^2 = 0.995$ to the linear fitted curve. Similarly, linear fit in the case of only AuNPs is intercept equals −2.58 and $R^2 = 0.987$ and sensitivity of 2.449 ΔA/RIU. Similarly, for the probe deposited with AuNPs (i.e., without encapsulation), the sensitivity is 2.449 ΔA/RIU having intercept equal to −2.58 and $R^2 = 0.987$ to the linear fitted curve. However, Cheng et al. (Cheng and Chau 2003) reported better performances with colloidal gold nanoparticles. The mismatch in the sensitivity with respect to proposed probe is due to the consideration of different fiber diameter, different immobilization technique, higher sensing length, a different mode of study, and different fiber location for immobilization. The absorbance peak rises by 75.78% for 0.0395 change in RI of sucrose.

Further, riding on the advantage of better signal quality and sensor performance, the transmission sensing probe has been used for the detection of immobilized BSA. Additionally, GO, as a unique inorganic material that binds proteins with a high degree of affinity, holds promise for use in biodevices (Guo and Wang 2007). Due to its structural similarity to human serum albumin, BSA has been a frequently investigated protein analyte (Carter and Ho 1994). It also plays an important role in disease- and drug-related peptides and proteins (Onaş et al. 2020). Therefore, a study on the optical fiber-based LSPR biosensor using GO for the immobilization detection of BSA has been carried out, which is discussed in the next section. To perform the experiment, AuNPs are synthesized as described by Turkevich et al. (Turkevich, Stevenson, and Hillier 1951) and GO by Hummer's method (Hummers and Offeman 1958). PCS fiber (200 μm core diameter with NA = 0.37) of length 15 cm is used as the sensing probe. Fiber is decladded at the center, and silica core is functionalized with silane treatment and coated with AuNPs (Sai, Kundu, and Mukherji 2009). GO is coated over the AuNPs-functionalized fiber with the help of some linking agent. The functional group −COOH of GO is activated using EDC/NHS solution. Here, 100 μM of EDC and 400 μM of NHS are mixed in 1:4 ratio to form EDC/NHS solution. The functionalized probe is used for further sensing purposes.

The in-house synthesized GO has been first characterized using UV-Vis spectrophotometer as shown in Figure 6.18. The two characteristic peaks occur at 230 nm and 301 nm due to $\pi \rightarrow \pi^*$ transition of C = C and $n \rightarrow \pi^*$ transition of the carbonyl groups, respectively. Further, the inset of Figure 6.19 shows the FESEM image of GO. In order to immobilize the GO on the functionalized

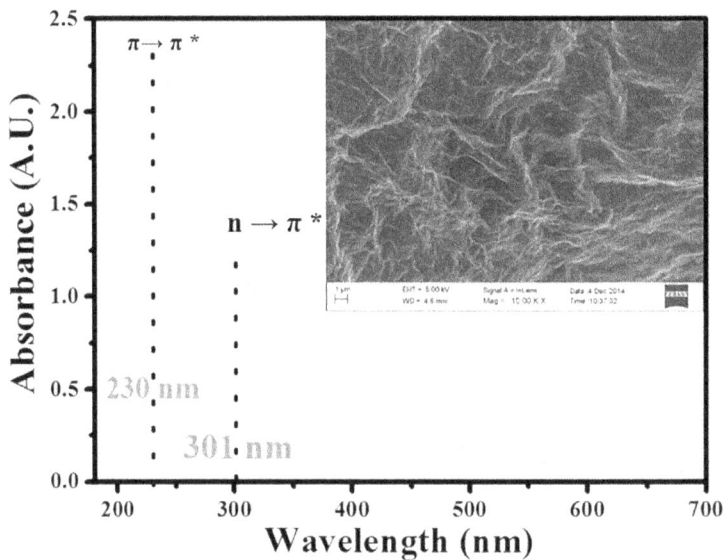

FIGURE 6.19 UV-Vis spectra of GO showing the characteristic peaks at 230 and 301 nm. Inset shows the FESEM image of GO.

fiber probe, the step-by-step procedure is pictorially shown in Figure 6.20. In the first step, the fiber is treated with sulfochromic acid. This step is required to create more Si-OH bond on the surface of the fiber. The fiber is further coated with amino-terminated silane (3-aminopropyltriethoxysilane, APTES), thus creating a chemical contrast of positively charged structures on the surface (step 1). Then, citrate-stabilized AuNPs (AuNP) 23 nm in diameter are coated on the surface through the electrostatic interaction between the negatively charged citrate and the positively charged amino groups of silanes (step 2).

The electrostatic attraction between the negatively charged AuNPs and the positively charged amino group causes the AuNPs to self-assemble on the fiber surface. This rendered the fiber's surface amphoteric. Again, positive charge on the surface of Au nanoparticle is introduced by modification with cysteamine (step 3). The modified fiber is washed with ethanol to remove excess cysteamine that is not adhered to the fiber surface. In the next step, modification with the help of cysteamine is required prior to the exposure of the fiber to negatively charged GO. As the modified fiber is dipped into the GO solution, GO is stacked on the fiber through electrostatic interaction between cysteamine and GO moiety (step 4). NH_2-containing BSA molecule can be immobilized onto carboxyl-containing GO-modified fiber via a covalent amide bond using a carbodiimide reagent. Because of the mild reaction conditions and high conversion efficiency observed in this study, the EDC/NHS activation approach has been employed. NHS is a type of activated ester that is both water soluble and stable in water, whereas EDC is amine-specific in nature and a type of activated ester. The EDC/NHS activated the carboxylic group of GO and also plays a role in amidation

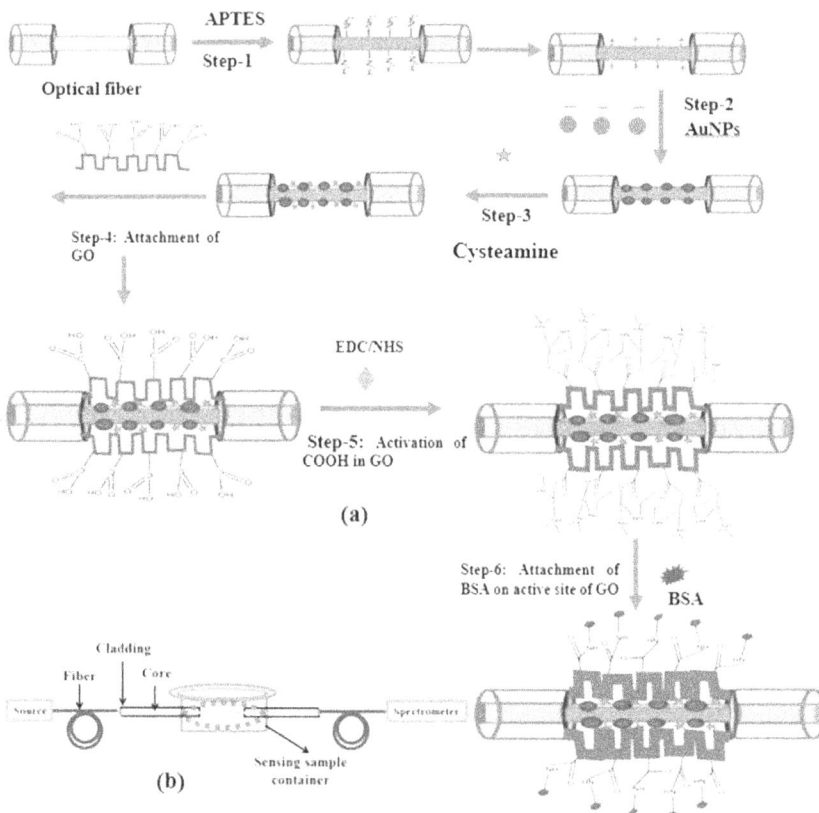

FIGURE 6.20 (a) Step-by-step process to immobilize the BSA molecules on optical fiber and (b) experimental setup.

reaction with BSA molecule; thus, it is more suitable for BSA immobilization. In step 5, the COOH group of the GO is activated by doping the probe in the EDC/NHS solution. The COOH group of the GO is changed to an active state by EDC that reacts with NHS and produces the stable amine-reactive NHS ester. Further, the amine group of the BSA molecule attaches with the NHS-ester to form an amide bond and leads to covalent bonding (step 6). Here, the functionalized optical fiber probe is used in sensing. The measurement setup depicted in Figure 6.20(b) is one in which an optical signal is launched at the input end of an optical fiber probe and collected at the other end of the probe, which is connected to a spectrometer. A beam of light from a broadband source is directed into a silane functionalized fiber probe where sensor probe has been dipped in AuNPs solution. The increase in peak absorbance with dip period is depicted in Figure 6.21.

The absorbance peak is increased due to immobilization of AuNPs over the fiber surface. To remove the unbound AuNPs, the probe is washed with DI water. Here, the first peak at the wavelength (λ) = 529 nm is predominant due to localized plasmons and second peak at λ = 655 nm results due to the aggregation of NPs (Norman et al. 2002) on the surface of the silane-treated fiber core. The immobilization of AuNPs is confirmed by the FESEM image as shown in Figure 6.22. Further, Figure 6.23 shows zoom in a portion of AuNPs immobilized fiber probe. From Figure 6.23, it has been observed that there are aggregates of NPs as well as nonaggregated NPs on the fiber probe. As a result, one can expect two LSPR peaks in the absorbance spectra, one for nonaggregated and another for aggregated NPs. The aggregation can be confirmed by comparing the absorbance spectra of freshly prepared AuNPs in solution form with the AuNPs immobilized fiber probe as shown in Figure 4.24.

In solution form, there is no aggregation of NPs and therefore only one LSPR peak occurs at λ = 529 nm. As the fiber probe contains both aggregated and nonaggregated NPs, two LSPR peaks have been observed in the absorbance spectra, one peak at λ = 529 nm is due to nonaggregation and another peak at λ = 655 nm due to these aggregated NPs. Further, confirmation of gold NPs is done by energy dispersive X-ray spectroscopy (EDX) spectra as shown in Figure 6.25. The presence of the Au peak clearly says that the immobilized particles are of gold. To immobilize GO, the AuNPs immobilized probe is dipped in cysteamine, which acts as a linking agent to GO. In order to see

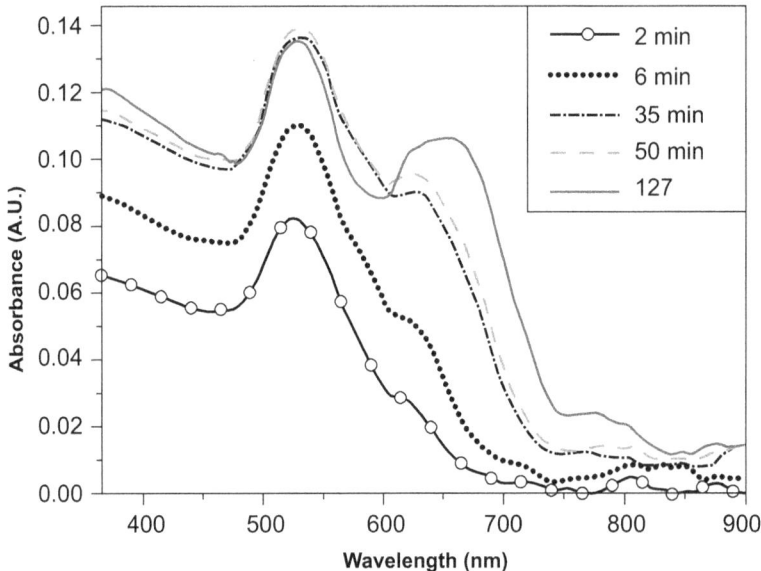

FIGURE 6.21 Absorbance variation with different dip period of AuNPs solution.

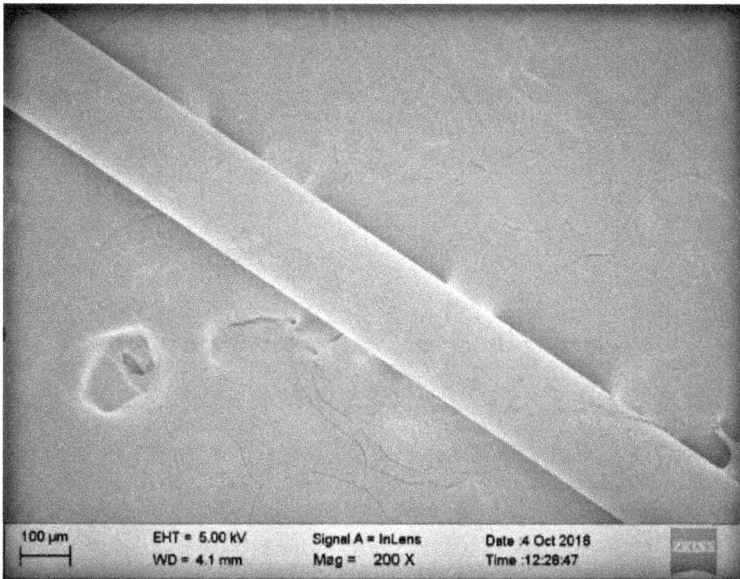

FIGURE 6.22 FESEM image of fiber probe immobilized with AuNPs.

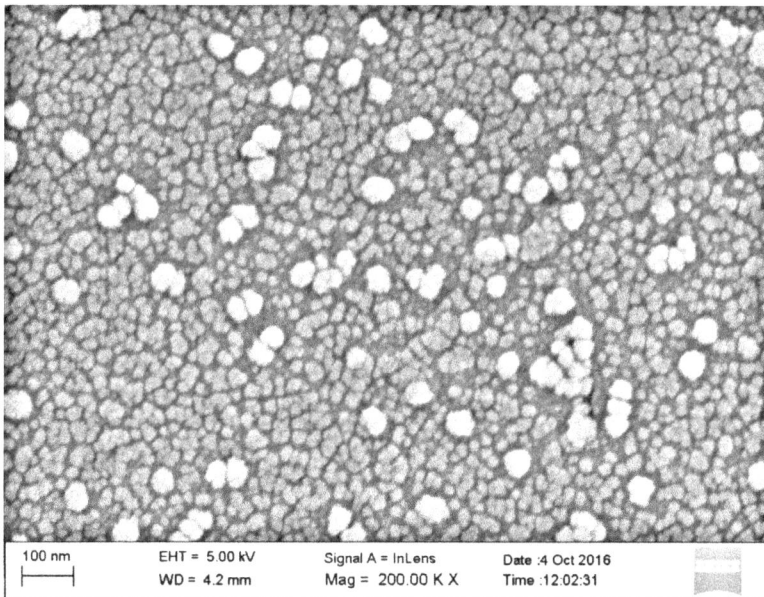

FIGURE 6.23 Zoom in picture of Figure 6.22, showing immobilization of AuNPs on the fiber probe.

the temporal response of cysteamine, Figure 6.26 shows the absorbance variation for different dip periods of cysteamine of 5 mM concentration.

It has been observed that the first peak absorbance decreases from 0.219 to 0.188 at $\lambda = 524$ nm, and the absorbance saturates within an hour, confirming the attachment of cysteamine on gold NPs. Similarly, the absorbance also decreases from 0.1825 to 0.1641 for second peak at $\lambda = 667$ nm. To attach the GO, the cysteamine-treated fiber probe is dipped in the GO solution, and it has been found that the absorbance saturates in around 100 minutes, as shown in Figure 6.27.

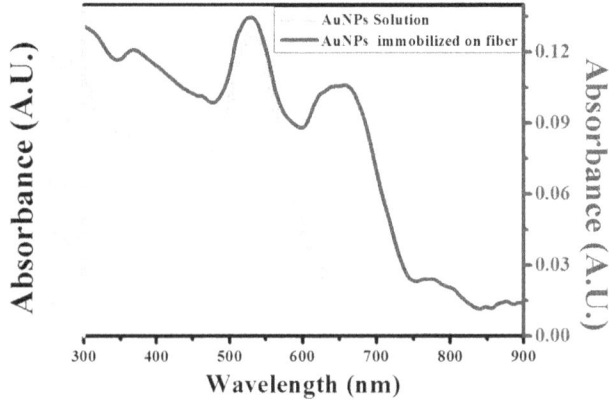

FIGURE 6.24 Shows variation of absorbance of AuNPs in solutions form by light grey line, and AuNPs immobilized on fiber by dark grey line.

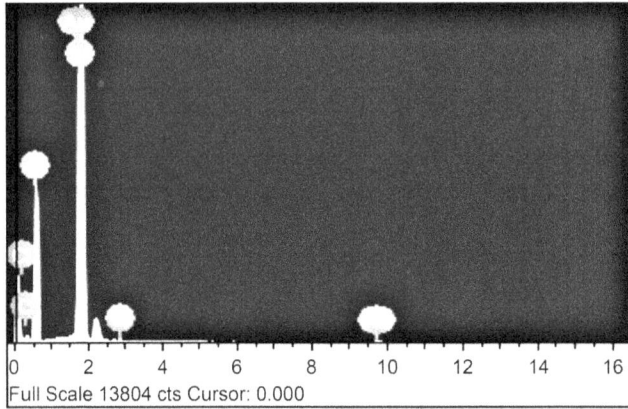

FIGURE 6.25 Shows the EDX spectra of the fiber probe immobilized with AuNPs.

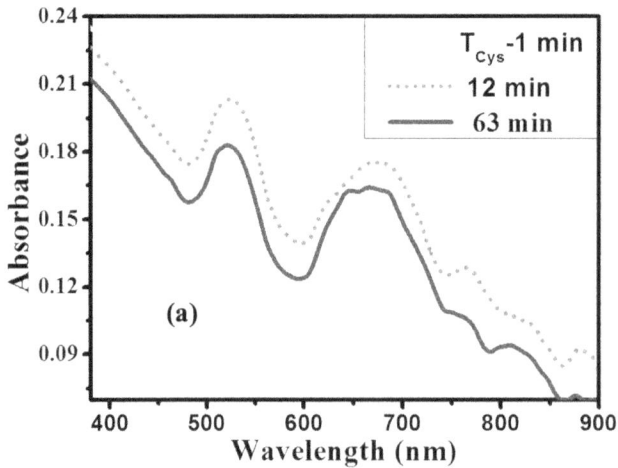

FIGURE 6.26 Absorbance variation for different dip period for 5 mM cysteamine.

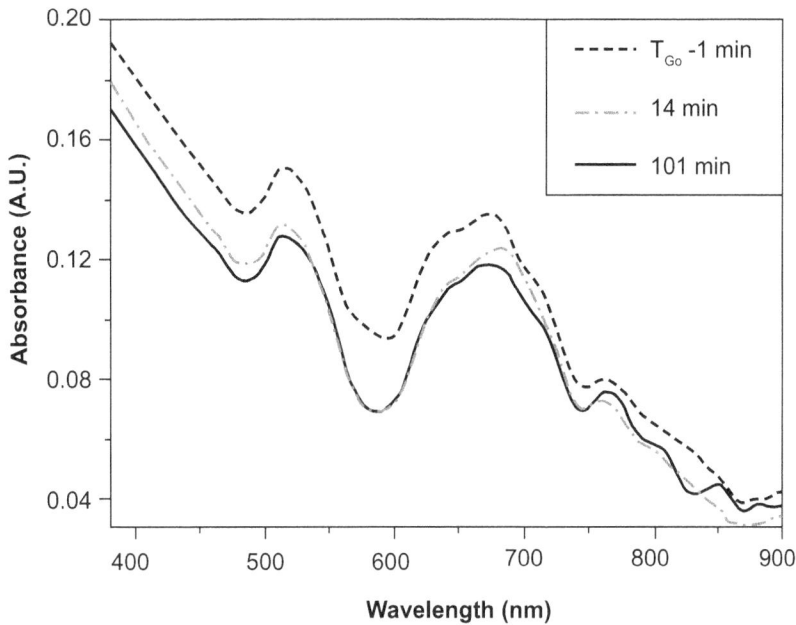

FIGURE 6.27 Absorbance variation for different dip period for GO.

The decrease in peak absorbance with time indicates the attachment of GO to the surface of the optical fiber. This is due to the immobilization of GO on the nanoparticle that causes the free electrons around the surface of the NPs to be damped, resulting in the absorbance decreasing with time.

Because of the active site of –COOH, the degree of interaction between BSA and GO is determined. Further, to activate the –COOH functional group, the fiber probe immobilized with GO is dipped in EDC/NHS solution. Here 100 μM of EDC and 400 μM of NHS are mixed in 1:4 ratio to form EDC/NHS solution. The temporal response of EDC/NHS on the GO immobilized probe has been observed for different dip periods in the EDC/NHS solution. It has been realized that the first peak absorbance decreases from 0.165 to 0.156 in around 15 minutes, depending on the conditions. Here the decrease in peak absorbance with time implies the activation of –COOH functional group of GO in the presence of EDC/NHS (Chiu and Huang 2014). Further, to compare the temporal response of cysteamine, GO and EDC/NHS of first and second peaks, Figure 6.28 shows the variation in absorbance with time for the whole process.

It has been observed that both peaks show a similar type of response with time. When cysteamine is used, it has been observed that first peak absorbance varies from 0.21951 to 0.18744, and second peak absorbance varies from 0.18526 to 0.16963 during the first hour of the experiment. For GO, the first and second peak absorbances decrease from 0.1519 to 0.13026 and from 0.13803 to 0.11932 from 64 minutes to 164 minutes, respectively. However, for EDC/NHS, the first and second peak absorbances vary from 0.16484 to 0.15672 and from 0.14663 to 0.14539 for the time variation from 165 minutes to 180 minutes, respectively. The decrease in peak absorbance in cysteamine, GO, and EDC/NHS is the clear indication of an interaction of cysteamine, GO, and EDC/NHS in subsequent steps. The investigation of the interaction between GO and biomolecules is extremely important, particularly for peptides and proteins that are associated with disease or drug development. Further, BSA protein is immobilized on the GO-coated fiber core. To study the interaction of different concentrations of BSA on GO-coated probe, the absorbance variation has been studied for different concentrations of BSA prepared in phosphate buffer solution (pH = 7.40): 1 ng/mL, 100 ng/mL, and 1 μg/mL.

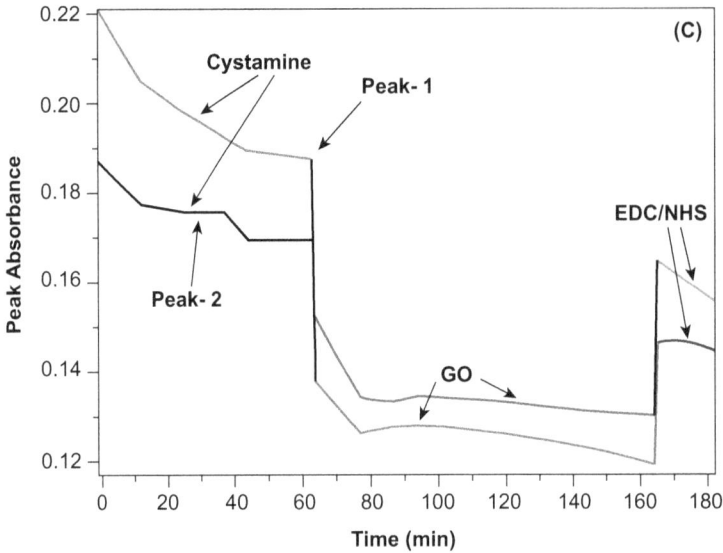

FIGURE 6.28 Variation of peak 1 and peak 2 absorbance with time for the entire chemical process (from cysteamine attachment to activation –COOH functional group of GO).

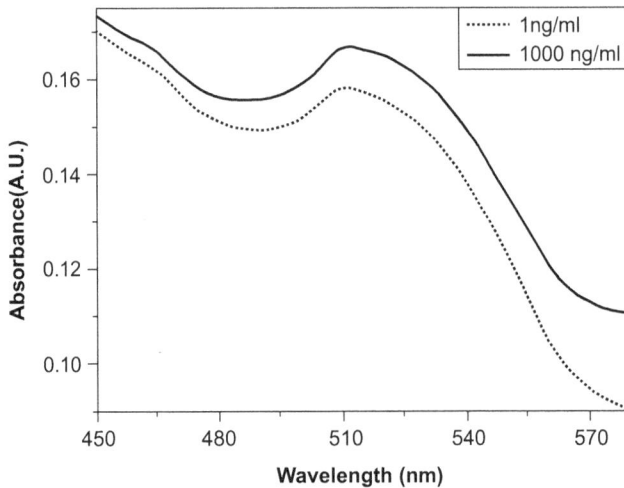

FIGURE 6.29 Absorbance variation for BSA concentration of 1 ng/mL and 1000 ng/mL.

The absorbance variation for BSA concentration of 1 ng/mL and 1 μg/mL is shown in Figure 6.29. Here the x-axis represents the incident wavelength, and the y-axis represents the corresponding absorbance values at the sensor output. In this study, it has been found that peak (here first peak) absorbance increases from 0.1598 to 0.16878 when the concentration increases from 1 ng/mL to 1 μg/mL. The increase in absorbance with the concentration of BSA can be attributed to its higher values of RI at higher concentration.

To study the interaction of BSA with different concentrations of GO, the peak absorbance with time has been plotted for 1 ng/mL, 100 ng/mL, and 1 μg/mL concentrations of BSA, as shown in Figure 6.30. The line with the squares is the peak absorbance with time for BSA concentration of 1 ng/mL, the line with circles and up triangles is for BSA concentration of 100 ng/mL and 1 μg/mL,

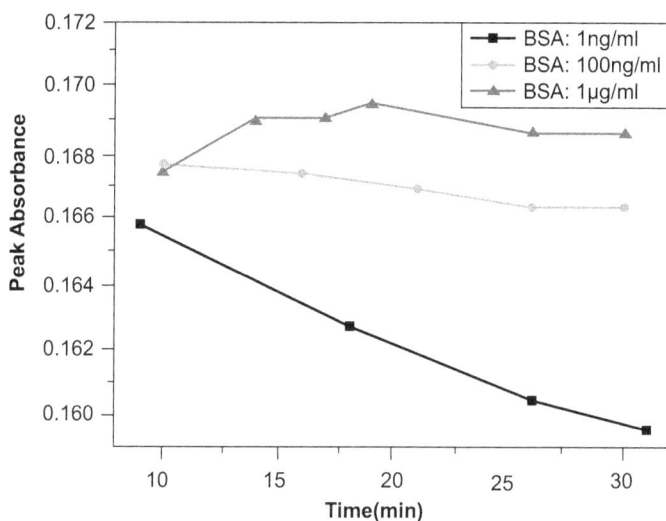

FIGURE 6.30 Absorbance variation with time for the different concentrations of BSA and the points with error bar are the experimental data.

TABLE 6.1
Limit of Detection for Different Analytes Using LSPR

Concept	Minimum limit of detection	Sample	Ref.
LSPR	0.8 nM	Anti-IgG	Sai, Kundu, and Mukherji 2009
LSPR	0.95 nM	Anti-DNP	Tang et al. 2006
LSPR	1.6 nM	Anti-human IgG	Cao et al. 2013
LSPR	100 μM	Methylene blue	Luo et al. 2013
LSPR	0.0289 nM	AFP in bovine (alpha-fetoprotein)	Li et al. 2014
LSPR	6.66 μM	Rabbit IgG	Wu et al. 2010
LSPR	10 pM	BSA	Nayak, Parhi, and Jha 2015

Note: AFP, alpha-fetoprotein; LSPR, localized surface plasmon resonance.

respectively. The decrease in peak absorbance from 0.1659 to 0.15961 with time confirms that BSA 1 ng/mL is interacting with the functional group (-COOH) of GO. For BSA concentration of 100 ng/mL, it has been seen that the peak absorbance reduces from 0.16765 to 0.16644 for the time variation from 10 to 30 minutes. However, for BSA concentration of 1 μg/mL, the absorbance versus time curve shows nearly saturation, as the active sites -COOH functional group of GO gets blocked in the presence of higher concentrations of BSA. This is in accordance with the report available in the literature (Wang et al. 2017). Further, the LoD of different biomolecules has been compared from the literature, and their values are given in Table 6.1. In the present case, the LoD is better than that reported in the literature with the advantage of fiber as an online system.

6.4 MICRO-BALL FIBER SENSOR PROBE BASED URIC ACID BIOSENSOR

In this section, an enzymatic biosensor based on LSPR was developed for the quantitative detection of uric acid (UA) from human serum. A special microsphere optical fiber with a diameter of 350 μm was made as the sensing system, which is designed as a sensing probe. Moreover, GO and AuNPs are selected as surface modifiers to improve the sensing performance. It shows excellent selectivity and high sensitivity in practical detection experiments. During the fabrication process of the proposed probes, the necessary immobilization materials of GO and AuNPs were synthesized by the well-known Hummer method and the Turkevich method, respectively. In order to determine their absorption properties in solution dispersions, the samples were thoroughly scanned using UV-Vis spectrophotometer. These two solutions about AuNPs and GO, separately, showed strong absorption peaks wavelengths at 519 and 230 nm. Moreover, a HRTEM was then employed to observe the surface micromorphology of the coating materials layer and to analyze the energy spectrum of existent elements. After that, uricase was then immobilized over coated material on the probe to enhance the specific perception of UA concentration. The sensitivity and detection limit of the developed sensor are 2.1% per mM and 65.60 µM, respectively, in a range of 10 µM–1 mM. Finally, an A5800 automatic biochemical analyzer was employed to detect the same UA samples, and compared to the proposed sensing system, the results were satisfactory with good consistency.

6.4.1 FABRICATION OF MICRO-BALL FIBER STRUCTURE

The discussed microsphere optical fiber structure was selected as a sensing probe due to the dual-beam interference that can be well realized. During this fabrication process, a standard single-mode fiber (SMF) without multimode-induced distortion and attenuation is processed by using an advanced fusion splicer machine (FSM) (Harun et al. 2013; Jasim et al. 2013; Song, Gehlbach, and Kang 2013). Here, in short, the end part of a bare fiber without a coating layer is fixed carefully between the V-grooves of the FSM, and the selected treatment procedure is then initiated. Finally, under the condition of the heating of the electrode and the cooperative rotation of the motor, the exposed end of the fiber will gradually become spherical (Jasim et al. 2013). Several key parameters here such as electrode gap, predischarge time, clean discharge time, and electrode adjustment are set as 2.2 mm, 0 sec, 150 ms, and 0 µm, respectively.

6.4.2 EXPERIMENTAL SETUP

A diagram of the experimental setup is presented in Figure 6.31. Here, the proposed spherical probe around 350 µm of diameter with compact nature, completely immersed in the UA sample solution, is connected to the tungsten-halogen light source and the spectrometer, respectively, by a bifurcated optical fiber. When the light source is turned on, the redox reaction of analyte and receptor occurs on the outer surface of the probe, and the related microscopic change of RI of the medium near the nanocoating is reflected in the signal. Meanwhile, the spectrometer will collect the reflected signal and send it to the computer to record the data. Here, UA samples of varying concentrations in a range of 0.01–1 mM are measured in the experiment. After each quantity test, the sensing region of the probe will follow by a full rinse with PBS solution.

6.4.3 CHARACTERIZATION OF GOLD NANOPARTICLES AND GRAPHENE OXIDE

It is crucial to evaluate the optical and physical properties of nanomaterials such as AuNPs and GO. Therefore, AuNPs solution and GO solution were well detected by UV-Vis spectrophotometer and HRTEM, respectively. As shown in Figure 6.32(a), the absorption spectrum of diluted AuNPs solution can be obtained by UV-Vis spectrophotometer. From the results, we can see that there is a strong absorption peak at 519 nm, which is called the peak of the SPR wavelength. Subsequently, with the help of HRTEM, the distribution of AuNPs in the solution was well studied. As illustrated in Figure 6.32(b), the AuNPs here are in spherical shape in the solution, and without cluster phenomenon, the spherical radius of the nanoparticles is around 11 nm.

Similarly, GO aqueous dispersion was characterized. As seen from Figure 6.33(a), the absorption curves have obvious peaks at 310 nm and 230 nm, respectively. This is due to

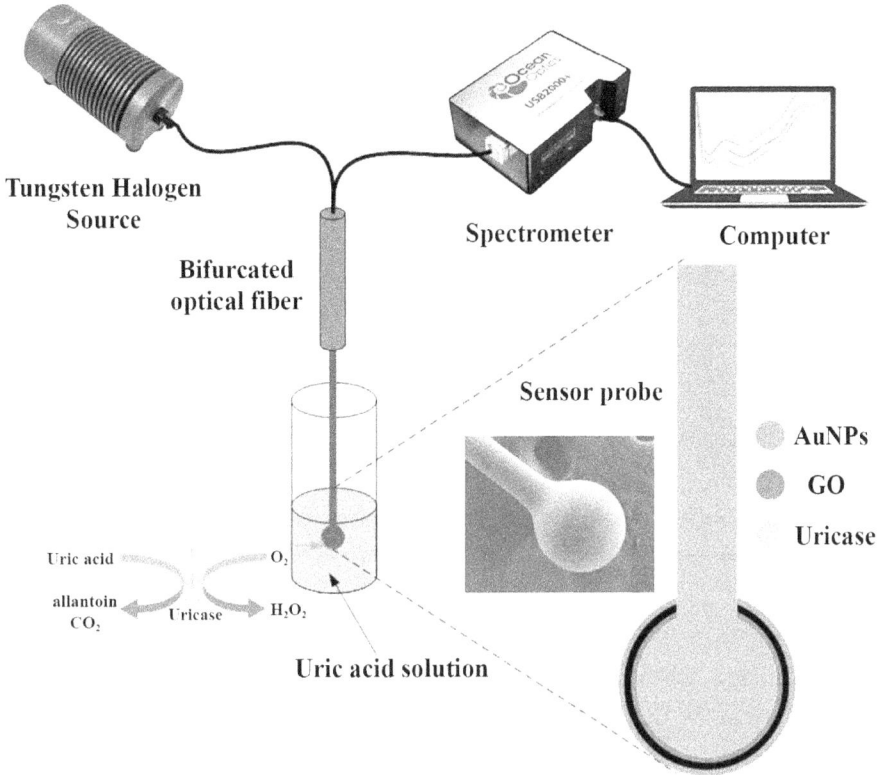

FIGURE 6.31 Experimental setup for uric acid detection using a micro-ball fiber structure.

Source: Reprinted with permission from *IEEE Transactions on NanoBioscience.* Copyright, 2020, IEEE (Kumar et al. 2020).

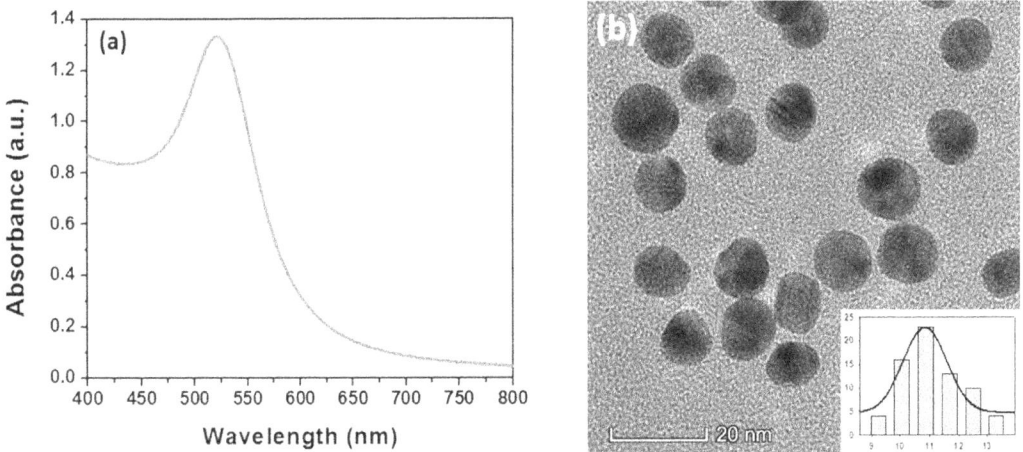

FIGURE 6.32 (a) Absorbance spectrum of gold nanoparticles, (b) high-resolution transmission electron microscopic image of synthesized gold nanoparticles.

Source: Reprinted with permission from *IEEE Transactions on NanoBioscience.* Copyright, 2020, IEEE (Kumar et al. 2020).

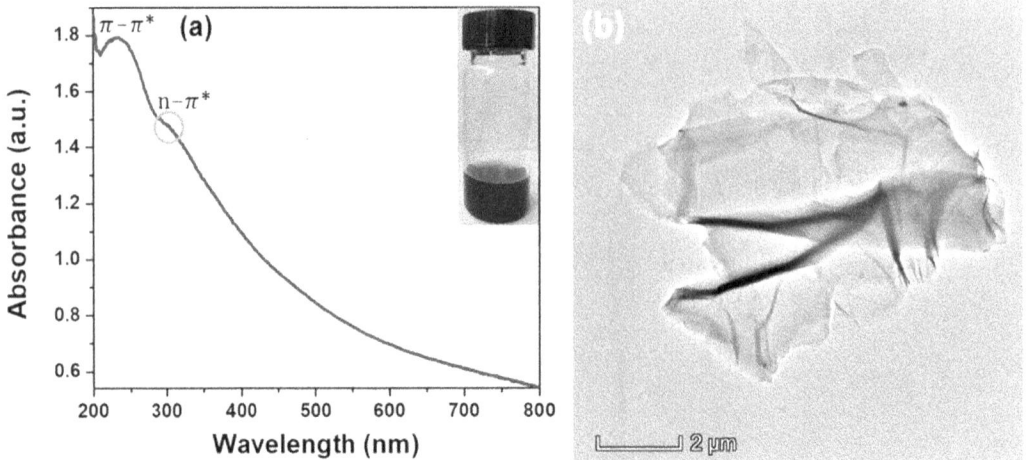

FIGURE 6.33   (a) Absorbance spectrum of GO, (b) HRTEM image of synthesized GO.

Source: Reprinted with permission from *IEEE Transactions on NanoBioscience.* Copyright, 2020, IEEE (Kumar et al. 2020).

the transitions of $n - \pi^*$ and $\pi - \pi^*$, as well as the sp^2 hybridization of carbon-oxygen bonds. The monolayer structure of the GO slice is clearly evident in Figure 6.33(b). Those characteristics may prove that the synthesized AuNPs and GO powders have good quality and are prepared for further use (Dissanayake et al. 2018).

6.4.4   DETECTION OF URIC ACID SOLUTIONS

The result in Figure 6.34(a) shows the detection of uric acid samples in a concentration range of 10 μM–1 mM based on a functional micro-ball fiber structure coated with uricase/AuNPs materials in the developed sensor system. From the result, the reflectivity intensity decreased with the increase of UA concentration. This is because different concentrations of UA in the sample solution are captured by uricase on the probe surface to produce a related concentration of allantoin, CO_2, and H_2O_2. This phenomenon will cause the RI of the dielectric near the nanocoating layer, which changes the reflectivity signal. Figure 6.34(b) shows the same experiment against the uricase/GO/AuNPs-based biosensing probe. It can be seen that with the help of GO, the range of reflectivity is wider (from 86.85%–86.76% to 95.39% to 93.38%), which means that the sensing performance of the proposed sensing system has improved.

6.4.5   SENSITIVITY, LINEARITY, AND DETECTION LIMIT OF SENSOR

Based on the results of Figure 6.35(a–b), the linear plots of reflectivity with UA concentration are plotted, and the regression equations of corresponding linear are calculated. The results show that the sensitivity is 0.005% and 2.1% per mM, respectively. The correlation coefficients (R^2) are 0.9928 and 0.9744, with the linear range of 0.05–1 mM and 0.01–1 mM, respectively. As can be seen, the GO/uricase/AuNPs-immobilized probes showed greater sensitivity and larger linearity range than the uricase/AuNPs-based probe without GO. At the same time, the corresponding blank standard deviation (SD) is observed as 0.045925 after 10 times repetition of PBS solution test. As for the sensor system based on the GO/uricase/AuNPs-optimized probe, the final detection limit, calculated as LoD = (3 × SD)/sensitivity (Rana et al. 2018), is 65.60 μM with the UA concentration in range of 10 μm–1 mM.

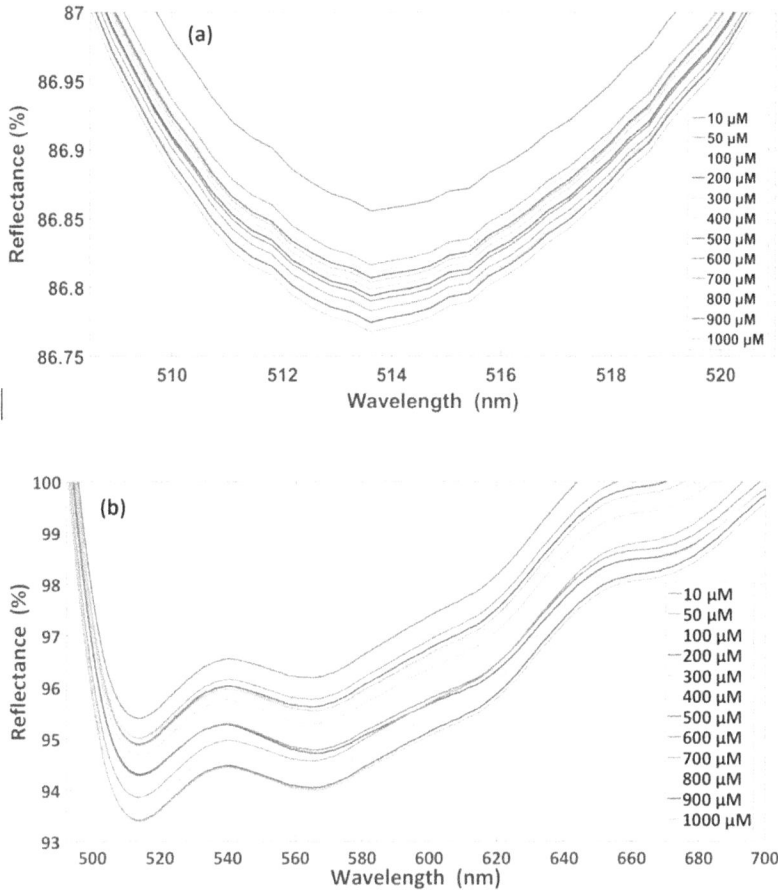

FIGURE 6.34 Variation of reflectance against the different solutions of UA concentrations: (a) uricase/ AuNPs-coated, (b) uricase/GO/AuNPs-coated micro-ball fiber structure.

Source: Reprinted with permission from *IEEE Transactions on NanoBioscience.* Copyright, 2020, IEEE (Kumar et al. 2020).

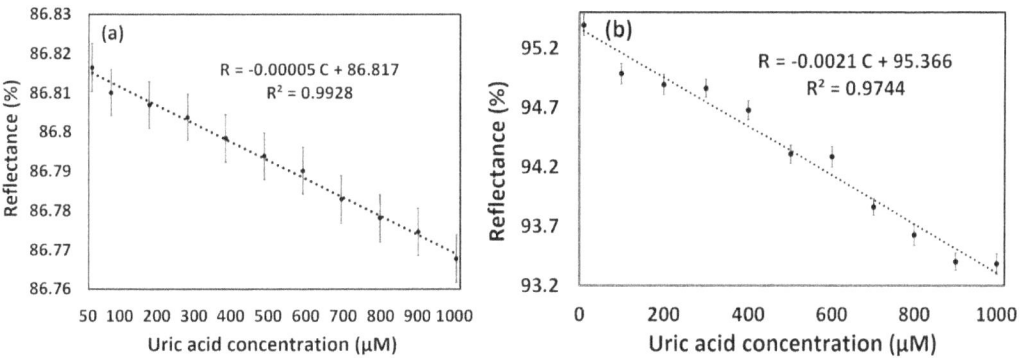

FIGURE 6.35 Variation of reflectance with respect to UA concentration: (a) uricase/AuNPs-, (b) uricase/ GO/AuNPs-coated micro-ball fiber structure.

Source: Reprinted with permission from *IEEE Transactions on NanoBioscience.* Copyright, 2020, IEEE (Kumar et al. 2020).

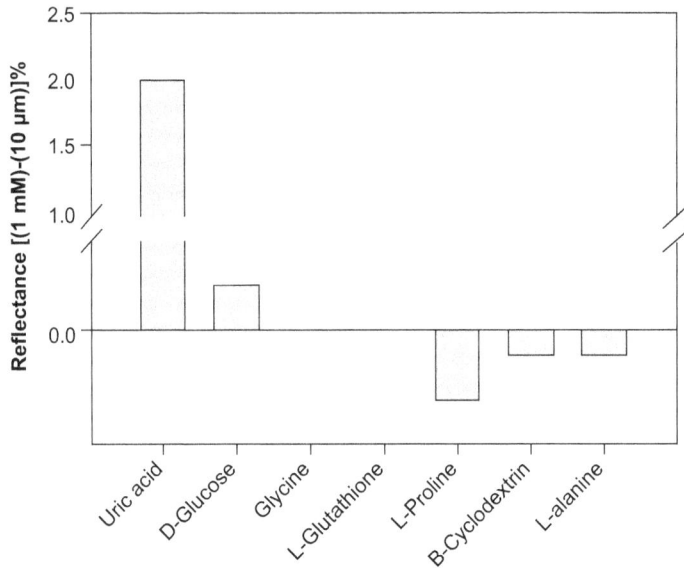

FIGURE 6.36 Selectivity analysis of the proposed UA sensor using different interferents found with the UA.

Source: Reprinted with permission from *IEEE Transactions on NanoBioscience.* Copyright, 2020, IEEE (Kumar et al. 2020).

6.4.6 SELECTIVITY OF SENSOR

In selectivity testing, common biological disruptors present in the serum or urine such as D-glucose, glycine, L-glutathione, L-proline, в-cyclodextrin, and L-alanine are determined to be tested compared to the UA samples. To this end, the minimum and maximum concentrations of each biomolecular sample are precisely prepared, and the correlative results are obtained by comparing the key gist, maximum reflection draft, as shown in Figure 6.36. From the data in that bar chart, it can be easily found that the developed biosensor system based on uricase/GO/AuNPs-functionalized probe performed the largest value of reflection drift to the UA analyte, which directly proves its specificity to UA analyte.

6.4.7 ANALYSIS OF URIC ACID IN HUMAN SERUM

For the evaluation of the practical detection effect to the actual samples, we extracted serum samples from five human serum samples, from Liaocheng People's Hospital associated with Medical College of LCU in China. We measured them directly using the developed probes (Misra et al. 2013; Xu et al. 2015; Wang et al. 2016; Wang et al. 2019). The extraction process is described simply as centrifuging the donated sample for 5 minutes at 4000 rpm, then carefully filtering the supernatant to produce a yellowish serum sample with the help of a 45 45-micron syringe (Misra et al. 2013). As a comparison to verify the reliability of the experimental results, similarly, an A5800 automatic biochemical analyzer was employed to quantitatively detect the concentration of UA in serum samples. Here, the normal range in the serum is 150–420 μM. The comparison results are shown in Figure 6.37. The experimental results show that the benchmark data of the A5800 machine are at 294 μM, 388 μM, 479 μM, 405 μM, and 214 μM, respectively; the relative errors (%) of the developed sensing system to five clinical samples here were 7.83, −8.98, 6.62, 5.15, and −0.94, respectively. It can be concluded that our method has high reliability, and the developed probe has great potential for clinical application in the future.

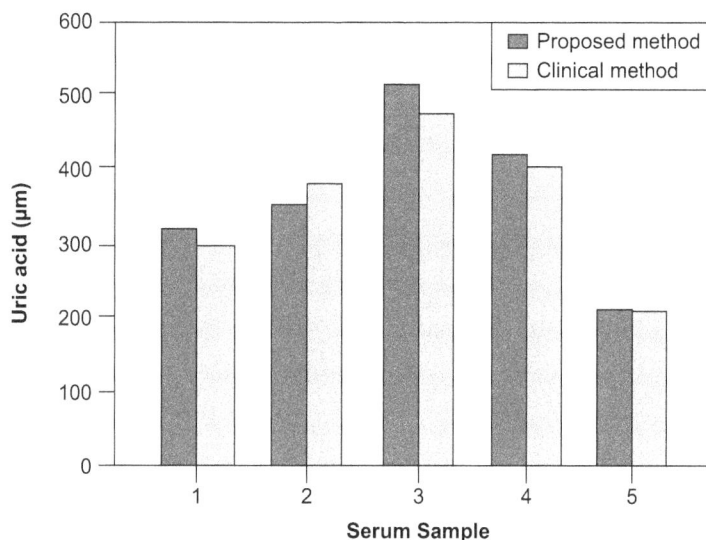

FIGURE 6.37 Analytical results of UA in human serum obtained using proposed uricase/GO/AuNPs-immobilized sensor and A5800 automatic biochemical analyzer.

Source: Reprinted with permission from *IEEE Transactions on NanoBioscience.* Copyright, 2020, IEEE (Kumar et al. 2020).

6.5 NOVEL PERIODICALLY TAPERED STRUCTURE-BASED SENSOR TO DETECT ASCORBIC ACID

As one of the most important components of human blood, ascorbic acid (AA) is closely related to the health of the central nervous system, organs, and tissues, as well as resisting aging, scavenging free radicals, and enhancing human immunity (Antonelli et al. 2002; Fu, Zheng, and Fu 2015; Mu et al. 2018). The normal range of AA in the central nervous system is 100–500 µM. In general, the necessity of that can be obtained easily from mashed homogenates of foods such as fruits and vegetables (Chauhan et al. 2011; Ferreira et al. 2015). In this section, an LSPR sensor based on a multitapered fiber structure is introduced for the determination of AA contented samples (Zhu et al. 2020). There are three different kinds of multitapered fiber with four, five, and eight of periods, which have been developed for the study of sensing performance. In the experiment, AuNPs (around 10 nm of particle size) were well immobilized on the surface of the sensing region of the developed fiber structure to stimulate stronger LSPR effects. After that, GO and functional ascorbate oxidase (AOx) were covered one after another to enhance sensing performance. The particles shape and size of AuNPs as well as the excellent sensing properties of GO are continuing throughout the whole book, and their role will not be repeated here. The results revealed that AuNPs/GO/AOx-functionalized sensing probes with five-period multitapered structure had the best sensing performance. The sensitivity, R^2, and LoD of the sensor are obtained as 8.3 nm/mM, 0.9724, and 51.94 µM, respectively.

6.5.1 DESIGN CONSIDERATION AND FABRICATION OF PROPOSED SENSORS

The periodic multitapered structure used in the experiment is based on the common single-mode fiber (SMF; 9 µm, 125 µm), which has low cost, as well as can effectively eliminate the mode compression (Villatoro, Monzón-Hernández, and Mejía 2003). The procedure as shown in Figure 6.38 is demonstrated as follows, the repeated times of the taper are set in the software, and the other important parameters such as the electrode discharge time, the translation speed, and translation

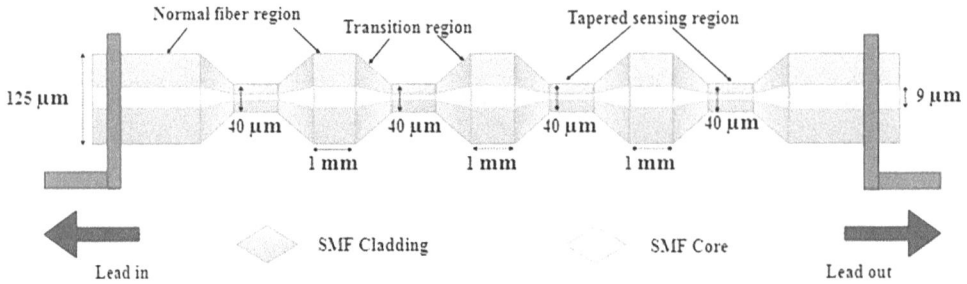

FIGURE 6.38 Bare fiber-tapered fiber structure.

Source: Reprinted with permission from *Optics & Laser Technology.* Copyright, 2020, Elsevier (Zhu et al. 2020).

time of the left and right motors are indispensable to modify the single taper of structure. The uncoated SMF is then carefully fixed between the electrodes. After clicking to run that program in software, the advanced FSM machine will perform repetitive taper processing on the fiber. Finally, four-, five-, and eight-segment tapered bare fiber structures were successfully obtained and named as probe 1, probe 2, and probe 3, respectively. In particular, the difficulty of program testing is that the structure shape and surface tension of the fiber will change after each taper treatment; thus, the fiber becomes more fragile as the number of taper segments increases, this is also the most important factor to limit the number of repetitions of tapering treatment. Figure 6.39(a–c) show the diameter scanning of multitapered fibers. From the related scan curves, it can be observed that the constant diameters of all probes' waist region are 40 µm and the interval between adjacent taper sections is 1000 µm. Figure 6.39(d) shows the SEM image about the partial of multitapered structure. It can be proved that the optical fiber structure has excellent symmetry and can be used in the follow-up experiments.

Before the experiment, AA contented samples with various concentrations (like 10 µM, 50 µM, 100 µM, 150 µM, 200 µM, 400 µM, 600 µM, 800 µM, and 1 mM) of AA, that is already covered at the normal level in the central nervous system, were diluted from high to low concentrations. Then, as shown in Figure 6.40(a), the biosensing platform was built, in which a tungsten-halogen light source, a sensing probe, and a spectrometer were directly connected in turn by using optical fiber jumpers. Here, the schematic of three different AuNPs/GO/AOx-functionalized sensing probes using probe 1, 2, and 3 are shown in Figure 6.40(b–d), respectively. Using a pipette gun, the analyte sample was then carefully dripped onto the surface of the probe for detection. After the reactions of different concentrations of AA are complete, the subtly varied RI of the medium around the probe will change the output wavelength gradually, so that it can be recorded by the software as the specific LSPR spectra.

With the help of SEM, the overall views of the sensing region of probes 1, 2, and 3 were imaged clearly as shown in Figure 6.41(a–c), to further prove the feasibility of the probe fabrication process. Then, Figure 6.41(d) displays the microscopic distribution of AuNPs/GO coating on the probe surface at a magnification of ×21.76 K (100 nm). As we can see, the GO slices are evenly spread over the AuNPs layer. In addition, EDX results shown in Figure 6.41(e) were used to analyze the element composition of the coating, and a large number of C and Au elements were found, which proved the feasibility of the coating technology.

6.5.2 Detection of Ascorbic Acid

In this experiment, two promising nanomaterials AuNPs and GO were selected to improve the sensing performance of biosensors. Further, by fully exploring the differences in the performance of the developed probes in even or odd numbers of taper regions, the sensing characteristic curves using individual probe 1, 2, 3 (taper periods are greater than three) are summarized and plotted as shown

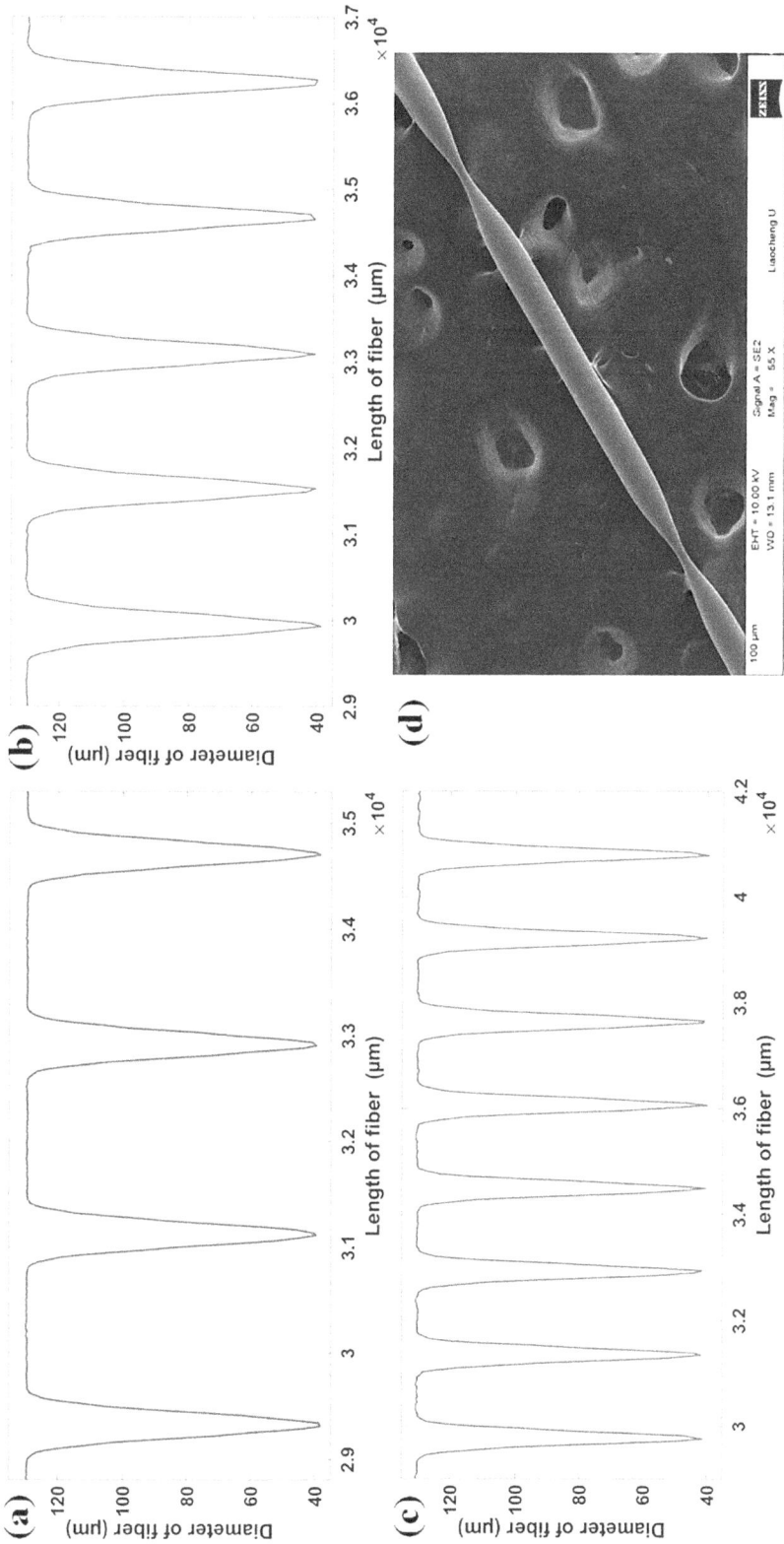

FIGURE 6.39 Probe configuration: length versus waist diameter: (a) probe 1, (b) probe 2, (c) probe 3, and (d) SEM image of tapered fiber.

Source: Reprinted with permission from *Optics & Laser Technology.* Copyright, 2020, Elsevier (Zhu et al. 2020).

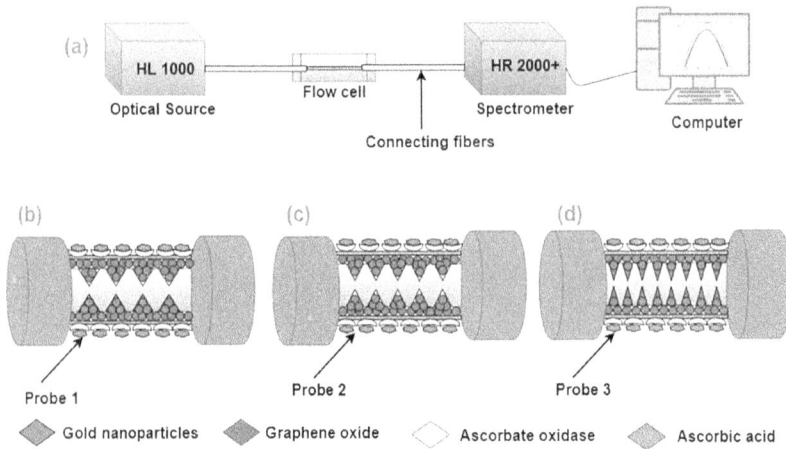

FIGURE 6.40   (a) Experimental setup, configurations, (b) probe 1, (c) probe 2, (d) probe 3.

Source: Reprinted with permission from *Optics & Laser Technology.* Copyright, 2020, Elsevier (Zhu et al. 2020).

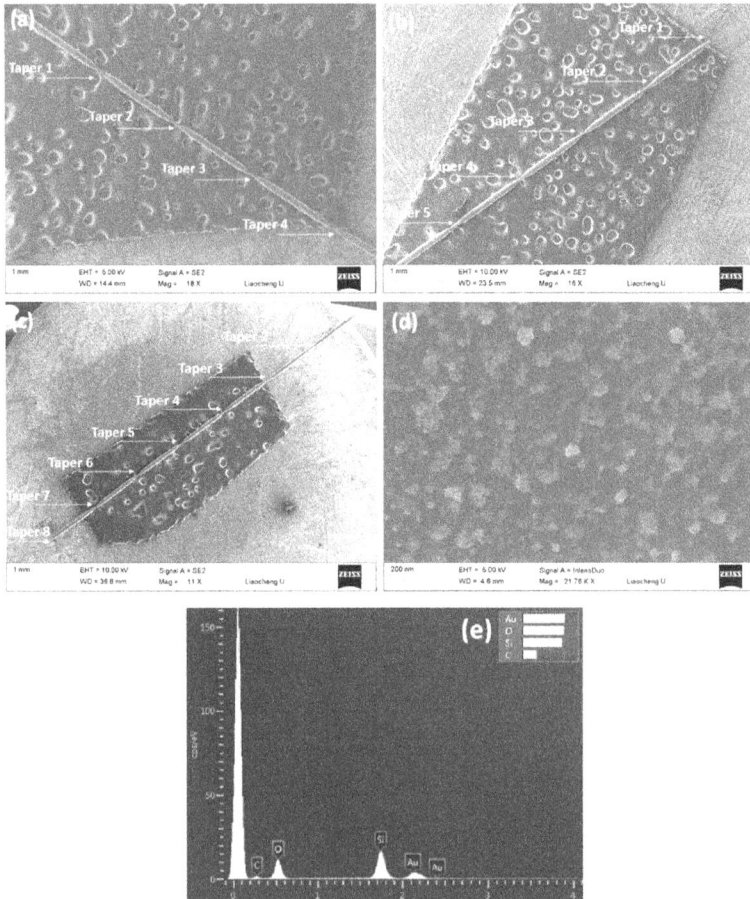

FIGURE 6.41   SEM image at lower magnification of (a) probe 1, (b) probe 2, (c) probe 3, (d) SEM image of proposed probe 2 at higher magnification, (e) EDX image of proposed probe 2.

Source: Reprinted with permission from *Optics & Laser Technology.* Copyright, 2020, Elsevier (Zhu et al. 2020).

in Figure 6.42(a–f). According to the results, probe 2 has the highest sensitivity, the largest wavelength shift, and the highest linear fit among the three fiber structures. In particular, the sensitivity of probe 2 at 8.3 nm/mM is much higher than that of the other two. This shows that probe 2 has more development value and is more suitable for quantitative detection of AA samples as a sensor probe. Therefore, the stability of the sensing probe with selected fiber structure was evaluated 10 times with PBS solution, and the final LoD was calculated to be 51.94 μM. For probe 3, the excessive number of taper structures can cause the high radiation loss of the sensing signal, which seriously affects the sensitivity and stability of the sensor. In the next step, to further optimize biosensor

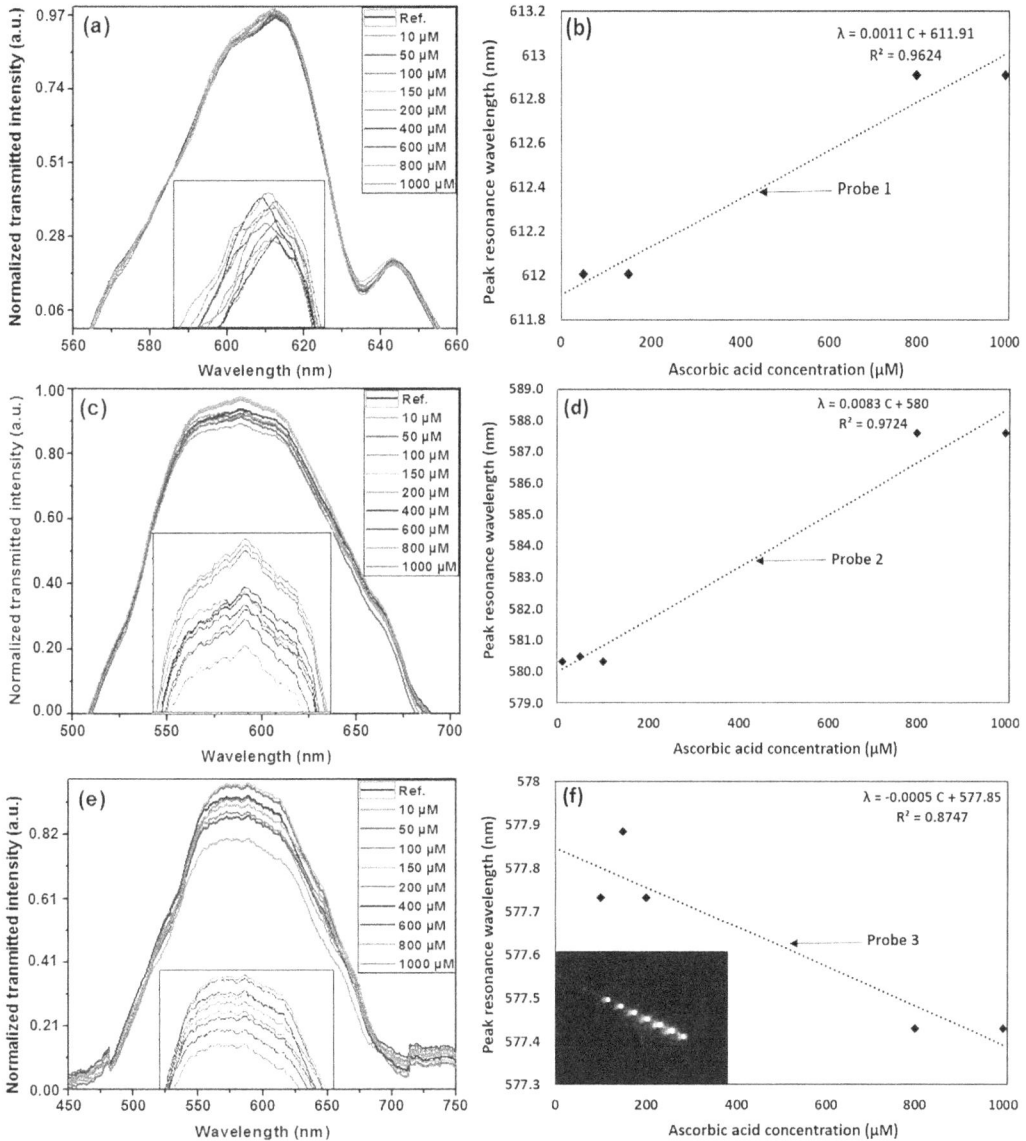

FIGURE 6.42 Analysis of sensor probe: (a) LSPR spectra for probe 1, (b) linear fitting curve for probe 1, (c) LSPR spectra for probe 2, (d) linear fitting curve for probe 2, (e) LSPR spectra for probe 3, and (f) linear fitting curve for probe 3.

Source: Reprinted with permission from *Optics & Laser Technology.* Copyright, 2020, Elsevier (Zhu et al. 2020).

systems for effective detection of AA in the application of a practical scenario, we can continue to explore the influence, like optimization of optical fiber structure and the selection of surface NMs, on the sensing performance.

6.6 SUMMARY AND CONCLUSION

In this chapter, a refractometer based on a fiber-optic tip sensor has been developed using the functionalization of GO encapsulated AuNPs (GOE-AuNPs). The tip sensor is easy to handle, can detect a minute amount of analyte solution due to the miniature size of the sensing tip, can work in harsh environmental conditions, and is simplified and economic in comparison to conventional fiber-assisted LSPR sensors. However, noisy and broad absorbance spectra make the system difficult to use for analysis. Therefore, the work has been extended from the reflection mode to the transmission mode. In transmission mode, better transmittance and narrower absorbance spectra have been observed. It has also been observed that encapsulation of AuNPs provides the stable performance of sensor. It keeps the AuNPs from agglomeration and broadens the absorbance spectra that reduce the sensor's performance. The sensitivity of the GOE-AuNPs-based sensor is 2.288 ΔA/ RIU. The developed sensor is economical, reusable, easier to fabricate, and provides label-free sensing and real-time detection with resolution of 8.7×10^{-5} RIU.

Further, a study has been carried out on an optical fiber biosensor for BSA detection using GO decorated AuNPs. The cysteamine linking agent has been used to immobilize the GO over AuNPs-coated fiber structure. The limit of detection for this reproducible probe is found to be 10 pM. Further increasing the concentration of BSA, the peak absorbance saturates, confirming no further interaction of BSA with GO. Such study will open a new avenue for production of low-cost optical fiber biosensors by riding on the advantages of 2D material oxides to study the kinetics of protein binding and different online biosensing applications.

In order to design and develop a low-cost optical fiber sensor, one can use silver nanoparticles (AgNPs) instead of AuNPs. Apart from being economical, Ag shows narrower absorbance due its lesser value of the imaginary part of RI. The narrower absorbance curve gives better detection accuracy. Also, the usage of GO will address the oxidation problem of AgNPs. Thereafter, the development process of a uric acid sensor and an ascorbic acid sensor has been discussed using AuNPs and GO. In the next chapter, a performance analysis of a GO-encapsulated AgNPs-based optical fiber LSPR sensor probe is elaborated.

REFERENCES

Antonelli, M. L., G. D'Ascenzo, A. Laganà, and P. Pusceddu. 2002. "Food analyses: A new calorimetric method for ascorbic acid (vitamin C) determination." *Talanta* 58 (5):961–967. https://doi.org/10.1016/ S0039-9140(02)00449-6.

Bekmurzayeva, Aliya, Zhannat Ashikbayeva, Zhuldyz Myrkhiyeva, Aigerim Nugmanova, Madina Shaimerdenova, Takhmina Ayupova, and Daniele Tosi. 2021. "Label-free fiber-optic spherical tip biosensor to enable picomolar-level detection of CD44 protein." *Scientific Reports* 11 (1):19583. DOI: 10.1038/s41598-021-99099-x.

Bharadwaj, Reshma, and Soumyo Mukherji. 2014. "Gold nanoparticle coated U-bend fibre optic probe for localized surface plasmon resonance based detection of explosive vapours." *Sensors and Actuators B: Chemical* 192:804–811. https://doi.org/10.1016/j.snb.2013.11.026.

Bohren, Craig F., and Donald R. Huffman. 2008. *Absorption and Scattering of Light by Small Particles*. John Wiley & Sons.

Brust, Mathias, Donald Bethell, Christopher J. Kiely, and David J. Schiffrin. 1998. "Self-assembled gold nanoparticle thin films with nonmetallic optical and electronic properties." *Langmuir* 14 (19):5425– 5429. DOI: 10.1021/la980557g.

Cao, Jie, Minh Hieu Tu, Tong Sun, and Kenneth T. V. Grattan. 2013. "Wavelength-based localized surface plasmon resonance optical fiber biosensor." *Sensors and Actuators B: Chemical* 181:611–619. https://doi. org/10.1016/j.snb.2013.02.052.

Carter, D. C., and J. X. Ho. 1994. "Structure of serum albumin." *Advances in Protein Chemistry* 45:153–203. DOI: 10.1016/s0065-3233(08)60640-3.

Chauhan, Nidhi, Jagriti Narang, Rachna Rawal, and C. S. Pundir. 2011. "A highly sensitive non-enzymatic ascorbate sensor based on copper nanoparticles bound to multi walled carbon nanotubes and polyaniline composite." *Synthetic Metals* 161 (21):2427–2433. https://doi.org/10.1016/j.synthmet.2011.09.020.

Chen, H., Y. S. Kim, J. Lee, S. J. Yoon, D. S. Lim, H. J. Choi, and K. Koh. 2007. "Enhancement of BSA binding on Au surfaces by calix[4]bisazacrown monolayer." *Sensors (Basel)* 7 (10):2263–2272. DOI: 10.3390/s7102263.

Cheng, Shu-Fang, and Lai-Kwan Chau. 2003. "Colloidal gold-modified optical fiber for chemical and biochemical sensing." *Analytical Chemistry* 75 (1):16–21. DOI: 10.1021/ac020310v.

Chiu, Nan-Fu, and Teng-Yi Huang. 2014. "Sensitivity and kinetic analysis of graphene oxide-based surface plasmon resonance biosensors." *Sensors and Actuators B: Chemical* 197:35–42. https://doi.org/10.1016/j.snb.2014.02.033.

Cittadini, Michela, Marco Bersani, Francesco Perrozzi, Luca Ottaviano, Wojtek Wlodarski, and Alessandro Martucci. 2014. "Graphene oxide coupled with gold nanoparticles for localized surface plasmon resonance based gas sensor." *Carbon* 69:452–459. https://doi.org/10.1016/j.carbon.2013.12.048.

Dissanayake, K. P. W., W. Wu, H. Nguyen, T. Sun, and K. T. V. Grattan. 2018. "Graphene-oxide-coated long-period grating-based fiber optic sensor for relative humidity and external refractive index." *Journal of Lightwave Technology* 36 (4):1145–1151. DOI: 10.1109/JLT.2017.2756097.

Ferreira, Danielle Cristhina Melo, Gabriela Furlan Giordano, Caio César dos Santos Penteado Soares, Jessica Fernanda Afonso de Oliveira, Renata Kelly Mendes, Maria Helena Piazzetta, Angelo Luiz Gobbi, and Mateus Borba Cardoso. 2015. "Optical paper-based sensor for ascorbic acid quantification using silver nanoparticles." *Talanta* 141:188–194. https://doi.org/10.1016/j.talanta.2015.03.067.

Fu, Li, Yu-Hong Zheng, and Zhu-Xian Fu. 2015. "Ascorbic acid amperometric sensor using a graphene-wrapped hierarchical TiO$_2$ nanocomposite." *Chemical Papers* 69 (5):655–661. DOI: 10.1515/chempap-2015-0079.

Gangopadhayay, Arun Kumar, and Animesh Chakravorty. 1961. "Charge transfer spectra of some Gold(III) complexes." *Journal of Chemical Physics* 35 (6):2206–2209. DOI: 10.1063/1.1732233.

Guo, Shaojun, and Erkang Wang. 2007. "Synthesis and electrochemical applications of gold nanoparticles." *Analytica Chimica Acta* 598 (2):181–192. https://doi.org/10.1016/j.aca.2007.07.054.

Haes, Amanda J., and Richard P. Van Duyne. 2002. "A nanoscale optical biosensor: Sensitivity and selectivity of an approach based on the localized surface plasmon resonance spectroscopy of triangular silver nanoparticles." *Journal of the American Chemical Society* 124 (35):10596–10604. DOI: 10.1021/ja020393x.

Harun, S. W., A. A. Jasim, H. A. Rahman, M. Z. Muhammad, and H. Ahmad. 2013. "Micro-ball lensed fiber-based glucose sensor." *IEEE Sensors Journal* 13 (1):348–350. DOI: 10.1109/JSEN.2012.2215958.

Henglein, Arnim. 1993. "Physicochemical properties of small metal particles in solution: 'Microelectrode' reactions, chemisorption, composite metal particles, and the atom-to-metal transition." *Journal of Physical Chemistry* 97 (21):5457–5471. DOI: 10.1021/j100123a004.

Huang, Xiaohua, Prashant K. Jain, Ivan H. El-Sayed, and Mostafa A. El-Sayed. 2007. "Gold nanoparticles: Interesting optical properties and recent applications in cancer diagnostics and therapy." *Nanomedicine* 2 (5):681–693. DOI: 10.2217/17435889.2.5.681.

Hummers, William S., and Richard E. Offeman. 1958. "Preparation of graphitic oxide." *Journal of the American Chemical Society* 80 (6):1339–1339. DOI: 10.1021/ja01539a017.

Jasim, A. A., A. Z. Zulkifli, M. Z. Muhammad, S. W. Harun, and H. Ahmad. 2013. "A new compact micro-ball lens structure at the cleaved tip of microfiber coupler for displacement sensing." *Sensors and Actuators A: Physical* 189:177–181. https://doi.org/10.1016/j.sna.2012.09.003.

Jian, A., L. Deng, S. Sang, Q. Duan, X. Zhang, and W. Zhang. 2014. "Surface plasmon resonance sensor based on an angled optical fiber." *IEEE Sensors Journal* 14 (9):3229–3235. DOI: 10.1109/JSEN.2014.2322124.

Jiang, Shouzhen, Zhe Li, Chao Zhang, Saisai Gao, Zhen Li, Hengwei Qiu, Chonghui Li, Cheng Yang, Mei Liu, and Yanjun Liu. 2017. "A novel U-bent plastic optical fibre local surface plasmon resonance sensor based on a graphene and silver nanoparticle hybrid structure." *Journal of Physics D: Applied Physics* 50 (16):165105. DOI: 10.1088/1361-6463/aa628c.

Kumar, S., R. Singh, G. Zhu, Q. Yang, X. Zhang, S. Cheng, B. Zhang, B. K. Kaushik, and F. Z. Liu. 2020. "Development of uric acid biosensor using gold nanoparticles and graphene oxide functionalized micro-ball fiber sensor probe." *IEEE Transactions on NanoBioscience* 19 (2):173–182. DOI: 10.1109/TNB.2019.2958891.

Kundu, T., Raghavendra Sai V, R. Dutta, S. Titas, P. Kumar, and S. Mukherjee. 2010. "Development of evanescent wave absorbance-based fibre-optic biosensor." *PRAMANA c Indian Academy of Sciences79.PW* 75. DOI: 10.1007/s12043-010-0193-6.

Li, Kaiwei, Guigen Liu, Yihui Wu, Peng Hao, Wenchao Zhou, and Zhiqiang Zhang. 2014. "Gold nanoparticle amplified optical microfiber evanescent wave absorption biosensor for cancer biomarker detection in serum." *Talanta* 120:419–424. https://doi.org/10.1016/j.talanta.2013.11.085.

Luo, Ji, Jun Yao, Yonggang Lu, Wenying Ma, and Xuye Zhuang. 2013. "A silver nanoparticle-modified evanescent field optical fiber sensor for methylene blue detection." *Sensors* 13 (3). DOI: 10.3390/s130303986.

Malinsky, Michelle Duval, K. Lance Kelly, George C. Schatz, and Richard P. Van Duyne. 2001. "Chain length dependence and sensing capabilities of the localized surface plasmon resonance of silver nanoparticles chemically modified with alkanethiol self-assembled monolayers." *Journal of the American Chemical Society* 123 (7):1471–1482. DOI: 10.1021/ja003312a.

Misra, Nilanjal, Virendra Kumar, Lalit Borde, and Lalit Varshney. 2013. "Localized surface plasmon resonance-optical sensors based on radiolytically synthesized silver nanoparticles for estimation of uric acid." *Sensors and Actuators B: Chemical* 178:371–378. https://doi.org/10.1016/j.snb.2012.12.110.

Mock, J. J., M. Barbic, D. R. Smith, D. A. Schultz, and S. Schultz. 2002. "Shape effects in plasmon resonance of individual colloidal silver nanoparticles." *Journal of Chemical Physics* 116 (15):6755–6759. DOI: 10.1063/1.1462610.

Mu, Chunlei, Haifeng Lu, Jie Bao, and Qunlin Zhang. 2018. "Visual colorimetric 'turn-off' biosensor for ascorbic acid detection based on hypochlorite-3, 3′, 5, 5′,-Tetramethylbenzidine system." *Spectrochimica Acta Part A: Molecular and Biomolecular Spectroscopy* 201:61–66.

Nayak, Jeeban Kumar, Purnendu Parhi, and Rajan Jha. 2015. "Graphene oxide encapsulated gold nanoparticle based stable fibre optic sucrose sensor." *Sensors and Actuators B: Chemical* 221:835–841. https://doi.org/10.1016/j.snb.2015.06.152.

Nayak, Jeeban Kumar, Purnendu Parhi, and Rajan Jha. 2016. "Experimental and theoretical studies on localized surface plasmon resonance based fiber optic sensor using graphene oxide coated silver nanoparticles." *Journal of Physics D: Applied Physics* 49 (28):285101. DOI: 10.1088/0022-3727/49/28/285101.

Norman, Thaddeus J., Christian D. Grant, Donny Magana, Jin Z. Zhang, Jun Liu, Daliang Cao, Frank Bridges, and Anthony Van Buuren. 2002. "Near infrared optical absorption of gold nanoparticle aggregates." *Journal of Physical Chemistry B* 106 (28):7005–7012. DOI: 10.1021/jp0204197.

Onaş, Andra Mihaela, Iuliana Elena Bîru, Sorina Alexandra Gârea, and Horia Iovu. 2020. "Novel bovine serum albumin protein backbone reassembly study: Strongly twisted β-sheet structure promotion upon interaction with GO-PAMAM." *Polymers* 12 (11):2603. DOI: 10.3390/polym12112603.

Ortega-Mendoza, J. Gabriel, Alfonso Padilla-Vivanco, Carina Toxqui-Quitl, Placido Zaca-Morán, David Villegas-Hernández, and Fernando Chávez. 2014. "Optical fiber sensor based on localized surface plasmon resonance using silver nanoparticles photodeposited on the optical fiber end." *Sensors (Basel, Switzerland)* 14 (10):18701–18710. DOI: 10.3390/s141018701.

Rana, Lokesh, Reema Gupta, Monika Tomar, and Vinay Gupta. 2018. "Highly sensitive love wave acoustic biosensor for uric acid." *Sensors and Actuators B: Chemical* 261:169–177. https://doi.org/10.1016/j.snb.2018.01.122.

Richardson, Hugh H., Zackary N. Hickman, Alexander O. Govorov, Alyssa C. Thomas, Wei Zhang, and Martin E. Kordesch. 2006. "Thermo-optical properties of gold nanoparticles embedded in ice: Characterization of heat generation and melting." *Nano Letters* 6 (4):783–788. DOI: 10.1021/nl0601051.

Roether, Johanna, Kang-Yu Chu, Norbert Willenbacher, Amy Q. Shen, and Nikhil Bhalla. 2019. "Real-time monitoring of DNA immobilization and detection of DNA polymerase activity by a microfluidic nanoplasmonic platform." *Biosensors and Bioelectronics* 142:111528. https://doi.org/10.1016/j.bios.2019.111528.

Ruddy, V., B. D. MacCraith, and J. A. Murphy. 1990. "Evanescent wave absorption spectroscopy using multimode fibers." *Journal of Applied Physics* 67 (10):6070–6074. DOI: 10.1063/1.346085.

Sai, V. V. R., Tapanendu Kundu, and Soumyo Mukherji. 2009. "Novel U-bent fiber optic probe for localized surface plasmon resonance based biosensor." *Biosensors and Bioelectronics* 24 (9):2804–2809. https://doi.org/10.1016/j.bios.2009.02.007.

Smitha, S. L., K. M. Nissamudeen, Daizy Philip, and K. G. Gopchandran. 2008. "Studies on surface plasmon resonance and photoluminescence of silver nanoparticles." *Spectrochimica Acta Part A: Molecular and Biomolecular Spectroscopy* 71 (1):186–190. https://doi.org/10.1016/j.saa.2007.12.002.

Song, Cheol, Peter L. Gehlbach, and Jin U. Kang. 2013. "Ball lens fiber optic sensor based smart handheld microsurgical instrument." *Proceedings of SPIE: The International Society for Optical Engineering* 8576:10.1117/12.2004947. DOI: 10.1117/12.2004947.

Song, Hang, Hongxin Zhang, Zhuo Sun, Ziyang Ren, Xiaoyu Yang, and Qi Wang. 2019. "Triangular silver nanoparticle U-bent fiber sensor based on localized surface plasmon resonance." *AIP Advances* 9 (8):085307. DOI: 10.1063/1.5111820.

Sperling, Ralph A., Pilar Rivera Gil, Feng Zhang, Marco Zanella, and Wolfgang J. Parak. 2008. "Biological applications of gold nanoparticles." *Chemical Society Reviews* 37 (9):1896–1908. DOI: 10.1039/B712170A.

Tagad, Chandrakant K., Sreekantha Reddy Dugasani, Rohini Aiyer, Sungha Park, Atul Kulkarni, and Sushma Sabharwal. 2013. "Green synthesis of silver nanoparticles and their application for the development of optical fiber based hydrogen peroxide sensor." *Sensors and Actuators B: Chemical* 183:144–149. https://doi.org/10.1016/j.snb.2013.03.106.

Tang, Jaw-Luen, Shu-Fang Cheng, Wei-Ting Hsu, Tsung-Yu Chiang, and Lai-Kwan Chau. 2006. "Fiber-optic biochemical sensing with a colloidal gold-modified long period fiber grating." *Sensors and Actuators B: Chemical* 119 (1):105–109. https://doi.org/10.1016/j.snb.2005.12.003.

Turkevich, John, Peter Cooper Stevenson, and James Hillier. 1951. "A study of the nucleation and growth processes in the synthesis of colloidal gold." *Discussions of the Faraday Society* 11 (0):55–75. DOI: 10.1039/DF9511100055.

Urrutia, Aitor, Javier Goicoechea, and Francisco J. Arregui. 2015. "Optical fiber sensors based on nanoparticle-embedded coatings." *Journal of Sensors* 2015:805053. DOI: 10.1155/2015/805053.

Villatoro, Joel, David Monzón-Hernández, and Efrain Mejía. 2003. "Fabrication and modeling of uniform-waist single-mode tapered optical fiber sensors." *Applied Optics* 42 (13):2278–2283. DOI: 10.1364/AO.42.002278.

Wang, Jian, Yong Chang, Wen Bi Wu, Pu Zhang, Shao Qing Lie, and Cheng Zhi Huang. 2016. "Label-free and selective sensing of uric acid with gold nanoclusters as optical probe." *Talanta* 152:314–320. https://doi.org/10.1016/j.talanta.2016.01.018.

Wang, Ruoyu, Xiaohong Zhou, Xiyu Zhu, Chao Yang, Lanhua Liu, and Hanchang Shi. 2017. "Isoelectric bovine serum albumin: Robust blocking agent for enhanced performance in optical-fiber based DNA sensing." *ACS Sensors* 2 (2):257–262. DOI: 10.1021/acssensors.6b00746.

Wang, Xiao-yan, Gang-bing Zhu, Wu-di Cao, Zhen-jiang Liu, Chang-gang Pan, Wen-jie Hu, Wan-ying Zhao, and Jian-fan Sun. 2019. "A novel ratiometric fluorescent probe for the detection of uric acid in human blood based on H_2O_2-mediated fluorescence quenching of gold/silver nanoclusters." *Talanta* 191:46–53. https://doi.org/10.1016/j.talanta.2018.08.015.

Wu, L., H. S. Chu, W. S. Koh, and E. P. Li. 2010. "Highly sensitive graphene biosensors based on surface plasmon resonance." *Optics Express* 18 (14):14395–14400. DOI: 10.1364/OE.18.014395.

Xu, Pingping, Ruiping Li, Yifeng Tu, and Jilin Yan. 2015. "A gold nanocluster-based sensor for sensitive uric acid detection." *Talanta* 144:704–709. https://doi.org/10.1016/j.talanta.2015.07.027.

Yang, Wen, Jing Yu, Xiangtai Xi, Yang Sun, Yiming Shen, Weiwei Yue, Chao Zhang, and Shouzhen Jiang. 2019. "Preparation of graphene/ITO nanorod metamaterial/U-bent-annealing fiber sensor and DNA biomolecule detection." *Nanomaterials* 9 (8). DOI: 10.3390/nano9081154.

Yonzon, Chanda Ranjit, Eunhee Jeoung, Shengli Zou, George C. Schatz, Milan Mrksich, and Richard P. Van Duyne. 2004. "A comparative analysis of localized and propagating surface plasmon resonance sensors: The binding of concanavalin A to a monosaccharide functionalized self-assembled monolayer." *Journal of the American Chemical Society* 126 (39):12669–12676. DOI: 10.1021/ja047118q.

Zangmeister, Christopher D. 2010. "Preparation and evaluation of graphite oxide reduced at 220°C." *Chemistry of Materials* 22 (19):5625–5629. DOI: 10.1021/cm102005m.

Zhu, Guo, Niteshkumar Agrawal, Ragini Singh, Santosh Kumar, Bingyuan Zhang, Chinmoy Saha, and Chandrakanta Kumar. 2020. "A novel periodically tapered structure-based gold nanoparticles and graphene oxide: Immobilized optical fiber sensor to detect ascorbic acid." *Optics & Laser Technology* 127:106156. https://doi.org/10.1016/j.optlastec.2020.106156.

7 Fiber-Optic LSPR Sensor Using Graphene Oxide Coated Silver Nanostructures

7.1 INTRODUCTION

Silver (Ag), a well-known noble metal, has been widely used in photonics (Zou and Schatz 2004), sensing (Luo et al. 2013), medicine (Singh and Singh 2008), catalysts (Rashid and Mandal 2007), antibacterial materials (Shrivastava et al. 2007), and kitchen utensils (Hussain and Schlager 2009) because at the nanometer level its metallic nanoparticles display uncommon optical (González and Noguez 2007), chemical (Evanoff and Chumanov 2005), and electronic properties (Kreibig 1974). Its optical properties can be modified by changing the morphology. Further, silver nanoparticles (AgNPs) help in the detection of certain chemical species that exhibit very weak signals that render them undetectable (Pande et al. 2007). This resulted in the magnification of the surface-enhanced Raman scattering (SERS). The excellent inhibition attributes of silver against numerous organisms, including bacteria, fungi, and viruses, just to name a few, have been well established according to Wen et al. (2007). Therefore, silver has seen a myriad of applications in the field of medicine and pharmaceuticals in areas such as scaffold, wound dressing, recipient sites, skin donation, medical catheters, sterilized materials in hospitals, contraceptive devices, bone prostheses, surgical instruments, bone coating, and artificial teeth (Liedberg, Nylander, and Lunström 1983). AgNPs have also been included in everyday consumer products including toothpaste, creams, lotions, cosmetics, soaps, laundry detergents, room sprays, surface cleaners, antimicrobial paints, toys, shoe insoles, brooms, washing machines and water filters, food storage containers, in addition to textiles (Liedberg, Nylander, and Lunström 1983).

Absorption-based optical fiber localized surface plasmon resonance (LSPR) sensors using AgNPs are very popular due to their unique properties, such as real-time response, easy fabrication, simple to implement, disposable, and economical (Nayak, Parhi, and Jha 2015; Luo et al. 2013; Bharadwaj and Mukherji 2014; Cheng and Chau 2003). The absorption band of AgNPs lies in the visible region, and its peak absorbance wavelength is around 420 nm. This absorption band is important due to the availability of cheaper optical sources and detectors. Further, AgNPs have been very popular for development of highly sensitive and selective chemical and biochemical sensors due to its enhanced surface activity (Haes and Van Duyne 2002; Ortega-Mendoza et al. 2014; Luo et al. 2013; Urrutia, Goicoechea, and Arregui 2015; Tagad et al. 2013; Mahmudin et al. 2015). Researchers have also reported the optical fiber-based ammonia sensor using AgNPs-doped silica nanocomposites (Guo and Tao 2007). However, some difficulties arise during the fabrication process, such as the inability to distribute NPs uniformly and the constraint of producing a very thin silica layer around AgNPs. In this case, if the NPs are very close together, the coupling of fields caused by adjacent NPs results in a resonance wavelength shift (Dutta, Singh, and Kundu 2013) and is a source of measurement errors that result in erroneous performance. This problem can be avoided by encapsulating AgNPs in graphene oxide (GO). This method avoids NPs from aggregating and also prevents AgNPs from oxidizing, as it inhibits AgNPs from coming into direct contact with sensing material.

DOI: 10.1201/9781003243199-7

Following that, various novel materials such as spherical gold nanoparticles (AuNPs)/AgNPs or nanorods with organic linkage were used to develop LSPR sensors based on optical fibers (Okamoto, Yamaguchi, and Kobayashi 2000). It has been found that these NPs or rods are not uniform in shape and occasionally form agglomerations, making it difficult to maintain the density. As a result, developed sensors exhibit low reproducibility and inaccurate measurement. Sometimes, people are using the Au/Ag-island films to develop wavelength interrogation-based LSPR sensors. Thus, metallic-island films are preferable to metallic NPs because they can be immobilized over the fiber surface using the thermal evaporation technique without agglomeration. Au-island assisted LSPR sensors have high sensitivity (Hosoki, Nisiyama, and Watanabe 2017; Meriaudeau et al. 1999). But, AgNPs have the unique properties of narrow bandwidth and strong plasmonic field with respect to gold. Also, this type of sensor is an economical and preferable choice for the development of optical fiber LSPR sensors.

Therefore, in this chapter, the theoretical and experimental performance of GO-encapsulated AgNPs (GOE-AgNPs) for RI sensing has been carried out using a simple fiber-optic probe. Also, a preliminary study on the optical fiber-based LSPR sensor using GOE Ag and AuNPs (GOE-AgNPs and GOE-AuNPs) has been carried out. By using one type of metallic nanoparticle, one can have only one LSPR band. Further, a multiple plasmon band is necessary to develop a multiparameter, multichannel detection system. This is a novel idea for immobilization of different novel NPs and respective bio-recognition molecules. This will help to develop the sensing zone for sensing different analytes together. This will help to detect the multiple analytes through a single sensor probe at the same time, which is quite demanding in the biotechnology field. Furthermore, by utilizing a single sensor, it is possible to examine relationships between analytes or screening analytes with the least amount of sample variation and the smallest amount of analyte-volume possible (Lin et al. 2012). Further, the work has been extended from an intensity-based to wavelength-based LSPR sensor by coating GO-coated Ag-island around the core of the optical fiber for RI sensing.

7.2 EXPERIMENTAL SECTION

7.2.1 Synthesis of AgNPs, GO, and Preparation of GO-Coated AgNPs

AgNPs synthesis protocol has been followed from Lee et al. (Lee and Meisel 1982). Then 90 mg of silver nitrate is dissolved in 500 mL of water and kept for boiling. Thereafter, 10 mL aqueous solution of 1% sodium citrate is added. Again, the solution is kept for boiling for the next 30 minutes.

GO can be synthesized with the help of Hummer's method as discussed in Chapter 6. Thereafter, GOE-AgNPs can be prepared with the mixture of aqueous GO solution (30 mL) and aqueous AgNPs (5 mL) in a reaction beaker. Then, the solution should be stirred using a magnetic stirrer for 30 minutes. Finally, the solution needs to be centrifuged at high speed to obtained the GOE-AgNPs. Its conversion procedure is shown in Figure 7.1.

7.2.2 Preparation of Fiber Sensing Probe

The method for the preparation of the fiber probe and immobilization of GO-coated AgNPs is similar to as discussed in Chapter 6, where AgNPs are used instead of AuNPs. The process of immobilization of GOE-AgNPs on the surface of optical fiber is shown in Figure 7.2.

7.3 RESULTS AND DISCUSSION

The prepared AgNPs/ GOE-AgNPs solution can be characterized using a UV-Vis spectrophotometer. The absorbance variation plot of AgNPs and GOE-AgNPs dispersed in water for measurement

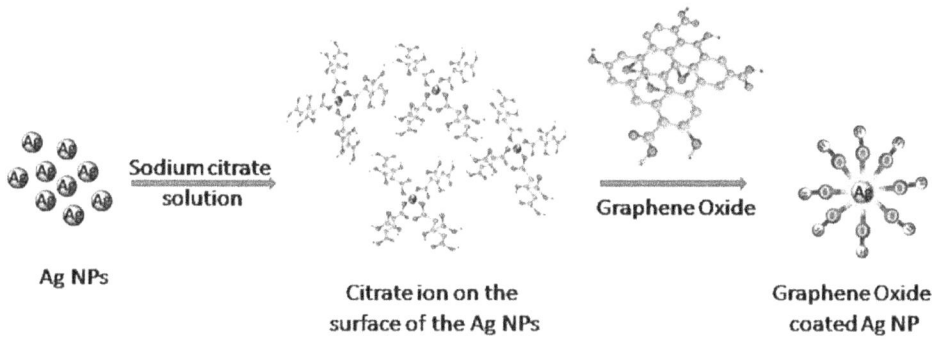

FIGURE 7.1   Fabrication process of GOE-AgNPs.

Source: Reprinted with permission from *Journal of Physics D: Applied Physics.* Copyright, 2016, IOP (Nayak, Parhi, and Jha 2016).

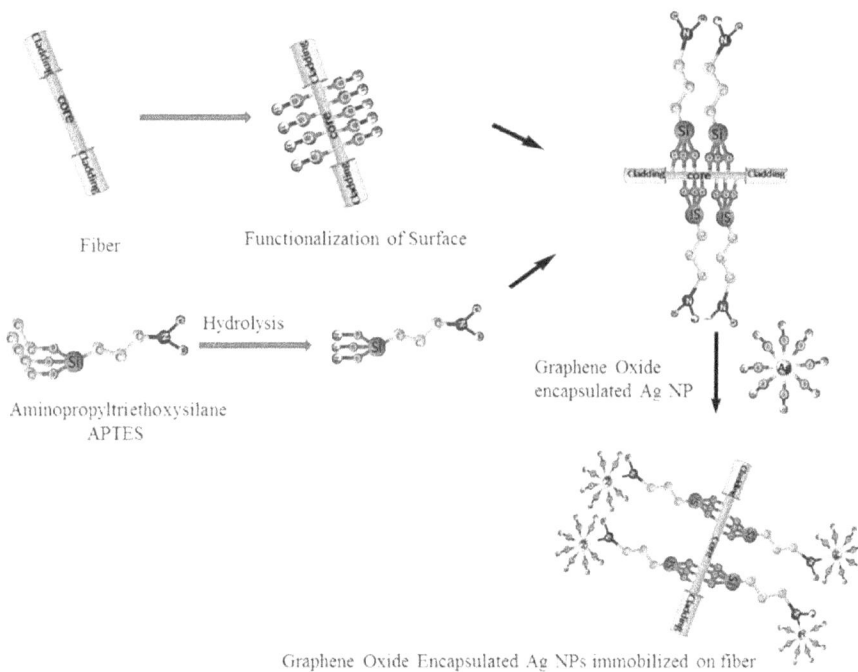

FIGURE 7.2   Coating process of GOE-AgNPs over optical fiber surface.

Source: Reprinted with permission from *Journal of Physics D: Applied Physics.* Copyright, 2016, IOP (Nayak, Parhi, and Jha 2016).

is shown in Figure 7.3. For AgNPs, the peak absorbance wavelength is 420.66 nm, and the absorbance value of synthesized AgNPs is 1.28 (Shrivastava et al. 2007; Pillai and Kamat 2004). The absorbance value and peak absorbance wavelength of GOE-AgNPs are 0.25 and 415.19 nm, respectively. Thus, the encapsulation process results in a 5.47-nm shift in the resonance wavelength. GO modifies the effective index of GOE-AgNPs in this process, thereby satisfying the resonance condition at different wavelengths. The width of the resonance curve also decreases in this case. The inset of Figure 7.3 depicts actual images of AgNPs and GOE-AgNPs synthesized, where the AgNPs

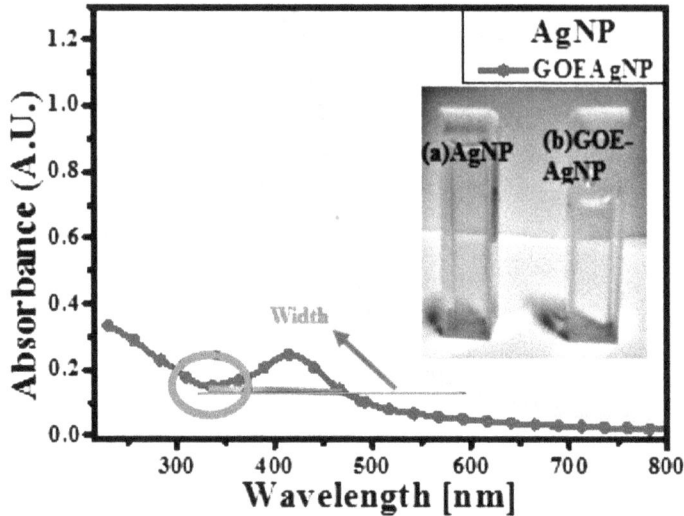

FIGURE 7.3 Absorbance variation for AgNPs and GOE-AgNPs. The actual images of synthesized solution are shown in the inset: (a) AgNPs and (b) GOE-AgNPs. The circle indicates the lowest absorbance value used to determine the curve's width; the extrapolated line also intersects the curve at this point.

Source: Reprinted with permission from *Journal of Physics D: Applied Physics.* Copyright, 2016, IOP (Nayak, Parhi, and Jha 2016).

solution is yellowish green in color and the mixed GOE-AgNPs solution is faded yellowish green in color. Further characterization of AgNPs was carried out using high-resolution transmission electron microscopy (HRTEM) at 200 kV, as shown in Figure 7.4(a). The diameter of individual AgNPs can be determined using the Image-J software, and its histogram is shown in Figure 7.4(b) to illustrate the AgNPs distribution in a solution. In this case, the average diameter of AgNPs is 35 nm. There is a concern regarding the long-term use or stability of AgNPs due to their susceptibility to oxidation.

To prevent AgNPs from oxidizing, GO was used as an encapsulant. After 2 months, the absorbance variation of three samples of GOE-AgNPs was determined, as shown in Figure 7.5(a). Even after a long period of time, the peak absorbance of GOE-AgNPs is clearly visible, and there is no aggregation of AgNPs due to oxidation. Due to the fact that this absorbance spectrum is nondeformable, it is useful for a variety of sensing applications, as illustrated in Figure 7.5(b). Following that, to verify the encapsulation of GOE-AgNPs, its morphology was analyzed using HRTEM and a Raman spectrometer.

The HRTEM images of GOE-AgNPs at various magnifications are shown in Figure 7.6(a and b). It is evident that a 1-nm layer of GO was deposited during GOE-AgNP binding, demonstrating GO encapsulation. Following that, Figure 7.6(c) illustrates the Raman spectra of GO and GOE-AgNPs with the sample retained on the silicon wafer for analysis. In GO samples, two peaks are observed at 1356 cm^{-1} and 1612 cm^{-1}, respectively. G-bands represent the bond stretching of sp^2 carbon pairs in both rings and chains in this case. The D-band is caused by aromatic rings with dangling bonds in plane terminations breathing. In this instance, a red shift of the G-peak was observed that corresponds to the degree of oxidation in GO (Kou, He, and Gao 2010). Additionally, the intensities of the D-peak (ID) and G-peak (IG) were observed to be comparable. This indicates that functional groups are present on the planar carbon backbones (Wang et al. 2020). The Raman-active mode in bulk silicon is represented by two sharp Raman peaks at 305 cm^{-1}, 521 cm^{-1}, and 970 cm^{-1}. Similarly, there are two peaks, D-peak and G-peak, at 1352 cm^{-1} and another at 1615 cm^{-1} in the

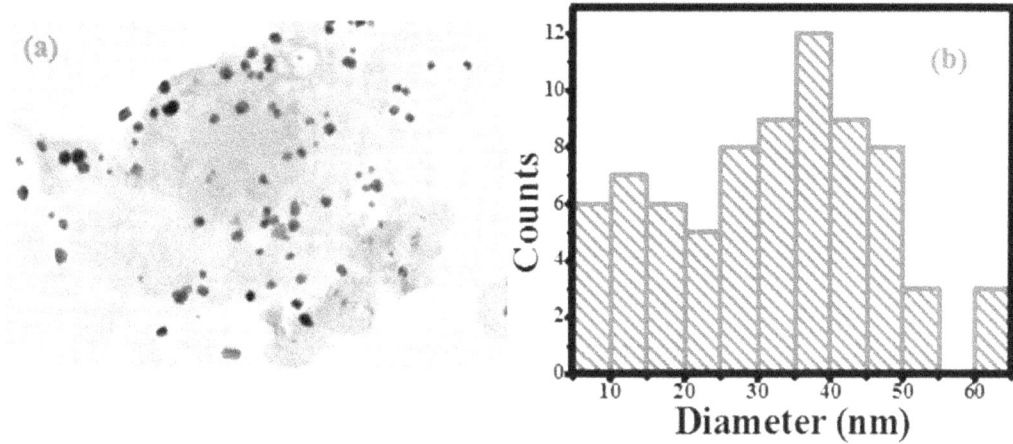

FIGURE 7.4 (a) HRTEM image of synthesized AgNPs solution, (b) histogram of AgNPs.

Source: Reprinted with permission from *Journal of Physics D: Applied Physics.* Copyright, 2016, IOP (Nayak, Parhi, and Jha 2016).

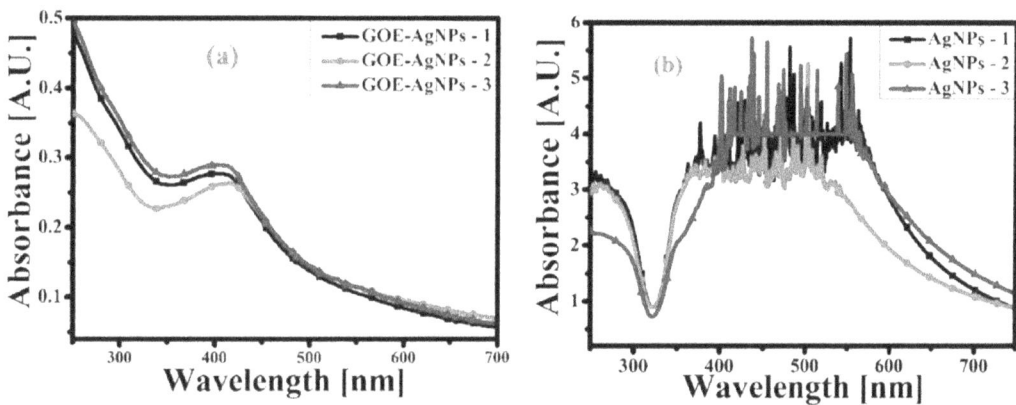

FIGURE 7.5 Absorbance variation for three different samples after 2 months of (a) GOE-AgNPs and (b) AgNPs.

Source: Reprinted with permission from *Journal of Physics D: Applied Physics.* Copyright, 2016, IOP (Nayak, Parhi, and Jha 2016).

case of GOE-AgNPs. When compared to GO and GOE-AgNPs, the D-peak appears at 1356 cm^{-1} and 1352 cm^{-1}, respectively. Similarly, G-peaks were found at 1612 cm^{-1} and 1615 cm^{-1} for GO and GOE-AgNPs, respectively. Thus, both peaks, D and G, are fairly similar for GO and GOE-AgNPs. Thus, the presence of GO in GOE-AgNPs has been confirmed. Additionally, there is a 64.72% and 52.91% increase in the intensity peak of D-peak and G-peak, respectively, when GOE-AgNPs is used instead of GO.

In this work, absorbance spectra were analyzed theoretically as well as experimentally to obtain reliable results. Theoretically, it has been simulated using MATLAB by using the Mie theory (Eq. [6.1]) as shown in Figure 7.7. The resolution of data in theoretical analysis is 0.1 nm, and its value is 0.3 nm during experimental analysis. Theoretically, the LSPR peak is placed at 404 nm with a full width at half maximum (FWHM) of 24 nm, while experimentally, it is located at 420.66 nm with

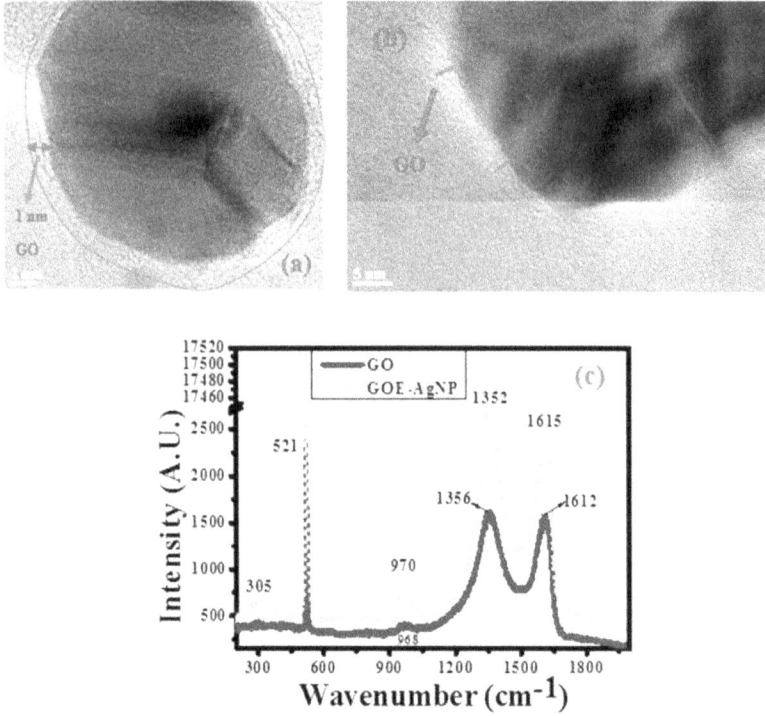

FIGURE 7.6   (a and b): HRTEM of GOE-AgNPs with different magnification, (c) Raman spectra of GO, and GOE-AgNPs.

Source: Reprinted with permission from *Journal of Physics D: Applied Physics*. Copyright, 2016, IOP (Nayak, Parhi, and Jha 2016).

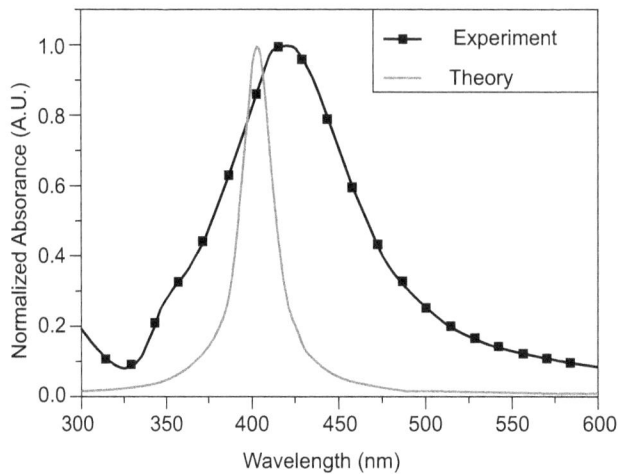

FIGURE 7.7   Results of absorbance spectra for AgNPs solution.

Source: Reprinted with permission from *Journal of Physics D: Applied Physics*. Copyright, 2016, IOP (Nayak, Parhi, and Jha 2016).

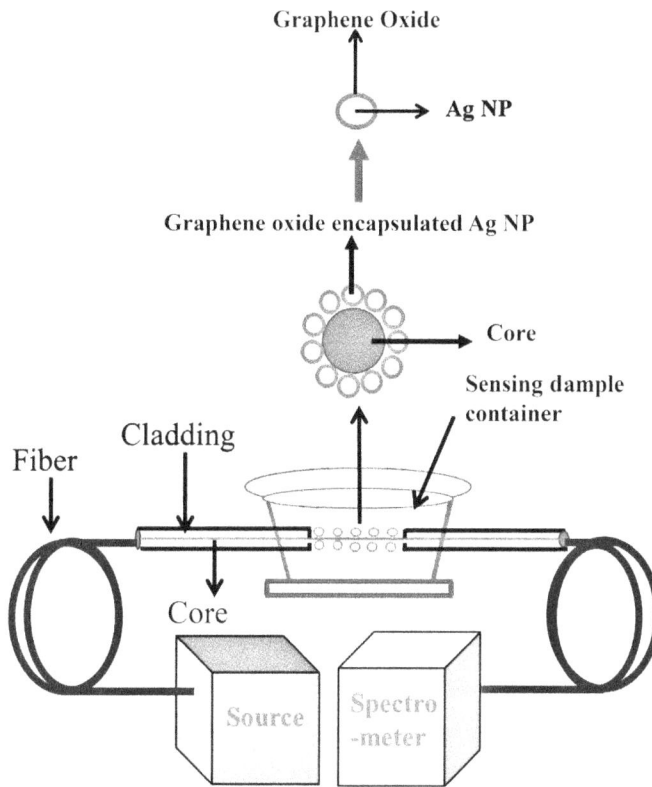

FIGURE 7.8 Experimental setup for measurement of sensing performance.

Source: Reprinted with permission from *Journal of Physics D: Applied Physics.* Copyright, 2016, IOP (Nayak, Parhi, and Jha 2016).

an FWHM of 88 nm, as shown in Figure 7.7. Due to the wide dispersion of the size and shape of the prepared NPs, the LSPR spectrum has a wider FWHM and a longer wavelength in this case (Pillai and Kamat 2004). The theoretical calculation considers spherical AgNPs with a diameter of 35 nm and a peak resonance wavelength of 404 nm. Figure 7.8 illustrates the experimental setup used to determine the sensor's performance. In this instance, one end of the sensor probe is connected to the source and the other end to the spectrometer.

In this case, a fiber probe immobilized with GOE-AgNPs is placed in the sample container. Prior to beginning the measurement, the dark spectrum and reference spectrum must be saved. To increase the SNR, absorbance mode is used with 100 spectra averaged. Following that, a functionalized sensor probe is immersed in the solution until the peak absorbance is obtained. After removing the sensor from the solution, it is rinsed with deionized (DI) water and allowed to air dry at room temperature. In this manner, the absorbance spectra of various analytes can be determined. Prior to measuring a new RI solution, the probe must be cleaned. The inset of Figure 7.9 depicts the transverse section of the fiber probe, which clearly demonstrates GOE-AgNP immobilization. Following that, the field emission scanning electron microscopy (FESEM) and scanning electron microscopy-energy dispersive X-ray spectroscopy (SEM-EDX) techniques were used to characterize the GOE-AgNPs-immobilized fiber structure. To accomplish this, NPs-immobilized fiber must first be placed on the carbon tape. The external high tension (EHT) is 5 KV during SEM characterization, and the lens magnification is ×100 K. The images in Figure 7.9(a–c) show different magnifications of GOE-AgNPs-immobilized fiber structures taken using FESEM.

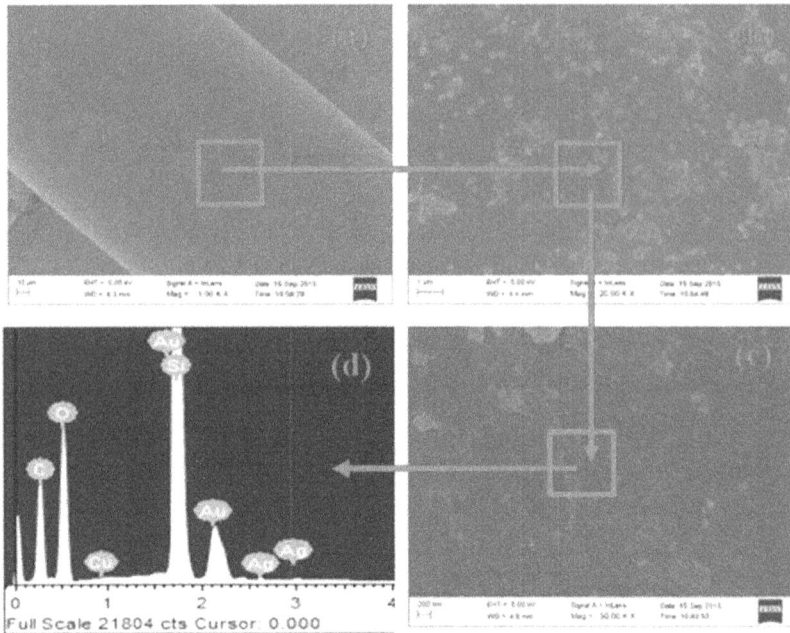

FIGURE 7.9 (a–c) FESEM image of the immobilized GOE-AgNPs fiber surface with different magnifications. (d) SEM-EDX of (c).

Source: Reprinted with permission from *Journal of Physics D: Applied Physics*. Copyright, 2016, IOP (Nayak, Parhi, and Jha 2016).

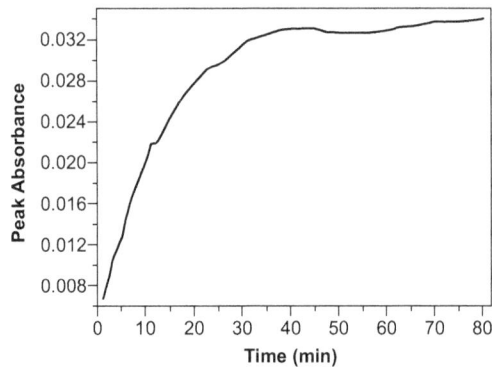

FIGURE 7.10 Absorbance variation with incubation time.

Source: Reprinted with permission from *Journal of Physics D: Applied Physics*. Copyright, 2016, IOP (Nayak, Parhi, and Jha 2016).

Figure 7.9(b) illustrates the proper attachment of the GOE-AgNPs to the fiber core surface. Following that, to confirm the material composition of the coating surface depicted in Figure 7.9(c), the SEM-EDX results are shown in Figure 7.9(d). Carbon (C) and oxygen (O) peaks indicate the presence of GO, while the silver (Ag) peak indicates the presence of GOE-AgNPs. Other than that, the silica (SiO_2) peak is due to the optical fiber's material composition, while the gold (Au) peak is due to the 2-nm coating of the gold layer. The immobilization of GOE-AgNPs on the surface of the fiber is time-dependent (incubation time). This type of analysis can also be performed by measuring the absorbance spectrum of the material during functionalization. Figure 7.10 illustrates the results obtained using a UV-Vis spectrophotometer after dipping a fiber probe in GOE-AgNPs for 80 minutes at the peak absorbance wavelength of 423.24 nm.

As shown in Figure 7.10, the maximum amount of immobilization occurs within 40 minutes, as peak absorbance increases rapidly during this time period. Following that, this absorbance curve reaches saturation within 80 minutes, indicating that the total absorbance variation caused by NPs immobilization occurs within 80 minutes. Take into consideration that this is not an analysis of the sensor's response time; rather, it is a calculation of the NPs' immobilization time. Following this procedure, the NPs-coated fiber structure should be removed from the GOE-AgNPs solution and rinsed three times with DI water. This procedure aids in the removal of unbounded NPs. Following functionalization, the GOE-AgNPs-immobilized probe is used to detect DI water (analyte, RI 1.3310), as illustrated in Figure 7.11. Theoretical absorbance variation is also calculated using Eq. (6.1) and is shown in Figure 7.11. As a result, it can be concluded that the experimental peak absorbance value is similar to the theoretical value obtained. Following that, to determine the response of the developed sensor in the presence of various RIs, the absorbance variation with wavelength for various RIs was determined. The peak absorbance changes from 0.0540 to 0.1014 in this case due to the RI changing from 1.3310 to 1.3810 at 423.24 nm (Figure 7.12). Sensitivity can be calculated in this case as the maximum absorbance shift caused by a small change in the analyte RI (Nayak, Parhi, and Jha 2016).

To determine the sensitivity, the absorbance variation was measured in the presence of various analytes RI (n_s) in Figure 7.13. Sensitivity is defined in this case as the slope of the linear fit to the curve, which is calculated as 0.9406 A/RIU with an intercept of −1.198 and an R^2 of 0.997. Similarly, another study (Luo et al. 2013) reported a sensitivity value of 0.402 A/concentration using immobilized AgNPs in the presence of methylene blue. A similar calculation has been made for another critical parameter, resolution (i.e., the smallest change in bulk RI causes detectable change on the sensor's output side). The resolution of a sensor is determined by the standard deviation (SD) of the noise at the sensor's output. Thus, in this work, the SD of the noise is 0.0012, and its sensitivity value is 0.9406 ΔA/RIU. The resolution of the sensor can be calculated as 12.8×10^{-4} RIU (refractive index unit). This value is similar to that obtained for resolution as 10.8×10^{-4} RIU with a standard deviation of 0.0012, theoretically.

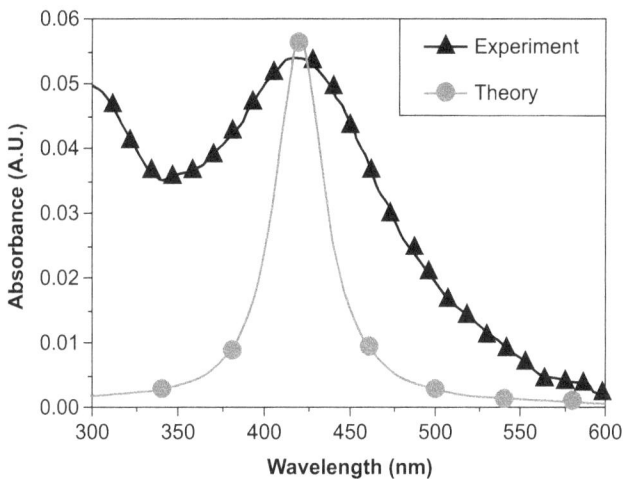

FIGURE 7.11 Experimental and theoretical absorbance variation for fiber sensor during GOE-AgNPs immobilization.

Source: Reprinted with permission from *Journal of Physics D: Applied Physics.* Copyright, 2016, IOP (Nayak, Parhi, and Jha 2016).

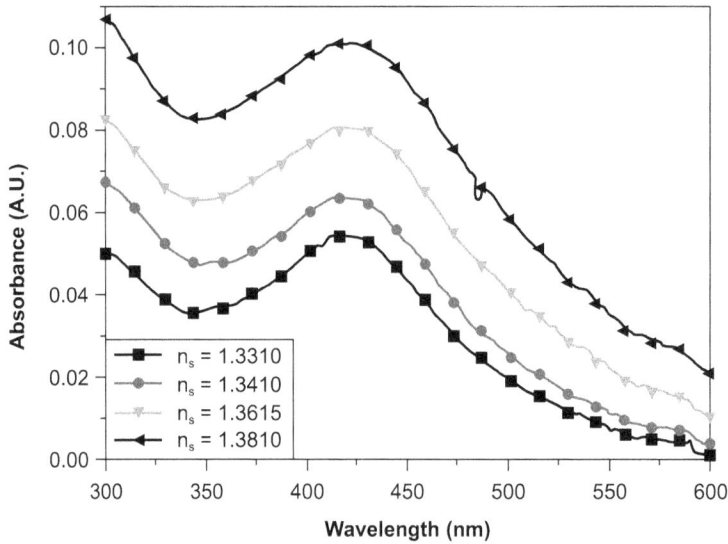

FIGURE 7.12 Absorbance variation measurement in the presence of different analyte RI.

Source: Reprinted with permission from *Journal of Physics D: Applied Physics.* Copyright, 2016, IOP (Nayak, Parhi, and Jha 2016).

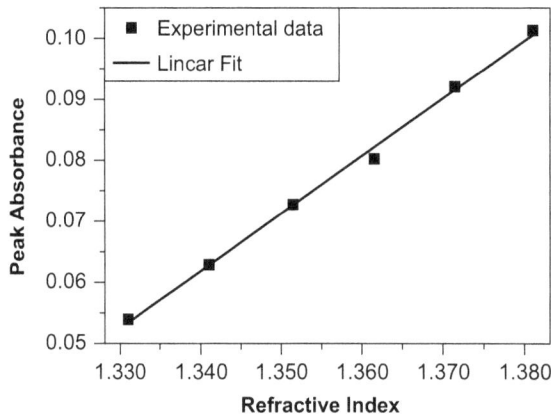

FIGURE 7.13 Absorbance variation in the presence of different analyte RI measured through developed sensor probe.

Source: Reprinted with permission from *Journal of Physics D: Applied Physics.* Copyright, 2016, IOP (Nayak, Parhi, and Jha 2016).

The absorbance spectrum was measured experimentally in the presence of DI water (RI of 1.3310) using a cyclic GOE-AgNPs-immobilized fiber sensor probe. Following that, the absorbance spectrum of the analyte RI 1.3410 is recorded, and the fiber surface is rinsed. Similarly, absorbance is determined in the presence of two additional RI analytes, namely, 1.3515 and 1.3615, as shown in Figure 7.14.

Following that, the change in absorbance peak with respect to different RI represents a cyclic measurement and is illustrated in Figure 7.15. The difference between the two absorbance levels is

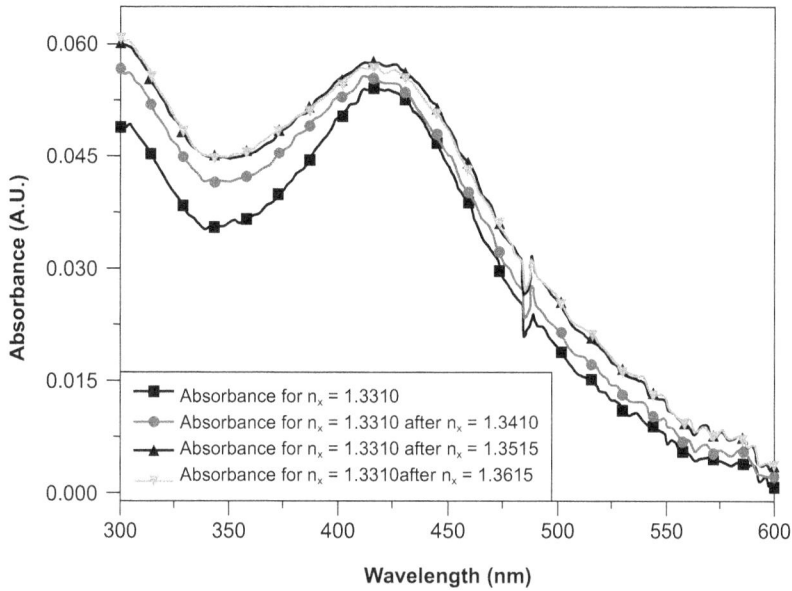

FIGURE 7.14 Absorbance variation for cyclic measurement of analyte.

Source: Reprinted with permission from *Journal of Physics D: Applied Physics.* Copyright, 2016, IOP (Nayak, Parhi, and Jha 2016).

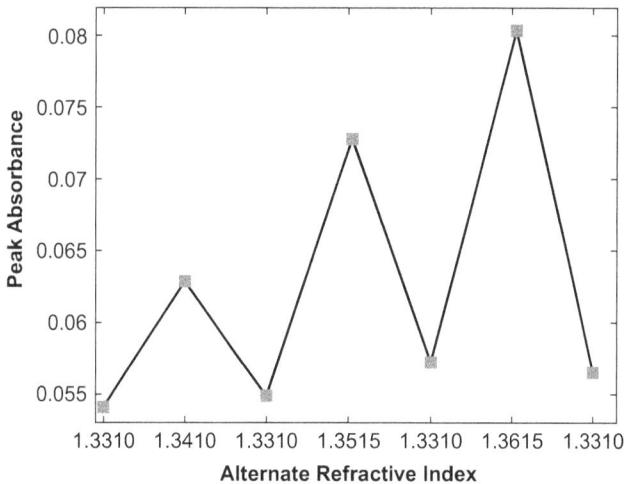

FIGURE 7.15 Peak absorbance measurement in the presence of different RI, showing cyclic measurement.

Source: Reprinted with permission from *Journal of Physics D: Applied Physics.* Copyright, 2016, IOP (Nayak, Parhi, and Jha 2016).

0.0031, indicating that the sensor is capable of multiple detection in the presence of different RI with high measurement accuracy.

Further, the LSPR band with A narrow frequency variation limits its application in the multiplex sensor or other multichannel systems. To have multiple plasmon bands, one has to expand the system from a single metal nanoparticle to a bimetallic system. However, when a sensor probe is functionalized with different NPs containing specific biorecognition molecules, it can be used as a sensing element for multiple analyte solution sensing. Due to the numerous sensing possibilities available today, this type of sensing technology is significant. Additionally, it can be advantageous for determining relationships between target analytes with minimal sample variation and a small sample volume via a single sensor (Lin et al. 2012). Thus, various biosensing applications such as molecular imaging and drug delivery can be accomplished using a specific biorecognition element and excellent nanomaterials assisted by AuNPs/AgNPs (Sperling et al. 2008).

Due to the presence of a strong absorption band of spherical AgNPs around 420 nm and AuNPs at 524 nm in the visible spectrum, designing NPs-based optical sensors as sources and detectors is economical. Therefore, immobilizing these NPs on the core of an optical fiber can lead to an efficient way to remotely detect two different analytes present in a solution. So here, a fiber-based LSPR sensor using GOE-AuNPs and AgNPs was analyzed. As discussed, by using the mixture of GOE-AuNPs and GOE-AgNPs, one can obtain two plasmon bands: one for GOE-AgNPs and another for GOE-AuNPs. Here the existence of two peaks in solution form has been theoretically shown. A preliminary study has been carried out using the fiber sensor immobilized with GOE-AuNPs and GOE-AgNPs.

To perform the experiment, AuNPs and AgNPs were prepared chemically as described in Chapter 6 and Chapter 7, respectively. The characterization of AuNPs and AgNPs has been done by HRTEM. Figure 7.16(a) shows a TEM image of AgNPs, with its average size found to be 28 nm. Figure 7.16(b) shows a TEM image of AuNPs having average diameter 30 nm.

Figure 7.17 shows the EDX of AgNPs-AuNPs, where EDX gives the elementary composition of the sample. In EDX spectra, the presence of peaks for both Ag and Au confirms the existence of both silver and gold. Figure 7.18(a) shows the experimental absorbance variation for AuNPs, AgNPs, and a mixture of AuNPs and AgNPs in solution form. The line with box represents the absorbance curve for AuNPs, and the dotted line is for that of AgNPs. For AuNPs, the LSPR peak occurs at 530.11 nm with an absorbance value of 1.05; for AgNPs, the LSPR peaks at 420.65 nm, having a peak absorbance value of 1.27. The continuous line represents the absorbance curve for the mixture of AgNPs and AuNPs. Here, two LSPR peaks occur at 418.07 nm with an absorbance value 1.118 and 525.36 nm with an absorbance value of 0.9030 for AuNPs and AgNPs, respectively. Figure 7.18(b) represents the theoretical absorbance variation with respect to wavelength for AgNPs, AuNPs, and a mixture of AgNPs and AuNPs. The absorbance calculations for AgNPs and AuNPs have been done using Eq. (6.1) with the help of MATLAB 2012A, and for a mixture of AgNPs and AuNPs Eq. (7.1) has been used:

$$A_{mixture\ of\ NPs} = \frac{\left(A_{AgNPs} + A_{AuNPs} \right)}{2} \tag{7.1}$$

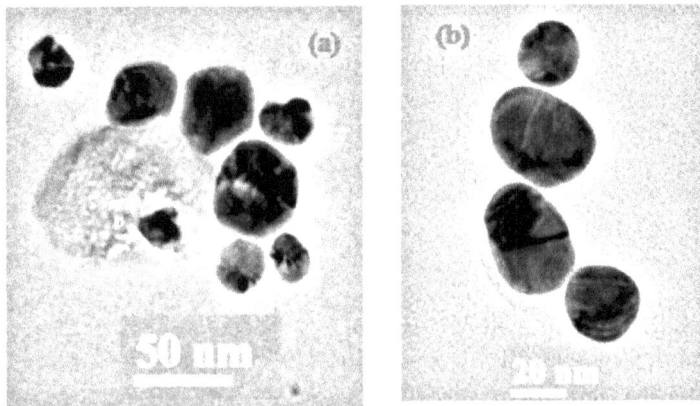

FIGURE 7.16 TEM image of (a) AgNPs and (b) AuNPs.

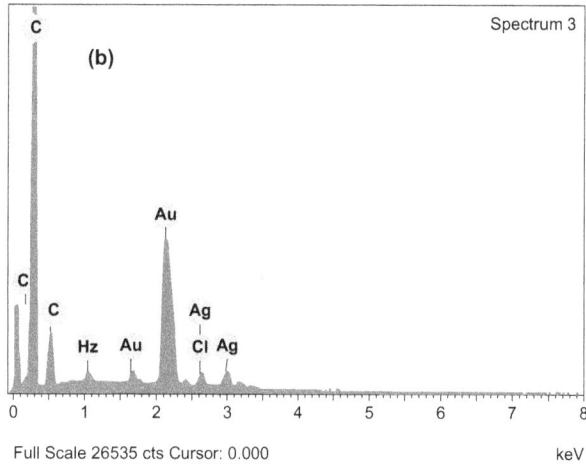

FIGURE 7.17 EDX spectra of AgNPs and AuNPs.

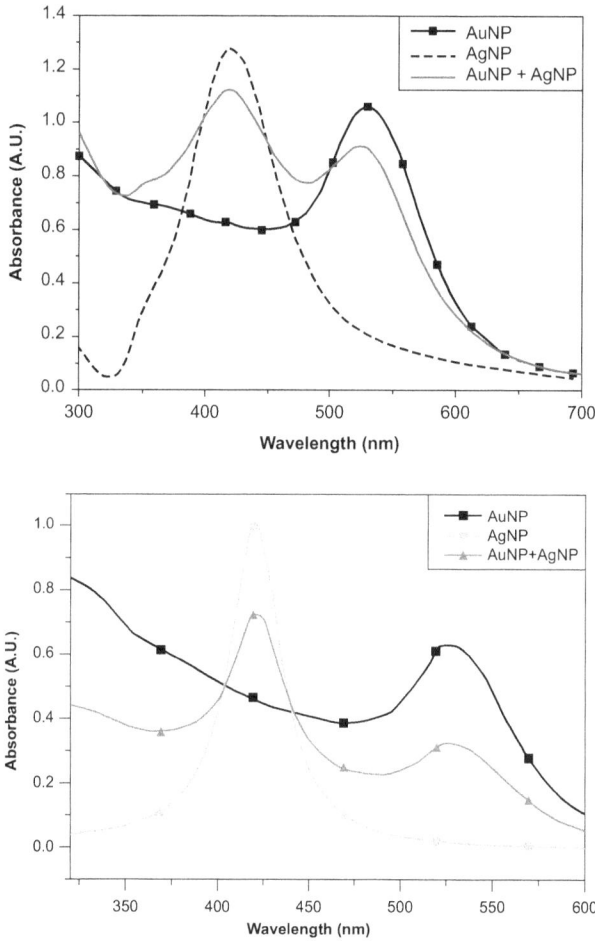

FIGURE 7.18 (a) Experimental and (b) theoretical absorbance change with respect to different wavelengths for AuNPs, AgNPs, and AuNPs/AgNPs.

Similarly, the absorbance of the mixture of GOE-AgNPs and GOE-AuNPs can be calculated. Additionally, theoretically, the performance of an LSPR-based optical fiber sensor dependents on the absorbance variation caused by an EW (Ruddy, MacCraith, and Murphy 1990) and has been calculated using Eq. (7.1). In order to perform the experiment, 50% of GOE-AuNPs and 50% of GOE-AgNPs are taken in a beaker separately. The mixture is sonicated for 20 minutes to get a mixture of GOE-AuNPs and GOE-AgNPs, which has been characterized using UV-Vis spectrophotometry.

Figure 7.19 shows the experimental variation of absorbance with wavelength for GOE-AuNPs and GOE-AgNPs. The continuous line shows the absorbance curve for GOE-AuNPs, and the dotted line is for that of GOE-AgNPs. For GOE-AuNPs, the LSPR peak occurs at 526.20 nm with absorbance of 0.222, and for GOE-AgNPs, the LSPR peaks at 407.12 nm with absorbance of 0.255. For the solution with GOE-AgNPs and GOE-AuNPs, two LSPR peaks have been observed. The peak at 528.72 nm with absorbance value of 0.164 and the peak at 407.986 nm with absorbance value of 0.231 were observed. Further, the encapsulation of GO on Ag and Au has been confirmed from TEM image, as shown in Figure 7.20(a and b), respectively. It has been found that approximately 1.5 nm and 1.7 nm of GO have been coated around the AgNP and AuNP, respectively. To compare this work with theoretical calculation, Figure 7.21(a) represents the theoretical absorbance variation with

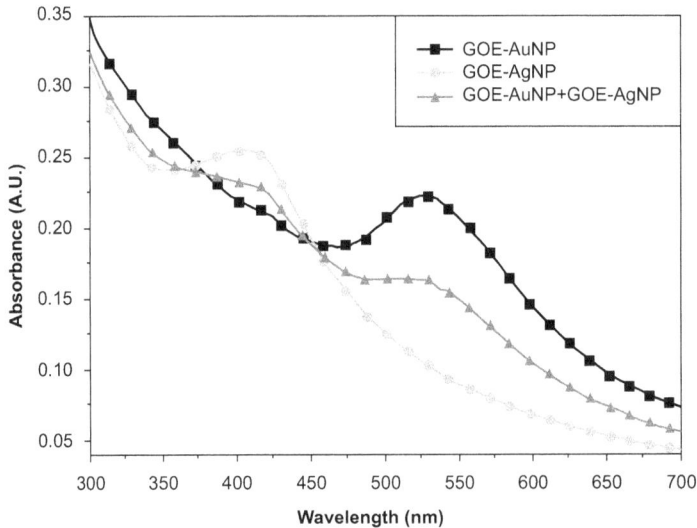

FIGURE 7.19 Experimental absorbance variation for GOE-AuNP, GOE-AgNPs, and mixture of GOE-AgNPs and GOE-AuNPs.

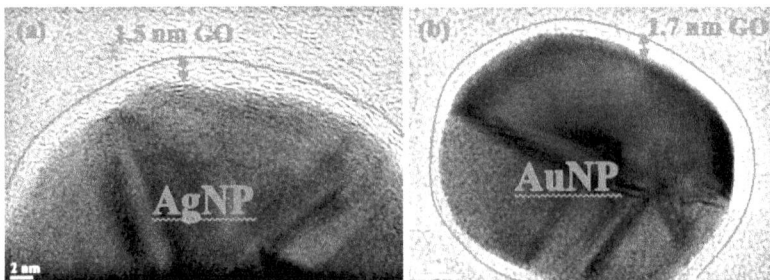

FIGURE 7.20 TEM image for (a) GOE-AgNP and (b) GOE-AuNP.

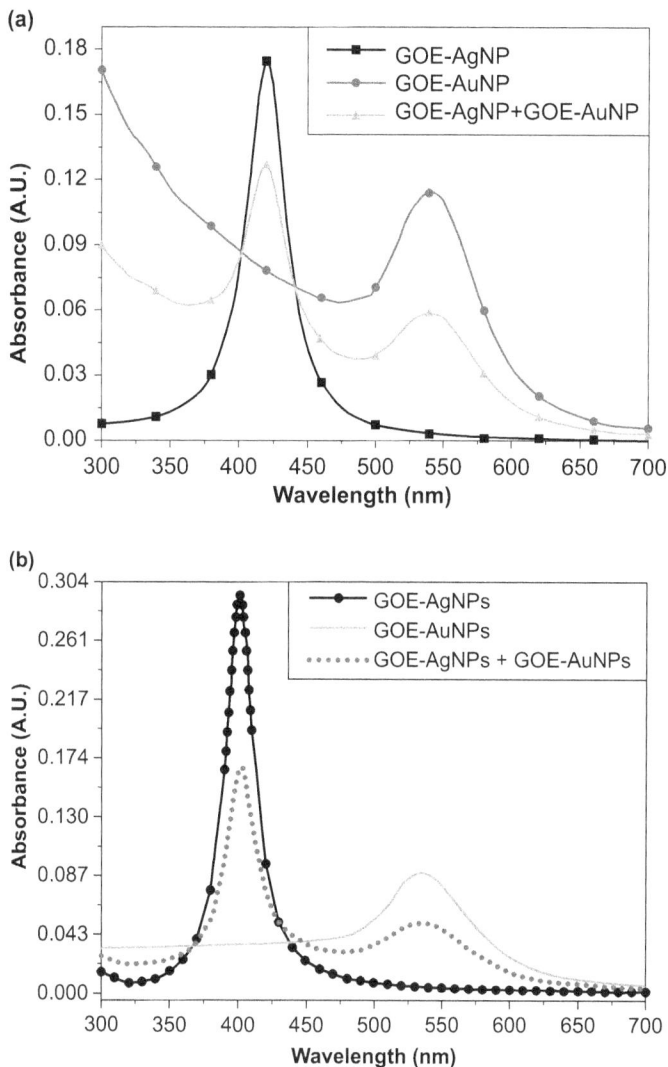

FIGURE 7.21 (a) Theoretical absorbance variation for GOE-AuNP, GOE-AgNPs, and GOE-AgNPs and GOE-AuNPs using MATLAB. (b) Theoretical absorbance variation with respect to wavelength for GOE-AuNP, GOE-AgNPs, and GOE-AgNPs and GOE-AuNPs using COMSOL Multiphysics.

respect to wavelength for GOE-AgNPs, GOE-AuNPs, and a mixture of GOE-AgNPs and GOE-AuNPs, which has been calculated using the partial wave equation (PWE) method. For theoretical calculation, MATLAB software has been used.

The peak absorbance for GOE-Ag NPs has been observed 420 nm; for GOE-AuNPs, the peak absorbance has been observed at 542 nm. The peak absorbance for GOE-AgNPs has been observed at 420 nm and for GOE-AuNPs at 542 nm. The small variation in resonance wavelength as compared to experimental results is due to nonuniformity in the GO film thickness around the metal nanoparticles and nonspherical nanoparticles. Further, similar results have been obtained using FEM as shown in Figure 7.21(b). Here, peak absorbance cross-section for GOE-AgNPs and GOE-AuNPs has been observed at 401 nm and at 536 nm, respectively. However, small variation in peak wavelength as shown in Figure 7.21(a and b) is due to different estimation methods (PWE and FEM) used in the calculation. With these particle sizes and GO thickness, the electric field distribution for GOE-AgNP (at 401 nm), GOE-AuNP (at 536 nm), and GOE-AgNP and GOE-AuNP (at 539 nm) surrounded with analyte (refractive index 1.330) are as shown in Figure 7.22 (a–c) respectively, as the electric field present around the nanoparticle is responsible for sensing analyte. For the electric field study across the nanoparticles, FEM has been used. During the study, a plane wave is incident along the z-direction, which have vector along the y-direction on the nanoparticles (GOE-AuNP and GOE-AgNP). Here the refractive index values for different wavelengths for Ag and Au have been obtained from the literature (Johnson and Christy 1972), the different refractive index values for different wavelengths are taken from (Jung et al. 2008), and the corresponding equation used is as follows:

$$n_{GO}(\lambda) = A1 \times exp\left(\frac{-\lambda}{w1}\right) + y_0 + 1i\left\{A2 \times exp\left(\frac{-\lambda}{w2}\right) + y_{01}\right\} \qquad (7.2)$$

where A1 = 2.86353, w1 = 92.45192, w2 = 112.6793, A2 = 3.81187, y0 = 1.83284, and y01 = 0.05044.

During the computation, scattering boundary condition has been used for the GOE-AuNP and GOE-AgNP domains. These domains are surrounded by the perfectly matched layer to avoid the effect of backscattering as shown in Figure 7.22(d) using finer mesh.

To perform the experiment, Figure 7.23 represents the measurement setup, in which light is provided at the one side of the fiber probe from a tungsten-halogen source, and the other side is connected to the detector.

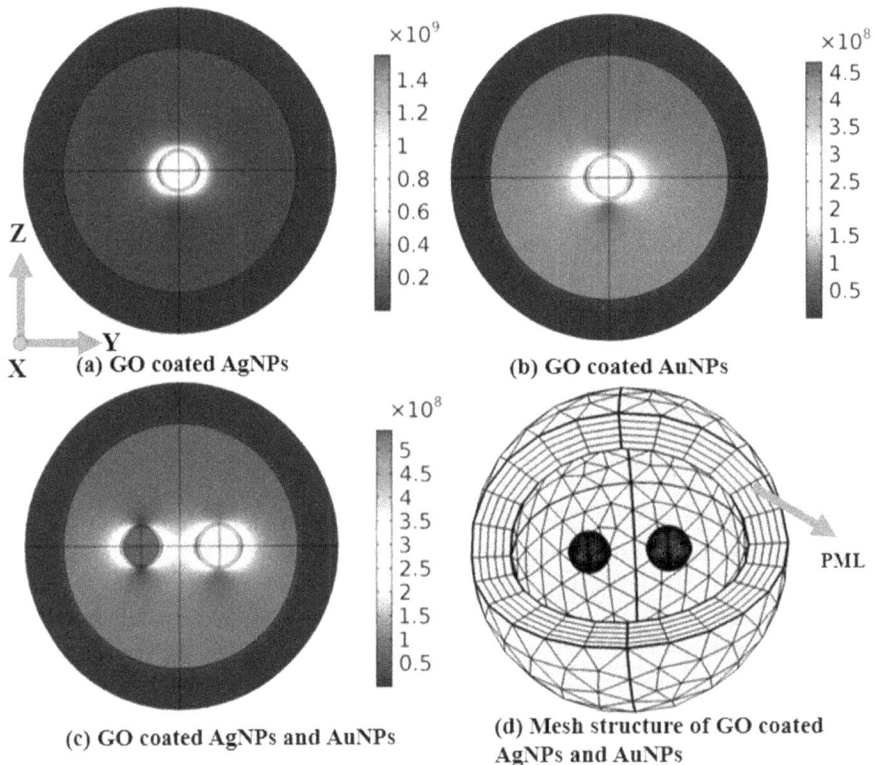

(a) GO coated AgNPs

(b) GO coated AuNPs

(c) GO coated AgNPs and AuNPs

(d) Mesh structure of GO coated AgNPs and AuNPs

FIGURE 7.22 Electric field distribution of (a) GOE-AgNP, (b) GOE-AuNP, and (c) GOE-AgNP and GOE-AuNP. (d) Mesh structure of and GOE-AgNP GOE-AuNP surrounded by perfectly matched layer.

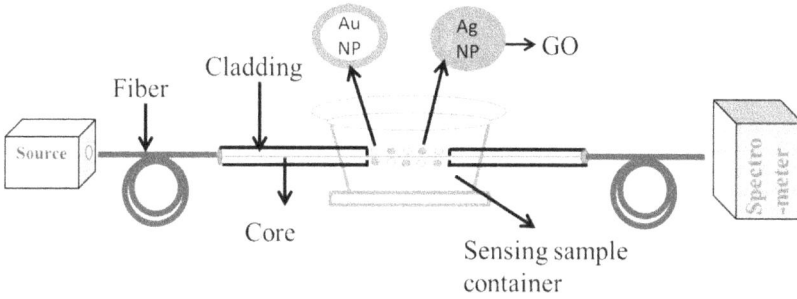

FIGURE 7.23 Experimental setup for sensing purposes.

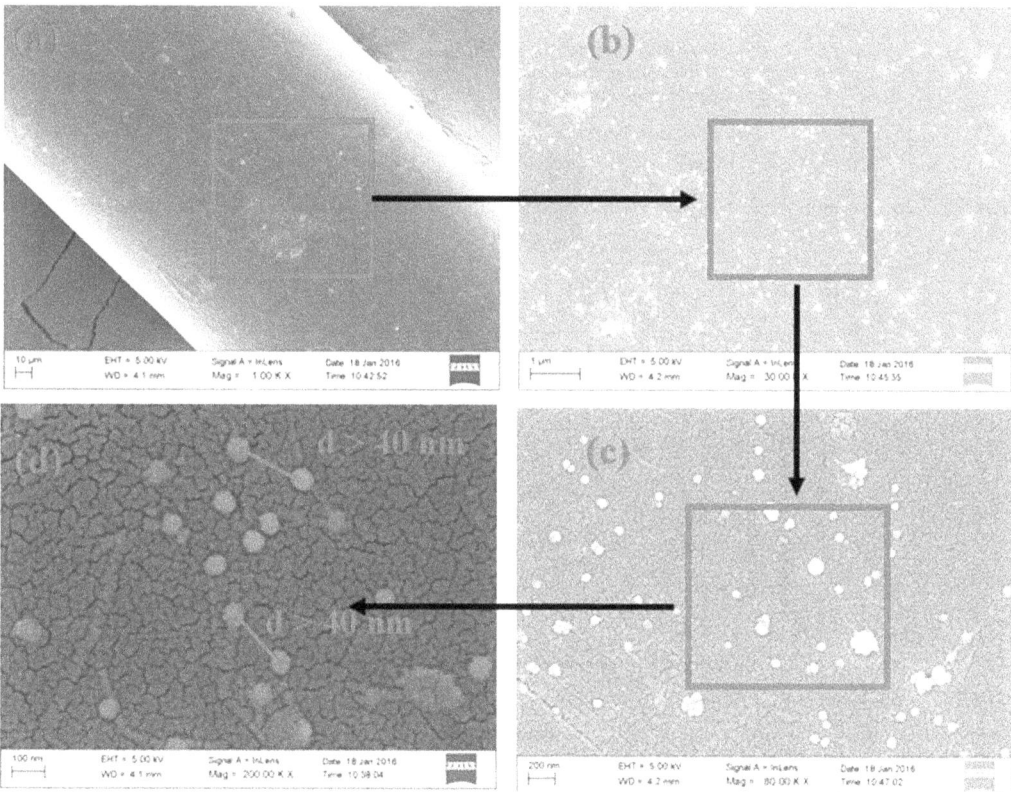

FIGURE 7.24 FESEM image of fiber probe immobilized with GOE-AgNPs and GOE-AuNPs.

Cladding at the central region of the fiber probe (PCS fiber) having 1-cm length is removed using KOH and methanol solution. At the decladded site, GOE-AgNPs and GOE-AuNPs are deposited after functionalizing the fiber core. To confirm the immobilization of GOE-Ag-AuNPs on the fiber probe, Figure 7.24 shows the FESEM image of the fiber probe immobilized with the different magnifications of GOE-AgNPs and GOE-AuNPs. Figure 7.25 shows the immobilization process of GO-coated AgNPs and GO-coated AuNPs on the functionalized core of the fiber.

To verify the sensing performance in the presence of different analyte RI, Figure 7.26 shows the peak absorbance variation with respect to wavelength for different RI of solution. Here, the peak absorbance also increases with increasing analyte RI. Here, two distinct absorbance peaks have

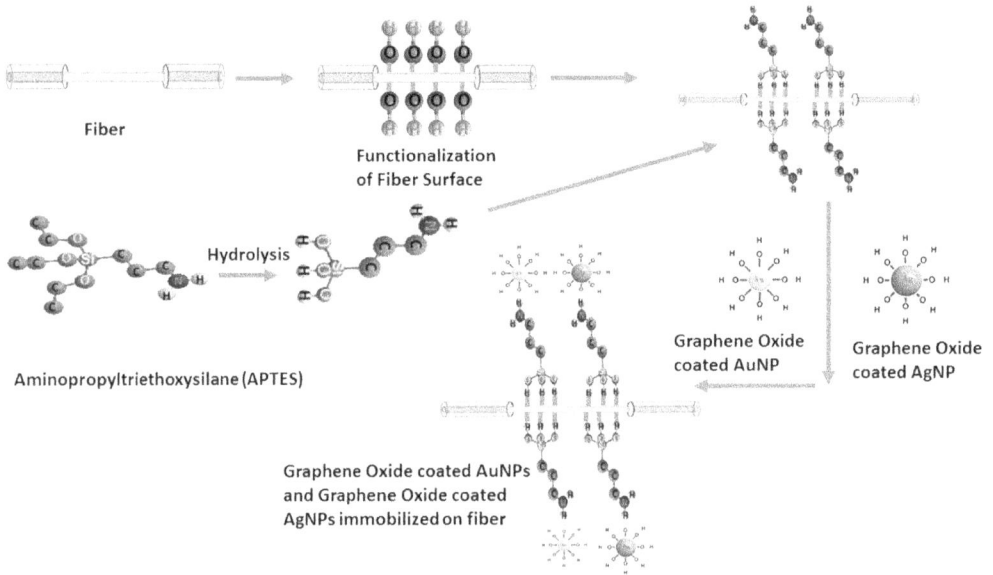

FIGURE 7.25 Immobilization of GO-coated AgNPs and GO-coated AuNPs on the functionalized surface of fiber.

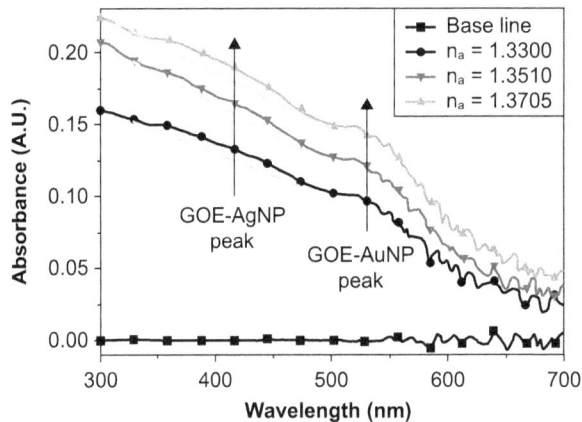

FIGURE 7.26 Absorbance variation with respect to wavelength for analyte (different RI) through GOE-AgNPs and GOE-AuNPs-based probe. The green dashed line can be considered as a base to realize the effect of GOE-AgNPs at $\lambda = 420$ nm.

been expected, one for GOE-AgNPs and another for GOE-AuNPs. However, the absorbance peak for GOE-AuNPs is prominent around 530 nm, and the absorbance peak can be noticed around 430 nm, which is due to GOE-AgNPs. Further, the intensity-based LSPR sensor suffers from power fluctuation problems. Also, the controlled deposition of metallic nanoparticles around the core of optical fiber is difficult. To address this issue, a wavelength-based LSPR sensor was proposed using GO-coated Ag-island.

The sensor probe was fabricated using a 15-cm-long polymer-cladded silica fiber with a core diameter of 600 μm and a NA of 0.37. Following that, 1 cm of polymer cladding is removed from the fiber's center using a KOH and methanol solution. Following that, the ends of the sensor probe should be polished with emery papers of varying roughness to ensure strong light coupling. In this case, an Ag-island film was coated over the declad portion of the fiber surface via vacuum thermal evaporation with the aid of a high Hind vacuum coating unit. A customized rotating system has been used in the deposition chamber to hold the fiber in place for uniform coating. Following that, using cysteamine as a linking agent, GO was coated over the Ag-coated fiber surface. As illustrated in Figure 7.27, this GO/Ag-coated fiber was used for sensing purposes.

The light was launched from one end of the fiber using a tungsten-halogen source and a microscope objective in this experiment. Following that, as illustrated in Figure 7.27, a spectrometer is connected to the other end of the fiber sensor to measure the transmitted spectrum. Just after that, the sensor probe was characterized by comparing its solutions to those of various RIs (sucrose solutions is considered in this case).

As shown in Figure 7.28, the transmission spectrum was initially measured in the presence of DI water (RI—1.330) using an Ag-island coated fiber probe (without GO). To improve the signal-to-noise ratio in this experiment, the reference spectrum and dark spectrum were saved and used to initialize the averaging of 100 spectra. In this case, resonance occurs at 445.60 nm, which corresponds to the theoretical computational result. Following that, the resonance wavelength (λ_R) for a fiber core coated with GO/AgNPs is defined as (Xu et al. 2003)

$$\lambda_R = \lambda_P \left[\frac{\varepsilon_{Av}}{(1-q)L} - \varepsilon_{Av} + \delta\varepsilon^b + 1 \right]^{1/2} \tag{7.3}$$

where, λ_p is the plasma wavelength and $\delta\varepsilon^b$ is the bound electron contribution to the dielectric constant of silver.

In simulation, the resonance wavelength for Ag-island is obtained using Eq. (7.3), and the different parameters are considered as $\lambda_p = 134.76$ nm, $\varepsilon_{water} = 1.7689$, $\varepsilon_{substrate (core)} = 2.1025$, ε_{Av} (inter-island dielectric constant) = 1.9357, L (depolarization factor for spherical particle) = 1/3, $\delta\varepsilon^b = 0$

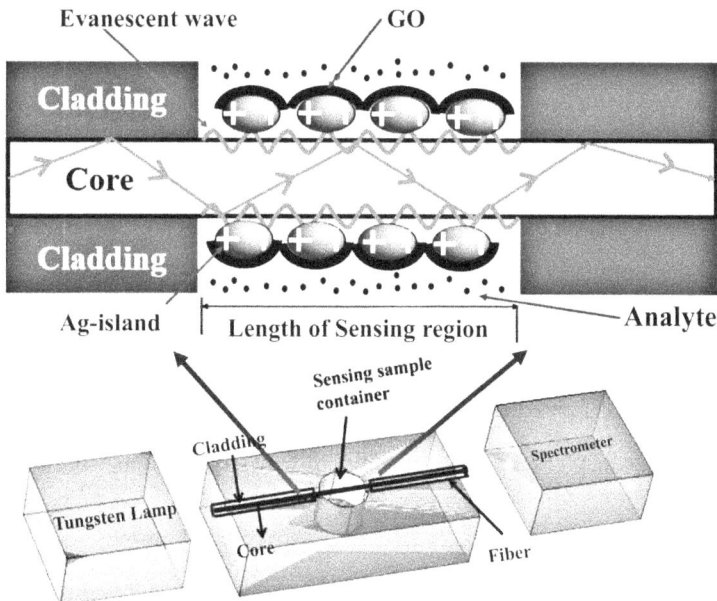

FIGURE 7.27 Measurement setup and the inset show the sensing region (Nayak and Jha 2018).

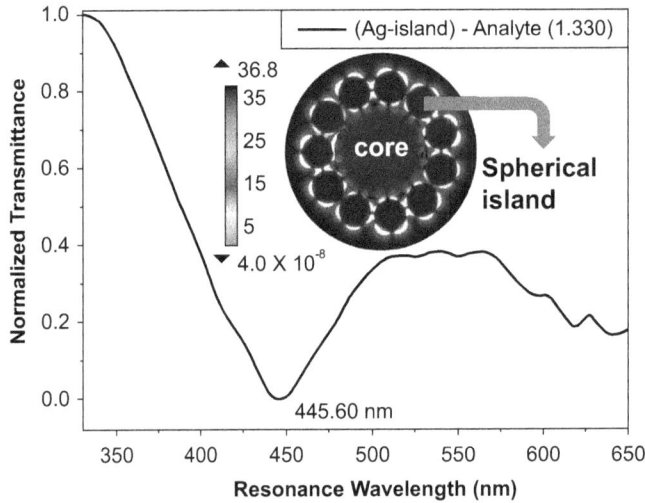

FIGURE 7.28 Normalized transmittance curve with Ag-island coated sensor probe in the presence of analyte (RI—1.330). The inset shows the electric field distribution obtained through FEM (Nayak and Jha 2018).

(excluded bound electron contribution), and q (average particle filling factor) = 0.5. The theoretical resonance wavelength (R) of 440.35 nm was obtained. The material parameters were chosen based on the materials specified for the experimental work, as well as the average value of q. The resonance wavelength obtained in this case confirms that the Ag material coated over the fiber surface is a component of the Ag-island as reported in the literature (Sreenivasan et al. 2013; Xu et al. 2005; Xu et al. 2003; Sreenivasan et al. 2013), where the Froehlich condition must be satisfied. As is well known, the electric field surrounding the system is critical to the operation of any plasmonic sensor. Figure 7.28 depicts the electric field distribution surrounding the immobilized Ag-island fiber surface in the presence of an analyte layer (DI water, RI—1.330). As a result of the electric field coupling between the fiber core and the Ag-island, the electric field surrounding the Ag-island is significantly strong. In this case, the electric field distribution is determined using the FEM-based COMSOL Multiphysics.

Figure 7.29 illustrates the FESEM image of an immobilized Ag-island fiber surface. This image clearly shows that immobilized silver appears as islands rather than as a continuous uniform thin film as expected at a lower resonance wavelength. If the resonance wavelength is around 550 nm, it should be in the form of a continuous film (Jorgenson and Yee 1993). Following that, a linking agent of 5 mM ethanolic cysteamine is used to immobilize the GO over the Ag-island. Figure 7.30 illustrates the normalized transmittance variation of an Ag-island immobilized fiber surface in cysteamine solution over a range of incubation times. Within 44 minutes, a shift in the LSPR spectrum occurs from 475.22 to 521.72 nm. This shift in resonance wavelength is caused by the presence of cysteamine that modifies the local RI. Additionally, no resonance wavelength shift occurs after 40 minutes, indicating that cysteamine is immobilized on the Ag-island. The functionalized fiber surface is then dried in the presence of nitrogen gas and maintained in an aqueous GO solution (concentration 1.1 mg/mL) prepared using a modified Hummer's method as previously discussed (Hummers and Offeman 1958).

In Figure 7.31, a blue shift in the resonance wavelength occurs with respect to time. This is because the effective RI decreases as a result of the GO coating on the fiber surface. Similarly, it has been reported that the resonance wavelength shift occurs as a result of functionalization of the self-assembled monolayer (SAM) dielectric layer on the metallic island (Jung et al. 2008). Due to the fact that the wavelength red or blue shift is dependents on the effective dispersion, the LSPR curve is

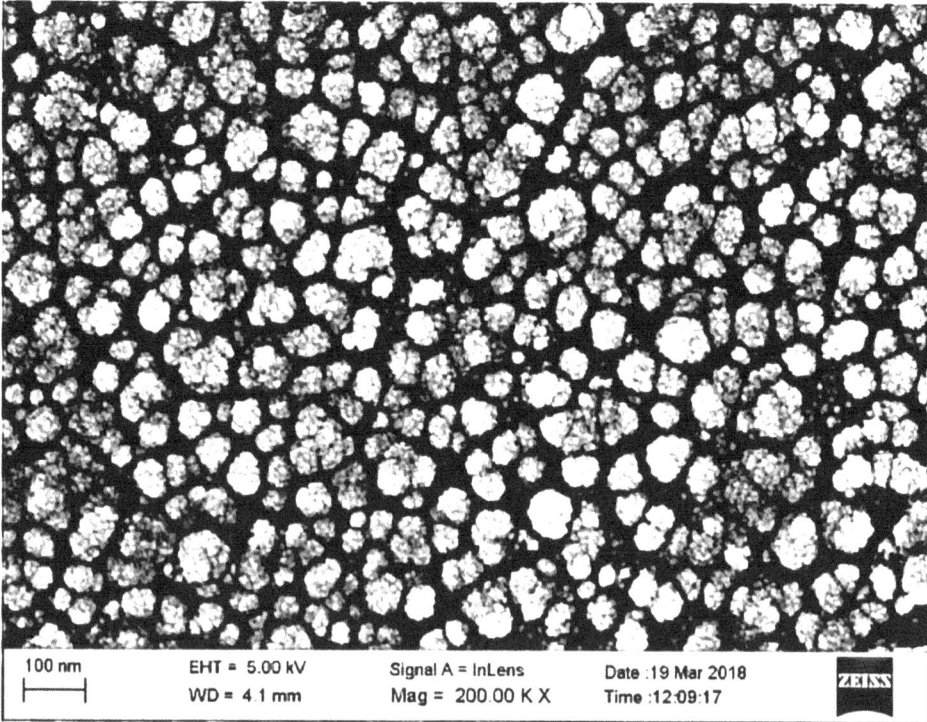

FIGURE 7.29 FESEM image of the Ag-island immobilized fiber surface (Nayak and Jha 2018).

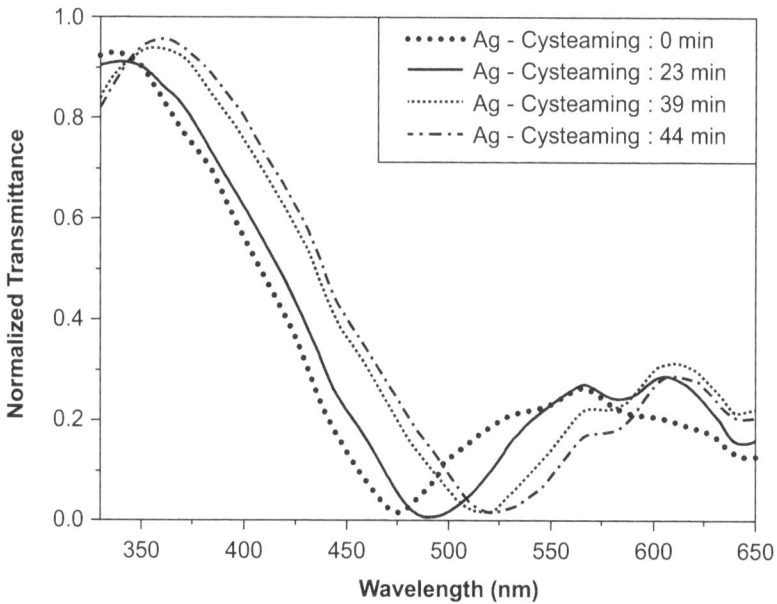

FIGURE 7.30 Variation of transmittance with wavelength at different dip period in cysteamine (Nayak and Jha 2018).

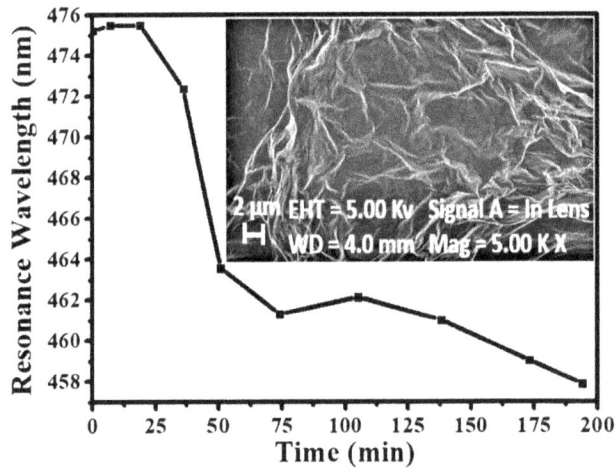

FIGURE 7.31   Resonance wavelength variation at different dip period in GO. The inset shows the FESEM image of GO (Nayak and Jha 2018).

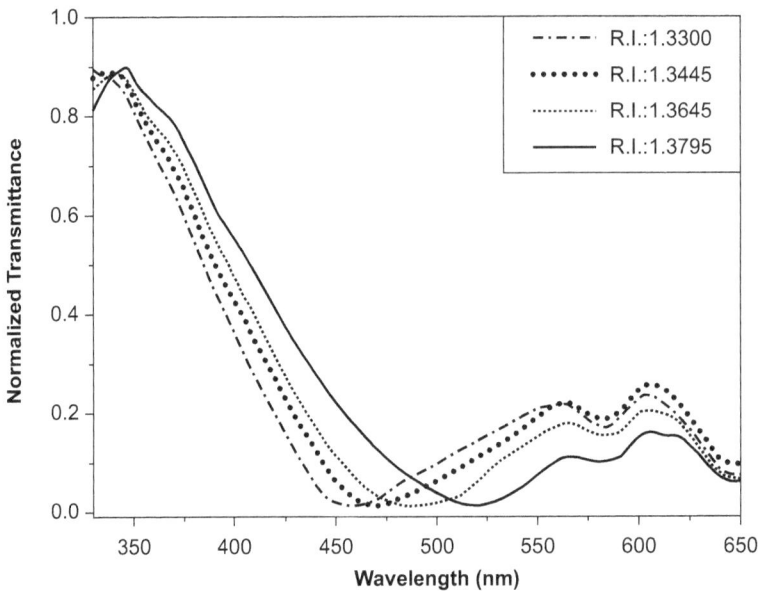

FIGURE 7.32   Transmittance variation at different analytes' refractive index (Nayak and Jha 2018).

widened with respect to time. The broadening of the LSPR spectrum indicates the presence of GO functionalized fiber sensor probes coated with cysteamine. As the incubation period lengthens, the GO thickness increases over the Ag-island, and the damping of the surface plasmon field results in the formation of a ring around the Ag-island, broadening the spectrum (Pockrand 1978).

Figure 7.31 shows a FESEM image of synthesized GO. The unbound GO was removed using a thrice-rinse with DI water. Following that, solutions of various RIs were maintained over the sensing area, and their respective transmission spectra were measured to determine the sensor's refractometer performance, as illustrated in Figure 7.32. There have been observed LSPR dip shifts between 460.36 and 521.72 nm for analyte RI variations between 1.3300 and 1.3795. With analyte

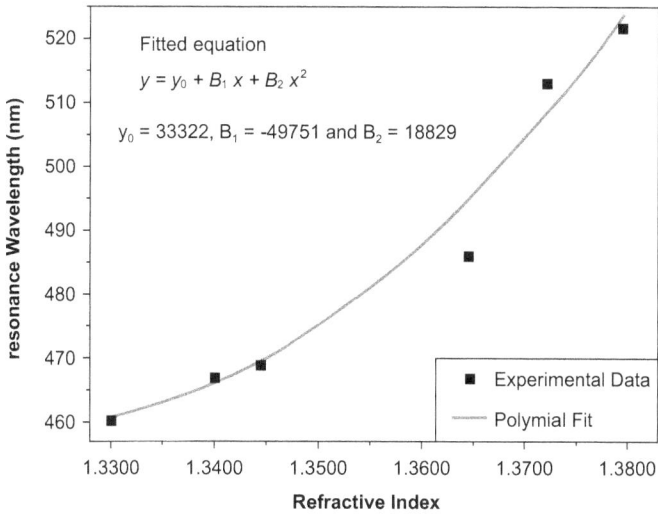

FIGURE 7.33 Resonance wavelength variation at different analytes' refractive index (Nayak and Jha 2018).

TABLE 7.1

Performance comparison for fiber-based LSPR sensor using metallic-island (Nayak and Jha 2018).

Island used	Refractive index range (RIU)	Sensitivity (nm/RIU)	Ref.
Gold	1–1.360	91.66	Meriaudeau et al. 1999
Gold	1.333–1.384	517	Hosoki, Nisiyama, and Watanabe 2017
Silver	1.330–1.3795	2217.04	Nayak, Parhi, and Jha 2016; Nayak and Jha 2018

RI, the LSPR wavelength is red-shifted as the resonance condition (Froehlich condition) is met at a higher wavelength (Willets and Van Duyne 2007).

The sensitivity can be calculated by measuring the resonance wavelength with corresponding RIs as shown in Figure 7.33. Slope in this plot gives the sensitivity of 2217.04 nm/RIU with an error of ± 0.9 nm. In this case, resolution of sensor is 4.05×10^{-4} RIU. Error has been calculated from standard deviation of data. The performance comparison of GO/Ag-island film immobilized optical fiber LSPR sensor is shown in Table 7.1. This shows that sensor discussed in this chapter shows that GO is a conducive platform for functionalization of biomolecules on its surface, and it opens a new window for biosensing applications.

7.4 AGNPS AND GO-BASED PLASMONIC SENSOR FOR L-CYSTEINE DETECTION

Biomarkers such as L-cysteine (L-Cys), glutathione (GSH), and homocysteine (Hcy) are abundant in the human physiological system (Fu et al. 2019; McCarty and DiNicolantonio 2015; Wang et al. 2019). The typical level of L-Cys in the human body is 240–360 μM, according to the literature. Glutathione is essential for not only maintaining or increasing the proper physiological function of human organs but also for establishing physiological activities in leukocytes and platelets. L-Cys, a component of glutathione, may boost human immunity and resistance while also assisting in the maintenance of a steady glutathione level and blood glucose regulation. Growth retardation, liver damage, cerebral thrombosis, human hematopoietic abnormalities, and other diseases/disorders may all be caused by an abnormal concentration of L-Cys.

To show the viability of sensors integrating taper and heteronuclear structures, the fiber structure based on conical single mode-multimode-single mode fiber (SMS) was employed to detect L-Cys in the present study. The taper fiber-based structure with a distinct core structure may significantly increase sensor sensitivity. To functionalize the sensor probe, biocompatible nanomaterials (NMs) (such as AgNPs and GO) were placed to the surface at the same time. GO has become the dominant material for functional sensor probes due to its large surface area, good optical transmittance, outstanding thermal conductivity, excellent additivity, and strong intrinsic mobility and electrical characteristics. Based on the aforesaid foundation, the taper SMS (TSMS)/AgNPs/GO L-Cys sensor (probe 2) is suggested, and a comparison with the basic taper multimode fiber-optic (TMMF)/AgNPs/GO L-Cys sensor (probe 1) is fabricated as shown in Figure 7.34. The sensor probe with the TSMS structure has a greater performance, according to the experimental data (Agrawal, Saha et al. 2020).

7.4.1 Synthesis of Silver Nanoparticles

An effective electrochemical technique was used to make AgNPs (Agrawal, Zhang et al. 2020). To begin, a 1-mM $AgNO_3$ solution was made by dissolving $AgNO_3$ in deionized water. $NaBH_4$ was dissolved in DI water to make a solution with a concentration of 1 mM. During the synthesis, a continual flow of 1-mM $AgNO_3$ solution was introduced to the $NaBH_4$ solution, and the solution became yellow green after 1 hour of continuous stirring. $NaBH_4$ is a reducing agent that also functions as a stabilizer.

7.4.2 Experimental Setup and Results

Figure 7.35 depicts an experimental measuring equipment for L-Cys detection based on a TSMS sensor probe. After the signal was steady, the sample L-Cys solution was injected into the antidish of the sensing probe, and the LSPR spectrum was recorded at the output end as shown in Figure 7.36. RI red-shifts the transmission strength and wavelength of LSPR. Total internal

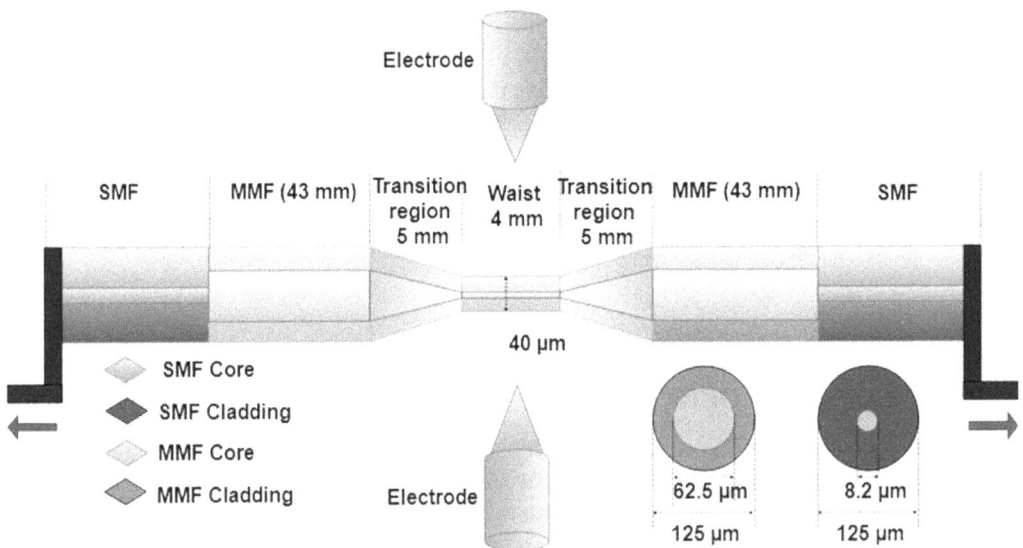

FIGURE 7.34 Schematic of proposed sensing probe.

Source: Reprinted with permission from *IEEE Sensors Journal.* Copyright, 2020, IEEE (Agrawal, Saha et al. 2020).

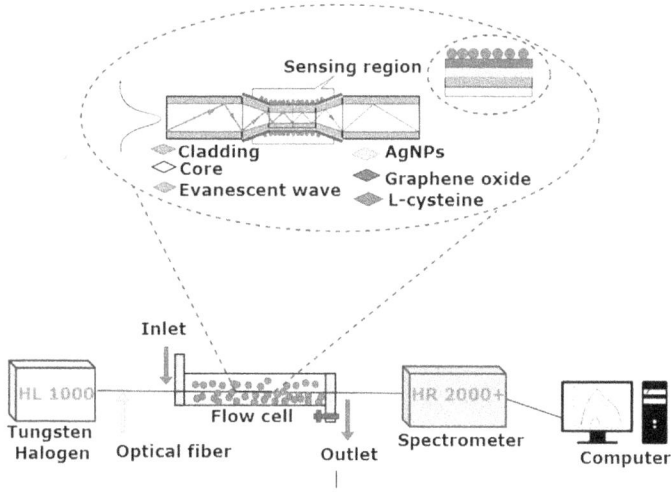

FIGURE 7.35 L-cysteine measurement setup.

Source: Reprinted with permission from *IEEE Sensors Journal*. Copyright, 2020, IEEE (Agrawal, Saha et al. 2020).

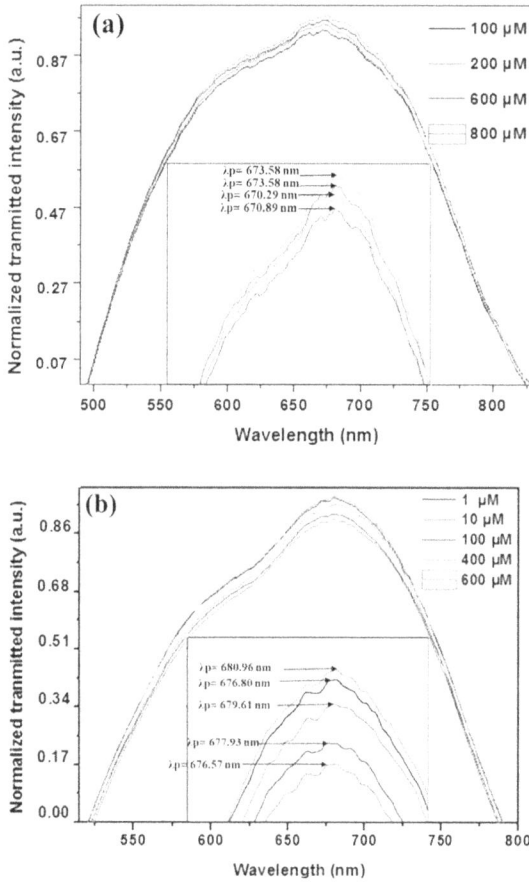

FIGURE 7.36 Sensing spectrum: (a) probe 1, (b) probe 2.

Source: Reprinted with permission from *IEEE Sensors Journal*. Copyright, 2020, IEEE (Agrawal, Saha et al. 2020).

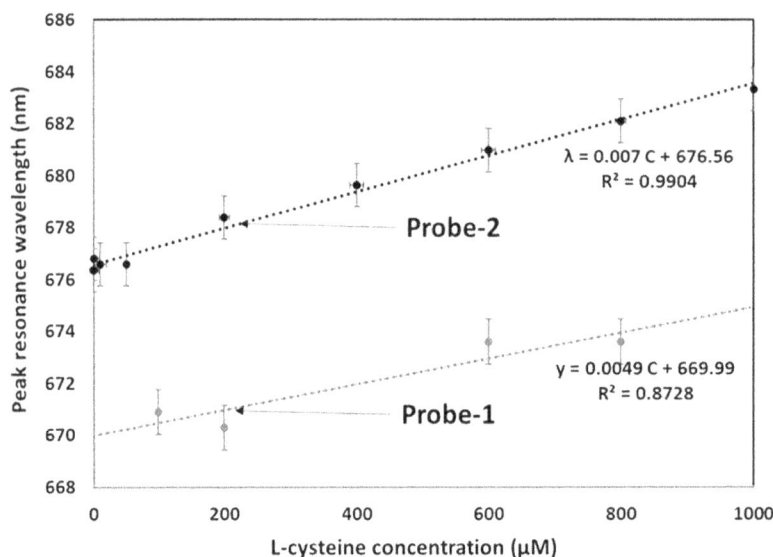

FIGURE 7.37   Linear plot of sensor probe 1 and probe 2.

Source: Reprinted with permission from *IEEE Sensors Journal.* Copyright, 2020, IEEE (Agrawal, Saha et al. 2020).

reflection transmits the transmitted light from the light source to the sensor probe. By tapering the detecting probe fiber to interact with external media, a portion of the light is efficiently transformed into EWs. An MMI structure offers a large measurement range, as well as high sensitivity and strong linearity (as shown in Figure 7.37), thanks to the combination of the TSMS conical structure and the hetero-core structure.

7.5   SUMMARY AND CONCLUSION

The GO coating forms a thin layer of encapsulation on top of the AgNPs that aids in controlling the interparticle distance and preventing AgNPs from aggregating. By isolating the AgNPs from direct contact with the aqueous medium, the GO encapsulation enhances colloidal stability and prevents AgNPs oxidation. The average size of AgNPs in this case is 35 nm, and they are encapsulated in a 1-nm-thick GO layer. UV-Vis spectrophotometer and Raman spectrometer are suitable instruments for characterizing GO and GOE-AgNPs. Raman spectroscopy reveals a 64.72% and 52.91% increase in the D-peak and G-peak intensities of GOE-AgNPs, respectively, when compared to GO. Then, GOE-AgNPs are synthesized and functionalized over the PCS fiber, as confirmed by FESEM. Peak absorbance is estimated to change by 87.55% with a 0.05 change in RI. The experimental results corroborate the simulation results in this work. This sensor is based on an optical fiber absorbance sensor functionalized with GOE-AgNPs. In this case, GO encapsulation is required to ensure the stability of AgNPs, as AgNPs have an inherent oxidation property that degrades sensor performance. Theoretically calculated resolution and sensitivity values agree with experimentally determined values. Additionally, a study was conducted on the GOE-AgNPs and GOE-AuNPs-based optical fiber LSPR sensor. The absorbance obtained experimentally was compared to the absorbance obtained theoretically. The absorbance of a mixture of GOE-AgNPs and GOE-AuNPs has been determined to be the average of the absorbance of the individual GOE-AgNPs and GOE-AuNPs. The GOE-AgNPs and GOE-AuNPs are coated on the optical fiber's functionalized surface. Two distinct absorbance peaks were observed. Two peak absorbance values have been observed to increase in proportion to the analyte RI.

Additionally, an experimental study on the performance of GO on an Ag-island coated optical fiber-based LSPR sensor has been presented. The presence of a 445-nm LSPR dip confirms the coating of Ag-island. Following that, GO was immobilized on the Ag-island using cysteamine as a linking agent. The proposed study discussed in this chapter will pave the way for new biosensing applications.

REFERENCES

Agrawal, N., C. Saha, C. Kumar, R. Singh, B. Zhang, R. Jha, and S. Kumar. 2020. "Detection of L-cysteine using silver nanoparticles and graphene oxide immobilized tapered SMS optical fiber structure." *IEEE Sensors Journal* 20 (19):11372–11379. DOI: 10.1109/JSEN.2020.2997690.

Agrawal, N., B. Zhang, C. Saha, C. Kumar, B. K. Kaushik, and S. Kumar. 2020. "Development of dopamine sensor using silver nanoparticles and PEG-functionalized tapered optical fiber structure." *IEEE Transactions on Biomedical Engineering* 67 (6):1542–1547. DOI: 10.1109/TBME.2019.2939560.

Bharadwaj, Reshma, and Soumyo Mukherji. 2014. "Gold nanoparticle coated U-bend fibre optic probe for localized surface plasmon resonance based detection of explosive vapours." *Sensors and Actuators B: Chemical* 192:804–811. https://doi.org/10.1016/j.snb.2013.11.026.

Cheng, Shu-Fang, and Lai-Kwan Chau. 2003. "Colloidal gold-modified optical fiber for chemical and biochemical sensing." *Analytical Chemistry* 75 (1):16–21. DOI: 10.1021/ac020310v.

Dutta, Rani, Bhanu P. Singh, and Tapenendu Kundu. 2013. "Plasmonic coupling effect on spectral response of silver nanoparticles immobilized on an optical fiber sensor." *Journal of Physical Chemistry C* 117 (33):17167–17176. DOI: 10.1021/jp401542a.

Evanoff, D. D., Jr., and G. Chumanov. 2005. "Synthesis and optical properties of silver nanoparticles and arrays." *Chemphyschem* 6 (7):1221–1231. DOI: 10.1002/cphc.200500113.

Fu, Xiaoyun, Shelby A. Cate, Melissa Dominguez, Warren Osborn, Tahsin Özpolat, Barbara A. Konkle, Junmei Chen, and José A. López. 2019. "Cysteine disulfides (Cys-ss-X) as sensitive plasma biomarkers of oxidative stress." *Scientific Reports* 9 (1):115. DOI: 10.1038/s41598-018-35566-2.

González, A. L., and Cecilia Noguez. 2007. "Optical properties of silver nanoparticles." *physica status solidi c* 4 (11):4118–4126. https://doi.org/10.1002/pssc.200675903.

Guo, Haiquan, and Shiquan Tao. 2007. "Silver nanoparticles doped silica nanocomposites coated on an optical fiber for ammonia sensing." *Sensors and Actuators B: Chemical* 123 (1):578–582. https://doi.org/10.1016/j.snb.2006.09.055.

Haes, Amanda J., and Richard P. Van Duyne. 2002. "A nanoscale optical biosensor: Sensitivity and selectivity of an approach based on the localized surface plasmon resonance spectroscopy of triangular silver nanoparticles." *Journal of the American Chemical Society* 124 (35):10596–10604. DOI: 10.1021/ja020393x.

Hosoki, Ai, Michiko Nisiyama, and Kazuhiro Watanabe. 2017. "Localized surface plasmon sensor using a hetero-core structured fiber optic with gold island films." *Journal of Physics: Conference Series* 922:012018. DOI: 10.1088/1742-6596/922/1/012018.

Hummers, William S., and Richard E. Offeman. 1958. "Preparation of graphitic oxide." *Journal of the American Chemical Society* 80 (6):1339–1339. DOI: 10.1021/ja01539a017.

Hussain, Saber M., and John J. Schlager. 2009. "Safety evaluation of silver nanoparticles: Inhalation model for chronic exposure." *Toxicological Sciences* 108 (2):223–224. DOI: 10.1093/toxsci/kfp032.

Johnson, P. B., and R. W. Christy. 1972. "Optical constants of the noble metals." *Physical Review B* 6 (12):4370–4379. DOI: 10.1103/PhysRevB.6.4370.

Jorgenson, R. C., and S. S. Yee. 1993. "A fiber-optic chemical sensor based on surface plasmon resonance." *Sensors and Actuators B: Chemical* 12 (3):213–220. https://doi.org/10.1016/0925-4005(93)80021-3.

Jung, Inhwa, Matthias Vaupel, Matthew Pelton, Richard Piner, Dmitriy A. Dikin, Sasha Stankovich, Jinho An, and Rodney S. Ruoff. 2008. "Characterization of thermally reduced graphene oxide by imaging ellipsometry." *Journal of Physical Chemistry C* 112 (23):8499–8506. DOI: 10.1021/jp802173m.

Kou, Liang, Hongkun He, and Chao Gao. 2010. "Click chemistry approach to functionalize two-dimensional macromolecules of graphene oxide nanosheets." *Nano-Micro Letters* 2 (3):177–183. DOI: 10.1007/BF03353638.

Kreibig, U. 1974. "Electronic properties of small silver particles: The optical constants and their temperature dependence." *Journal of Physics F: Metal Physics* 4 (7):999–1014. DOI: 10.1088/0305-4608/4/7/007.

Lee, P. C., and D. Meisel. 1982. "Adsorption and surface-enhanced Raman of dyes on silver and gold sols." *Journal of Physical Chemistry* 86 (17):3391–3395. DOI: 10.1021/j100214a025.

Liedberg, Bo, Claes Nylander, and Ingemar Lunström. 1983. "Surface plasmon resonance for gas detection and biosensing." *Sensors and Actuators* 4:299–304. https://doi.org/10.1016/0250-6874(83)85036-7.

Lin, Hsing-Ying, Chen-Han Huang, Chia-Chi Huang, Yu-Chia Liu, and Lai-Kwan Chau. 2012. "Multiple resonance fiber-optic sensor with time division multiplexing for multianalyte detection." *Optics Letters* 37 (19):3969–3971. DOI: 10.1364/OL.37.003969.

Luo, Ji, Jun Yao, Yonggang Lu, Wenying Ma, and Xuye Zhuang. 2013. "A silver nanoparticle-modified evanescent field optical fiber sensor for methylene blue detection." *Sensors* 13 (3). DOI: 10.3390/s130303986.

Mahmudin, Lufsyi, Edi Suharyadi, Agung Utomo, and Kamsul Abraha. 2015. "Optical properties of silver nanoparticles for surface plasmon resonance (SPR)-based biosensor applications." *Journal of Modern Physics* 06:1071–1076. DOI: 10.4236/jmp.2015.68111.

McCarty, M. F., and J. J. DiNicolantonio. 2015. "An increased need for dietary cysteine in support of glutathione synthesis may underlie the increased risk for mortality associated with low protein intake in the elderly." *Age (Dordrecht)* 37 (5):96. DOI: 10.1007/s11357-015-9823-8.

Meriaudeau, F., T. Downey, A. Wig, A. Passian, M. Buncick, and T. L. Ferrell. 1999. "Fiber optic sensor based on gold island plasmon resonance." *Sensors and Actuators B: Chemical* 54 (1):106–117. https://doi.org/10.1016/S0925-4005(98)00318-9.

Nayak, J. K., and R. Jha. 2018. "Graphene-oxide coated Ag-island-based inline LSPR fiber sensor." *IEEE Photonics Technology Letters* 30 (19):1667–1670. DOI: 10.1109/LPT.2018.2865491.

Nayak, Jeeban Kumar, Purnendu Parhi, and Rajan Jha. 2015. "Graphene oxide encapsulated gold nanoparticle based stable fibre optic sucrose sensor." *Sensors and Actuators B: Chemical* 221:835–841. https://doi.org/10.1016/j.snb.2015.06.152.

Nayak, Jeeban Kumar, Purnendu Parhi, and Rajan Jha. 2016. "Experimental and theoretical studies on localized surface plasmon resonance based fiber optic sensor using graphene oxide coated silver nanoparticles." *Journal of Physics D: Applied Physics* 49 (28):285101. DOI: 10.1088/0022-3727/49/28/285101.

Okamoto, Takayuki, Ichirou Yamaguchi, and Tetsushi Kobayashi. 2000. "Local plasmon sensor with gold colloid monolayers deposited upon glass substrates." *Optics Letters* 25 (6):372–374. DOI: 10.1364/OL.25.000372.

Ortega-Mendoza, J. Gabriel, Alfonso Padilla-Vivanco, Carina Toxqui-Quitl, Placido Zaca-Morán, David Villegas-Hernández, and Fernando Chávez. 2014. "Optical fiber sensor based on localized surface plasmon resonance using silver nanoparticles photodeposited on the optical fiber end." *Sensors (Basel, Switzerland)* 14 (10):18701–18710. DOI: 10.3390/s141018701.

Pande, Surojit, Sujit Kumar Ghosh, Snigdhamayee Praharaj, Sudipa Panigrahi, Soumen Basu, Subhra Jana, Anjali Pal, Tatsuya Tsukuda, and Tarasankar Pal. 2007. "Synthesis of normal and inverted gold-silver core-shell architectures in β-cyclodextrin and their applications in SERS." *Journal of Physical Chemistry C* 111 (29):10806–10813. DOI: 10.1021/jp0702393.

Pillai, Zeena S., and Prashant V. Kamat. 2004. "What factors control the size and shape of silver nanoparticles in the citrate ion reduction method?" *Journal of Physical Chemistry B* 108 (3):945–951. DOI: 10.1021/jp037018r.

Pockrand, I. 1978. "Surface plasma oscillations at silver surfaces with thin transparent and absorbing coatings." *Surface Science* 72 (3):577–588. https://doi.org/10.1016/0039-6028(78)90371-0.

Rashid, Md Harunar, and Tarun K. Mandal. 2007. "Synthesis and catalytic application of nanostructured silver dendrites." *Journal of Physical Chemistry C* 111 (45):16750–16760. DOI: 10.1021/jp074963x.

Ruddy, V., B. D. MacCraith, and J. A. Murphy. 1990. "Evanescent wave absorption spectroscopy using multimode fibers." *Journal of Applied Physics* 67 (10):6070–6074. DOI: 10.1063/1.346085.

Shrivastava, Siddhartha, Tanmay Bera, Arnab Roy, Gajendra Singh, P. Ramachandrarao, and Debabrata Dash. 2007. "Characterization of enhanced antibacterial effects of novel silver nanoparticles." *Nanotechnology* 18 (22):225103. DOI: 10.1088/0957-4484/18/22/225103.

Singh, Dr Mritunjai, and S. Singh. 2008. "Nanotechnology in medicine and antibacterial effect of silver nano particles." *Journal of Nanomaterials and Biostructures* 3:115–122.

Sperling, Ralph A., Pilar Rivera Gil, Feng Zhang, Marco Zanella, and Wolfgang J. Parak. 2008. "Biological applications of gold nanoparticles." *Chemical Society Reviews* 37 (9):1896–1908. DOI: 10.1039/B712170A.

Sreenivasan, M. G., Shweta Malik, Srikanth Thigulla, and Bodh Raj Mehta. 2013. "Dependence of plasmonic properties of silver island films on nanoparticle size and substrate coverage." *Journal of Nanomaterials* 2013:247045. DOI: 10.1155/2013/247045.

Tagad, Chandrakant K., Sreekantha Reddy Dugasani, Rohini Aiyer, Sungha Park, Atul Kulkarni, and Sushma Sabharwal. 2013. "Green synthesis of silver nanoparticles and their application for the development of optical fiber based hydrogen peroxide sensor." *Sensors and Actuators B: Chemical* 183:144–149. https:// doi.org/10.1016/j.snb.2013.03.106.

Urrutia, Aitor, Javier Goicoechea, and Francisco J. Arregui. 2015. "Optical fiber sensors based on nanoparticle-embedded coatings." *Journal of Sensors* 2015:805053. DOI: 10.1155/2015/805053.

Wang, Hui, Letian Wang, Shanyu Meng, Hanxue Lin, Melanie Correll, and Zhaohui Tong. 2020. "Nanocomposite of graphene oxide encapsulated in polymethylmethacrylate (PMMA): Pre-modification, synthesis, and latex stability." *Journal of Composites Science* 4 (3). DOI: 10.3390/jcs4030118.

Wang, N., M. Chen, J. Gao, X. Ji, J. He, J. Zhang, and W. Zhao. 2019. "A series of BODIPY-based probes for the detection of cysteine and homocysteine in living cells." *Talanta* 195:281–289. DOI: 10.1016/j. talanta.2018.11.066.

Wen, Hua-Chiang, Yao-Nan Lin, Sheng-Rui Jian, Shih-Chun Tseng, Ming-Xiang Weng, Yu-Pin Liu, Po-Te Lee, Pai-Yen Chen, Ray-Quan Hsu, Wen-Fa Wu, and Chang-Pin Chou. 2007. "Observation of growth of human fibroblasts on silver nanoparticles." *Journal of Physics: Conference Series* 61:445–449. DOI: 10.1088/1742-6596/61/1/089.

Willets, Katherine A., and Richard P. Van Duyne. 2007. "Localized surface plasmon resonance spectroscopy and sensing." *Annual Review of Physical Chemistry* 58 (1):267–297. DOI: 10.1146/annurev. physchem.58.032806.104607.

Xu, G., M. Tazawa, P. Jin, S. Nakao, and K. Yoshimura. 2003. "Wavelength tuning of surface plasmon resonance using dielectric layers on silver island films." *Applied Physics Letters* 82 (22):3811–3813. DOI: 10.1063/1.1578518.

Xu, G., M. Tazawa, Puyang Jin, and Setsuo Nakao. 2005. "Surface plasmon resonance of sputtered Ag films: Substrate and mass thickness dependence." *Applied Physics A* 80:1535–1540. DOI: 10.1007/ s00339-003-2395-y.

Zou, Shengli, and George C. Schatz. 2004. "Narrow plasmonic/photonic extinction and scattering line shapes for one and two dimensional silver nanoparticle arrays." *Journal of Chemical Physics* 121 (24):12606– 12612. DOI: 10.1063/1.1826036.

8 Novel Nanomaterials Assisted Optical Fiber-Based Plasmonic Biosensors

8.1 INTRODUCTION

In the preceding chapter, design technology, material synthesis, and characterizations are discussed. Several novel nanomaterials are employed in this chapter for the detection of important biomolecules found in the human body. Creatinine is a by-product of muscle metabolism that is removed primarily by the glomerulus in the human body. It is an important biomarker for a variety of renal functional diseases (Jacobi et al. 2008; Polinder-Bos et al. 2017). Serum creatinine concentration in a healthy individual is 140 µM; however, if a person's serum creatinine level exceeds 800 µM, it indicates serious kidney disease, which in severe cases can lead to death. Therefore, serum creatinine levels in patients with chronic kidney disease can achieve early prevention and treatment (Coresh et al. 2003; Reddy and Gobi 2013; Hanif et al. 2016). To estimate creatinine concentration, some researchers formerly relied primarily on colorimetric (Jaffe reaction) or enzyme colorimetric approaches (Tymecki et al. 2013; Kuster et al. 2012). Sharma et al. created an optic fiber creatinine biosensor on MoS_2/SnO_2 nanocomposites molecular imprinting technique (Sharma, Shrivastav, and Gupta 2020). However, colorimetric analysis has its complex preparation process and strict requirements on the compatibility of biological materials. The development of enzyme colorimetric detection creatinine sensor needs great cost, so the cost performance is very low (Ciou et al. 2020; Lewińska et al. 2021). Kumar et al. constructed an enhanced amperometric biosensor for the detection of creatinine levels in humans and achieved desirable results (Kumar, Jaiwal, and Pundir 2017). This method has been used to detect blood creatinine levels in healthy people as well as those with renal and muscular problems. Menon et al. developed a surface plasmon resonance (SPR) sensor based on Kretschmann principle for creatinine detection using nanocomposite gold sheet as substrate material (Menon et al. 2018). Topçu et al. developed a sensor based on SPR principle by using molecular imprinting technology, which can detect creatinine without a label (Arif Topçu et al. 2019). Therefore, this chapter discusses the development of a biosensor based on localized surface plasmon resonance (LSPR) to detect human creatinine concentration. The goal of this chapter is also to create a biosensor that uses Nb_2CTx MXene to improve the LSPR impact of AuNPs for detecting creatinine levels.

Similarly, alanine aminotransferase (ALT) is a serum transaminase that can be used as a marker for liver function diseases. Clinical studies and laboratory tests have shown that slightly elevated ALT levels may predict when certain metabolic problems such as obesity and other diseases develop in the body. Alanine aminotransferase is found in other organs and tissues such as adipose tissue, liver, and intestines. Among them, the active content of ALT in liver is the highest compared with other organs in human body. Therefore, when functional liver disease occurs, it will lead to the increase of ALT level in blood, resulting in the significant increase of alanine aminotransferase activity. The ratio of liver enzyme activity to serum enzyme activity is about 3000:1. Meanwhile, the ALT enzyme's typical activity level in blood is 5–40 U/L (Liu et al. 2014). Because the ALT enzyme in the blood acts as a barometer of liver health, abnormal ALT enzyme levels may indicate liver damage (Hsueh et al. 2012). Thus, clinical trials may be used to establish if the liver is badly damaged by looking at the amount of ALT activity in blood samples (Nanji, French, and Freeman 1985). Despite these obstacles, scientists' institutions have made significant progress in recent years

DOI: 10.1201/9781003243199-8

in developing tools for clinical surveillance of patients with liver disease. For example, colorimetric analysis requires calculating and plotting calibration curves for the number of products produced and the number of substrates consumed during enzyme reactions, and then using these curves to get the concentration of the analyte (Liu, Ma, and Zhang 2010). For biomolecular detection of glutamic-pyruvate transaminase, biosensor based on LSPR not only has the advantages of high sensitivity and labeling free, but also has the advantages of real-time and rapid detection.

Similarly, phenol wastewater, as one of the industrial wastewaters, not only seriously polluted the environment, but also seriously damaged water resources. Drinking water with phenol might result in muscular spasms, walking difficulties, and even death (Michałowicz and Duda 2007). When these phenolic compounds are burned, they generate poisonous fumes that may be detrimental to human health if inhaled. Catechol, 4-chlorophenol, m-cresol, o-cresol, phenol, p-cresol, and other phenolic compounds are members of the phenolic compound family. Due to its hydrophobicity and biotransformation properties, this leads to the formation of reactive conjugated molecules (meth-ylquinone) or free radicals, P-cresol and seriously affect the health of the body (Usha and Gupta 2018). Apart from its existence in tea, oil, and tap water, p-cresol may enter the human body in a variety of ways. It is employed as a flavoring ingredient in foods and as a precursor in certain tradi-tional treatments (Usha and Gupta 2018). Furthermore, p-cresol is created by protein breakdown or microbial activity in the intestines, both of which produce a small quantity of p-cresol. The body's capacity to absorb nutrients and discharge them, mostly via urine, improves as a protein accumu-lates (Agrawal, Saha et al. 2020). Because of its significance, p-cresol has been discovered in human feces and urine using both qualitative and quantitative methods. In the literature, many techniques for detecting p-cresol have been published, the most common of which is high-performance liq-uid chromatography (HPLC) (Singh, Mishra, and Gupta 2013), fluorescence (Harper et al. 2009), and gas chromatography-mass spectrometry (Kovács et al. 2008). Optical sensors, on the other hand, are small and dependable, with basic construction, quick detection time, great sensitivity, and high dependability. As a result, optical sensors are seen to be the best choice for high sensitivity, label-free detection, quick response, compact size, and flexibility in sensor systems. Tyrosinase is widely utilized for p-cresol detection to address the sensor's specificity (Li et al. 2006). Tyrosinase (polyphenol oxidase) catalyzes the o-hydroxylation of phenol to produce o-diphenol, which is then oxidized to o-quinone (Adamski, Nowak, and Kochana 2010).

Similarly, acute myocardial infarction (AMI) has become a cause of death across the earth. AMI may cause irreversible heart muscle injury and blood troponin release (Abdolrahim et al. 2015; Nigam 2007). Cardiac troponin I (cTnI) is an important biomarker for AMI, with a normal value of 30–80 pg/mL in human serum. Following 12 hours of an AMI, cTnI levels in the blood rise and remain high for 5–9 days after the infarction (Chekin et al. 2018). When the concentration surpasses 100 pg/mL, however, it signals a cardiovascular disease risk (CVD). Long-term exposure to high concentrations is linked to an increased risk of life-threatening incidents (Maynard, Menown, and Adgey 2000). As a result, developing a biosensor for the detection of cTnI is critical. cTnI has been detected using a variety of sensors, including photoelectrochemical immunosensors (Liao et al. 2021), molecular imprinted polymers (Mokhtari et al. 2020), and lateral flow immunoassay (Lee et al. 2020). These approaches, however, have disadvantages such as limited linear range, high cost, and low sensitivity. As a consequence, in order to overcome these flaws, a highly sensitive, low-cost, and portable cTnI sensor is required. Compact size, mobility, simplicity of fabrication, great sensi-tivity, and outstanding antinoise performance are just a few of the benefits of fiber-optic biosensors (He et al. 2021; Kumar and Singh 2021).

CVDs are a major cause of death worldwide. The mortality rate from CVDs is gradually increas-ing due to increased social pressure, excessive obesity, long-term smoking and drinking, lack of physical activity, and other bad living habits (Çimen et al. 2020; Kim et al. 2016; Negahdary and Heli 2019). cTnI is a biomarker with high sensitivity for an AMI compared with the other two (Dhara and Mahapatra 2020). cTnI is considered to be the most obvious and direct indicator for myocardial injury, so it acts as a specific biomarker, a label, for early detection of AMI (Perrone et al. 2021; Kim et al. 2017; Abdolrahim et al. 2015). Thus, there is an urgent requirement to develop a label-free, more efficient, effective, and easier method for rapid and specific detection of cTnI (Dhawan et al. 2018). cTnI has established itself as the aim standard for the detection of AMI. In normal human serum, cTnI concentrations range between 30 and 80 pg/mL. This increases quickly after the onset of AMI, reaching a high of about 200 ng/mL about a day later (Dhara and Mahapatra 2020). At present, antigen-antibody interaction is one of the major promising methods for the development of biosensors in general. Antibody-antigen interaction possesses high selectivity and specificity activity and thus is mainly used for the determination of specific low concentration biomarkers (Liu et al. 2011). Various assay methods, like electrochemical immunoassay (Sun et al. 2019), electrochemiluminescence immunosensor (Wang et al. 2020), fluorescence immunoassay (Liu et al. 2018), photoelectrochemical (Fan et al. 2018), and mass spectrometry (Onwuli et al. 2019), were developed for the detection of cTnI. These traditional methods have limitations: low sensitivity or high cost or poor selectivity and complex chemical processing. In this chapter, the controlled etched single-mode fiber–multimode fiber–single-mode fiber (SMS) fiber structure is used as a processed substrate, which not only helps in guiding the light but at the same time facilitates the strong interaction of the higher-order modes of multimode fiber that allows fast and easier detection of cTnI.

A steady level of bioactive chemicals in a specified range is required for a healthy human body. Each biomolecule has the potential to be out of balance, resulting in catastrophic sickness. Acetylcholine (ACh) was the first neurotransmitter to be discovered and may be present in the central and peripheral nervous systems of humans (Lee et al. 2009). Due to active neurotransmitters, it also plays a crucial function in the neurological system. In recent years, the metabolic pathway of ACh has gotten a lot of attention (Lee et al. 2009). By attaching to cholinergic receptors, ACh, for example, stimulates a variety of signaling pathways. However, ACh deficiency is significantly associated with many illnesses (Tunç, Aynacı Koyuncu, and Arslan 2016). Therefore, a high-throughput assay for quantitative determination of acetylcholine is needed. In recent years, with the improvement of sensor performance, various nanomaterials have been widely used in the preparation of ACh sensors (Sattarahmady, Heli, and Vais 2013; Boruah and Biswas 2018; Martín-Barreiro et al. 2018). Light can now be routed and manipulated on a nanoscale thanks to the development of plasmon-based devices (Singh, Kumar et al. 2020). Furthermore, noble nanoparticles (NPs) have been thoroughly investigated and put to use. Gold nanoparticles (AuNPs) are preferred because of their superb optical characteristics, surfactant capabilities, and chemical durability (Saha et al. 2012; Tu, Sun, and Grattan 2012; Nayak, Parhi, and Jha 2015; Qiao and Qi 2021; Rampazzi et al. 2016).

Similarly, cholesterol is one of the main components of the human body and can be used as a biomarker for diabetes, cardiovascular disease, hypertension, stroke, and heart attack (Alexander et al. 2017). Various biosensing techniques, such as (i) electrochemical (Pundir et al. 2018), (ii) conductometric (Guan, Miao, and Zhang 2004), (iii) ion-sensitive (Krishnamurthy, Monfared, and Cornell 2010), (iv) piezoelectric (Bunde, Jarvi, and Rosentreter 1998), (v) optical (Vizzini et al. 2019), etc., have been used to detect a variety of analytes. In recent study, an effective LSPR-based approach is used among many optical techniques (Agrawal, Zhang, Saha, Kumar, Pu et al. 2020).

Glutathione (GSH) is critical for maintaining and/or improving the detoxification functions of the lungs, brain, and liver (McCarty and DiNicolantonio 2015). L-Cys is a part of glutathione, which boosts the body's glutathione level and helps the body recover from surgery (Wani, Singh, and Upadhyay 2017). It improves the patient's immune system and reduces the side effects of toxic chemicals and drugs, improves sperm quality, and regulates blood sugar levels in men (Wani, Singh, and Upadhyay 2017). Typical levels of L-Cys in humans are thought to be between 240 and 360 micrograms per milliliter (Wang et al. 2019). Disorders caused by abnormal levels of L-Cys include growth retardation, thrombosis, neuropsychiatric disorders, liver damage, muscle loss, and skin damage (Fu et al. 2019). In this chapter, tapered and hetero-core structure-based sensors are used to show an exceedingly effective approach for detecting L-Cys (Singh, Singh et al. 2020).

Collagen is a protein found in the connective tissue and internal organs of animals in the form of fibers (Di Lullo et al. 2002; Sivaguru et al. 2010). Amino acid sequence affects the quality and significance of collagen fibrils, resulting in a wide variety of collagen fibrils. Collagen-IV exists in the base of cell membranes and is the focus of this study. The accumulation of collagenous IV can lead to the development of scleroderma, keloids, or tumors, as well as glaucoma, among other catastrophic conditions (Maruyama et al. 2010; Park et al. 2009). Given this, a number of strategies have been developed to identify its presence as soon as possible. Yasmin et al. presented an enzymatic detection of collagen based on a fluorescence approach. Compared to quick response surface plasmon (SPR) methods, the detection period of 60 minutes may reduce the dependability of the job (Yasmin et al. 2014). Kim et al. suggested employing red dye in picric acid to calorimetrically detect collagen, although the protocol's efficacy is limited by its poor specificity (Kim et al. 2010). Therefore, a quantitative, low-cost method for the detection of type collagen IV is still in high demand. Collagenase produced by *Clostridium histolyticum* maintains its biological characteristics in the normal pH range of the human body (Kleber 1991). Therefore, samples for enzymatic testing are usually produced within the pH range described earlier. In vitro, collagen can be detected by preparing samples in phosphate-buffer saline (PBS). In vivo, it can be detected by using nanogels containing human cells (Breul et al. 1980). According to Breul et al., most soft tissue fibroblasts produce no more than 100 ng of collagen IV per milligram of total protein, but less than 5% of collagen per milligram of protein in bone fibroblasts and tendon cells (Breul et al. 1980).

As a consequence, choosing a technique that is cost effective, simple, quick, highly selective, and sensitive is essential. Biosensors have the following benefits over traditional technologies: quick reaction time, simplicity of use, great sensitivity, and cheap cost of analysis (Yadav, Kumar, and Pundir 2011; Yadav et al. 2011; Kumar, Jaiwal, and Pundir 2017; Do, Chang, and Tsai 2018). In addition to optical, electrochemical, spectrophotometer, and chromatographic sensors, biosensors are available in a wide range of shapes and methods. Chromatography demands the employment of advanced measurement tools as well as sample handling methods (Li et al. 2015; Pei and Li 2000). The electrode fabrication process for electrochemical types is time consuming. Optical sensors are favored by researchers because of their labeling free detection capability, fast response time, and high sensitivity (Kumar and Singh 2021; Willets and Van Duyne 2007). In addition, strong anti-electromagnetic interference ability, small volume, and high sensitivity are the requirements of optical fiber sensors based on SPR technology. However, since the SPR fiber sensor signal relies on a uniform metal layer, precisely controlling the thickness and homogeneity of the metal film on a non-planar substrate is difficult (Homola, Yee, and Gauglitz 1999). Due to these limitations of the traditional SPR sensor, its application is limited. In recent years, the rapid development of nanomaterials (NMs) manufacturing technology and the emergence of nano-photon technology have promoted the development of LSPR sensors. Drug detection, cell markers, bioassays, molecular dynamics studies, and site-specific diagnostics are all possible applications of LSPR sensors (Kumar et al. 2021; Singh, Kumar, et al. 2020; Gish et al. 2007; Niedziółka-Jönsson et al. 2010). With the development of metal NMs and nanostructure preparation technology and the development of advanced characterization instruments, LSPR technology is developing steadily on the basis of SPR technology. When light is incident on NPs composed of precious metals, if the incident photon frequency matches the overall vibration frequency of precious metal NMs or metal conduction electrons, NMs will have a strong absorption of photon energy, and LSPR will occur (Willets and Van Duyne 2007). When the frequency of the incident light matches the frequency of the free electron oscillation of the NPs, the surface electrons collectively oscillate (Gish et al. 2007; Niedziółka-Jönsson et al. 2010).

8.2 NANOMATERIAL SYNTHESIS PROCESS

8.2.1 Synthesis Process of AuNPs

AuNPs with diameters of 10 nm were synthesized mainly using Turkevich procedures (Turkevich, Stevenson, and Hillier 1951). The synthesis steps are as follows: First, 15 mL $HAuCl_4$ solution (150 µL, 100 mM) was $HAuCl_4$ dissolved in 14.85 mL DI water and heated to boiling to 110°C in a clean container. Then 1.8 mL 38.8 mM sodium citrate solution was added, and this was heated at 110 °C for 5 minutes and stop heating and continue stirring for 10 minutes. In this way, the AuNPs solvent can be synthesized. The solution of the produced AuNPs showed good stability, allowing it to be kept for 3 months in a cold, dry environment without aggregation (Li et al. 2021).

8.2.2 Synthesis of AgNPs Solution

The electrochemical technique was used to make the AgNPs solution (Agrawal, Zhang, Saha, Kumar, Kaushik et al. 2020). A steady flow of ice-cooled 1 mM $AgNO_3$ solution was introduced to an ice-cooled 1 mM $NaBH_4$ solution. After 1 hour of continual vigorous stirring, the final solution was greenish-yellow in color. A UV-Vis spectrophotometer demonstrated that AgNPs had a peak absorbance wavelength of 395 nm.

8.2.3 Synthesis Process of MXene

MXene has a continuous tunable electronic structure from metal to semiconductors, as well as different surface chemistry, making it useful in a variety of fields including energy storage (Aghamohammadi, Eslami-Farsani, and Castillo-Martinez 2022), catalysis (Sharma et al. 2022), biology (Liu et al. 2021), electronics (Tan et al. 2021), and sensing (Li et al. 2021). Because of its unique physical and chemical features, MXene has been widely employed in biosensing. Its layered structure makes MXene have a wide surface area and increases the landing sites of external substances. The surface of MXene is rich in hydrophilic functional groups such as O,–OH, and –F, which helps to improve the adsorption of water-soluble biomolecules on MXene, so as to improve the performance results. The high surface area and superior hydrophilicity of MXene help to adsorb more biomolecules and thus improve the detection sensitivity (Li et al. 2021). It has a great degree of control over its physical qualities and causal functions due to the variety of its chemical makeup and crystal structure. Nb_2CTx MXene has better light absorption qualities than noble metals, and its surface may be readily covered with various functional groups while maintaining metal conductivity (Li et al. 2021; Yin et al. 2021; Arif et al. 2021). Nb_2CTx MXene has significant LSPR effect and high hydrophilicity. Because Nb_2CTx MXene readily forms chemical bonds with other ions and macromolecules, the NMs can be attached to the component under test. Furthermore, an ultrasonic machine was used for 1 hour to achieve Nb_2CTx MXene dispersion (Yin et al. 2021; Pandey et al. 2020).

8.2.4 Synthesis Process of MoS_2-NPs

The MoS_2-NPs solution was made using a liquid-phase exfoliation process (Kumar et al. 2021). To put it simply, MoS_2 powder was soaked and dissolved in 10 mL NMP solution to form a suspension, which was ultrasonically crushed for 20 minutes on the bath machine of an ultrasonic cell crusher. The mixture was poured into the ultrasonic probe and removed for another 10 minutes. The treated solution was centrifuged at 4000 rpm for 1 hour to obtain the desired synthetic solution.

8.2.5 Synthesis Process of CeO_2-NPs

Cerium oxide nanoparticles (CeO_2-NPs) are nontoxic NMs with good biocompatibility. They have been used in chemical and biosensing fields for their excellent electrical conductivity, chemical stability, and strong electron transport capacity. Therefore, CeO_2-NPs has great potential as a biosensor. CeO_2-NPs were obtained by placing 0.1 g of $Ce(NO_3)_3$ into a container, adding 49 mL of DI water, and then gently dropping 1 mL of 3wt % H_2O_2 solution. Due to redox, the color of the solution will gradually turn pale yellow after these steps. Finally, the resulting solution is left for 3 weeks, during which time the color of the solution gradually fades.

8.2.6 Synthesis Process of GO

GO was synthesized by modified Hummer's method. First, 11.5 mL (98%) was mixed with 0.5 g graphite powder and 0.25 g NaNO$_3$ for 1 hour. Then 1.5 g KMnO$_4$ powder was slowly and carefully added to the combined solution under ice bath condition. Then, add 250mL DI water and place in the oven at 98°C for 15min. Then add 250mL warm water and 2.5mL H$_2$O$_2$. After full reaction, the supernatant was filtered and 5% HCl solution was added to remove impurities in the mixture. In addition, the centrifugal precipitates were roasted at 70°C to produce graphite oxide powder for further use.

8.2.7 Synthesis Process of Colloidal CuO-NPs Solution

CuO nanopowder (1 mg) was placed into 10 mL DI water and vigorously stirred using a magnetic stirrer for 20 minutes to make the CuO-NPs solution. To make the suspension even more uniform, it was sonicated for 10 minutes with a high-power ultra-sonicator with a 1000 W output power. In each cycle of sonication, the ON and OFF times are 9 and 6 seconds, respectively. A cooling technique was implemented to keep the sample temperature at roughly 32°C during ultrasonication to prevent temperature variations. After that, the dispersed solution was centrifuged for another 20 minutes at 3000 rpm.

8.3 CHARACTERIZATION OF NANOPARTICLES

Characterization of the synthesized nanoparticles (NPs) is illustrated in this section. The primary confirmation of synthesis of NPs can be done by observing their color appearance. The color confirmation is not very reliable to assure the exact size and distribution of NPs inside the solutions. The water dispersions of GO, AuNPs, and MoS$_2$-NPs solutions were characterized by UV-Vis spectrophotometer and HRTEM. Absorption peaks of the three NMs can be seen in the UV-Vis region. Absorption spectra of the three NMs are shown in Figure 8.1(a), Figure 8.2(a), and Figure 8.3(a). This ensures that the peak of the transmission spectrum of the sensor probe is in the visible region. TEM images of the three NMs are shown in Figure 8.1(b), 8.2(b), and 8.3(b), respectively, to observe the distribution and morphology of the three NMs in aqueous solution.

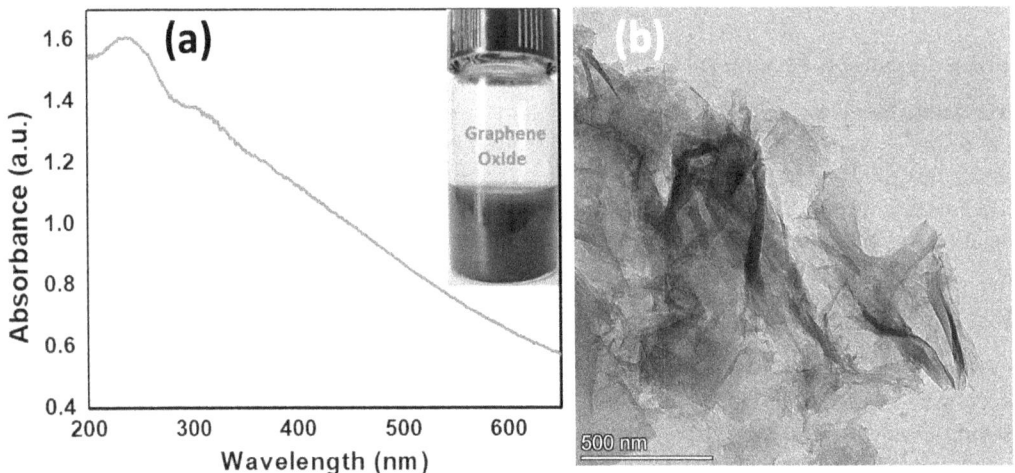

FIGURE 8.1   GO (a) absorbance spectrum, (b) TEM image.

Source: Reprinted with permission from *Optics Express.* Copyright, 2022, Optica (Li et al. 2021).

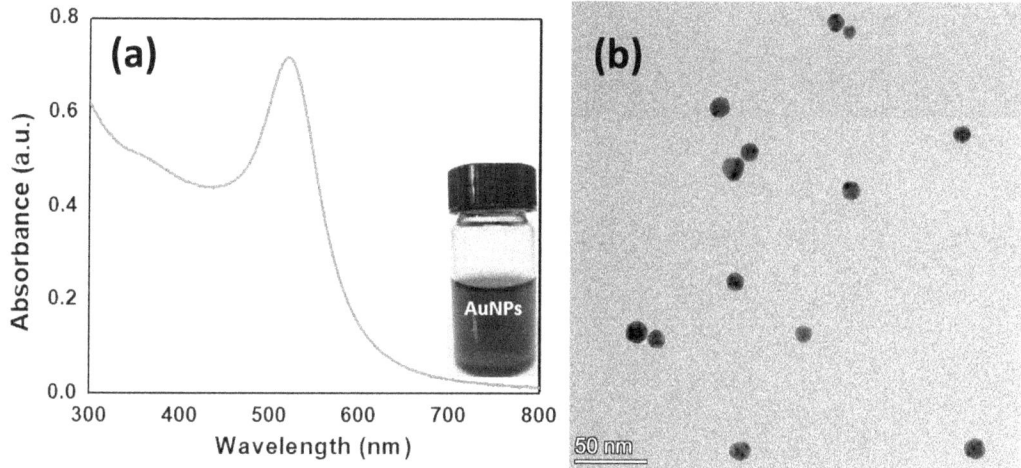

FIGURE 8.2 AuNPs (a) absorbance spectrum, (b) TEM image.

Source: Reprinted with permission from *Optics Express*. Copyright, 2022, Optica (Li et al. 2021).

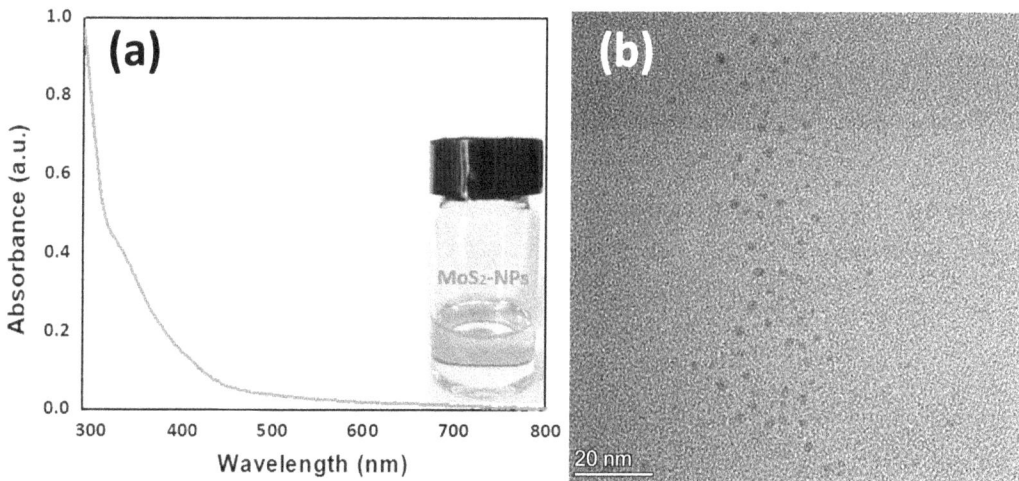

FIGURE 8.3 MoS_2-NPs (a) absorbance spectrum, (b) TEM image.

Source: Reprinted with permission from *Optics Express*. Copyright, 2022, Optica (Li et al. 2021).

HR-TEM was also utilized to describe Nb_2CTx MXene, and it was discovered that its geometric shape is a layered structure, as shown in Figure 8.4.

As illustrated in Figure 8.5(a), the absorbance wavelength peak of CeO_2-NPs solutions was measured at 253 nm using a UV-Vis spectrophotometer. HRTEM was employed to describe the morphology of CeO_2-NPs at the same time. Figure 8.5(b) shows a TEM picture of CeO_2-NPs.

Figure 8.6(a) shows the absorbance spectrum of AgNPs, and Figure 8.6(b) shows the absorbance spectrum of CuO-NPs. Figures 8.6(c) and 8.6(d) show TEM images of AgNPs and CuO-NPs, respectively.

As shown in Figure 8.7(a), the absorption spectra of AuNPs with diameters of 10 and 30 nm are shown, and the corresponding absorption peak wavelength positions are 519 and 527 nm,

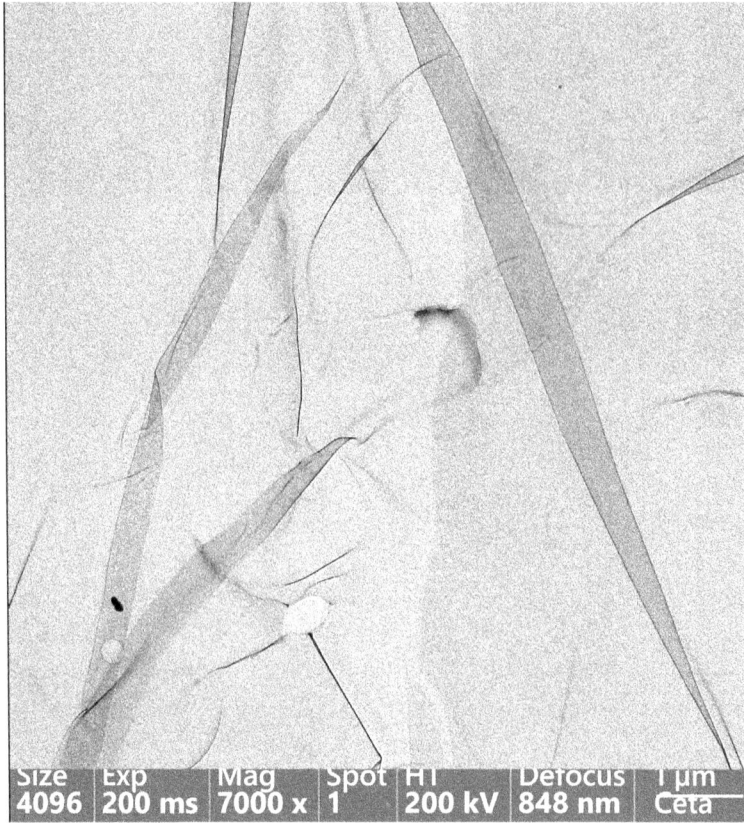

FIGURE 8.4 HRTEM image of MXene.

Source: Reprinted with permission from *Optics Express.* Copyright, 2022, Optica (Li et al. 2022).

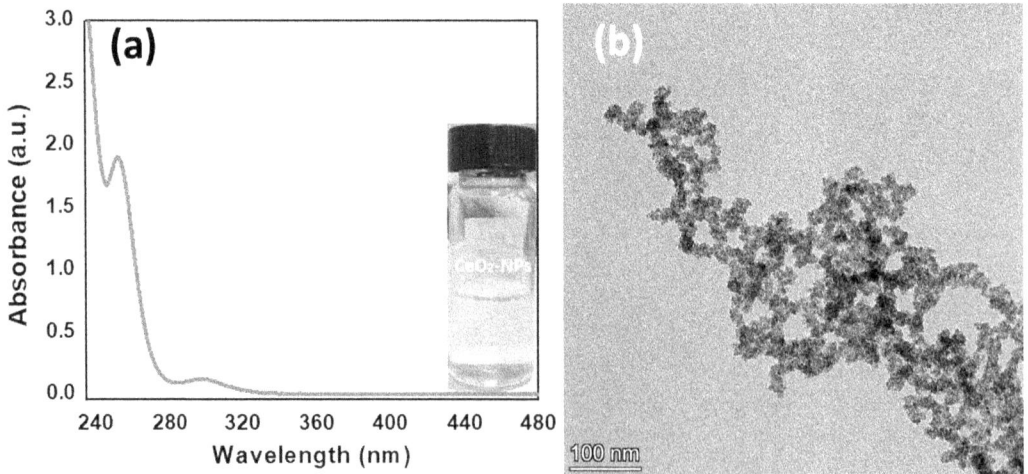

FIGURE 8.5 (a) Absorbance spectra of CeO_2-NPs and (b) HRTEM images of CeO_2-NPs.

Source: Reprinted with permission from *Optics Express.* Copyright, 2021, Optica (Wang, Singh et al. 2021).

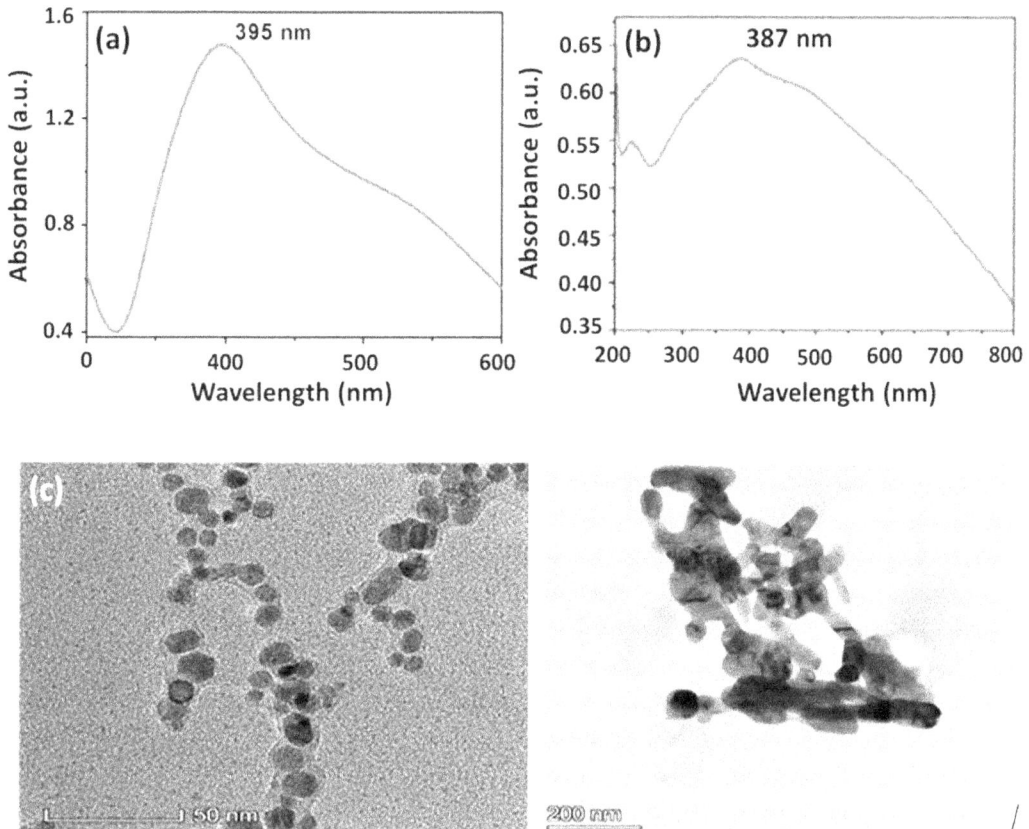

FIGURE 8.6 Absorbance spectra of (a) AgNPs and (b) CuO-NPs. HRTEM images of (c) AgNPs and (d) CuO-NPs.

Source: Reprinted with permission from *IEEE Transactions on Instrumentation & Measurement.* Copyright, 2020, IEEE (Agrawal, Saha et al. 2020).

respectively. The prepared AuNPs were also observed with its color properties, reddish and dark reddish, respectively. The optical signal passing through the sensor probe reacts with the ZnO-NPs/ AuNPs immobilized. The absorbance spectrum of ZnO-NPs was observed at 370 nm as shown in Figure 8.7(b). The size and shape of prepared NPs observed though HR-TEM for AuNPs (10 and 30 nm), and ZnO-NPs are shown in Figure 8.7(c), Figure 8.7(d), and Figure 8.7(e), respectively. Further, the morphology of ZnO-NPs was observed with atomic force microscopy (AFM), as shown in Figure 8.7(f). The distribution of AuNPs and its mean was further investigated using ImageJ software.

We measured the absorption peak wavelengths of PVA-AgNPs and ZnO-NPs using UV-Vis spectrophotometer to determine the size of NMs. The distribution of particles in the solution was observed by HRTEM. The synthesis of AgNPs was stabilized using PVA; therefore, the absorbance spectrum was measured for both PVA solution and PVA-AgNPs as shown in Figure 8.8(a). The absorbance spectrum of PVA solutions reflects a peak wavelength below 300 nm, and almost no absorbance appeared in visible wavelength range. The absorbance peak wavelength of PVA-AgNPs was observed at 424 nm. The obtained peak also shows the characteristic surface plasmon resonance absorbance of AgNPs. Thereafter, the EDS and TEM image was taken to ensure the

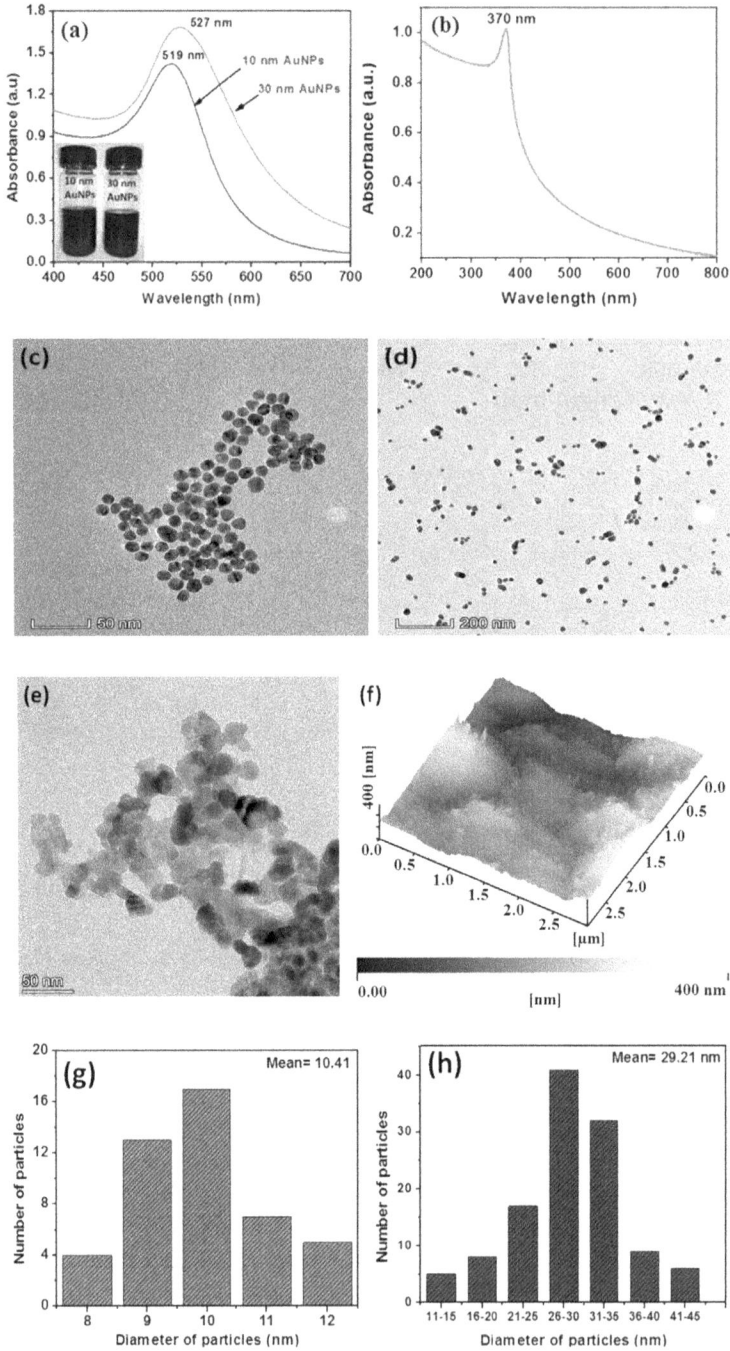

FIGURE 8.7 Analysis of NPs absorbance spectrum of (a) 10 and 30 nm AuNPs and (b) ZnO-NPs. HRTEM image of (c) 10 nm AuNPs, (d) 30 nm AuNPs, and (e) ZnO-NPs. AFM image of (f). ZnO-NPs, histogram of (g) 10 nm AuNPs and (h) 30 nm AuNPs.

Source: Reprinted with permission from *Journal of Lightwave Technology.* Copyright, 2020, IEEE (Agrawal, Zhang, Saha, Kumar, Pu et al. 2020).

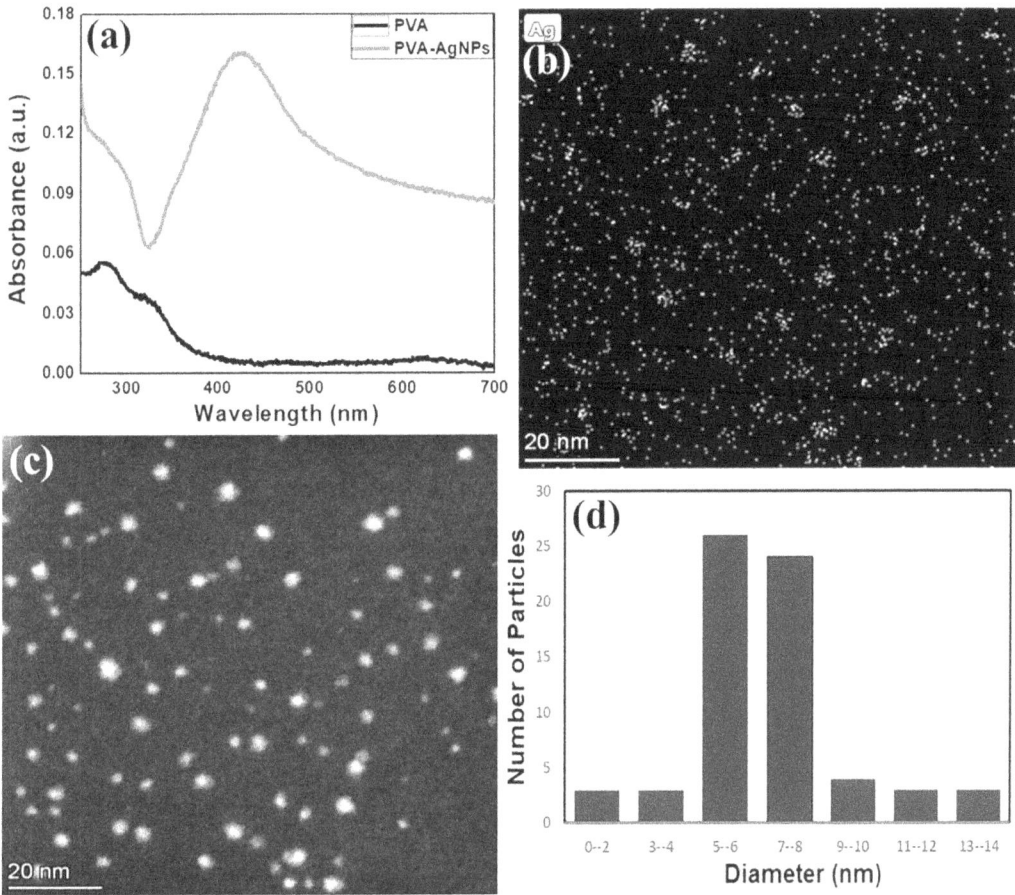

FIGURE 8.8 Characterization of PVA-AgNPs: (a) absorbance spectrum, (b) EDS image, (c) HRTEM image, and (d) histogram.

Source: Reprinted with permission from *IEEE Transactions on NanoBioscience.* Copyright, 2020, IEEE (Kaushik et al. 2020).

charge polarity and distribution of AgNPs as shown in Figure 8.8(b and c), respectively. In the EDS image, the bright green color dots depict the presence of AgNPs. Afterward, an average size of 5–6 nm of PVA-AgNPs was estimated through TEM image by plotting the histogram as shown in Figure 8.8(d).

The 20% wt. ZnO-NPs aqueous solution was dissolved in deionized water for absorbance determination, see Figure 8.9(a). The appearance of an absorbance peak at 370 nm indicates the formation of ZnO-NPs with diameter of 50 nm. Thereafter, to ensure the particle distribution, a TEM image was taken and presented in Figure 8.9(b). In a TEM image, a uniform distribution of particles can be observed. The high concentration of ZnO solution utilized for the experiment caused the particle clusters. As illustrated in Figure 8.9(c), the surface morphology of ZnO-NPs was studied by collecting an image using the AFM method. The AFM picture was used to investigate the rough surface morphology of ZnO-NPs, which may give a greater surface area for molecule adsorption and promote contact with increased bonding strength.

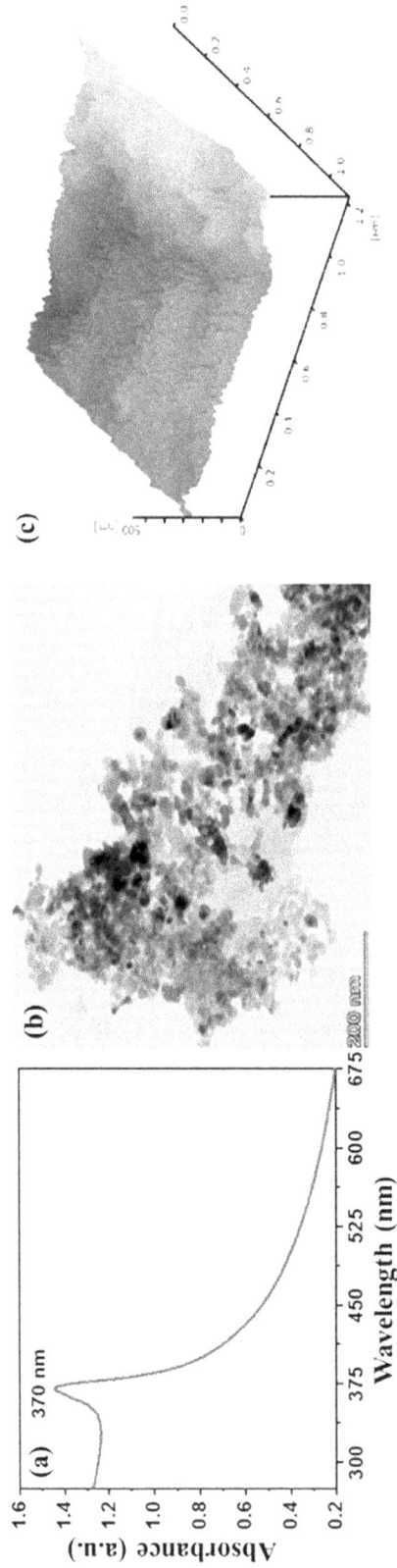

FIGURE 8.9 Characterization of ZnO-NPs: (a) absorbance spectrum, (b) HRTEM image, and (c) AFM image.

Source: Reprinted with permission from *IEEE Transactions on NanoBioscience.* Copyright, 2020, IEEE (Kaushik et al. 2020).

8.4 IMMOBILIZATION OF NANOPARTICLES OVER THE OPTICAL FIBER PROBE

8.4.1 FABRICATION OF AuNPs/ZnO-NPs-BASED OPTICAL FIBER PROBE

The schematic of AuNPs and ZnO-NPs immobilization process on the surface of the sensing probe is shown in Figure 8.10. Initially, a bare fiber structure, cleaned with acetone, is used to remove the unbound dust. In the next step, to activate the –OH group and to remove the unbounded particles on the surface, the bare probe was dipped in the piranha solution for 30 minutes (The volume ratio is 3:7). Then the probes were coated with 1% ethanolic (3-mercaptopropyl) trimethoxysilane (MPTMS) solution, which acts as a hydrophobic silane agent. Finally, AuNPs were immobilized on the surface of the salinized probe using the dip-coating method for 48 hours. AuNP immobilized probes were further coated with ZnO-NPs. For this, suspension of ZnO-NPs (4 wt.%) was prepared by titration method. The AuNP immobilized probe was immersed in ZnO-NPs suspension for 10 minutes and then dried in the oven for 20 minutes. The process was repeated three times to make the probe uniformly coated with ZnO-NPs.

8.4.2 FABRICATION OF CuO-NPs-BASED OPTICAL FIBER PROBE

The sensing region of probes was dipped in a freshly prepared aqueous solution of CuO-NPs (1 mg/mL) for 7 minutes and dried for 30 minutes. To prepare the CuO-NPs solution (1 mg/mL), the available CuO-NPs powder was dissolved in DI water through tip sonication. The sonication process was done for 4 minutes with ON time of 9 seconds and OFF time of 6 seconds at the power of 900 W. The CuO-NPs coating process was repeated three times to ensure uniform fixation of the NPs. The CuO-NP-coated fibers were kept at room temperature for 24 hours before carrying any test in order to stabilize the CuO-NPs film.

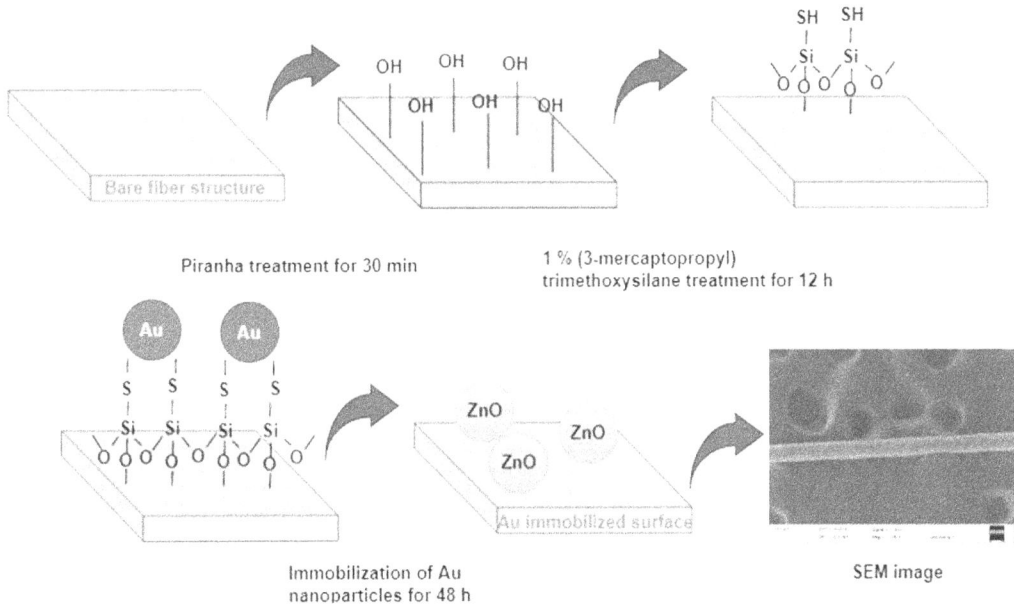

FIGURE 8.10 Immobilization process of ZnO/AuNPs and SEM image of attached nanocoating.

Source: Reprinted with permission from *Journal of Lightwave Technology.* Copyright, 2020, IEEE (Agrawal, Zhang, Saha, Kumar, Pu et al. 2020).

8.4.3 Fabrication of ZnO-NPs/PVA-AgNPs-Based Optical Fiber Probe

In another set of probes, PVA-AgNPs was used as a metallic layer between the fiber surface and a layer of ZnO-NPs. First, the sensing region of fiber probes was cleaned as previously discussed. After depositing a layer of SH group, sensing regions of probes were immersed in a synthesized aqueous solution of PVA-AgNPs. After 48 hours, the sensing region of probes was thoroughly rinsed by ethanol and dried using N_2 gas. Thereafter, ZnO-NPs were deposited over the PVA-AgNP-coated sensor probe.

8.4.4 Fabrication of MoS₂-NPs/AuNPs-Based Optical Fiber Probe

Following the production of the tapered or etched optical fiber structure, the Turkevich technique was used to synthesis AuNPs and MoS_2-NPs according to the methodology described in Section 8.2. The optical fiber structure was functionalized with AuNPs and MoS_2-NPs using the dip coating process. The AuNPs-immobilized fiber probes were then coated with MoS_2 by dipping them eight times in a 5-mL newly produced MoS_2-NPs solution.

8.5 DETECTION OF VARIOUS BIOMOLECULES

8.5.1 SMF-MCF-MMF-SMF Structure Based LSPR Biosensor for Creatinine Detection

The goal of research is to develop a simple, portable, and sensitive biosensor structure for detecting creatinine in the human body. To create strong evanescent waves (EWs), chemical etching was employed to reduce the diameter of the probe about 90 μm. GO, AuNPs, MoS_2-NPs, and the creatininase (CA) enzyme are used to functionalize the sensor probe. EWs were used to stimulate the LSPR effect of AuNPs, two-dimensional materials were used to enhance biocompatibility, and CA-enhanced probe specificity was used to develop biosensors for creatinine concentration detection. Experimental settings for detecting creatinine solution are shown in Figure 8.11. The light

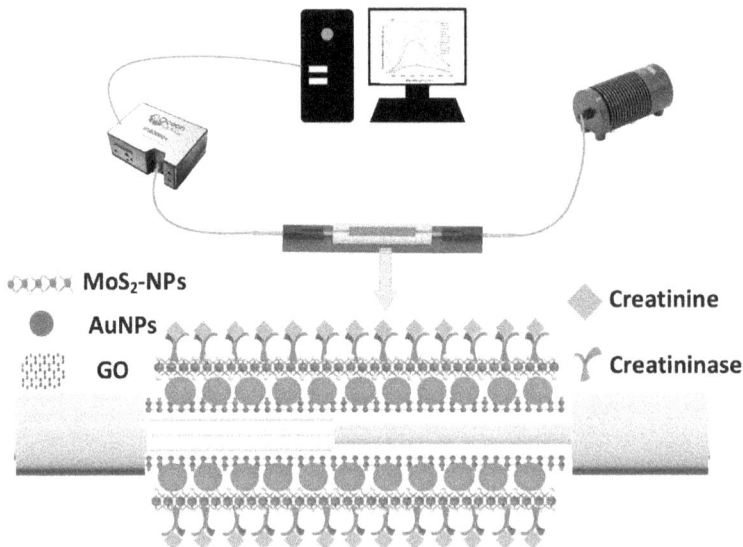

FIGURE 8.11 Experimental setup for the estimation of creatinine solution.

Source: Reprinted with permission from *Optics Express.* Copyright, 2021, Optica (Li et al. 2021).

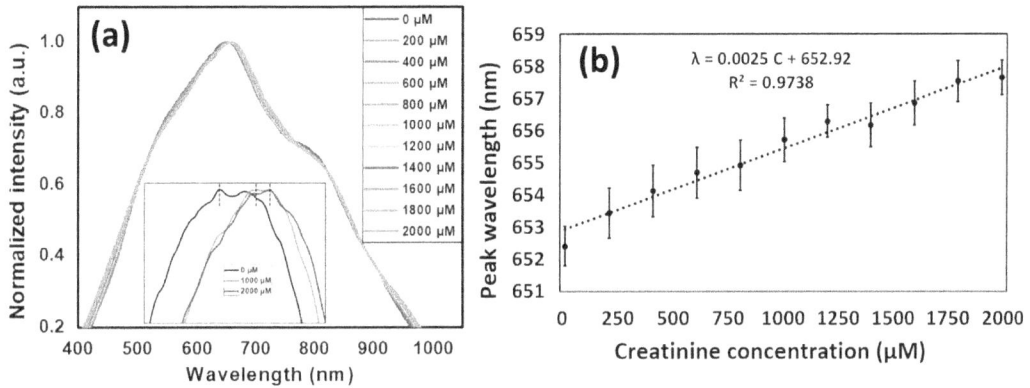

FIGURE 8.12 (a) LSPR sensing spectra, (b) linearity plot of proposed sensor.

Source: Reprinted with permission from *Optics Express.* Copyright, 2021, Optica (Li et al. 2021).

source and the spectrometer are connected to the sensor probe, and the spectrometer transmits the signal to a computer for detection.

The LSPR effect of AuNPs was stimulated using a tungsten-halogen light source. Creatinine was decomposed into creatine and sarcosine under the catalytic decomposition of CA enzyme on the probe surface, resulting in the change of RI around AuNPs. In this case, the red shift of absorption peak of LSPR spectrum is also different, and the concentration of creatinine sample can be further detected by the wavelength shift. Using the experimental setup shown in Figure 8.12, the LSPR spectrum was measured by reaction tests on creatinine samples at different concentrations. In order to reduce experimental error and eliminate contingency, the experiment employed three different sensing probes to measure responsiveness.

The LSPR spectra shown in Figure 8.12(a) were obtained by averaging three separate sensor probes. With the increase of creatinine concentration, the peak wavelength of the detection spectrum moved to higher wavelength. The probe sensitivity, linearity, and other associated performance criteria were also evaluated by examining the test data from the three sensor probes. The linear fitting results for the sensor probe are shown in Figure 8.12(b). This shows that the constructed sensor probe is linearly accurate.

8.5.2 MULTICORE TAPERED FIBER STRUCTURE-BASED SENSOR FOR CREATININE DETECTION IN AQUACULTURE

Here, researchers present an optical fiber sensor probe for the detection of creatinine in aquaculture, based on the LSPR approach. AuNPs, Nb_2CTx MXene, and a creatinase enzyme are used in the functionalization of the sensing probe. A heterogeneous core mismatch and tapering probe structure (convex fiber-tapered seven core fiber-convex fiber [CTC] structure) are used to modify the intrinsic total internal reflectance (TIR) mechanism in order to boost the EWs field intensity. The LSPR effect, which increases probe sensitivity, may be induced by strong evanescent fields that excite AuNPs. Nb_2CTx MXene adsorbs more active CA enzymes, which improves the specific recognition.

The investigations were carried out using a functioning sensor probe. Figure 8.13 depicts the study's equipment. A solution of creatinine sample was placed in a reaction dish with the sensor probe. The sensor probe received an optical signal from a light source. When the functional sensor probe outputs its spectrum, the spectrometer captures it and delivers it to the computer for additional data processing so that the LSPR spectra may be acquired.

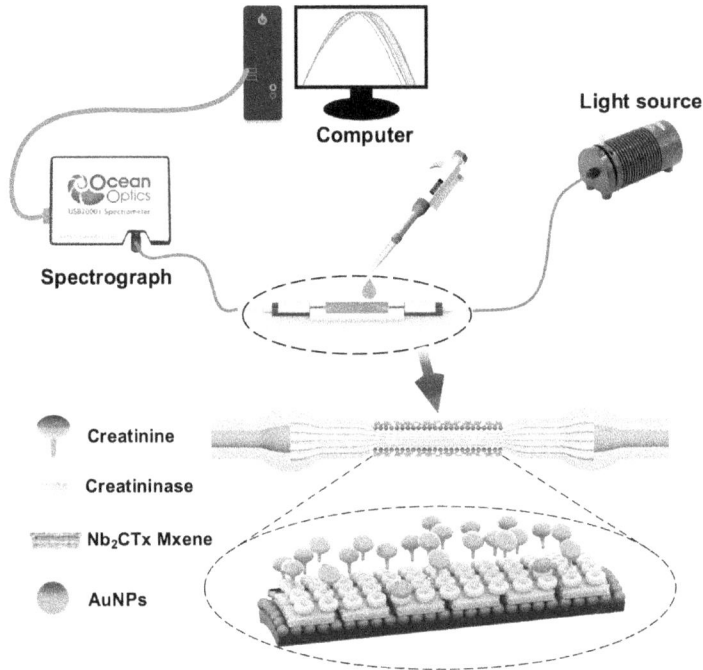

FIGURE 8.13 Proposed sensing probe is used as an experimental device for creatinine-level detection.

Source: Reprinted with permission from *Optics Express.* Copyright, 2022, Optica (Li et al. 2022).

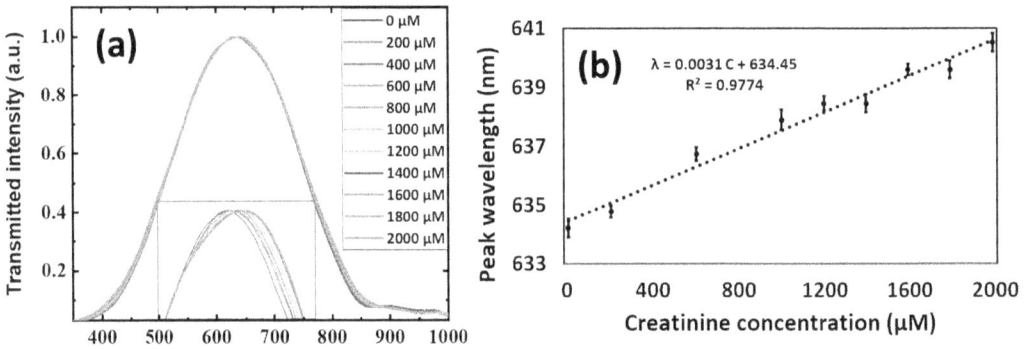

FIGURE 8.14 (a) LSPR sensing spectrum, (b) linearity plot of the developed sensor.

Source: Reprinted with permission from *Optics Express.* Copyright, 2022, Optica (Li et al. 2022).

Experimental settings are shown in Figure 8.13. With the increase of adding time of creatinine solution, the resonant wavelength red-shifted stably to obtain LSPR spectra of different concentrations of creatinine solution. Wavelength shift increases with creatinine concentration increasing. During the whole experiment, the researcher used three probes to reduce the measurement error brought by the test process and accurately evaluate the sensor performance. The results of the three groups of tests were averaged, as shown in Figure 8.14(a). LSPR sensor spectra are shown. After evaluation of test data, the relationship between sample solution concentration and resonance wavelength is shown in Figure 8.14(b). The linear regression fitting equation of the relationship between solution concentration and resonance wavelength is as follows:

$$\lambda = 0.0031c + 634.45$$

where c is the level of creatinine samples. Within the effective detection range, the linear fitting coefficient of the proposed probe is $R^2 = 0.9774$. The chemical reaction equation for creatinine combining with oxygen at an exponential rate catalyzed by the CA enzyme is as follows:

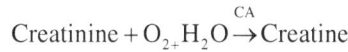

$$\text{Creatinine} + O_{2+}H_2O \xrightarrow{\text{CA}} \text{Creatine}$$

Creatinine degradation into creatine and other chemicals catalyzed by the CA enzyme alters the RI of the surrounding medium. Changes in RI will cause a considerable shift in the excitation resonance peak of the LSPR sensor. The peak wavelength of the LSPR spectrum is red-shifted when creatinine content rises, as seen in the inset of Figure 8.14(a). The experiment employed the wavelength sensing approach, and the sensitivity was determined to be 3.1 nm/mM using the formula:

$$S = \frac{\Delta s}{\Delta c}$$

where Δs is the wavelength offset, and Δc indicates the effective detection range from the highest to the lowest.

8.5.3 TAPER-IN-TAPER FIBER STRUCTURE-BASED LSPR SENSOR FOR ALANINE AMINOTRANSFERASE DETECTION

The enzyme alanine aminotransferase (ALT), which is found in every human blood cell, is intrinsically linked to liver damage. The current study aims to create a novel biosensor based on LSPR principle for ALT analyte detection. This is the first sensor probe designed in a conical fiber structure for biosensing applications. It was constructed by three-electrode semi-vacuum taper method and described by a combinator production system. To boost sensing performance, AuNPs, MoS_2-NPs, and CeO_2-NPs are immobilized on the sensing area. HRTEM and a UV-Vis spectrophotometer are used to evaluate these nanoparticles prior to application. AuNPs are used to excite LSPR phenomena, while MoS_2-NPs/CeO_2-NPs contribute to biocompatibility and stability of sensor probes. Glutamate oxidase (GluOx) is used to functionalize sensing probes to achieve specific selectivity. In subsequent experiments, there was a strong linear correlation between the probes and ALT levels.

A halogen light source produces a specified quantity of light, which travels through the core to the detecting probe. On the reaction platform, the probe was then submerged in the sample solution. The analyte produced will bind particularly to the surface-immobilized enzyme, creating a change in the RI near the metal immobilization layer. A spectrometer is used to record the transmitted signals, and the data collected are displayed on a computer. The sensor experimental setup is shown in Figure 8.15.

In order to reliably detect abnormal ALT levels in human serum. ALT enzymes in the range of 10 ~ 1000 U/L were selected. ALT analytes can be calculated after the experimental equipment is integrated according to Figure 8.15. First, 5 mL PBS solution was poured into the ALT substrate tube to dissolve sample 1. The optical signal of sample 1 was collected 20 minutes after entering the reaction cell. In the other substrate tube, 10 U/L ALT enzyme solution was added and reacted for 3 minutes to obtain sample 2. LSPR spectrum was recorded by computer after sample 2 was introduced into the measurement unit. Finally, other samples were tested to generate LSPR spectra corresponding to the remaining ALT concentrations.

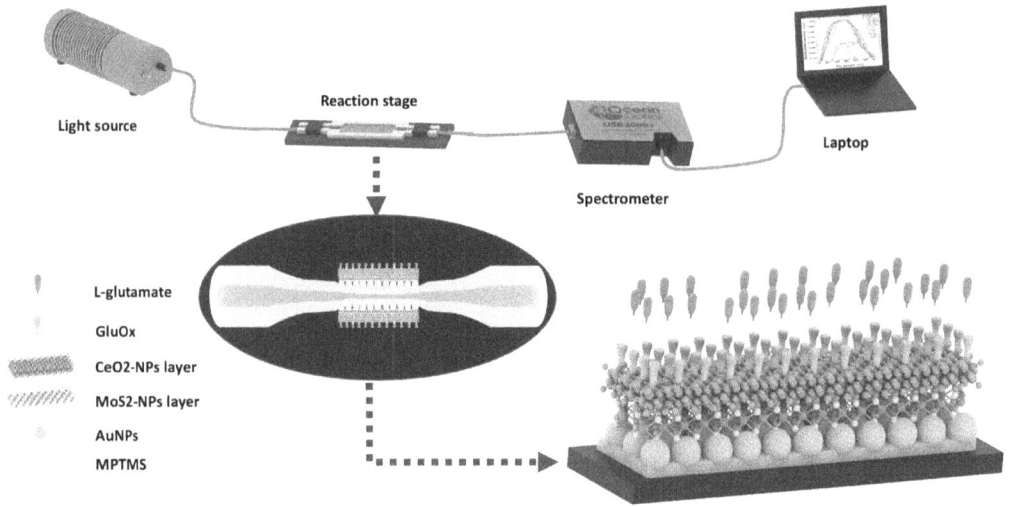

FIGURE 8.15 Experimental setup for ALT detection.

Source: Reprinted with permission from *Optics Express.* Copyright, 2022, Optica (Wang, Singh et al. 2021).

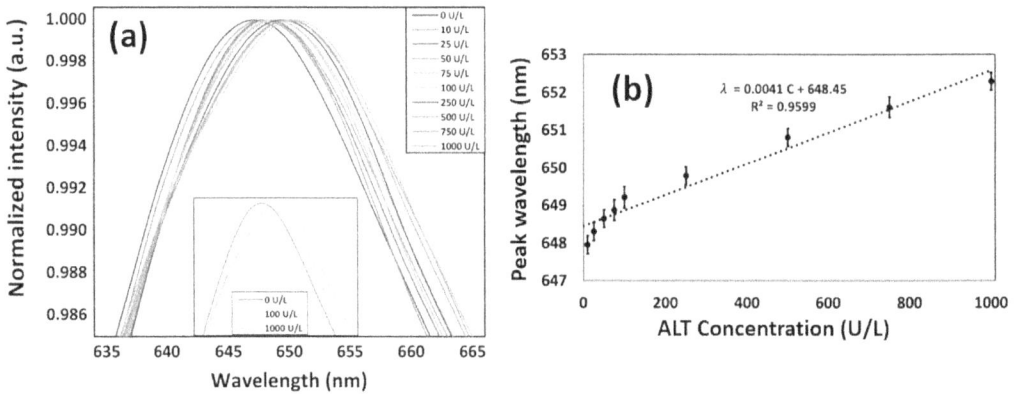

FIGURE 8.16 (a) LSPR measured spectrum, (b) linearity plot of sensor.

Source: Reprinted with permission from *Optics Express.* Copyright, 2022, Optica (Wang, Singh et al. 2021).

Figure 8.16(a) shows the mean values of normalized wavelength spectra of three groups from different fiber-optic probes at different ALT concentrations. Figure 8.16(b) shows the sensor's linearity response. The curve displays a linearity of 0.9562, suggesting that the shift of the resonant peak grows linearly as the ALT enzyme concentration increases from 10 to 1000 U/L. Furthermore, the sensitivity and limit of detection (LoD) of the ALT sensor are the most important factors in determining its performance. Data analysis determined that the sensor's sensitivity is 4.1 pm/(U/L). The LoD values were calculated using the SD of the probe's stability test. As a consequence, the probe's LOD for short is set at 10.61 U/L. The suggested sensor is successful in diagnosing human liver damage, according to the data analysis.

8.5.4 Taper Fiber-Based Sensor for Water Pollutants p-Cresol Detection

In this section, a simple biosensor based on AuNPs/Zno-NPs functionalized tapered optical fiber (TOF) has been developed to accurately assess the concentration of p-cresol in urine samples

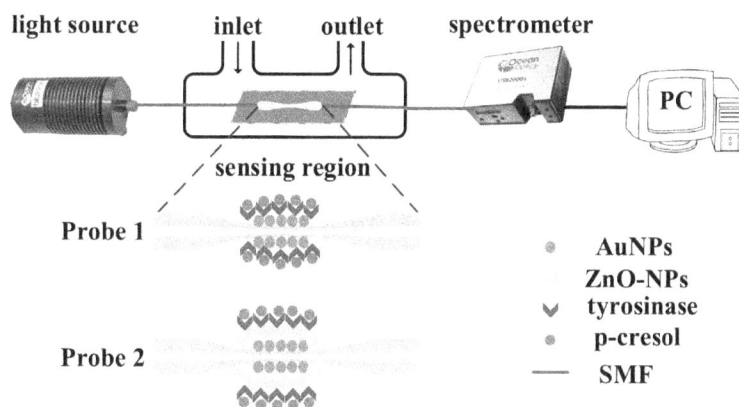

FIGURE 8.17 Experimental setup for detection of p-cresol solutions.

Source: Reprinted with permission from *IEEE Transactions on NanoBioscience*. Copyright, 2021, IEEE (Wang, Zhu et al. 2021).

(Wang, Zhu et al. 2021). The sensor is designed to detect p-cresol in urine solution at concentrations ranging from 0 to 1 mM, covering the entire range of p-cresol concentrations found in humans. The p-cresol solutions changed the RI surrounding the sensor in this study, and the change in the transmitted spectrum was recorded. The sensing region of probe 1 was fixed with AuNPs, and the sensing region of probe 2 was fixed with AuNPs/ZnO-NPs. After that, tyrosinase functionalization was performed on the sensitive area covered by NPs to ensure that the sensor had high specificity for p-cresol detection.

The surface plasmon is stimulated by a light source with a visible peak wavelength. A spectrometer was used to record the transmitted intensity of an optical signal at the end of TOF probes. OceanView software was used to gather the results. Using a fusion splicer, the sensing probe was linked into the spectrometer and the light source to establish a full optical route. The instrumentation for detecting p-cresol solution is shown in Figure 8.17.

The sensor probe functionalized by the enzyme measures the change of p-cresol concentration from 0 to 1 mM by recording the transmission intensity spectrum. Use PBS solution activation sensor probe at room temperature 15 minutes before. In order to reduce the data contingency, the emission intensity spectrum of the sensor probe is measured sequentially. Similarly, Figures 8.18(a) and 8.18(c) show the mean values of normalized transmission intensity spectra of probe 1 and probe 2. Obviously, due to the catalytic action of tyrosinase on p-cresol oxidation, the peak wavelength moves to a higher wavelength. The presence of by-products in the oxidation process changes the RI of the sensitive region and causes the wavelength red shift. The linear curve-fitting diagram of sensor probe 1 and error bar are shown in Figure 8.18(b). In this case, the linear fitting equation of peak wavelength fluctuation with p-cresol solution is

$$\lambda = 0.0072\ C + 645.33$$

where λ is the wavelength position of the absorption peak, and C is the level of a p-cresol sample solution. Similarly, the linear fitting equation for probe 2 is

$$\lambda = 0.0056\ C + 659.49$$

As shown in Figure 8.18(d), the sensitivity of probe 2 was 5.6 nm/mM, and the correlation coefficient was 0.9808. Compared with probe 1, probe 2 has better performance parameters.

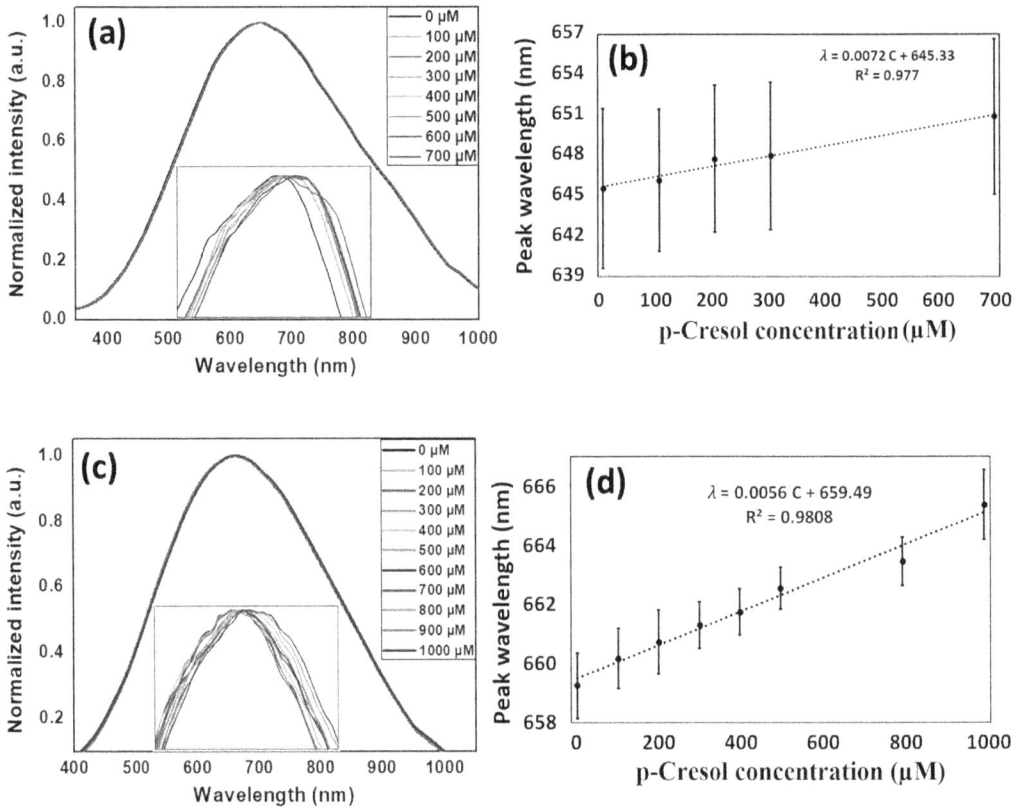

FIGURE 8.18 Normalized sensing spectrum and linear fitting curve of (a, b) probe 1, (c, d) probe 2, respectively.

Source: Reprinted with permission from *IEEE Transactions on NanoBioscience*. Copyright, 2021, IEEE (Wang, Zhu et al. 2021).

8.5.5 MPM FIBER STRUCTURE SENSOR PROBE FOR cTnI

In this study, LSPR technology was used to fabricate a fiber-optic sensor for cTnI detection (Wang et al. 2022). A multimode-photosensitive-multimode (MPM) fiber structure was adopted. Then, NMs are fixed on the etched MPM surface. The selectivity is improved by functionalizing the probe surface with antibodies. The sensing probe is coupled to the optical signal generated by the light source. It is attached to a spectrometer that runs in the visible light wavelength region, and the data were collected using OceanView software which can then be studied on computer. A full measurement apparatus is shown in Figure 8.19.

The sensor was put to the test by recording the sensor spectrum of various cTnI solution levels. cTnI sample solution concentrations of 0 ng/mL–1000 ng/mL may all be measured using the sensor probe. First, 1 mL solution containing 25 ng/mL was examined, after which the solution was withdrawn, and the biosensor probe of cTnI was dried. The procedures for measuring different concentrations of solution are the same as those described previously. As shown in Figure 8.20(a), check the other two sensor probes in the same way and use the average of the three tests to reduce experimental errors. The peak wavelength increases linearly with the increase of solution concentration, as shown in Figure 8.20(b). The linear fitting equation is as follows:

$$\lambda = 0.0034 \, C + 631.12$$

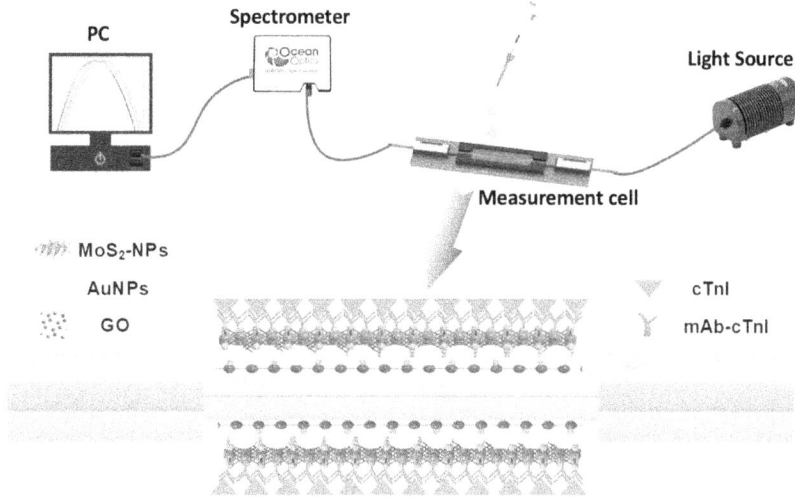

FIGURE 8.19 Experimental setup to measure the spectrum of cTnI solution.

Source: Reprinted with permission from *IEEE Transactions on Instrumentation & Measurement.* Copyright, 2022, IEEE (Wang et al. 2022).

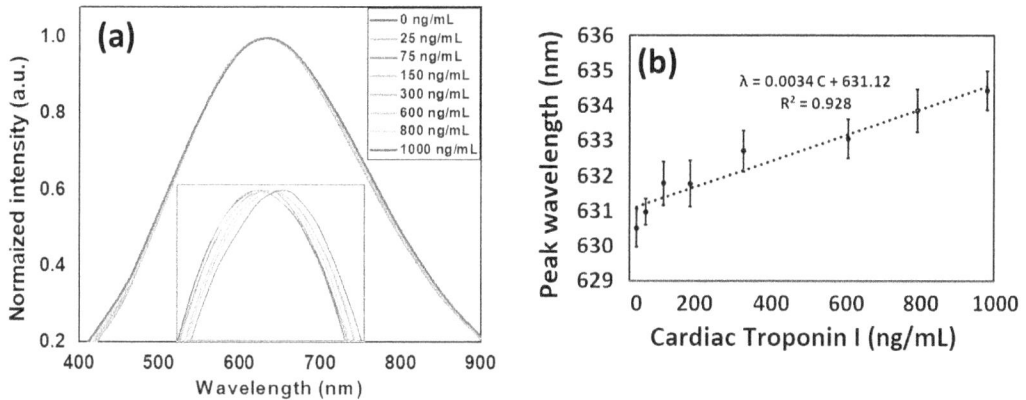

FIGURE 8.20 (a) Sensing result of cTnI and (b) linearity plot of proposed MSM-based sensor probe.

Source: Reprinted with permission from *IEEE Transactions on Instrumentation & Measurement.* Copyright, 2022, IEEE (Wang et al. 2022).

The probe's sensitivity is 3.4 pm/(ng/mL), and the fitting coefficient is 0.928. Similarly, the change of RI of surrounding medium caused by oxidation reaction of cTnI solution with different concentration and mAb-cTnI is reflected in the peak wavelength red shift.

8.5.6 Hetero-Core Fiber Structure-Based Cardiac Troponin I Detection

The development of a hetero-core optical fiber sensing structure based on LSPR for the detection of cTnI solution is described in this chapter. A single-mode fiber–multimode fiber–single-mode fiber (SMS) structure was used to achieve this structure. To increase the sensor's detecting capabilities, AuNPs and CeO$_2$-NPs were used to immobilize it.

A set of effective optical measuring equipment for detecting cTnI is shown in Figure 8.21. The optical signals were generated using a tungsten-halogen light source, and the final transmitted spectrum was received using a spectrograph with a spectral range of 200–1000 nm. The FSM was used to link the probe to the detecting optical route. After the current sensing spectrum had stabilized, the concentration of the produced cTnI solution was injected into the measuring cell in order from low to high, and the current sensing spectrum was recorded. The measuring cell was repeatedly washed with 1 × PBS before assessing the new sample.

Quantitative analysis of the proposed sensor was carried out by measuring the different concentrations of cTnI solutions (0–1000 ng/mL). Figure 8.22(a) shows the transmitted intensity spectrum of biosensors for different concentrations of cTnI. Figure 8.22(b) shows the peak resonance wavelength variation with the concentration of cTnI. It is apparent from the plot that wavelength shift exhibits a linear relationship with cTnI concentration within the range of 0–1000 ng/mL. The linearity expression is $\lambda = 0.003\ C + 652.49$ (unit of C is ng/mL), and accuracy is 0.9898. Thus, its sensitivity is 3 pm/(ng/mL), and LoD can be obtained through formulae. The SD is the value calculated by measuring 10 times blank sample (PBS) with the same sensing probe, and its obtained value is 0.108. The LoD of the proposed sensor is 108.15 ng/mL with the linear range. LoD is

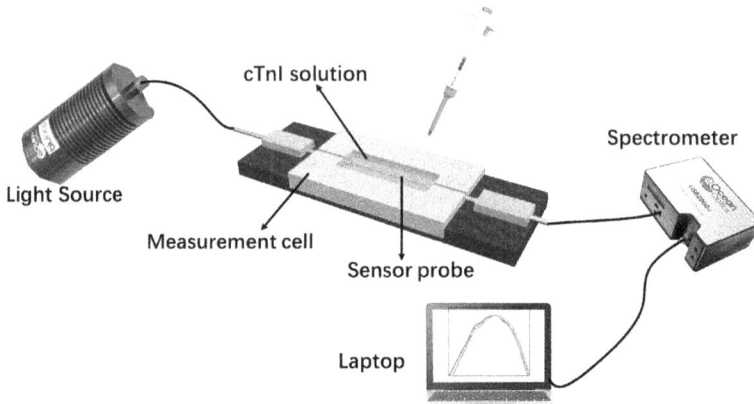

FIGURE 8.21   Experimental setup for detection of cTnI solution.

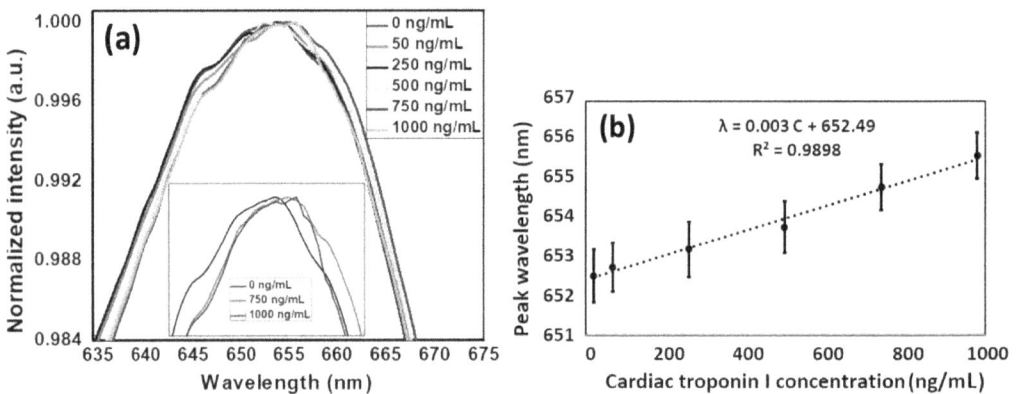

FIGURE 8.22   (a) Sensing spectrum during measurement of different concentrations of cTnI solutions, (b) linearity plot of proposed sensor.

defined as the minimum detectable signal (spectral change) due to the interaction. By definition, this indicator is determined by two factors: the change in spectral size due to the interaction of the analyte and the spectrum of the resolution device used for detection. The sensor will be used in a practice to detect AMI.

8.5.7 MULTICORE FIBER BIOSENSOR FOR ACETYLCHOLINE DETECTION

To fabricate the sensor structure in the study, tapered/etched MCF probes are spliced with MMF (Zhu et al. 2022). Both probes are immobilized using AuNPs and MoS_2-NPs to boost sensitivity. The peak absorption wavelengths of synthesized AuNPs and MoS_2-NPs are 519 nm and 330 nm, respectively. Subsequently, the sensor probe functionalized by acetylcholinesterase has specific selectivity. Finally, the performance of the sensor probe was tested by detecting different levels of acetylcholine. A spectrometer was used to record the LSPR spectrum of the sensor probe, as shown in Figure 8.23.

   Both probe 1 and probe 2 are based on the taper MCF fiber structure, which was created using the CMS machine. The etched MMF-MCF-MMF structure is shown in Figure 8.23. Probes 1 and 2, MMF, and MCF were linked by an FSM during the manufacturing of the probe's bare structure. The fiber was then severed with a precision cleaver, leaving a 2-cm piece of MCF on the MMF. On the opposite end of the MCF, another MMF was spliced. As illustrated in Figure 8.23, a tapered fiber was created on the middle section of the MCF using the CMS instrument. The ends of MMF and MCF are spliced together to become probe 3, as previously indicated. At a separate time, the MCF was etched with HF solution, and the reduced fiber diameter to 75 μm was observed at etching time 25 minutes. The outer MCF cores were destroyed by further etching of the fiber; therefore, the probe 3 structure was constructed with a 25-minute etching period.

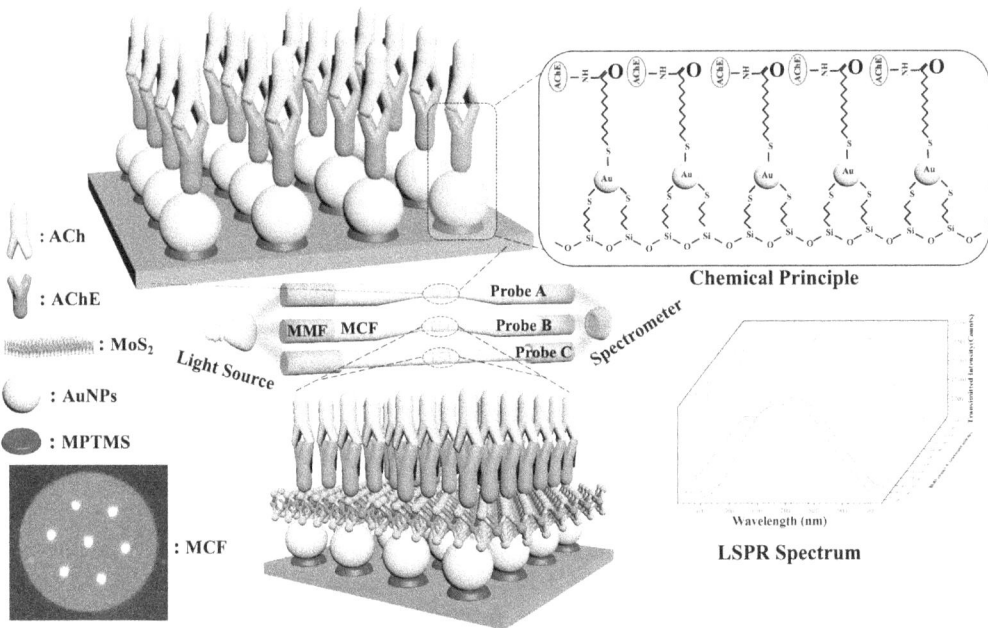

FIGURE 8.23   Multicore optical fiber based LSPR sensor.

Source: Reprinted with permission from *IEEE Transactions on Instrumentation & Measurement.* Copyright, 2022, IEEE (Zhu et al. 2022).

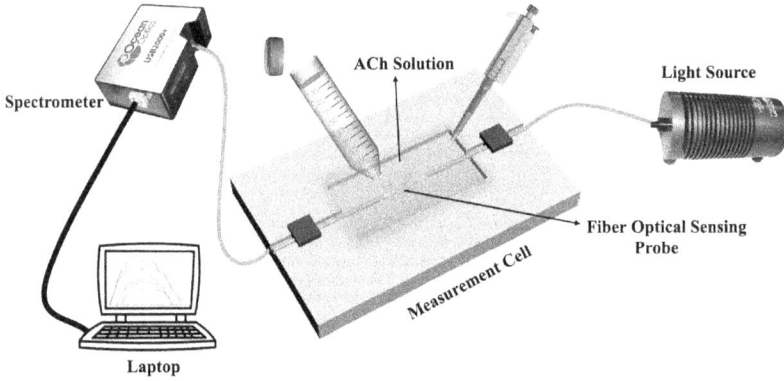

FIGURE 8.24   Setup for measuring the response of an LSPR sensor.

Source: Reprinted with permission from *IEEE Transactions on Instrumentation & Measurement.* Copyright, 2022, IEEE (Zhu et al. 2022).

The sensor probes' experimental setup is shown in Figure 8.24. The optical signal was launched, and the variation during the chemical reaction surrounding the sensing zone was analyzed using a light source. LSPR spectral data were recorded using a spectrometer. Various ACh concentrations were utilized to evaluate the sensor probe. The LSPR sensor probe was investigated using acetylcholine solutions of various concentrations ranging from 0 to 1 mM. The experimental error was calculated using three different sensors of the same kind. The target acetylcholine (Ach) interacts with the functionalized acetylcholinase (AChE) on the sensor probe to change the RI around the sensor probe, resulting in the wavelength red-shift of LSPR spectrum. LSPR spectrum of sensing probes 1, 2, and 3 (and its linear graph) are given in Figure 8.25 (a, c, e) and (b, d, f). The sensitivity of the developed acetylcholine sensor probe is 0.062 nm/μM in the detection range of 0–1 mM

8.5.8   TAPERED OPTICAL FIBER BASED LSPR BIOSENSOR FOR ASCORBIC ACID DETECTION

Ascorbic acid (AA) is an important biomarker that can be used for surveillance and identification of scurvy, and cardiovascular disease (Zhu et al. 2020). A sensor model based on the principle of LSPR was established to detect the presence of AA samples (Zhu et al. 2021). The prepared AuNPs and ZnO were fixed in the conical region. Two different biosensor probes are created based on NP designs. AuNPs are fixed and called probe 1. The AuNP fixed layer is covered by ZnO-NPs layer, called probe 2. The sensor probe is functionalized by ascorbate oxidase, which oxidizes AA to decompose it in the presence of oxygen to improve selectivity.

The responsiveness of the designed sensor probe was tested using a broad range of AA concentrations. For the propagation of an optical signal, the experimental device includes a halogen light source. The spectrometer then records the emitted signal. The sensor probe is fused between the source and the detector through the splicer, as shown in Figure 8.26. An extended view of the two sensor probes created is also shown in the illustration in Figure 8.26.

The designed sensor probes were utilized to detect AA solutions with concentrations ranging from 0.5 to 1 mM. This range encompasses both the highest and lowest levels of AA seen in humans. All of the concentrations were tested in progressive order. The probe was cleaned with a PBS solution before feeling a concentration solution of AA. Following the drying of the sensor probe, the transmission intensity and wavelength were measured. The probe was then washed with a base solution and dried before being used to measure the other AA concentration solution. Similarly, all of the samples were sensed with both of the created sensor probes, with the findings

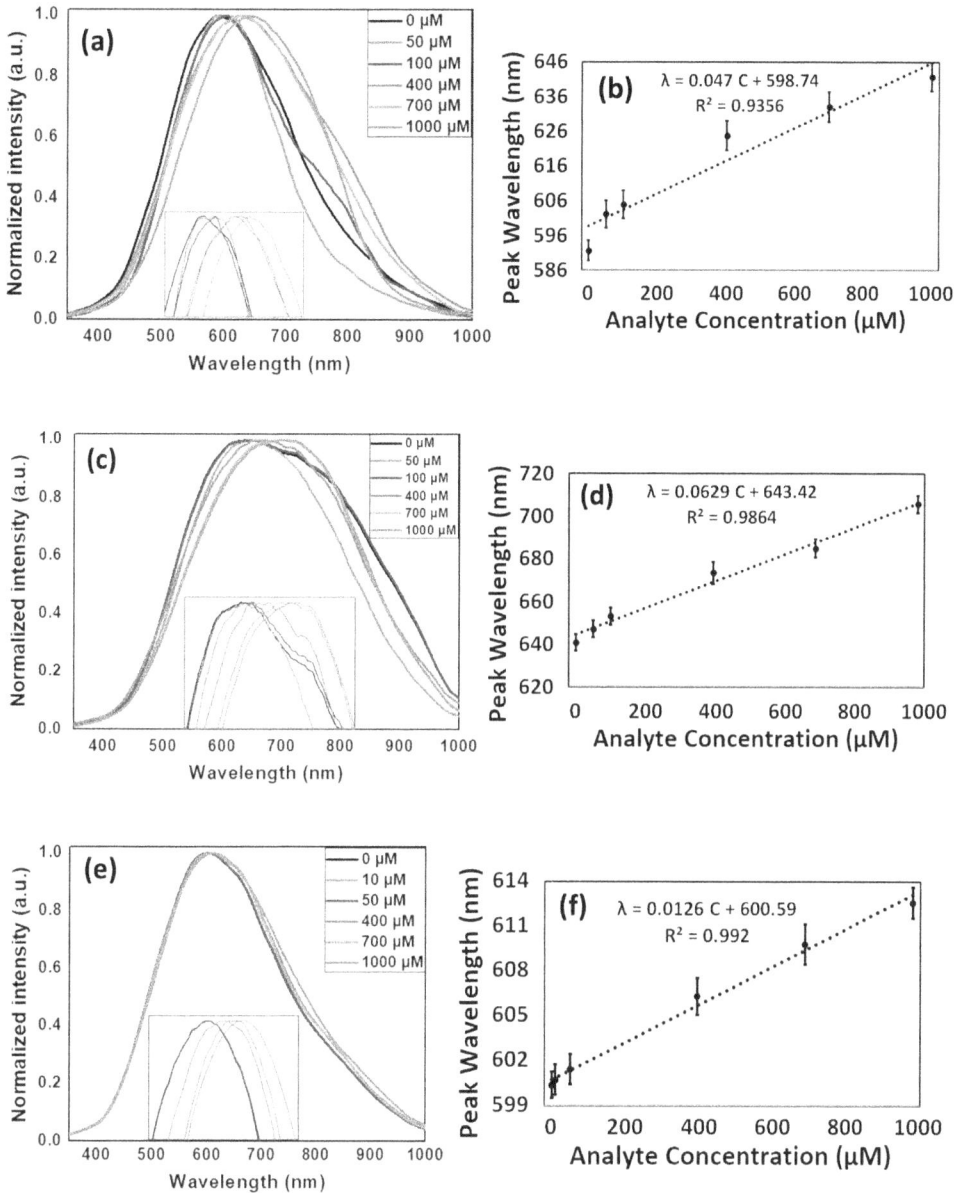

FIGURE 8.25 LSPR spectrum with different acetylcholine level and its linearity plot for (a,b) probe 1 (MMF-tapered MCF-MMF/AuNPs/AChE), (c,d) probe 2 (MMF-tapered MCF-MMF/AuNPs/MoS$_2$-NPs/AChE), (e,f) probe 3 (MMF-etched MCF-MMF/AuNPs/MoS$_2$-NPs/AChE).

Source: Reprinted with permission from *IEEE Transactions on Instrumentation & Measurement.* Copyright, 2022, IEEE (Zhu et al. 2022).

being displayed as transmission intensity spectra. By injecting a 0.5 μM AA solution near the sensor probe, LSPR spectrum was acquired. The LSPR spectral mean of each solution was calculated after three tests. The LSPR spectrum of probe 1 is shown in Figure 8.27(a). When can be observed from the data, when the concentration analytical rises, the transmitted intensity decreases. The peak resonance wavelength, on the other hand, displays the reverse reaction, rising as the concentration of

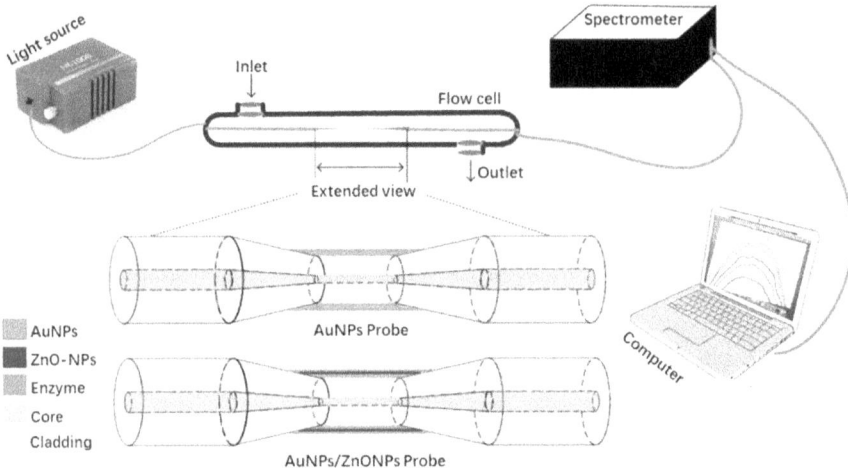

FIGURE 8.26 Experimental setup for the sensing of ascorbic acid through tapered fiber sensor probe (Zhu et al. 2021).

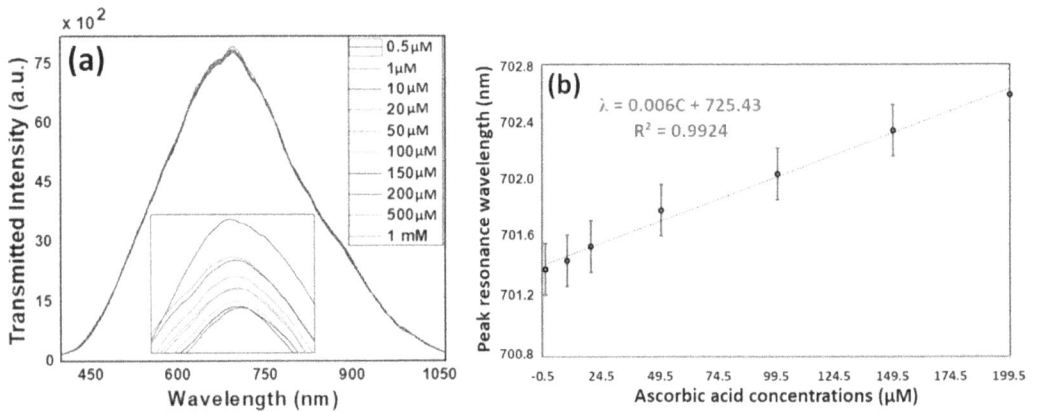

FIGURE 8.27 LSPR of probe 1: (a) transmitted intensity spectra, (b) linearity response of sensor (Zhu et al. 2021).

analytical increases. The experiment was done three times with three separate sensor probes to plot the curves. After that, the total spectra were displayed by normalizing each experiment's graphs. The strange behavior might be the result of various readings from separate studies. However, the linear range curve is used to determine the experiment's overall outcomes, such as the linear range and sensitivity. The linear range graph clearly shows that the wavelength rises as the concentration of AA solution increases. This antibehavior is caused by a decrease in the imaginary component of RI in the perception layer. Within the concentration range of 1–200 µM, the response of probe 1 was linear, as shown in Figure 8.27(b), and the autocorrelation fitting rate was 99.24%. As shown in Figure 8.28(a). the performance of probe 2 was assessed by detecting all concentrations and creating average LSPR spectrograms. This is due to the development of chemical by-products, which might alter the sensor layer's effective RI. Higher concentration observations are skipped in the findings supplied due to the nonlinearity of the data.

The formant wavelength is basically proportional to AA concentration, as shown in Figure 8.28(b). This red-shift response is caused by the rise of the actual profile RI of the sensing layer. The response of probe 2 was also linear in the range of 10–200 µM.

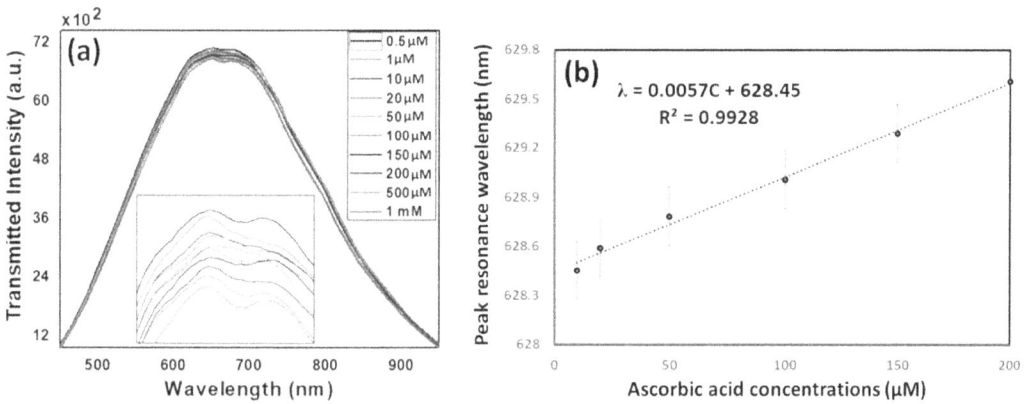

FIGURE 8.28 LSPR of probe 2: (a) transmitted intensity spectra, (b) linearity response of sensor (Zhu et al. 2021).

When fitted with an autocorrelation curve, sensor probes have a linearity response of 99.28%. The LoD is an important characteristic to consider when assessing a sensor's performance. The SD of the blank measurement result may be evaluated by multiplying it three times (3 blank) using the calibration curve. From the slope of the linear curve, it can be seen that the sensitivity of probe 1 to the concentration of 1–200 μM is 6 nm/mM. When the concentration range is 10–200 μM, the LoD of probe 2 is 25.78 μM, which is similar to that of probe 1. The sensitivity response of probe 2 is about 5.7 nm/mM according to the fitting of the autocorrelation curve. The response of the sensor probe was tested by detecting AA samples in the range of 500 nM to 1 mM, which covers the range of AA found in humans.

8.5.9 CORE MISMATCH MPM/SPS PROBE-BASED SENSOR FOR CHOLESTEROL DETECTION

A new biosensor for the detection of human cholesterol based on LSPR effect was proposed and designed (Agrawal et al. 2020). The sensor performs well in a wide range of cholesterol concentrations (0.1–10 mM), covering cholesterol values in human blood (Agrawal, Zhang, Saha, Kumar, Pu et al. 2020). By designing and making the core mismatch structure, multimode photosensitive multimode (MPM) and single-mode photosensitive single-mode optical fiber (SPS) structures were fabricated for the study of cholesterol biosensor probe. The proposed sensor was modified with AuNPs (10 nm and 30 nm) with different diameters and ZnO-NPs to improve the sensitivity.

Cholesterol is normally found in human serum at a quantity of 5.17 mM. As a result, a broad variety of test samples range from 0.1 to 10 mM were generated. In a 5% Triton X–100 aqueous solution, 96.7 mg cholesterol was dissolved to make a 25 mL stock solution. Cholesterol was heated at 70°C to thoroughly dissolve it to its waxy nature. Figure 8.29 shows the optical test setup for effective cholesterol detection, and Figure 8.30(a), Figure 8.30(b), and Figure 8.30(c) illustrate the alternative structural designs for probes 1, 2, and 3, respectively.

In this part, the performance of the optical fiber sensor based on LSPR phenomenon is studied in depth. During the measurement process, experimental results in the spectral form of LSPR were detected, as shown in Figure 8.31. The spectral wavelength shift was caused, as predicted, by changes in cholesterol concentration. The enzymatic process is responsible for the change in resonance wavelength (ChOx-Cholesterol). Before adding the prepared cholesterol sample, clean the sensor probe with PBS solution. LSPR spectrum (ChOx-Cholesterol) was obtained after the output signal was stabilized to assist the enzymatic reaction. The mean values of three independent observations are considered when plotting the linear calibration curve (Figure 8.32).

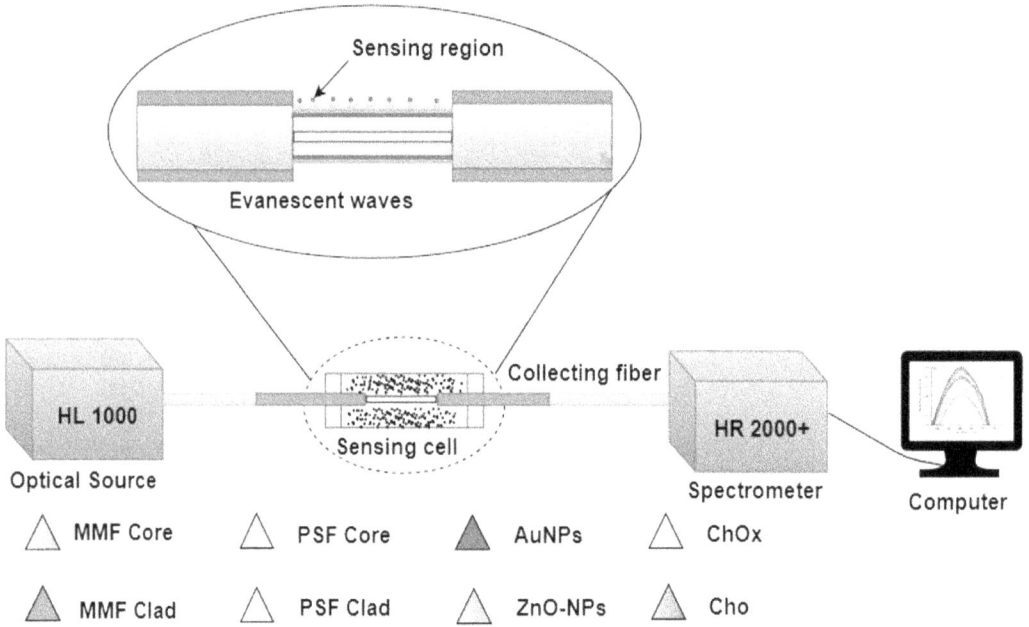

FIGURE 8.29 Experimental setup for the detection of cholesterol.

Source: Reprinted with permission from *Journal of Lightwave Technology.* Copyright, 2020, IEEE (Agrawal, Zhang, Saha, Kumar, Pu et al. 2020).

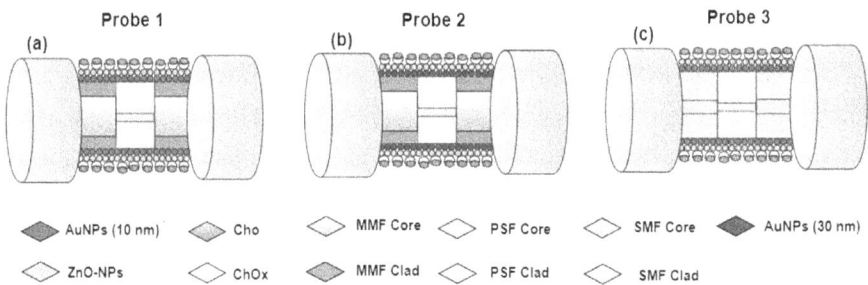

FIGURE 8.30 Configurations of probes: (a) probe 1, (b) probe 2, (c) probe 3.

Source: Reprinted with permission from *Journal of Lightwave Technology.* Copyright, 2020, IEEE (Agrawal, Zhang, Saha, Kumar, Pu et al. 2020).

Probe 1: Figures 8.30(a), 8.31(a), and 8.32(a) illustrate the schematic design, LSPR spectra, and linear calibration curve for probe 1, respectively. In this situation, the highest wavelength shift measured is 7.18 nm. For probe 1, the linear curve equation is

$$\lambda = 0.6898\ C + 691.71$$

where C is the cholesterol concentration. The sensitivity is 0.69 nm/mM, a correlation coefficient is 0.97, and the LoD is 0.61 mM, respectively.

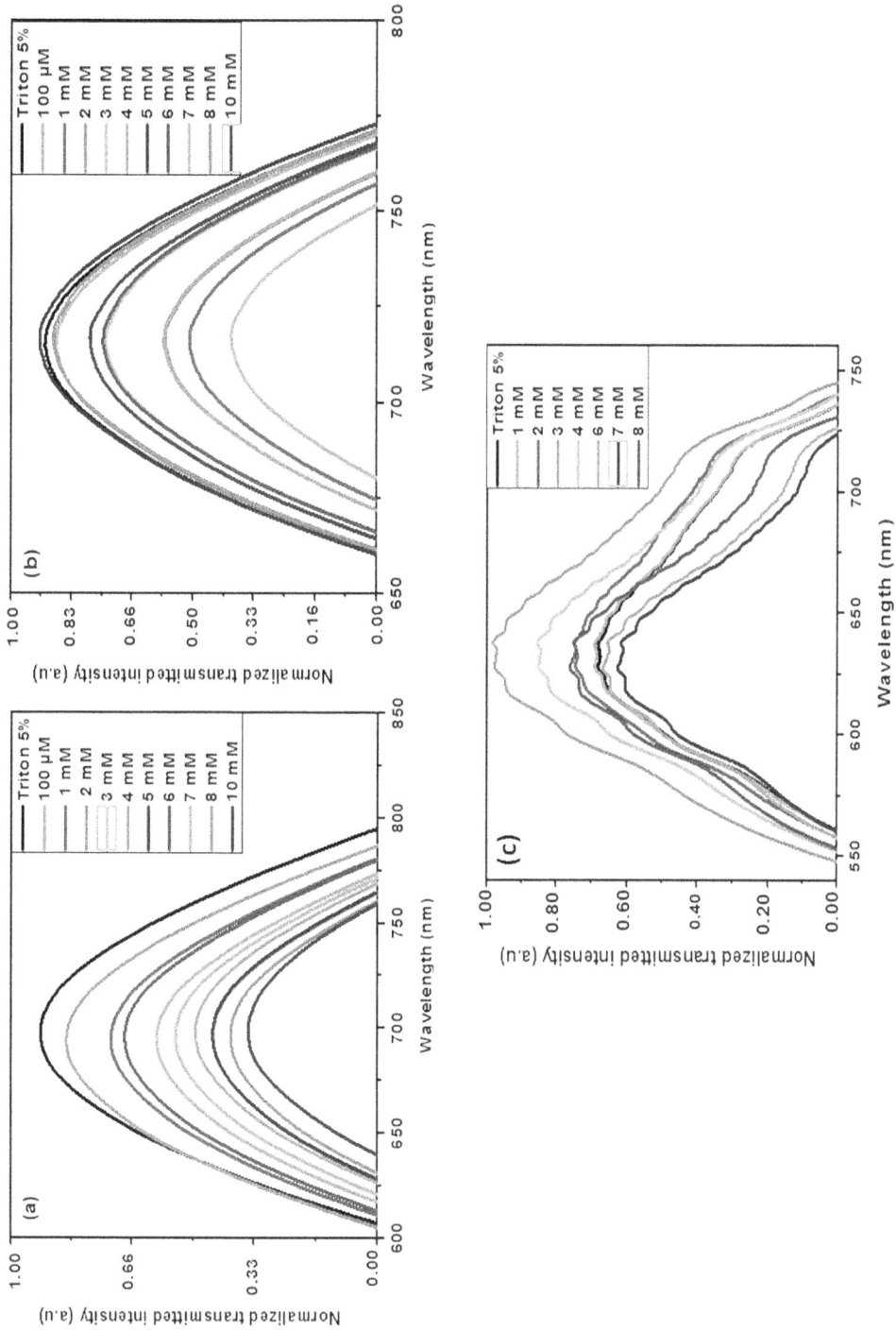

FIGURE 8.31 LSPR spectra of (a) probe 1, (b) probe 2, (c) probe 3.

Source: Reprinted with permission from *Journal of Lightwave Technology.* Copyright, 2020, IEEE (Agrawal, Zhang, Saha, Kumar, Pu et al. 2020).

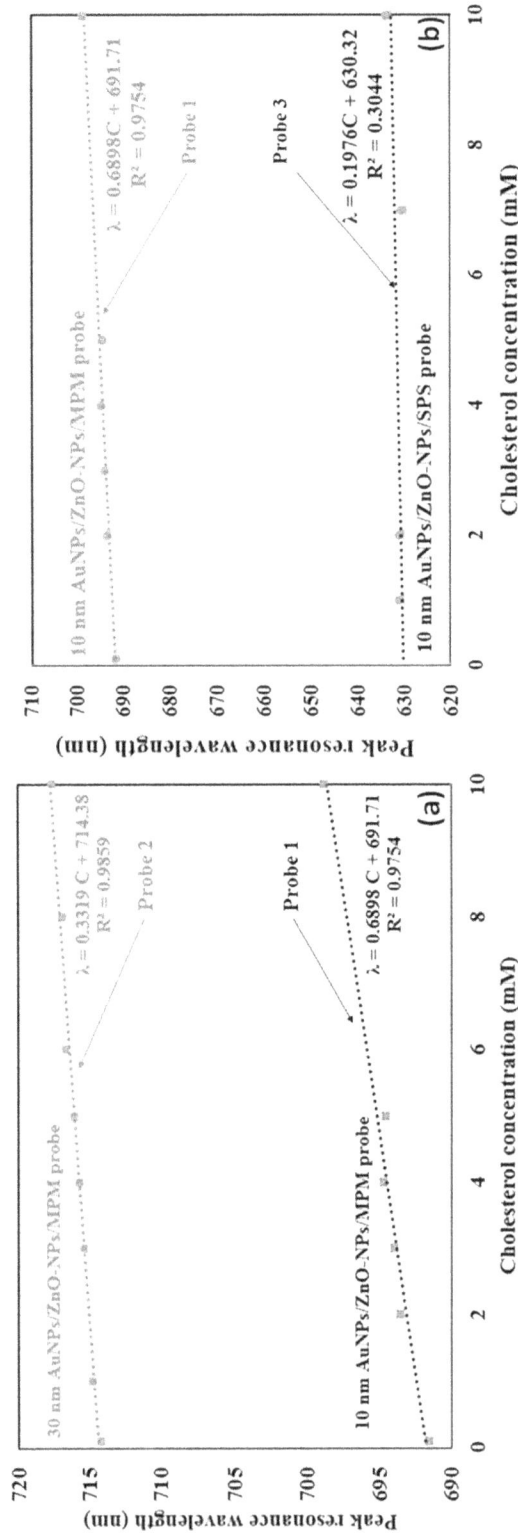

FIGURE 8.32 Linearity calibration curve: (a) probe 1 versus probe 2, (b) probe 1 versus probe 3.

Source: Reprinted with permission from *Journal of Lightwave Technology.* Copyright, 2020, IEEE (Agrawal, Zhang, Saha, Kumar, Pu et al. 2020).

Probe 2: Figures 8.30(b), 8.31(b), and 8.32(a) illustrate the schematic setup, LSPR spectra, and linear calibration curve of probe 2, respectively. In this study, the greatest wavelength shift is 3.425 nm, and the relevant linear curve equation is

$$\lambda = 0.3319 \, C + 714.38$$

In this situation, the sensitivity was 0.3319 nm/mM, the correlation coefficient was 0.986 mM, and the LoD was 1.28 mM.

Probe 3: Figures 8.30(c), 8.31(c), and 8.32(b) illustrate the schematic setup, LSPR spectra, and linear calibration curve for probe 3, respectively, where $\lambda = 0.1976 \, C + 630.32$ is the linear curve equation. In this comparative test, probe 3 has been used as a baseline (structural comparison). The linear equation clearly shows the sensitivity of probe 1. Since the normal value in human serum is 5.17 mM, the linear range of probe 1 is 0.1–10 mM, which is suitable for biomedical applications. In the immunobinding process of cholesterol to a ChOx functional probe, all the key sensing properties of the proposed sensor are greatly enhanced, including the sensitivity, linear range, LoD, and correlation coefficient of the probe.

8.5.10 CuO and AgNPs Modified SMSMS Structure Probe for Uric Acid Detection

The Mach-Zehnder interferometer (MZI) fiber-optic structure sensor was fabricated by LSPR technology and immobilized by AgNPs and CuO-NPs as shown in Figure 8.33 (Agrawal et al. 2020). AgNPs and CuO-NPs are employed to increase the sensor's biocompatibility and sensitivity. For the detection of uric acid (UA), the suggested optimized structure-based optical fiber sensors (OFSs) have high sensitivity, good specificity, and LoD (Agrawal, Saha et al. 2020). Furthermore, the proposed sensor has a linear profile across a broad range of concentrations: serum UA is tested at 10 µm–1 mM, with a normal range of 100–400 µM, and urine UA is measured at 0.4–10 mM, with a typical range of 1.5–4.4 mM. The sensor also has several unique features, such as multicompatibility UA serum and urine detection, as well as strong selectivity, reusability, repeatability, and low LoD. The suggested LSPR sensor immobilized SMSMS structure using AgNPs and CuO-NPS, as well as the LSPR sensor functionalized SMSMS structure using uricase, are more compatible and offer a wider range of medical applications.

The experimental device shown in Figure 8.34 is used to evaluate the performance of the proposed sensor for UA detection. According to the literature, the normal concentration of UA in human serum and urine is 100–400 µM and 1.5–4.4 mM, respectively. The excitation and output LSPR spectra of white light source was recorded by optical spectrometer. According to the LSPR

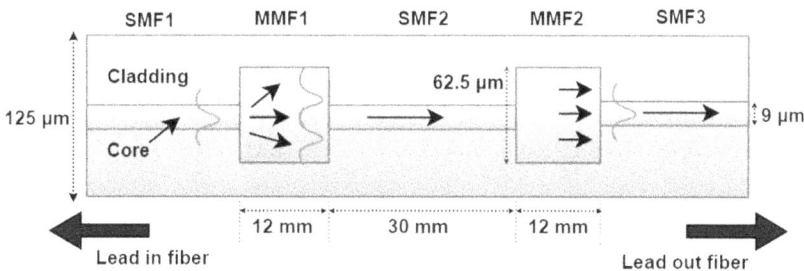

FIGURE 8.33 The optical signal is propagated through the proposed structure.

Source: Reprinted with permission from *IEEE Transactions on Instrumentation & Measurement.* Copyright, 2020, IEEE (Agrawal, Saha et al. 2020)

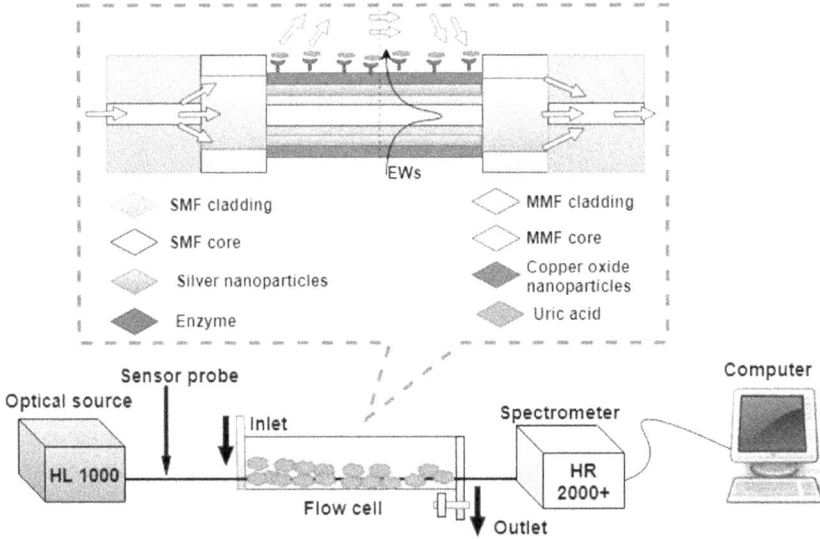

FIGURE 8.34 Experimental setup for the detection of UA.

Source: Reprinted with permission from *IEEE Transactions on Instrumentation & Measurement.* Copyright, 2020, IEEE (Agrawal, Saha et al. 2020).

principle, the change of the propagation constant is caused by the change of RI of the medium, which leads to wavelength red shift. The prepared UA solutions with different concentrations were dropped into the reaction dish with the sensor probe to obtain the LSPR spectra of different UA samples.

The SMF2 part of the SMSMS structure proposed by the LSPR phenomenon is most obvious. Recording the results only after the spectrum signal is stable can effectively demonstrate the better performance of the proposed LSPR-based sensor. Each experiment was performed three times to confirm that the achieved sensor was reproducible. In addition, spectra between resonance wavelength and normalized intensity were recorded in a wide range of UA samples to examine spectral fluctuations of the input optical signal.

Figure 8.35(a) shows the changes of probe 1's LSPR spectrum, while Figure 8.35(b) shows the changes of probe 2's LSPR spectrum. In addition, the results show that the resonance wavelength has a high fitting linear relationship with UA concentration. The experimentally verified linear correlation of UA in serum and urine was shown in Figure 8.36(a and b), respectively.

The sensitivity, correlation coefficient, and LoD of probe 1 and probe 2 were systematically determined by linear correlation diagram. The expression of probe 1 in serum was $\lambda = 4.03C + 661.22$, the sensitivity was 4 nm/mM, the correlation coefficient was 0.9539, and the LoD is 162.17 μM, $\sigma = 0.2178$. The sensitivity, correlation coefficient, and LoD of urine samples were 0.67 nm/mM, 0.98 and 0.98 mM, respectively. For probe 2, the sensitivity, correlation coefficient, and LoD of serum samples were 6.15 nm/mM, 0.94 and 69.26 μM, and the sensitivity, correlation coefficient, and LoD of urine samples were 1.23 nm/mM, 0.97 and 0.35 mM, respectively.

8.5.11   STRUCTURE OF OPTICAL FIBER MACH-ZEHNDER INTERFEROMETER FOR COLLAGEN IV DETECTION

In this section, a Mach-Zehnder interferometer (MZI) sensing probe based on photosensitive fiber (PSF) is introduced to detect the presence of type IV collagen in the human body (Kaushik et al. 2020). As shown in Figure 8.37, MZI is composed of SMF-MMF-PSF-MMF-SMF (SMPMS)

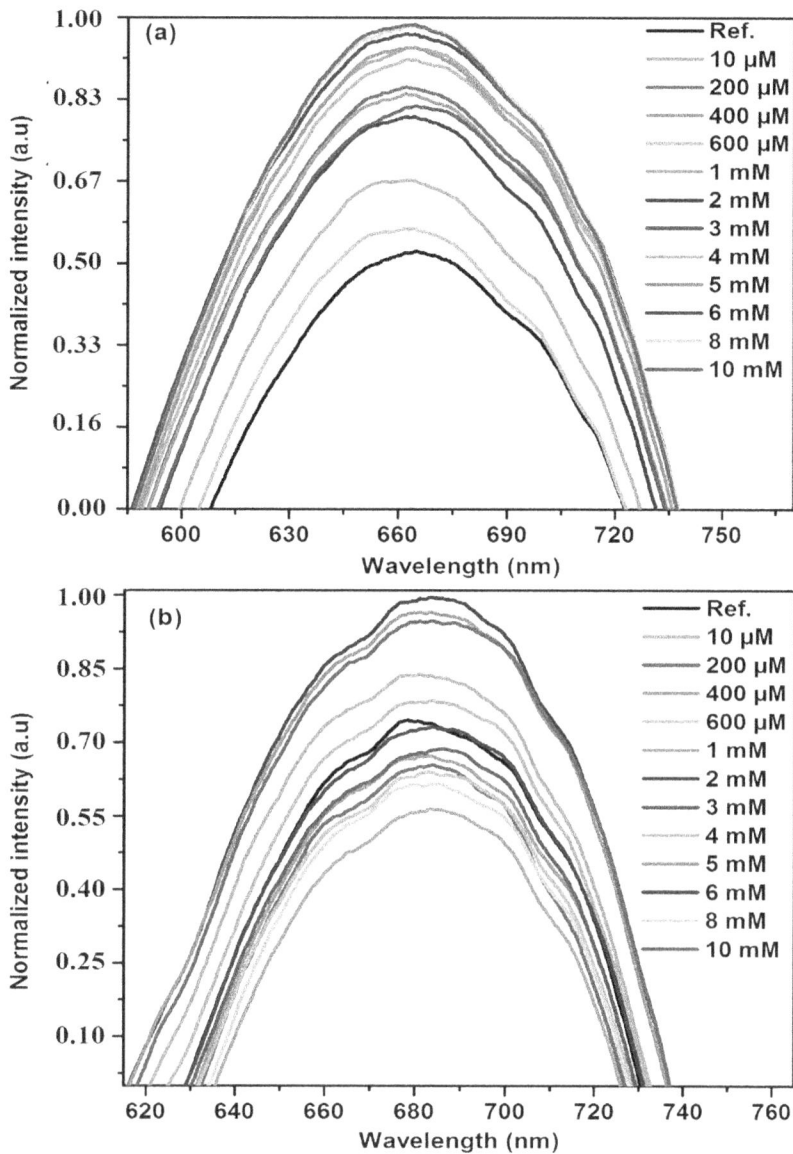

FIGURE 8.35 LSPR spectra (a) CuO fixed sensor probe, (b) AgNPs/CuO-NPs fixed sensor probe.

Source: Reprinted with permission from *IEEE Transactions on Instrumentation & Measurement.* Copyright, 2020, IEEE (Agrawal, Saha et al. 2020).

segments (Kaushik et al. 2020). The sensing region of MZI structure is a sensing probe of LSPR by etching the photosensitive optical fiber coating with 40%HF acid, and then depositing a layer of metal nanoparticles (NPs) on the surface of the sensing region. Polyvinyl alcohol stabilized AgNPs (PVA-AgNPs) were used. The sensor probe is functionalized with a collagenase to prevent other biomolecules from interfering with collagen-IV detection, thus providing the probe with excellent specific selectivity. The probe's sensing capacity is tested by detecting a broad range of collagen solution concentrations from 0 to 1 μg/mL. It has been discovered that immobilizing the probe using PVA-AgNPs and ZnO-NPs improves its sensing capability significantly.

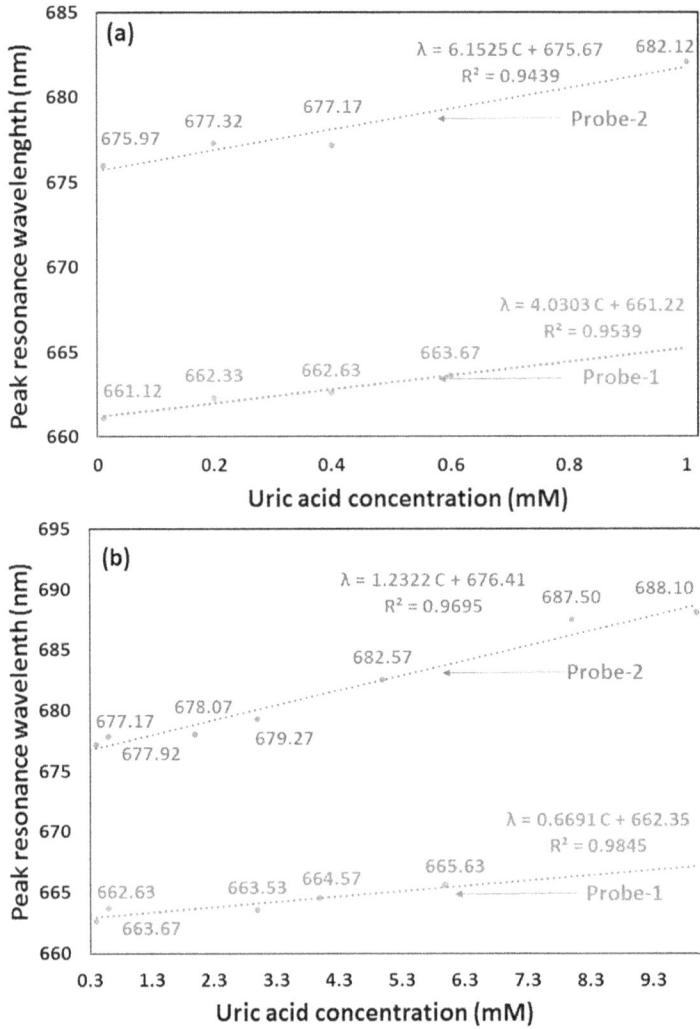

FIGURE 8.36 Linear analysis of the UA sensor probe: detect in the (a) serum and (b) urine.

Source: Reprinted with permission from *IEEE Transactions on Instrumentation & Measurement.* Copyright, 2020, IEEE (Agrawal, Saha et al. 2020).

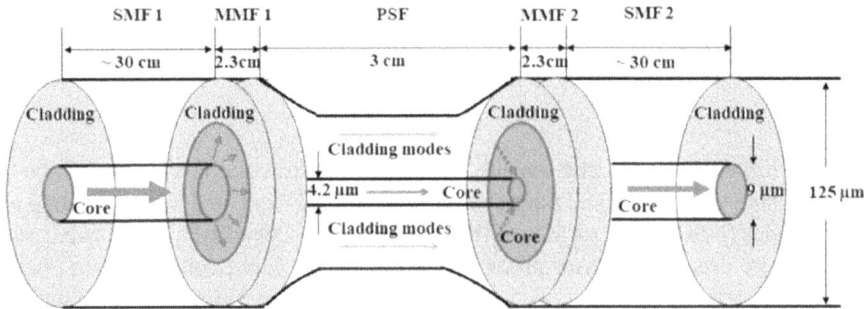

FIGURE 8.37 Photosensitive fiber-based MZI structure.

Source: Reprinted with permission from *IEEE Transactions on NanoBioscience.* Copyright, 2020, IEEE.

The measuring device uses light sources with wavelengths ranging from 200 to 1100 nm. Accordingly, spectrometers with spectral response of 200–1100 nm were used for spectral detection and collection. The probe of the optical fiber sensor is connected to the light source and the detector using an optical fiber jumper, as shown in Figure 8.38. An enlarged view of both sensor probes can be seen in the illustration.

The optimized probe was used to test collagen solutions of different concentrations (10 ng/mL). PBS is used to wash the sensor head to remove adsorbed impurities in the sensing area before testing a concentration of solution. Different sensors were used to measure the same concentration three times to reduce experimental error. Figure 8.39(a) shows the average LSPR spectrum for all observations. LSPR spectrum shows that the transmission intensity decreases gradually with the increase of collagen concentration.

Binding of collagen molecules has the opposite effect in the active part of the sensing layer functionalized by enzymes. The real and virtual components of dielectric constant/refractive index change when the analyte molecule is combined with collagen hydrolase. Changes in the real and

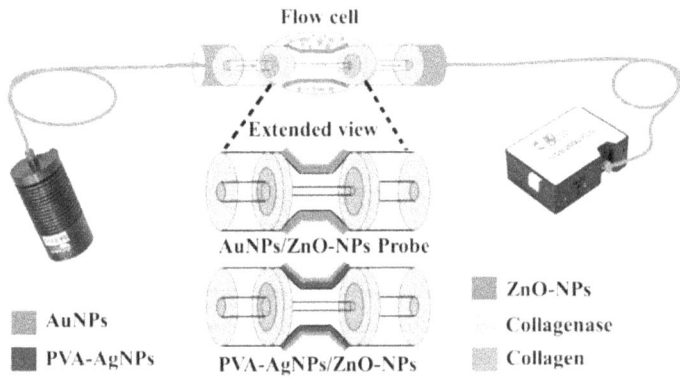

FIGURE 8.38   Device for measuring collagen solutions.

Source: Reprinted with permission from *IEEE Transactions on NanoBioscience*. Copyright, 2020, IEEE (Kaushik et al. 2020).

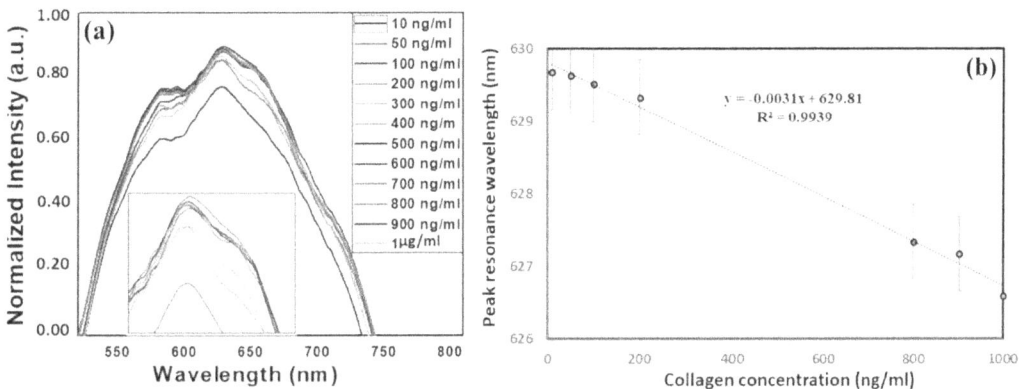

FIGURE 8.39   Probe 1: (a) LSPR spectra, (b) calibration curve.

Source: Reprinted with permission from *IEEE Transactions on NanoBioscience*. Copyright, 2020, IEEE (Kaushik et al. 2020).

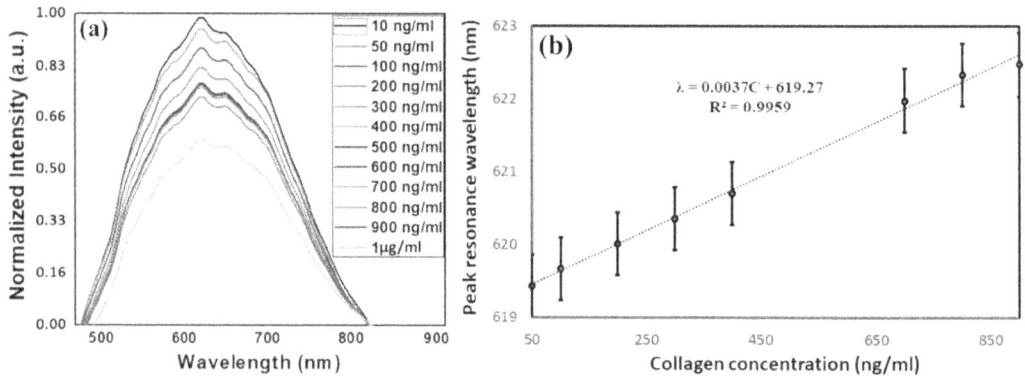

FIGURE 8.40   Probe 2: (a) LSPR spectra, (b) calibration curve.

Source: Reprinted with permission from *IEEE Transactions on NanoBioscience.* Copyright, 2020, IEEE (Kaushik et al. 2020).

imaginary parts correspond to wavelength and spectral displacement, respectively. This has been detailed in a previous work that used a silicon substrate to construct an LSPR-based electro-optic modulator. The observed blue shift in probe 1 has been interpreted as a decrease in a real fraction of the RI. Figure 8.39(b) shows the calibration of the curve. Due to the restricted binding sites accessible on the sensing layer, the wavelength becomes saturated at greater concentrations. As the concentration of analytes rises, the number of accessible sites for collagenase molecules decreases. The sensitivity value obtained from the calibration curve is 0.0031 ng/mL. Some measurements were skipped in the calibration curve to identify the best performance of the created probe. The linear fitting curve shows that the developed sensor probe has strong linearity in the detection of collagen with low concentration. Therefore, the proposed probe can be suitable for the detection of lower concentrations of analytes. In this case, PBS was used as blank solution and tested 10 times. SD was 0.32474, and LoD was calculated to be 314.04 ng. Similarly, Figure 8.40 shows the (a) LSPR spectra and (b) calibration curve of probe 2.

8.6   SUMMARY AND CONCLUSION

In order to stimulate LSPR phenomenon and generate strong evanescent wave, the fiber structure was etched with HF acid to make its diameter reach 90 μm. GO, AuNP, and MoS_2-NP are fixed on the sensing probe from bottom to top to modify the detection area to improve the sensing efficiency of LSPR. When the concentration of creatinine solution was within the linear range (0–2 mM), the sensitivity of the probe was 2.5 nm/mM, SD was 0.107, and LoD was 128.4 μM. The proposed creatinine biosensor can completely cover the creatinine concentration level that the human body can bear. It allows rapid measurement of creatinine levels and can be used for early identification and prevention.

In addition to breaking the inherent total reflection transmission mode, it is recognized that the evanescent field intensity can be improved by the combination of hetero-core fiber and conical structure. Using AuNPs, Nb_2CTx, MXene, and CA enzyme, the sensing probe can obtain good sensitivity and specificity identification. In the linear range of 0 ~ 2 mM, the sensitivity of the probe is 3.1 nm/mM, the LoD is 86.12 μM, and the R^2 is 0.9974. This indicates that the wavelength of the formant appears red-shift in the whole linear range with the gradual increase of the test concentration. These promising experimental data suggest that LSPR-based creatinine biosensors have potential applications in aquaculture.

A biosensor probe based on LSPR effect modified by multiple NMs was proposed to detect ALT enzyme. The quantitative concentration of ALT enzyme activity was accurately matched by measuring the change of resonance absorption peak wavelength. The results showed that the concentration of glutamate pyruvate aminotransferase was linearly correlated with the wavelength of the resonance peak. The results show that in the effective detection range of 10 ~ 1000 U/L, the curve-fitting value of the sensor is 95.62%, LoD is 10.61 U/L, and the sensitivity is 4.1 pm/(U/L). The results show that the sensor probe can effectively identify ALT enzyme and has a certain ability to identify liver injury.

In this study, the development process of a biosensor for monitoring p-cresol solution was also discussed. The proposed sensor probes detect p-cresol solutions in artificial urine at different concentrations, with selected measurements ranging from 0 to 1000 µM. Compared with the sensor probe 1 with only AuNPs fixed, the sensor probe with AuNPs and ZnO-NPs fixed at the same time has a larger detection range, and then the sensitivity is slightly worse than that of probe 1 with LoD.

A variety of NMs is used to attach to the surface of the sensing probe structure, including GO, AuNPs, and MoS_2-NPs. A sensitivity of 3.4 pm /(ng/mL), a correlation value of 0.928, and the LoD is 96.26 ng/mL in detection range of 0–1 µg/mL for fiber-optic biosensing specifically designed to detect cTnI solutions.

The goal of the research was to create an LSPR-based hetero-core sensor for monitoring cTnI concentrations. By immobilizing AuNPs and CeO_2-NPs on the sensing region, the sensor probe's performance and stability can be considerably increased while maintaining its biocompatibility. The sensor's specific identification is aided by an antibody-functionalized sensing area. Analysis of the transmitted intensity spectrum at values ranging from 0 to 1000 ng/mL was used to create the sensor probe. Finally, cTnI solutions had a LoD of 108.15 ng/mL and a sensitivity of 3 pm/(ng/mL), respectively.

The newly developed sensor will be able to identify acute myocardial infarction in people. The goal of this project is to create three different kinds of MMF/MCF structure sensor probes for ACh biomolecule detection. Probes 1 and 2 structures operate on the core-mismatch and tapering basis. Probe 1 is immobilized with AuNPs; however, it is unclear if probe 2 is immobilized with both AuNPs and MoS_2-NPs. It aids in observing the improvement in sensing owing to the addition of 2D material (MoS_2-NPs). Similarly, in probe 3, tapered MCF was compared to etched MCF, which is based on MMF-MCF splicing and MCF etching (i.e., operates on core-mismatch and etched EW phenomena). As a result of the tapered fiber and incorporation of 2D material, probe 2 is found to be superior to probe 1 and probe 3. Immobilization of acetylcholinesterase onto the nanosphere sensor probes improves the specific selectivity of the sensor probes developed in all situations. The proposed sensor ball for Achi detection has a linear detection range of 0 ~ 1 mM, the sensitivity is 0.062 nm/µM, and the LoD is 14.28 µM. Because of the increase of EWs fraction power, tapered fiber sensor is more suitable for sensors than corroded fiber sensor. The sensor detects the biological molecule acetylcholine in the body, which could be very helpful in treating Alzheimer's disease.

AuNPs and ZnO-NPs were immobilized in the sensing region of the 40-µm probe in the waist region to stimulate the LSPR of the probe and improve its biocompatibility, respectively. Two types of probes were designed based on two distinct NPs setups. The detection of AA in the first probe was accomplished by scattering AuNPs throughout the sensing zone. In addition, the specificity of the probe was improved by using AOx, which only oxidizes AA. The sensor response of the created probe was recorded by monitoring the change of peak wavelength in AA solutions with different concentrations. Probes were also authenticated by looking at their reusability, reproducibility, and selectivity. Probe 1 and probe 2 achieved curve-fitting and LoD values of 0.9924 and 0.9928, respectively, and 12.56 µM and 25.78 µM. For the linearity ranges of 1–200 µM and 10–200 µM, the obtained values for probe 1 and probe 2 sensitivity are 6 nm/mM and 5.7 nm/mM, respectively. As a consequence of the obtained data, it was determined that probe 1's response is superior in terms of linearity range and LoD.

The ultrasensitive new sensor based on the LSPR phenomenon is suggested in this work for detection of cholesterol. The new sensors' potential is being evaluated across a broad variety of cholesterol. For the first time, a cholesterol sensor based on LSPR has a wide linear range and low

LoD. A wide detection range can be ensured using biocompatible AuNPs with different surface functions. The AuNPs increases the effective range and sensitivity of detection.

An LSPR-based UA biosensor developed by AgNPs/CuO functionalized SMSMS fiber structure can be used to detect UA efficiently. Comprehensive experimental studies and measurements have given reliable results for the detection of UA in serum and urine. The probe 2 performance parameter of the sensor was proposed to detect serum UA: the sensitivity was 6.15 nm/mM, the LoD was 69.26 nM, the fitting coefficient was 0.9439, and the linear range was 10 µM–1 mM. The LSPR-based UA sensor is not only suitable for specific determination of UA but also for determination of UA concentration in serum or urine. According to the report, due to its improved performance and good selectivity, the sensor has great application potential in the field of UA detection in routine diagnostics.

MZI has fabricated using a PSF-based structure for detecting collagen in human bodies in this study. The performance of the generated probes was evaluated by evaluating collagen sample at different concentrations. The stability, LoD, and sensitivity of the constructed sensor probe were verified. The results showed that probe 2 performed better than probe 1 in LoD and sensitivity.

REFERENCES

Abdolrahim, M., M. Rabiee, S. N. Alhosseini, M. Tahriri, S. Yazdanpanah, and L. Tayebi. 2015. "Development of optical biosensor technologies for cardiac troponin recognition." *Analytical Biochemistry* 485:1–10.

Adamski, Juliusz, Paweł Nowak, and Jolanta Kochana. 2010. "Simple sensor for the determination of phenol and its derivatives in water based on enzyme tyrosinase." *Electrochimica Acta* 55 (7):2363–2367.

Aghamohammadi, Hamed, Reza Eslami-Farsani, and Elizabeth Castillo-Martinez. 2022. "Recent trends in the development of MXenes and MXene-based composites as anode materials for Li-ion batteries." *Journal of Energy Storage* 47:103572.

Agrawal, N., C. Saha, C. Kumar, R. Singh, B. Zhang, and S. Kumar. 2020. "Development of uric acid sensor using copper oxide and silver nanoparticles immobilized SMSMS fiber structure-based probe." *IEEE Transactions on Instrumentation and Measurement* 69 (11):9097–9104.

Agrawal, N., B. Zhang, C. Saha, C. Kumar, B. K. Kaushik, and S. Kumar. 2020. "Development of dopamine sensor using silver nanoparticles and PEG-functionalized tapered optical fiber structure." *IEEE Transactions on Biomedical Engineering* 67 (6):1542–1547.

Agrawal, N. K., B. Zhang, C. Saha, C. Kumar, X. Pu, and S. Kumar. 2020. "Ultra-sensitive cholesterol sensor using gold and zinc-oxide nanoparticles immobilized core mismatch MPM/SPS probe." *IEEE/OSA Journal of Lightwave Technology* 38 (8):2523–2529.

Alexander, Sheeba, P. Baraneedharan, Shriya Balasubrahmanyan, and S. Ramaprabhu. 2017. "Modified graphene based molecular imprinted polymer for electrochemical non-enzymatic cholesterol biosensor." *European Polymer Journal* 86:106–116.

Arif, Nimrah, Sundus Gul, Manzar Sohail, Syed Rizwan, and Mudassir Iqbal. 2021. "Synthesis and characterization of layered Nb$_2$C MXene/ZnS nanocomposites for highly selective electrochemical sensing of dopamine." *Ceramics International* 47 (2):2388–2396.

Arif Topçu, Aykut, Erdoğan Özgür, Fatma Yılmaz, Nilay Bereli, and Adil Denizli. 2019. "Real time monitoring and label free creatinine detection with artificial receptors." *Materials Science and Engineering: B* 244:6–11.

Boruah, Bijoy Sankar, and Rajib Biswas. 2018. "Localized surface plasmon resonance based U-shaped optical fiber probe for the detection of Pb^{2+} in aqueous medium." *Sensors and Actuators B: Chemical* 276:89–94.

Breul, S. D., K. H. Bradley, A. J. Hance, M. P. Schafer, R. A. Berg, and R. G. Crystal. 1980. "Control of collagen production by human diploid lung fibroblasts." *Journal of Biological Chemistry* 255 (11):5250–5260.

Bunde, R. L., E. J. Jarvi, and J. J. Rosentreter. 1998. "Piezoelectric quartz crystal biosensors." *Talanta* 46 (6):1223–1236.

Chekin, Fereshteh, Alina Vasilescu, Roxana Jijie, et al. 2018. "Sensitive electrochemical detection of cardiac troponin I in serum and saliva by nitrogen-doped porous reduced graphene oxide electrode." *Sensors and Actuators B: Chemical* 262:180–187.

Çimen, Duygu, Nilay Bereli, Serdar Günaydın, and Adil Denizli. 2020. "Detection of cardiac troponin-I by optic biosensors with immobilized anti-cardiac troponin-I monoclonal antibody." *Talanta* 219:121259.

Ciou, Ding-Siang, Pei-Hsuan Wu, Yu-Cheng Huang, Ming-Chang Yang, Shuenn-Yuh Lee, and Chia-Yu Lin. 2020. "Colorimetric and amperometric detection of urine creatinine based on the ABTS radical cation modified electrode." *Sensors and Actuators B: Chemical* 314:128034.

Coresh, J., B. C. Astor, T. Greene, G. Eknoyan, and A. S. Levey. 2003. "Prevalence of chronic kidney disease and decreased kidney function in the adult US population: Third national health and nutrition examination survey." *American Journal of Kidney Diseases* 41 (1):1–12.

Dhara, Keerthy, and Debiprosad Roy Mahapatra. 2020. "Review on electrochemical sensing strategies for C-reactive protein and cardiac troponin I detection." *Microchemical Journal* 156:104857.

Dhawan, S., S. Sadanandan, V. Haridas, N. H. Voelcker, and B. Prieto-Simón. 2018. "Novel peptidylated surfaces for interference-free electrochemical detection of cardiac troponin I." *Biosensors and Bioelectronics* 99:486–492.

Di Lullo, G. A., S. M. Sweeney, J. Korkko, L. Ala-Kokko, and J. D. San Antonio. 2002. "Mapping the ligand-binding sites and disease-associated mutations on the most abundant protein in the human, type I collagen." *Journal of Biological Chemistry* 277 (6):4223–4231.

Do, Jing-Shan, Yu-Hsuan Chang, and Ming-Liao Tsai. 2018. "Highly sensitive amperometric creatinine biosensor based on creatinine deiminase/Nafion®-nanostructured polyaniline composite sensing film prepared with cyclic voltammetry." *Materials Chemistry and Physics* 219:1–12.

Fan, Dawei, Chunzhu Bao, Malik Saddam Khan, et al. 2018. "A novel label-free photoelectrochemical sensor based on N,S-GQDs and CdS co-sensitized hierarchical Zn_2SnO_4 cube for detection of cardiac troponin I." *Biosensors and Bioelectronics* 106:14–20.

Fu, Xiaoyun, Shelby A. Cate, Melissa Dominguez, et al. 2019. "Cysteine disulfides (Cys-ss-X) as sensitive plasma biomarkers of oxidative stress." *Scientific Reports* 9 (1):115.

Gish, Douglas A., Francis Nsiah, Mark T. McDermott, and Michael J. Brett. 2007. "Localized surface plasmon resonance biosensor using silver nanostructures fabricated by glancing angle deposition." *Analytical Chemistry* 79 (11):4228–4232.

Guan, Jian-Guo, Yu-Qing Miao, and Qing-Jie Zhang. 2004. "Impedimetric biosensors." *Journal of Bioscience and Bioengineering* 97 (4):219–226.

Hanif, Saima, Peter John, Wenyue Gao, Muhammad Saqib, Liming Qi, and Guobao Xu. 2016. "Chemiluminescence of creatinine/H_2O_2/Co^{2+} and its application for selective creatinine detection." *Biosensors and Bioelectronics* 75:347–351.

Harper, Jason C., Susan M. Brozik, Jeb H. Flemming, et al. 2009. "Fabrication and testing of a microneedles sensor array for p-cresol detection with potential biofuel applications." *ACS Applied Materials & Interfaces* 1 (7):1591–1598.

He, Chenyang, Serhiy Korposh, Ricardo Correia, Liangliang Liu, Barrie R. Hayes-Gill, and Stephen P. Morgan. 2021. "Optical fibre sensor for simultaneous temperature and relative humidity measurement: Towards absolute humidity evaluation." *Sensors and Actuators B: Chemical* 344:130154.

Homola, Jiří, Sinclair S. Yee, and Günter Gauglitz. 1999. "Surface plasmon resonance sensors." *Sensors and Actuators B: Chemical* 54 (1–2):3–15.

Hsueh, Chang-Jung, Joanne H. Wang, Liming Dai, and Chung-Chiun Liu. 2012. "Development of an electrochemical-based aspartate aminotransferase nanoparticle Ir-C biosensor for screening of liver diseases." *Biosensors* 2 (2):234–244.

Jacobi, D., C. Lavigne, J. M. Halimi, et al. 2008. "Variability in creatinine excretion in adult diabetic, overweight men and women: Consequences on creatinine-based classification of renal disease." *Diabetes Research and Clinical Practice* 80 (1):102–107.

Kaushik, B. K., L. Singh, R. Singh, et al. 2020. "Detection of collagen-IV using highly reflective metal nanoparticles: Immobilized photosensitive optical fiber-based MZI structure." *IEEE Transactions on NanoBioscience* 19 (3):477–484.

Kim, Hee Jung, Seok Bean Song, Jung Min Choi, et al. 2010. "IL-18 downregulates collagen production in human dermal fibroblasts via the ERK pathway." *Journal of Investigative Dermatology* 130 (3):706–715.

Kim, K. R., H. J. Chun, Y. D. Han, et al. 2017. "A time-resolved fluorescence immunosensing platform for highly sensitive detection of cardiac troponin I." Paper read at 2017 19th International Conference on Solid-State Sensors, Actuators and Microsystems (TRANSDUCERS), 18–22 June.

Kim, Kihyun, Chanoh Park, Donghoon Kwon, et al. 2016. "Silicon nanowire biosensors for detection of cardiac troponin I (cTnI) with high sensitivity." *Biosensors and Bioelectronics* 77:695–701.

Kleber, H.-P. 1991. D. Schomburg and M. Salzmann (Editors), Enzyme Handbook Volume 1, Class 4: Lyases. 810 S., Loose-Leaf-Binder. Berlin 1990. Springer-Verlag. DM 248, 00. ISBN: 3-540-52579-3. Wiley Online Library.

Kovács, Ágnes, Anikó Kende, Mária Mörtl, Gábor Volk, Tamás Rikker, and Kornél Torkos. 2008. "Determination of phenols and chlorophenols as trimethylsilyl derivatives using gas chromatography-mass spectrometry." *Journal of Chromatography A* 1194 (1):139–142.

Krishnamurthy, Vikram, Sahar Moradi Monfared, and Bruce Cornell. 2010. "Ion-channel biosensors—Part I: Construction, operation, and clinical studies." *IEEE Transactions on Nanotechnology* 9 (3):303–312.

Kumar, P., R. Jaiwal, and C. S. Pundir. 2017. "An improved amperometric creatinine biosensor based on nanoparticles of creatininase, creatinase and sarcosine oxidase." *Analytical Biochemistry* 537:41–49.

Kumar, S., Z. Guo, R. Singh, et al. 2021. MoS_2 functionalized multicore fiber probes for selective detection of *Shigella* bacteria based on localized plasmon." *Journal of Lightwave Technology* 39 (12):4069–4081.

Kumar, Santosh, and Ragini Singh. 2021. "Recent optical sensing technologies for the detection of various biomolecules: Review." *Optics & Laser Technology* 134:106620.

Kuster, N., A. S. Bargnoux, G. P. Pageaux, and J. P. Cristol. 2012. "Limitations of compensated Jaffe creatinine assays in cirrhotic patients." *Clin Biochem* 45 (4–5):320–325.

Lee, Kyung Won, Ka Ram Kim, Hyeong Jin Chun, et al. 2020. "Time-resolved fluorescence resonance energy transfer-based lateral flow immunoassay using a raspberry-type europium particle and a single membrane for the detection of cardiac troponin I." *Biosensors and Bioelectronics* 163:112284.

Lee, Seung-Ro, Mohammed Muzibur Rahman, Makoto Ishida, Kazuaki Sawada, Makoto Ishida, and Kazuaki Sawada. 2009. "Development of a highly-sensitive acetylcholine sensor using a charge-transfer technique on a smart biochip." *TrAC Trends in Analytical Chemistry* 28 (2):196–203.

Lewińska, Izabela, Mikołaj Speichert, Mateusz Granica, and Łukasz Tymecki. 2021. "Colorimetric point-of-care paper-based sensors for urinary creatinine with smartphone readout." *Sensors and Actuators B: Chemical* 340:129915.

Li, Muyang, Ragini Singh, Carlos Marques, Bingyuan Zhang, and Santosh Kumar. 2021. "2D material assisted SMF-MCF-MMF-SMF based LSPR sensor for creatinine detection." *Optics Express* 29 (23):38150–38167.

Li, Muyang, Ragini Singh, Maria Simone Soares, Carlos Marques, Bingyuan Zhang, and Santosh Kumar. 2022. "Convex fiber-tapered seven core fiber-convex fiber (CTC) structure-based biosensor for creatinine detection in aquaculture." *Optics Express* 30 (8):13898–13914.

Li, Xi-Ling, Gao Li, Ying-Zi Jiang, et al. 2015. "Human nails metabolite analysis: A rapid and simple method for quantification of uric acid in human fingernail by high-performance liquid chromatography with UV-detection." *Journal of Chromatography B* 1002:394–398.

Li, Y. F., Z. M. Liu, Y. L. Liu, Y. H. Yang, G. L. Shen, and R. Q. Yu. 2006. "A mediator-free phenol biosensor based on immobilizing tyrosinase to ZnO nanoparticles." *Anal Biochem* 349 (1):33–40.

Liao, X. J., H. J. Xiao, J. T. Cao, S. W. Ren, and Y. M. Liu. 2021. "A novel split-type photoelectrochemical immunosensor based on chemical redox cycling amplification for sensitive detection of cardiac troponin I." *Talanta* 233:122564.

Liu, Chunlan, Rui Wang, Yabin Shao, et al. 2021. "Detection of GDF11 by using a Ti_3C_2-MXene-based fiber SPR biosensor." *Optics Express* 29 (22):36598–36607.

Liu, Dongkui, Xing Lu, Yiwen Yang, Yunyun Zhai, Jian Zhang, and Lei Li. 2018. "A novel fluorescent aptasensor for the highly sensitive and selective detection of cardiac troponin I based on a graphene oxide platform." *Analytical and Bioanalytical Chemistry* 410 (18):4285–4291.

Liu, H. L., Y. N. Ma, and P. Zhang. 2010. Diagnostic value of AFP, TBA, GGT, ALT joint detection on hepatocarcinoma. *Laboratory Medicine and Clinic* 7 (2):122–123.

Liu, J. T., C. J. Chen, T. Ikoma, et al. 2011. "Surface plasmon resonance biosensor with high anti-fouling ability for the detection of cardiac marker troponin T." *Analytica Chimica Acta* 703 (1):80–86.

Liu, Zhengtao, Shuping Que, Jing Xu, and Tao Peng. 2014. "Alanine aminotransferase-old biomarker and new concept: A review." *International Journal of Medical Sciences* 11 (9):925–935.

Martín-Barreiro, Alba, Susana de Marcos, Jesús M. de la Fuente, Valeria Grazú, and Javier Galbán. 2018. "Gold nanocluster fluorescence as an indicator for optical enzymatic nanobiosensors: Choline and acetylcholine determination." *Sensors and Actuators B: Chemical* 277:261–270.

Maruyama, S., J. Cheng, M. Yamazaki, et al. 2010. "Metastasis-associated genes in oral squamous cell carcinoma and salivary adenoid cystic carcinoma: A differential DNA chip analysis between metastatic and nonmetastatic cell systems." *Cancer Genetics and Cytogenetics* 196 (1):14–22.

Maynard, S. J., I. B. Menown, and A. A. Adgey. 2000. "Troponin T or troponin I as cardiac markers in isch-aemic heart disease." *Heart* 83 (4):371–373.

McCarty, M. F., and J. J. DiNicolantonio. 2015. "An increased need for dietary cysteine in support of gluta-thione synthesis may underlie the increased risk for mortality associated with low protein intake in the elderly." *Age (Dordrecht)* 37 (5):96.

Menon, P. Susthitha, Fairus Atida Said, Gan Siew Mei, et al. 2018. "Urea and creatinine detection on nano-laminated gold thin film using Kretschmann-based surface plasmon resonance biosensor." *PloS One* 13 (7):e0201228.

Michałowicz, J., and W. Duda. 2007. "Phenols: Sources and toxicity." *Polish Journal of Environmental Studies* 16 (3).

Mokhtari, Zaynab, Habibollah Khajehsharifi, Sedigheh Hashemnia, Z. Solati, R. Azimpanah, and Saeed Shahrokhian. 2020. "Evaluation of molecular imprinted polymerized methylene blue/aptamer as a novel hybrid receptor for cardiac troponin I (cTnI) detection at glassy carbon electrodes modified with new biosynthesized ZnONPs." *Sensors and Actuators B: Chemical* 320:128316.

Nanji, A. A., S. W. French, and J. B. Freeman. 1985. "Relationship between arterial oxygen tension and serum aminotransferases in morbidly obese patients with fatty liver." *Clinical Chemistry* 31 (9):1571–1572.

Nayak, Jeeban Kumar, Purnendu Parhi, and Rajan Jha. 2015. "Graphene oxide encapsulated gold nanoparticle based stable fibre optic sucrose sensor." *Sensors and Actuators B: Chemical* 221:835–841.

Negahdary, M., and H. Heli. 2019. "An electrochemical troponin I peptisensor using a triangular icicle-like gold nanostructure." *Biochemical Engineering Journal* 151:107326.

Niedziółka-Jönsson, Joanna, Fatiha Barka, Xavier Castel, et al. 2010. "Development of new localized sur-face plasmon resonance interfaces based on gold nanostructures sandwiched between tin-doped indium oxide films." *Langmuir* 26 (6):4266–4273.

Nigam, P. K. 2007. "Biochemical markers of myocardial injury." *Indian Journal of Clinical Biochemistry: IJCB* 22 (1):10–17.

Onwuli, D. O., S. F. Samuel, P. Sfyri, et al. 2019. "The inhibitory subunit of cardiac troponin (cTnI) is modified by arginine methylation in the human heart." *International Journal of Cardiology* 282:76–80.

Pandey, Ravi P., P. Abdul Rasheed, Tricia Gomez, et al. 2020. "Effect of sheet size and atomic struc-ture on the antibacterial activity of Nb-MXene nanosheets." *ACS Applied Nano Materials* 3 (11):11372–11382.

Park, H. J., D. H. Cho, H. J. Kim, et al. 2009. "Collagen synthesis is suppressed in dermal fibroblasts by the human antimicrobial peptide LL-37." *Journal of Investigative Dermatology* 129 (4):843–850.

Pei, Jianhong, and Xiao-yuan Li. 2000. "Xanthine and hypoxanthine sensors based on xanthine oxidase immobilized on a CuPtCl6 chemically modified electrode and liquid chromatography electrochemical detection." *Analytica Chimica Acta* 414 (1):205–213.

Perrone, M. A., F. Spolaore, M. Ammirabile, et al. 2021. "The assessment of high sensitivity cardiac tropo-nin in patients with COVID-19: A multicenter study." *International Journal of Cardiology: Heart and Vasculature* 32:100715.

Polinder-Bos, H. A., H. Nacak, F. W. Dekker, S. J. L. Bakker, Cajm Gaillard, and R. T. Gansevoort. 2017. "Low urinary creatinine excretion is associated with self-reported frailty in patients with advanced chronic kidney disease." *Kidney International Reports* 2 (4):676–685.

Pundir, C. S., R. Deswal, V. Narwal, and J. Narang. 2018. "Quantitative analysis of metformin with special emphasis on sensors: A review." *Current Analytical Chemistry* 14 (5):438–445.

Qiao, Juan, and Li Qi. 2021. "Recent progress in plant-gold nanoparticles fabrication methods and bio-applications." *Talanta* 223:121396.

Rampazzi, S., G. Danese, F. Leporati, and F. Marabelli. 2016. "A localized surface plasmon resonance-based portable instrument for quick on-site biomolecular detection." *IEEE Transactions on Instrumentation and Measurement* 65 (2):317–327.

Reddy, K. Koteshwara, and Kauveri Vengatajalabathy Gobi. 2013. "Artificial molecular recognition mate-rial based biosensor for creatinine by electrochemical impedance analysis." *Sensors and Actuators B-Chemical* 183:356–363.

Saha, Krishnendu, Sarit S. Agasti, Chaekyu Kim, Xiaoning Li, and Vincent M. Rotello. 2012. "Gold nanopar-ticles in chemical and biological sensing." *Chemical Reviews* 112 (5):2739–2779.

Sattarahmady, N., H. Heli, and R. D. Vais. 2013. "An electrochemical acetylcholine sensor based on lichen-like nickel oxide nanostructure." *Biosensors and Bioelectronics* 48:197–202.

Sharma, S., A. M. Shrivastav, and B. D. Gupta. 2020. "Lossy mode resonance based fiber optic creatinine sensor fabricated using molecular imprinting over nanocomposite of MoS$_2$/SnO$_2$." *IEEE Sensors Journal* 20 (8):4251–4259.

Sharma, Sunil Kumar, Amit Kumar, Gaurav Sharma, et al. 2022. "MXenes based nano-heterojunctions and composites for advanced photocatalytic environmental detoxification and energy conversion: A review." *Chemosphere* 291:132923.

Singh, L., R. Singh, B. Zhang, B. K. Kaushik, and S. Kumar. 2020. "Localized surface plasmon resonance based hetero-core optical fiber sensor structure for the detection of L-cysteine." *IEEE Transactions on Nanotechnology* 19:201–208.

Singh, Ragini, Santosh Kumar, Feng-Zhen Liu, et al. 2020. "Etched multicore fiber sensor using copper oxide and gold nanoparticles decorated graphene oxide structure for cancer cells detection." *Biosensors and Bioelectronics* 168:112557.

Singh, Sarika, Satyendra K. Mishra, and Banshi D. Gupta. 2013. "SPR based fibre optic biosensor for phenolic compounds using immobilization of tyrosinase in polyacrylamide gel." *Sensors and Actuators B: Chemical* 186:388–395.

Sivaguru, M., S. Durgam, R. Ambekar, et al. 2010. "Quantitative analysis of collagen fiber organization in injured tendons using Fourier transform-second harmonic generation imaging." *Optics Express* 18 (24):24983–24993.

Sun, D., Z. Luo, J. Lu, et al. 2019. "Electrochemical dual-aptamer-based biosensor for nonenzymatic detection of cardiac troponin I by nanohybrid electrocatalysts labeling combined with DNA nanotetrahedron structure." *Biosensors and Bioelectronics* 134:49–56.

Tan, Dongchen, Chengming Jiang, Nan Sun, et al. 2021. "Piezoelectricity in monolayer MXene for nanogenerators and piezotronics." *Nano Energy* 90:106528.

Tu, M. H., T. Sun, and K. T. V. Grattan. 2012. "Optimization of gold-nanoparticle-based optical fibre surface plasmon resonance (SPR)-based sensors." *Sensors and Actuators B: Chemical* 164 (1):43–53.

Tunç, Ayşe Tuğçe, Elif Aynacı Koyuncu, and Fatma Arslan. 2016. "Development of an acetylcholinesterase: Choline oxidase based biosensor for acetylcholine determination." *Artificial Cells, Nanomedicine, and Biotechnology* 44 (7):1659–1664.

Turkevich, John, Peter Cooper Stevenson, and James Hillier. 1951. "A study of the nucleation and growth processes in the synthesis of colloidal gold." *Discussions of the Faraday Society* 11:55–75.

Tymecki, Ł., J. Korszun, K. Strzelak, and R. Koncki. 2013. "Multicommutated flow analysis system for determination of creatinine in physiological fluids by Jaffe method." *Analytica Chimica Acta* 787:118–125.

Usha, Sruthi P., and Banshi D. Gupta. 2018. "Urinary p-cresol diagnosis using nanocomposite of ZnO/MoS$_2$ and molecular imprinted polymer on optical fiber based lossy mode resonance sensor." *Biosensors and Bioelectronics* 101:135–145.

Vizzini, P., M. Braidot, J. Vidic, and M. Manzano. 2019. "Electrochemical and optical biosensors for the detection of campylobacter and listeria: An update look." *Micromachines (Basel)* 10 (8).

Wang, L., B. Xing, X. Ren, et al. 2020. "Mo$_2$C combined with carbon material nanosphere as an electrochemiluminescence super-enhancer and antibody label for ultrasensitive detection of cardiac troponin I." *Biosensors and Bioelectronics* 150:111910.

Wang, N., M. Chen, J. Gao, et al. 2019. "A series of BODIPY-based probes for the detection of cysteine and homocysteine in living cells." *Talanta* 195:281–289.

Wang, Y., R. Singh, S. Chaudhary, B. Zhang, and S. Kumar. 2022. "2-D nanomaterials assisted LSPR MPM optical fiber sensor probe for cardiac troponin I detection." *IEEE Transactions on Instrumentation and Measurement* 71:1–9.

Wang, Y., G. Zhu, M. Li, et al. 2021. "Water pollutants p-cresol detection based on Au-ZnO nanoparticles modified tapered optical fiber." *IEEE Trans Nanobioscience* 20 (3):377–384.

Wang, Zhi, Ragini Singh, Carlos Marques, Rajan Jha, Bingyuan Zhang, and Santosh Kumar. 2021. "Taper-in-taper fiber structure-based LSPR sensor for alanine aminotransferase detection." *Optics Express* 29 (26):43793–43810.

Wani, A. Basit, Joginder Singh, and Niraj Upadhyay. 2017. "Synthesis and characterization of transition metal complexes of para-aminosalicylic acid with evaluation of their antioxidant activities." *Oriental Journal of Chemistry* 33:1120–1126.

Willets, Katherine A., and Richard P. Van Duyne. 2007. "Localized surface plasmon resonance spectroscopy and sensing." *Annual Review of Physical Chemistry* 58:267–297.

Yadav, S., R. Devi, A. Kumar, and C. S. Pundir. 2011. "Tri-enzyme functionalized ZnO-NPs/CHIT/c-MWCNT/ PANI composite film for amperometric determination of creatinine." *Biosensors and Bioelectronics* 28 (1):64–70.

Yadav, S., A. Kumar, and C. S. Pundir. 2011. "Amperometric creatinine biosensor based on covalently coim- mobilized enzymes onto carboxylated multiwalled carbon nanotubes/polyaniline composite film." *Analytical Biochemistry* 419 (2):277–283.

Yasmin, Hasina, Tsutomu Kabashima, Mohammed Shafikur Rahman, Takayuki Shibata, and Masaaki Kai. 2014. "Amplified and selective assay of collagens by enzymatic and fluorescent reactions." *Scientific Reports* 4 (1):4950.

Yin, J., S. Pan, X. Guo, et al. 2021. "Nb_2C MXene-functionalized scaffolds enables osteosarcoma photo- therapy and angiogenesis/osteogenesis of bone defects." *Nano-Micro Letters* 13 (1):30.

Zhu, G., N. K. Agrawal, B. Zhang, C. Saha, C. Kumar, and S. Kumar. 2020. "A novel periodically tapered structure-based gold nanoparticles and graphene oxide – Immobilized optical fiber sensor to detect ascorbic acid." *Optics & Laser Technology* 127:106156.

Zhu, Guo, Lokendra Singh, Yu Wang, et al. 2021. "Tapered optical fiber-based LSPR biosensor for ascorbic acid detection." *Photonic Sensors* 11 (4):418–434.

Zhu, Guo, Y. Wang, Z. Wang, et al. 2022. "Localized plasmon-based multicore fiber biosensor for acetylcho- line detection." *IEEE Transactions on Instrumentation and Measurement* 71:1–9.

9 Optical Sensors for Detection of Microorganisms

9.1 INTRODUCTION

We have previously discussed the design, fabrication, and measurement of optical biosensors used to detect a variety of biomolecules found in the human body. This chapter is extremely essential because it discusses optical sensors for microorganism detection, particularly cancer and bacterial cells. As we know that there are numerous advantages in optical biosensing such as real-time detection, low response time, low detection limit, highly sensitive, portable, and specific for analytes, those have bright prospects for monitoring the abnormal state of bacterial cells and cancer. In a general way, conventional sensors required milliard orders of magnitude of tumor tissue with a cell diameter around 7–10 nm; however, optical biosensors have the ability to identify the lesions in fewer tumor cells. In addition, traditional detection techniques have certain limitations including expense, complex in nature, need for experts, and time-consuming. As a result, in this chapter, plasmonic optical sensing techniques for early detection microorganism detection are discussed and presented at length, and primarily, they focus on advanced methods in the excogitation of different biosensors like reflectance, interference, luminescence, chemiluminescence, resonance, scattering, and absorbance. Meanwhile, the rapid flourishing of the optical sensing platform against the diagnosis toward several acute diseases, for the most part, is promoted by using two-dimensional (2D) materials with excellent photometric characteristics, like biocompatibility, field enhancement, large-space extensibility, and advanced microfabrication techniques.

The single molecule can be detected through the surface-enhancing Raman spectroscopy techniques with high specificity. In this regard, terahertz waves also play a vital role especially in cancer detection. The fast growth of optical sensors is also benefits from peculiar optical properties like miniaturization, remote sensing capabilities, anti-electromagnetic interference, and multiplexing. This chapter discusses the merits and demerits of existing and advanced optical sensing techniques for diagnosis of cancer cells and other microorganisms. Also, the current and potential status of advance optical fiber biosensors applied to a clinical and fast-response realizable system will be investigated in detail.

Cancer, as an inevitable challenge to human life and health, is an insurmountable barrier to modern medicine, causing 10 million deaths worldwide in 1 year (2020) alone (Sung et al. 2021). Among them, according to the literature (Yang et al. 2019), mammary and lung cancers are seen as most lethal for men and women as the two most common cancers, respectively. Some tumor diseases, such as melanoma, sarcoma, lymphoma, and leukemia, can be concealed in specific organs or tissue and invade the health of organs everywhere. Current knowledge about the pathological causes of these conditions is limited; some of the known potential carcinogenic factors are cellular aging, radiation exposure, chemicals, excessive smoking, viral infections, and hormonal disorders (Wu et al. 2018). In the early stage of cell disease, its basic cell structure will be changed, its shape is abnormal, and it has many nuclei (Ramanujam et al. 2019; Fischer 2020). Due to such characteristics of cancer cells, like infinitely multiplying, metastasizing, and transmutable, modern standard cancer screening is like a time war. For this, clinical protocols such as biopsy, polymerase chain reaction, roentgenography, enzyme-linked immunosorbent assays (ELISA), molecular imaging, and magnetic resonance imaging can accurately detect cancerous organs. Unfortunately, it is also accompanied by a number of practical problems to be improved, such as sample collection, expensive costs, complex equipment, and operator expertise. It is worth mentioning that the early samples of cancer patients generally do not have enough cancerous cells (million order of magnitude) to be ignored, and puts the human race at a disadvantage (Mittal et al. 2017). As we can see, researchers have been working hard to develop more sensitive, fast-test sensors that could seize valuable time for human health and early cancer detection.

At present, the technique of noninvasive optical biosensing system is developing like a raging fire in cancer cell detection experiments. Most optical sensing systems consist of a detection sample, a marker, a recognition receptor, and a physical chemistry detection module (Jayanthi, Das, and Saxena 2017). Analyte samples can be obtained from serum, saliva, or urine. Biomarkers, as a biochemical indicators of pathological characteristics, are usually selected for microRNAs, circulating tumor cells (CTCs), proteins, exosomes, and DNA (Underwood et al. 2020). With the widespread use of nanotechnology and noble metals materials in biosensing, it seems to bring a new perspective for discovering a method for detecting precancer. A phenomenon of surface plasmon resonance (SPR) at the dielectric boundary related NMs to surroundings has drawn a lot of attention. When the incident light satisfies the total internal reflection condition on the NM surface, the surface evanescent wave will be produced, and when the evanescent wave and the surface plasma wave of the NMs layer satisfy the resonance condition, the intensity of the reflected light will be substantially decreased. This phenomenon, known as the SPR, has extensive use in biosensing to obtain the perception of biomolecular interactions by detecting the sensing media refractive index (RI) reflected on the exploratory shifts of wavelength or angular. The field distribution is rigorously limited around the surface of nanoparticles (NPs) which is a well-known phenomenon called as the localized surface plasmon resonance (LSPR) (Hammond et al. 2014). At this point, the absorption peak of LSPR is strongly linked to the RI around NPs.

With the wide application of nanotechnology and NMs in biosensing, it seems to bring a new vitality to the incipient detection of carcinoma cell lines. However, the problem is that the adsorption effect of NPs on biomolecules is not ideal, and that causes a serious effect on the specificity and sensitivity of the sensor. For this, people try to use various NMs with biocompatibility to increase the enzyme attachment sites over the sensor probe and enhance the sensing performance (Chocarro-Ruiz et al. 2017; Kumar, Singh et al. 2021). Based on this idea, a CuO/GO-based LSPR biosensor platform was designed for cancer cell detection. Here, CuO is an excellent semiconductor oxide (Wang et al. 2019), and GO has excellent biocompatibility, and large surface ratio, that are conducive to enzyme immobilization and sensing properties (Kumar, Singh et al. 2021; Agrawal, Saha et al. 2020).

The plasma optical biosensor is based on a special optical fiber structure such as U-bent optical fiber (Luo et al. 2019), tapered fiber-optic structure (Arjmand et al. 2017), multicore fiber (MCF) (May-Arrioja and Guzman-Sepulveda 2017), etc. Obviously, they have the characteristics of economy, remote access, high sensitivity, strong corrosion resistance, strong robustness, and so on. In the future, it is expected that a highly sensitive biomolecular sensor with remote access, that is easy to operate, has strong portability, and has fast response for various microorganisms like cancerous cells will be developed (Luo et al. 2019; Alizadeh et al. 2019; Martucci et al. 2015; Lin et al. 2019; Ravikumar et al. 2018; Yuan et al. 2018; Punjabi, Satija, and Mukherji 2015; Janik et al. 2018; Zhou et al. 2018).

As for special fiber-optic structure, in particular, Luo et al. have found the excellent sensing performance of the U-shaped fiber, and based on the specific structure, successfully applied it to detect cancer cells by evaluating N-glycan expression (Luo et al. 2019). However, it is difficult to overcome bending loss and radiation loss in the application of similar structures. Subsequently, researchers need to turn their attention to some new optical fiber structures, typical of which is multicore optical fiber (MCF). This fiber structure is more favorable for the coupling of light waves due to smaller fiber spacing that is helpful to enhance the response signal of the sensing probe. Meanwhile, owing to its special structure, it is possible to make a more complex fiber fusion structure. For example, an SMF-MCF structure is very sensitive to the limited supermodes excited by the light field on account of its axial symmetry that provides the basis for the fabrication of supersensitive biosensing probes. In other practical detection, applications like vibration (Villatoro et al. 2017), bending (Villatoro et al. 2016), as well as RI (Zhang et al. 2017) also play a significant role.

This chapter introduces a micro-platform based on MCF structure for detecting microorganisms. There are two kinds of probes, MCF and SMF are fused together as probe 1, and probe 2 is treated with hydrofluoric acid on the basis of probe 1. By comparing with the sensing performance of the two probes mentioned, the results show that probe 2 presents stronger sensing characteristics after being etching due to the reduction of the cladding diameter, and the coupling efficiency of the supermodel is greatly enhanced. To this end, as for probe 2, the sensing region was modified with NMs to make an LSPR probe for detection of various live cancer cells from, like MCF-7 (human breast), A549 (human lung), HepG2 (human liver), Hepa1 6 (mouse liver), as well as normal cells like NCF cell lines (a kind of canine fibroblasts), and LO2 (in human liver) for comparison. The results showed excellent selectivity and sensitivity to specific analytes.

Similarly, in this chapter, *Shigella*, also famous for a kind of gram-negative bacteria, is one of the main causes of intestinal infections in human beings, along with stomach cramps, vomiting, nausea, and diarrhea. There is a high incidence of *Shigella* in countries and regions where there is poor sanitation and people are suffering with several diseases (Xiao et al. 2014).

There are various detection methods for bacteria, such as serological detection, bacterial culture, polymerase chain reaction (PCR), which is a traditional detection method, has been popular and widely promoted for many decades (Huang et al. 2011; Mao et al. 2006; Mokhtari et al. 2013; Wu et al. 2012; Xiao et al. 2014). But, with the development of clinical trials, its application is limited due to many different conditions. First, the detection response time is too long, which will undoubtedly have a bad effect on the progress of follow-up diagnosis, and even on the early treatment. Second, because of the complexity of the process and the need to provide large equipment, professionals will increase the cost of the regional testing, although it is already very high. Additionally, the sensitivity and specificity need to be further improved. Therefore, it is a task for researchers to develop a simple, self-testing, time-consuming, high-sensitivity detection method for *Shigella* and other bacteria, and the optical fiber-based biosensor seems to be a step in the right direction (Srinivasan et al. 2017; Xiao et al. 2014; Zainuddin et al. 2018). By the fluorescence labeling method, Xiao et al. (2014) have proven that the detection signal is related to the specific hybridization reaction of the probe to the surface, showing that the sensing principle is feasible.

On the one hand, the fiber-optic local surface plasmon resonance (LSPR) sensing platform on the grounds of absorption has a bright future by combining the concept of plasma with optical fiber, because it is economical, disposable, cost-effective, and real-time responsive, and can be put into practice. With the development of nanotechnology, the biosensing technique has widespread use in pioneering and interdisciplinary research, containing the real sample test of bacterial cells. In biosensing applications, nanoparticles such as AuNPs and molybdenum disulfide (MoS_2-NPs) as an intensive study have been investigated thoroughly. On the other hand, because the superior properties of MoS_2-NPs, such as electron mobility, high spacing volume ratio and thermal stability, low toxicity, free sulfur group with hydrophobic effect, etc., they have attracted the scientific community's interest in the application of its lower full width at half maximum (FWHM) for biosensing (Zeng et al. 2015) (Nayak, Maharana, and Jha 2017). Based on that, Kaushik et al. reported a MoS_2-NPs characterized optical fiber SPR biosensor for specificity control against *Escherichia coli* (Kaushik et al. 2019). The immunosensor was prepared by probing the wavelength and fixing the *E. coli* monoclonal antibody, and the connection between the sensor and the quantity of *E. coli* was linear. It is nonspecific to other bacteria and has shown practical applications in real samples such as water and orange juice. In addition, Halkare and others have developed AuNPs-based LSPR biosensors that detect *E. coli* using phages as recognition units (Halkare et al. 2015). Because bacteriophages react with specific strains, the sensor can only be used to detect specific strains.

Plasma technology has been gaining prevalence in the field of sensing over the past few decades and has shown great research vitality and potential (Maharana, Bharadwaj, and Jha 2013; Maharana, Srivastava, and Jha 2014). In the last decade, as an important branch of plasma technology, the combination of LSPR and optical fiber technology has attracted much attention (Nayak, Parhi, and Jha 2016; Ben Haddada et al. 2017; Jans and Huo 2012; Agrawal, Saha et al. 2020; Jans and Huo 2012). To further explore the potential of this cross-technology, nanotechnology was introduced subsequently. Nanotechnology, as a golden key to biotech, has been studied as various nanoparticles are used in biosensing technology. For instance, molybdenum disulfide (MoS_2) has good hydrophilicity, heat stability, high surface volume ratio, and conductivity (Kaushik et al. 2019; Zeng et al. 2015; Nayak, Maharana, and Jha 2017). Based on that, Kaushik et al. (2019) have reported a biosensor platform using SPR to quantitively test *Escherichia coli*. Similarly, Halkare et al. (2015) have developed a new type of LSPR sensor using phage as a specific receptor for detection of *E. coli*.

In this chapter, a plasma-based biosensor platform for quantitative *Shigella* detection has been discussed properly. According to the splicing treatment toward the MCF and SMF, the specific fiber structure was composed to a basic guided wave system as the sensor probe. On this basis, NMs like AuNPs and MoS_2 are fixed over the fiber surface in order to improve the sensing property. The results of quantitative detection toward *Shigella* were satisfying, and in reaction time (less than 5 minutes) there was a rapid decrease of the detection limit (1.56 CFU/mL) within a linear range of $1 \sim 10^9$ CFU/mL.

9.2 SPR-BASED SENSORS

Based on SPR technology, various kinds of multifunctional cancer detection platforms have been developed that have strong robustness and can be reused. For example, for detecting prostate antigens, a microcontact imprinted biosensor chip has been successfully developed. The researchers used α-α′-azoiso-butyronitrile and ethylene glycol dimetharylate as cross-linking agents to successfully modify the methacrylic acid functional monomers on the surface of the sensing region, which can be stored stably for a long time. Concerning the quantity test of cancer mammary cells 916delTT and 6174delT from the exosome, a graphene oxide (GO)-layer-coated fiber-optic biosensor platform was designed based on SPR. The optical fiber sensing platform is prepared by sequentially fixing gold nanoparticles (AuNPs), graphene oxide layer, and analyte layer with the help of high RI prism (Dilsiz 2020; Hossain et al. 2020). In addition, a fiber-optic platform based on SPR has been developed for the detection of cancer mammary cells, according to the biomarker like HER2, and immobilized on 50 nm of Au layer (Loyez et al. 2021).

9.3 LSPR-BASED SENSORS

LSPR technique has been widely used in cancer cell detection toward various types of cancer cells, like cervical cell lines, hepatocellular carcinoma, prostate carcinoma, and colon that can be realized through the interaction of noble materials like AuNPs, Ag-NPs and NMs such as GO (Macfarlane and Murphy 2010; Wang et al. 2016), and two-dimensional nanocomposites like carbon nitride (g-C_3N_4), zinc oxide (ZnO) nanowires (Kim, Park, and Lee 2019). According to the LSPR technique, the researchers successfully functionalized Au nanorods and oligonucleotide aptamers into a biosensor system that can monitor the overexpression of Mucin-1 protein in a variety of cancers (Li et al. 2016). The LSPR colorimetric aptasensor using AuNPs modifies specific protein biomarkers to detect disparate cancer mammary cells, such as MCF-7 and MDA-MB-231 (Ahirwar and Nahar 2016), PSA, CEA, and α-fetoprotein (Xiao et al. 2017).

Guo et al. used a metal organic framework (MOF) combined with Ag nanoclusters and electrochemical (EC) analysis to quantitatively detect carcinoembryonic antigen (CEA), as shown in Figure 9.1(a). It is found that the porous material with MOF Zr-uio-66 has thermal stability, including high spacing volume ratio, and shows good RSD value (less than 5%) (Guo et al. 2017).

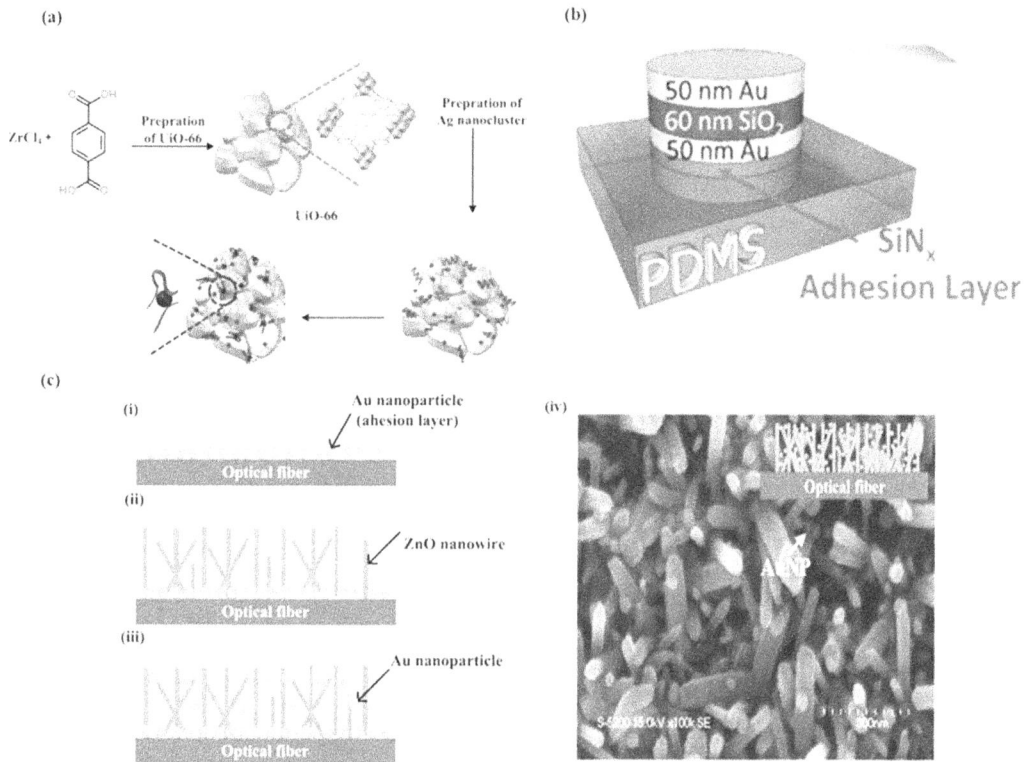

FIGURE 9.1 LSPR-based biosensing platform configuration: (a) flow of work about the AgNCs@Apt@UiO-66-immobilization of the aptasensor (Guo et al. 2017); (b) central device using MIM nanodisk for A549 detection, discussed in Chang et al, (2018); (c) synthesizing steps about ZnO nanowires including (i) monodispersed AuNPs on silica fiber surface, (ii) ZnO nanowire over AuNPs layer, (iii) ZnO nanowires functionalized using AuNPs, and (iv) SEM images of AuNPs immobilized over ZnO nanowires referred from Kim et al. (2019).

Source: Reprinted with permission from *Biosensors & Bioelectronics.* Copyright, 2022, Elsevier (Kaur, Kumar, and Kaushik 2022).

Polydimethylsiloxane, which has excellent transparency, acid resistance and bio-inertia, was used to create a metal insulated sandwich LSPR sensing platform for detection of lung cancer in A549 cancerous cells (Chang et al. 2018). Two-dimensional nanocomposite of carbon nitride (g-C_3N_4), as an excellent 2D material, has a structure similar to GO. Duan et al. synthesized a kind of nanocomposite material composed of g-C_3N_4, MoS_2-QDs and AuNPs stabilized by chitosan through experiments and found its plasma properties. The sensor based on the composite nanomaterial is used for PSA-specific detection (Duan et al. 2018).

Other innovative methods, such as the use of a switch connector in the sensor system, help to achieve the corresponding signal amplification (Hahn et al. 2019). Novel channels of microfluidic (MF) are added to enhance the sensing performance. Core-shell semiconductor quantum dots composed of cadmium sulfide and cadmium selenide are designed to be composed with some other NMs (Sasi et al. 2021). Besides the application of novel functional materials, the design of the basic structure of the probe is also a potential direction. The U-shaped optical fiber sensor, demonstrated in Figure 9.2(a), is designed for detection for N-glycan levels (Luo et al. 2019). Figure 9.2(b) shows a special optical fiber LSPR system with seven hexagonal cores based on multicore fiber. Copper oxide nanoflowers (CuO-NFs), AuNPs, and GO were modified on the surface of the sensing region, and then 2-deoxy-D-glucose was used as the sensing receptor to detect the cancer cells (Singh et al.

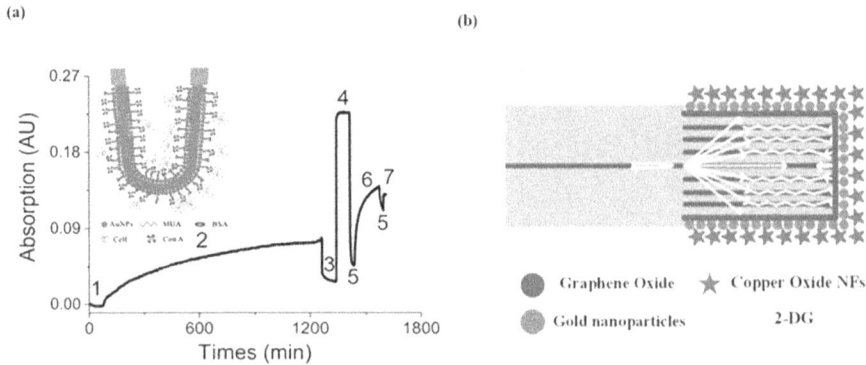

FIGURE 9.2   (a) Cytosensing-based U-shaped LSPR sensor using AuNPs for cancer cell lines (Luo et al. 2019), (b) multicore fiber sensor (Singh et al. 2020).

Source: Reprinted with permission from *Biosensors & Bioelectronics.* Copyright, 2022, Elsevier (Kaur, Kumar, and Kaushik 2022).

2020). Loyez et al. showed a special tilted grating structure for specific detection of the mammaglobin protein on the outer layer of cancer mammary cells (Loyez et al. 2020).

9.4   MULTICORE FIBER SENSOR FOR CANCER CELLS DETECTION

9.4.1   Material and Method

9.4.1.1   Material

In order to fabricate a SMF-MCF fiber structure, conventional single-mode fiber (SMF) and MCF are used for further splicing treatment. All NMs, like AuNPs, GO, and CuO-NFs, can be synthesized in the lab. According to the Turkevich method, which is very well-known, for the synthesis of AuNPs, trisodium citrate and gold (III) chloride trihydrate (hydrogen tetrachloroaurate) are used. As for the synthesis of CuO-NFs, copper(II) nitrate, sodium hydroxide (NaOH), and ethanol are employed. To synthesize GO powder by Hummer's method, graphite flakes, sodium nitrate, sulfuric acid, and potassium permanganate ($KMnO_4$) are mainly used. Here, three steps of cleaning are using acetone, piranha solution (H_2O_2 mixed with H_2SO_4, 3:7), and water. Then 3-(trimethoxysilyl)propyl methacrylate solution (silane agent), and (3-mercaptopropyl)trimethoxy silane (MPTMS) act as coupling reagents for the process of coating of CuO-NFs, AuNPs, and GO over SMF-MCF fiber structure. To functionalize the 2-DG over NMs-coated optical fiber structure, used the 11-mercaptoundecanoic acid (MUA), N-(3-Dimethylaminopropyl)-N′-ethylcarbodiimide hydrochloride (EDC), N-Hydroxysuccinimide (NHS), and phosphate-buffered saline (PBS).

9.4.1.2   Fabrication of the Sensor Probe

This section shows a schematic for the fabrication of a bioprobe through an SMF-MCF structure, as shown in Figure 9.3. The main distribution of MCF is particularly beneficial to the modulation of coupling coefficient of the coupling cores, which is composed of an intermediate core and six identical cores arranged in a hexagonal pattern (May-Arrioja and Guzman-Sepulveda 2017; Villatoro et al. 2016). In the following part, the development process for fiber fusion splicing is briefly described. The MCF and SMF are cut to approximately 1 mm ~ 5 mm by precision cutting machine. Then MCF and SMF are spliced together through a fusion splicer machine. It should be noted that the splicing loss should be less than 0.1 dB to ensure the efficiency of coupling.

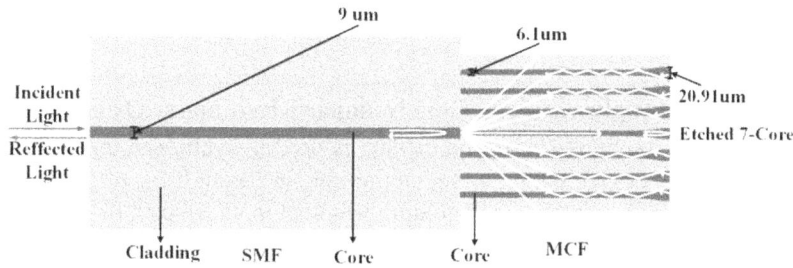

FIGURE 9.3   Splicing and etching of SMF-MCF-based sensor structure.

Source: Reprinted with permission from *Biosensors & Bioelectronics.* Copyright, 2020, Elsevier (Singh et al. 2020).

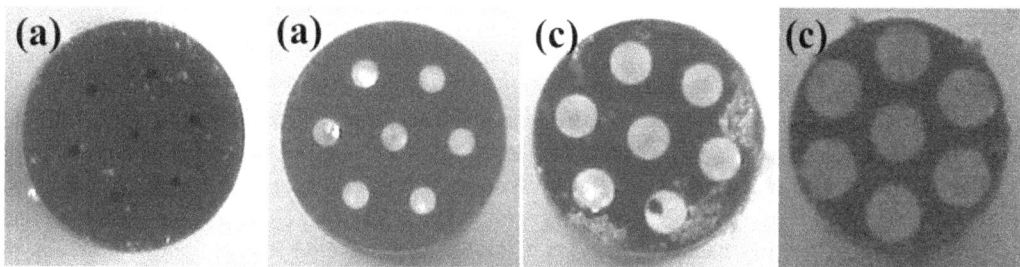

FIGURE 9.4   Cross section of multicore fiber (a) before etching, etching treated (b) 6 minutes, (c) 10 minutes, and (d) 15 minutes.

Source: Reprinted with permission from *Biosensors & Bioelectronics.* Copyright, 2020, Elsevier (Singh et al. 2020).

9.4.1.3   Etching of SMF-MCF Structure

During the fabrication process of the SMF-MCF structure (sensor probe), the polymer coating is removed with the help of fiber stripper. Thereafter for etching at room temperature, the SMF-MCF structure was soaked in a 48% HF solution for the purpose of removing the cladding part and widening the cores of MCF fiber. It helps in the coupling of modes as well as exposes the EWs outside the cladding. The MCF fiber was immersed in a glass beaker containing an HF solution for 6 minutes, 10 minutes, and 15 minutes. Care should be taken such that only the cladding end facet of MCF fiber should be in contact with the acid. Then, the fiber is removed from the acid and rinsed by ethanol. The CCD images about before and after etching of a cross section of an MCF structure are illustrated in Figure 9.4. It can be observed that the material (germanium) of the fiber core is first washed into HF acid. The diameter of the core of the MCF structure is widened, and the diameter of the outer cladding has been reduced due to etching. The MCF structure of the sparsely placed core is more appropriate for the coupling of modes. The modes of SMF are coupled into seven cores of MCF structure. The integrity of the optical fiber structure is ensured by controlling the etching treatment.

9.4.1.4   Characterization

The AuNPs solution was diluted and then put into a quartz cuvette. The absorption spectra of AuNPs can be determined by UV-Vis spectrophotometer. The microscopic shape and distribution of AuNPs in solution can be observed and recorded by transmission electron microscopy (TEM), while the energy distribution can be observed by TEM-energy-dispersive spectroscopy (EDS). The TEM image illustrated the shape and size, and the AuNP dimension can be analyzed by using

ImageJ software. The analysis method of GO, CuONFs is similar to AuNPs and can be followed accordingly.

9.4.1.5 Synthesis of Graphene Oxide/Gold Nanoparticles/Copper Oxide Nanoflowers

According to protocol, modified Hummer's method is used to synthesize the GO (Kumar et al. 2020). For the synthesis of GO, 0.25 g of sodium nitrate, included, 0.5 g of graphite flakes were mixed in 11.5 mL of H_2SO_4 solution. This mixture was kept in an ice bath (0–5°C) with 1 hour of stirred treatment. Afterward, 1.5 g of potassium permanganate was added carefully as a mixture solution under vigorous stirring. The solution was mixed in an ice bath at 15°C or lower. The ice bath was removed after the addition of oxidant, and further solution was treated for stirring at 35°C for 2 hours. Then, solution was diluted with 250 mL of ultrapure water. Next, it was kept at 98°C for 15 minutes. The brownish color appears after 15 minutes. To stop the reaction, 2.5 mL of H_2O_2 and 250 mL of deionized (DI) water were slowly injected. Then the solution turns brown to yellowish, which primarily affirms the synthesis of GO. The prepared solution was given a filtration using the centrifugation process (4000 rpm/min for 2 minutes). During centrifugation, GO particles were settled down, and excess water was removed from solution. Thereafter, the remaining solution was washed twice with 5% HCl and the same processing with ultrapure water to dispose the sulfate and chloride ions to get the neutral gel-like substance. Further, after 6 hours of baking processing at 60°C, the gel-like substance was obtained, and GO powder was obtained using pestle mortar.

The Turkevich method is widely used to synthesize AuNPs colloidal solution (Turkevich et al. 1951). The chloroauric acid (150 μL, 100 mM) is mixed with DI water (14.85 mL) in glassware and heated using magnetic stirrer until reaching a boil. When the solution starts to boil, 1.8 mL of 38 mM trisodium citrate are added into a boiled solution under stirring for the reduction process. The resultant solution appears red after 5–10 minutes, which primarily confirms the synthesis of 10 nm AuNPs. Similarly, 30 nm, 50 nm, and 70 nm AuNPs were synthesized per protocol discussed in Shah et al. (2015). For 30-nm AuNPs, trisodium citrate with 1 mL of 38.8 mM was used, and the synthesized solution's color appeared as dull red after synthesis. For 50-nm AuNPs, use 700 μL of 19.4 mM trisodium citrate, and then the resultant solution's color appears after synthesis. Thereafter, 70-nm AuNPs were synthesized by using 450 μL of 19.4 mM trisodium citrate, and the color of the solution appears as pink-purple after synthesis.

We synthesized CuO-NFs with the help of protocol as discussed in Sun et al. (2013). First, copper(II) nitrate (0.12 mM) was dissolved in 2 mL of ultrapure water using a magnetic stirrer at ambient temperature. Thereafter, 30 mL ethanol was added into the dissolved copper(II) nitrate solution and heated at 75°C for 2 minutes. Afterward, NaOH ethanolic solution (0.02 M) was added drop-wise under constant stirring. After 15 minutes, the generative solution was chilled at ambient temperature. Thereafter, the solution was centrifuged for 2 minutes at 10,000 rpm to get the CuO-NFs, and it was washed with ethanol and ultrapure water, twice using the centrifugation process. Then, precipitates were allowed to dry at 60°C, overnight. The following chemical reaction occurred during synthesis of CuO-NFs (Sun et al. 2013):

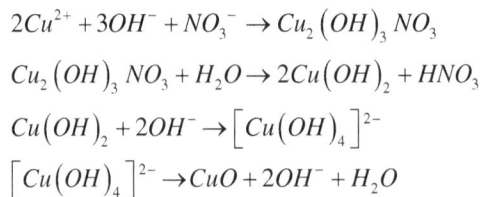

$$2Cu^{2+} + 3OH^- + NO_3^- \rightarrow Cu_2\left(OH\right)_3 NO_3$$

$$Cu_2\left(OH\right)_3 NO_3 + H_2O \rightarrow 2Cu\left(OH\right)_2 + HNO_3$$

$$Cu\left(OH\right)_2 + 2OH^- \rightarrow \left[Cu\left(OH\right)_4\right]^{2-}$$

$$\left[Cu\left(OH\right)_4\right]^{2-} \rightarrow CuO + 2OH^- + H_2O$$

9.4.1.6 Immobilization of GO/AuNPs/CuO-NFs Over SMF-MCF Structure

In simple terms, the GO aqueous solution is fully dispersed in an ultrasonic pulverizer to form a 1 mg/mL aqueous solution. The cleaned, uncoated fiber is then immersed in 5% ethanol silane for

30 minutes, and then it is placed in a drying chamber at 70°C for 30 minutes. Next, by the point dip method, the bare fibers are placed for 5 minutes in an aqueous solution of GO and baked for 30 minutes. Besides, the above-mentioned point dipping method is repeated three times, and the optical fiber is cleaned with DI water for further treatment.

The AuNPs-immobilization steps were laid out in detail in the previous chapters. For this, it is necessary to pay attention that after the immobilization process, the treated region of the probe needs to be thoroughly washed with ethanol for cluster protection between the unbonded AuNPs and immobilized AuNPs to affect the sensing performance (Kumar, Singh et al. 2021).

Wang et al. developed a technology for CuO-NFs immobilization (Wang et al. 2019). First, 1.5 mg/mL of CuO-NFs aqueous solution was prepared with solvent DI water as the dipping solution. Second, the GO/AuNPs-coated area was immersed in the dipping solution for 6 minutes, and next for 30 minutes was heated by being placed in a 70°C oven, and these steps were repeated three times. Finally, the unattached CuO-NFs were carefully cleaned from the fiber surface with DI water.

The steps of enzymatic functionalization have been described in detail in Chapter 8. The 2-DG solution is prepared with a concentration of (200 mg/mL) and dissolving by 1X PBS as the buffer solution.

9.4.1.7 Cell Culture

There were six kinds of normal cells and cancer cells including NCF, LO2, HepG2, Hepa 1–6, MCF-7, A549 in a humus environment with 5% CO_2, 10% fetal bovine serum, and 1% antibiotics. It is worth noting that Hepa 1–6 cells do not need 1% antibiotics because of their specificity. The cell count was obtained by diluting the 1X PBS solution from high to low concentrations from 1×10^2 to 1×10^6 cells/mL.

9.4.1.8 Experimental Setup

Figure 9.5 depicts the experimental setup. The fixed sensor probe is immersed in the sample and connected via bifurcated optical fiber to a spectrometer and light source. When the light source is

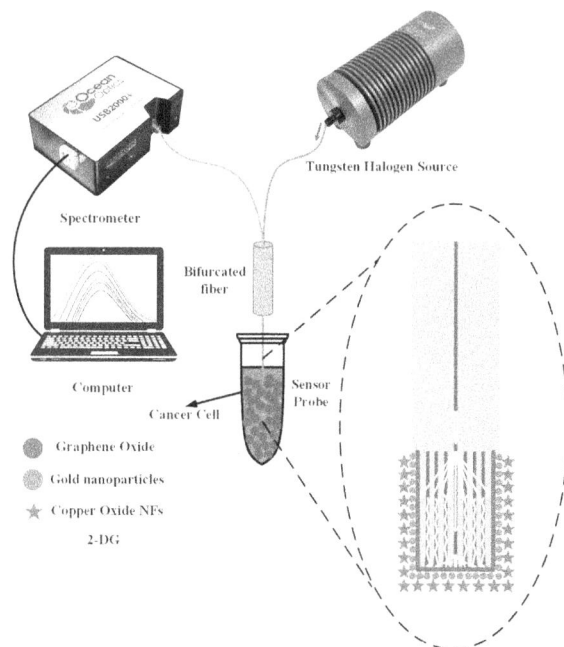

FIGURE 9.5 Experimental components for the quantity analysis of cancer cells.

Source: Reprinted with permission from *Biosensors & Bioelectronics.* Copyright, 2020, Elsevier (Singh et al. 2020).

turned on, the spectrometer collects the detected LSPR-based response signals from the sensing region and sends them to the computer in real time in the form of a reflection spectrum.

9.4.2 Results and Discussion

9.4.2.1 Optimization of Bare Sensor Structure

To improve the sensing probe's performance, the influencing factors such as the length of the MCF and the etching treatment time were investigated. As illustrated in Figure 9.6(a), as the MCF length increases, the effective path of the sensing area increases, resulting in an increase in reflected signal loss that is detrimental to the sensor's sensitivity enhancement. As a result, the etching time was determined using a 1-mm MCF detecting probe. In the reaction depicted in Figure 9.6(b), the reflection strength increases linearly with increasing etching time, owing to the reduction in cladding thickness. However, the enhancement effect of transmission intensity is very weak when the etching time exceeds 10 minutes, making 10 minutes the more economical and efficient etching time standard. On the basis of the experimental results, to complete the optical fiber probe structure, a length of 1-mm MCF can be selected as well as etching treatment for 10 minutes.

9.4.2.2 Characterization of Nanomaterials

With the help of the UV-Vis spectrophotometer, the energy spectra of the diluted gold nanoparticles of four particle sizes (~10 nm, 30 nm, 45 nm, and 70 nm) were obtained, and the absorption peaks visualized at 519 nm, 526 nm, 532 nm, and 550 nm, respectively, as shown in Figure 9.7. According to these results, GO and CuO-NFs with noninterfering absorption wavelength have excellent biocompatibility with immobilized AuNPs. Then, their microscopic distribution and nanometer size were investigated in the solution by using TEM and ImageJ software. From the results in Figure 9.8(a–d) and Figure 9.9, it can be seen clearly that the spherical nanoparticles have a smooth shape and a good diameter distribution. Figure 9.10(a) described the absorption spectra of GO. It was found that the absorption peaks appeared at ~230 and 310 nm. This indicates that $C = C$ bond transition absorption occurs at 230 nm, and $C = O$ bond energy transition occurs at 310 nm (Arumugam and Kim 2018). From 9.10(b), we can see that the GO nanopatch has obvious layer structure. At the same time, the micromorphology distribution of flower-shaped CuO-NFs can be clearly obtained from Figure 9.11. Finally, with the help of TEM-EDS, AuNPs, GO, and CuO-NFs were analyzed. The results in Figure 4.12(a–c) showed the presence of Au, C, and Cu, which means the coating method of AuNPs, GO, and CuO-NFs is successful.

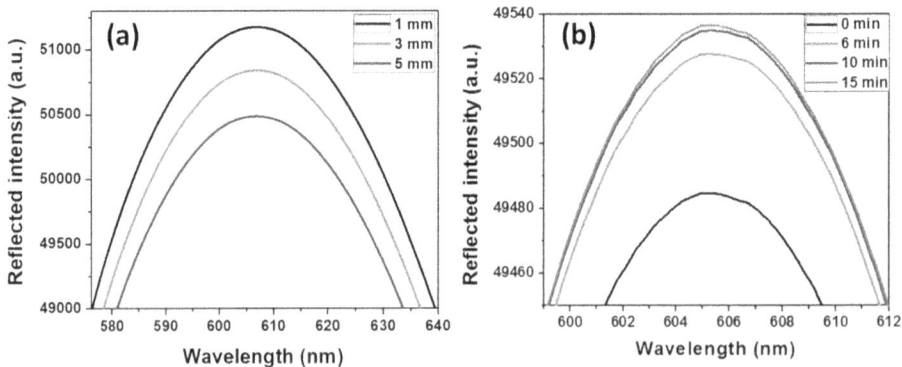

FIGURE 9.6 Variation of reflected intensities with respect to (a) length and (b) etching time of multicore fiber in SMF-MCF structure.

Source: Reprinted with permission from *Biosensors & Bioelectronics.* Copyright, 2020, Elsevier (Singh et al. 2020).

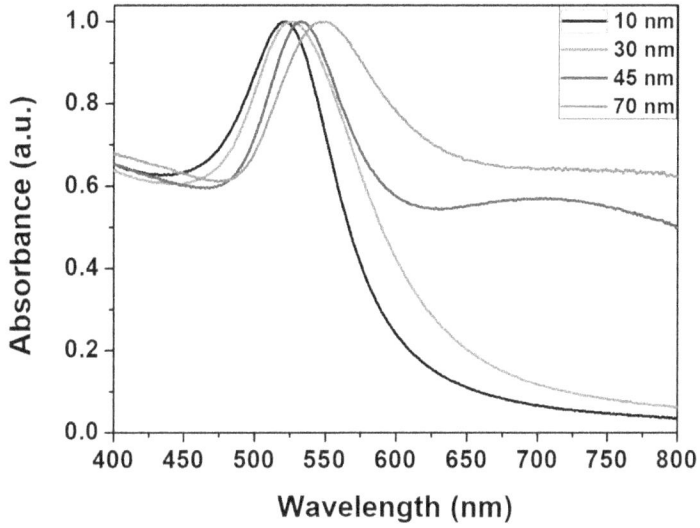

FIGURE 9.7 Absorbance spectrum of AuNPs.

Source: Reprinted with permission from *Biosensors & Bioelectronics.* Copyright, 2020, Elsevier (Singh et al. 2020).

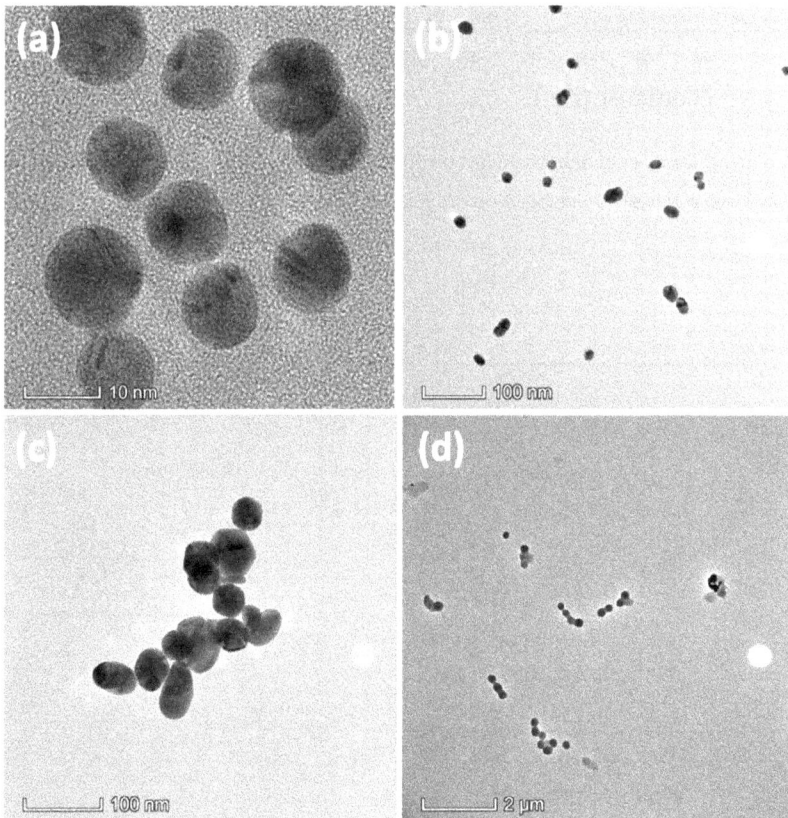

FIGURE 9.8 HRTEM images show AuNPs at different sizes: (a) 10 nm, (b) 30 nm, (c) 45 nm, and (d) 70 nm.

Source: Reprinted with permission from *Biosensors & Bioelectronics.* Copyright, 2020, Elsevier (Singh et al. 2020).

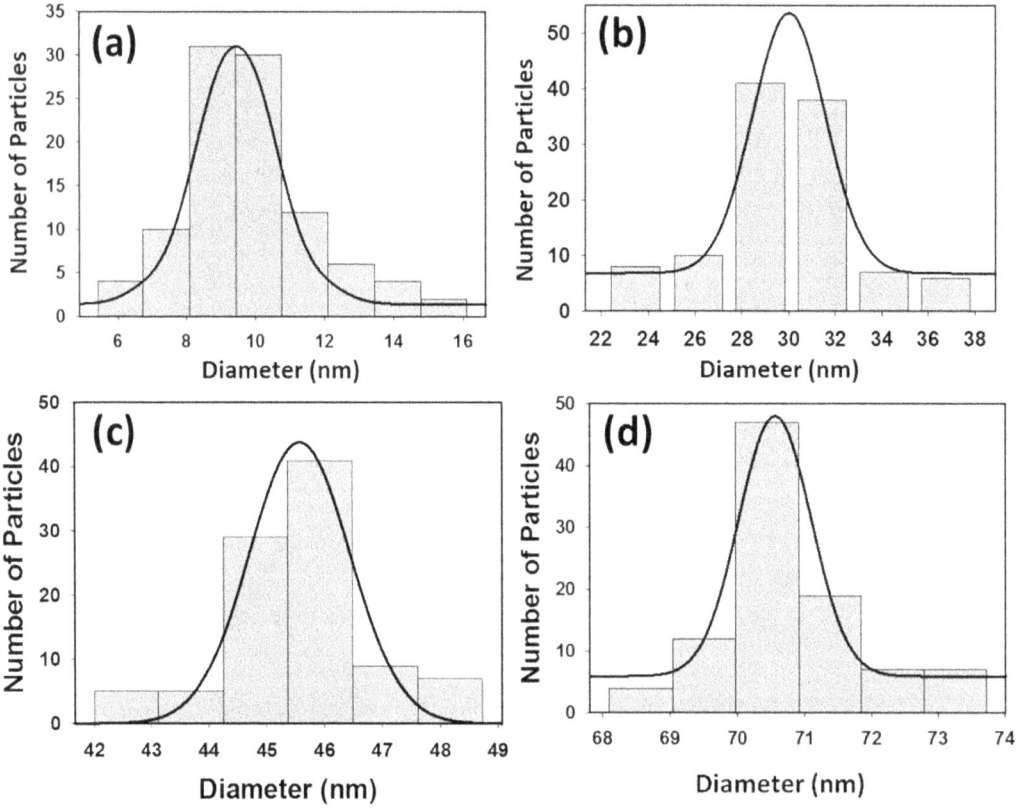

FIGURE 9.9 Histogram of gold nanoparticles: (a) 10 nm, (b) 30 nm, (c) 45 nm, and (d) 70 nm AuNPs.

Source: Reprinted with permission from *Biosensors & Bioelectronics.* Copyright, 2020, Elsevier (Singh et al. 2020).

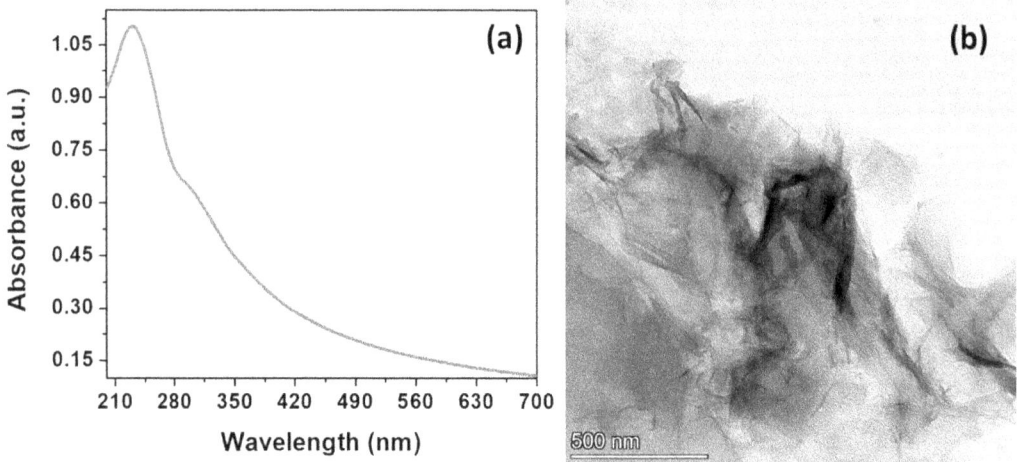

FIGURE 9.10 (a) Absorbance spectrum, (b) HRTEM image of graphene oxide.

Source: Reprinted with permission from *Biosensors & Bioelectronics.* Copyright, 2020, Elsevier (Singh et al. 2020).

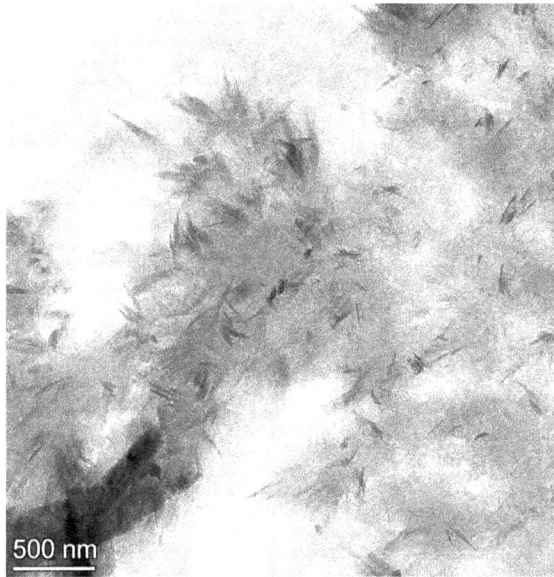

FIGURE 9.11 HRTEM image of copper oxide nanoparticles.

Source: Reprinted with permission from *Biosensors & Bioelectronics*. Copyright, 2020, Elsevier (Singh et al. 2020).

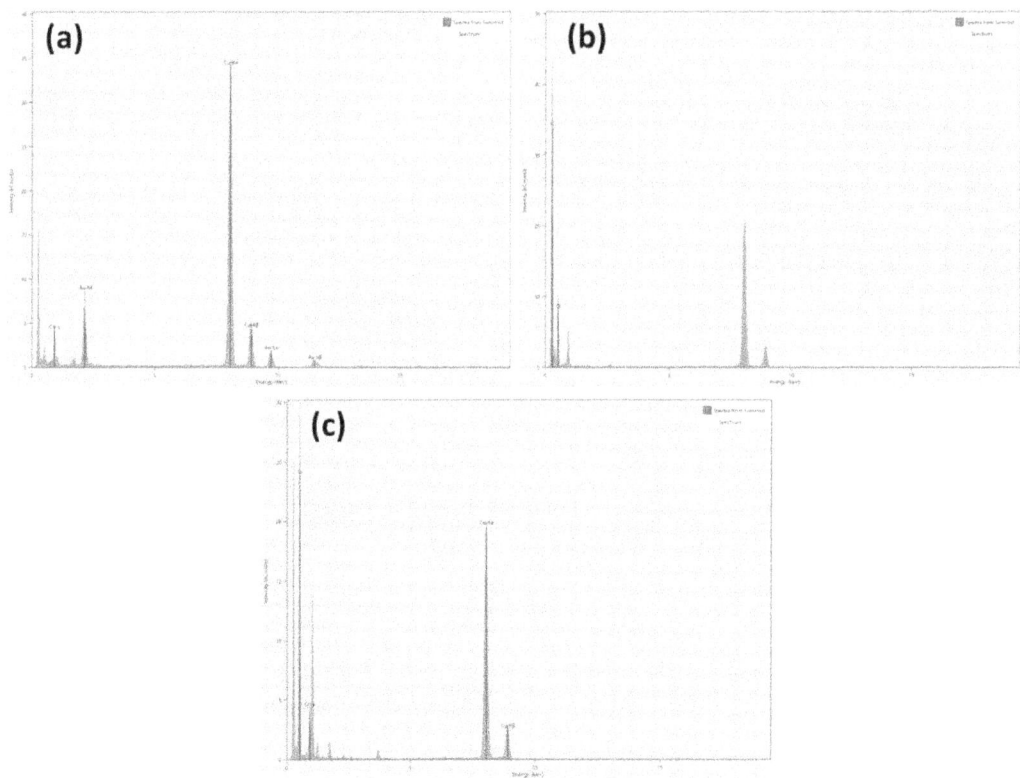

FIGURE 9.12 TEM-EDS analysis of (a) AuNPs, (b) GO, and (c) CuONFs nanomaterials clearly show the presence of Au, C, and Cu, respectively.

Source: Reprinted with permission from *Biosensors & Bioelectronics*. Copyright, 2020, Elsevier (Singh et al. 2020).

9.4.2.3   Characterization of Nanoparticles Coated Sensor Probes

Figures 9.13 and 9.15 show the high-resolution images of the SMF-MCF probe before and after etching, respectively. Figure 9.13 illustrates the surface of the sensing region. Figure 9.14 reveals the micromorphology of the SMF-MCF structure splicing process and the splicing loss evaluation from the fusion splicer. The morphologies of MCF after etching treatment can be visualized in Figure 9.15. Figure 9.15(c and d) show the surface morphology of the probe after NMs immobilization. Figure 9.15(e) is a SEM-EDS scan result to demonstrate the immobilization of NMs. The presence of Au, C, and Cu indicate AuNPs, and some kinds of NMs such as GO, and CuO-NFs over the probe surface.

To further optimize the fabrication process of the sensor, the nanoscale of AuNPs is selected. Four kinds of AuNPs sensors based on particle size of 10 nm, 30 nm, 45 nm, and 70 nm were used for quantitative determination of glucose. The results of four kinds of probes for detection of glucose concentration are shown in Figure 9.16(a–d). After statistical analysis, the absorbance efficiency of the four probes was summarized in Figure 9.17. We can obviously see that AuNPs bio-probes with particle size of 10 nm have better sensing performance; thus, 10 nm of AuNPs is chosen as the standard NMs for the coating process.

9.4.2.4   Detection of Cancerous Cells

The LSPR-based probe can achieve high sensitivity due to the specific coupling of the receptor to the specific analyte that results in a significant change in the peripheral RI. As a result, it is critical

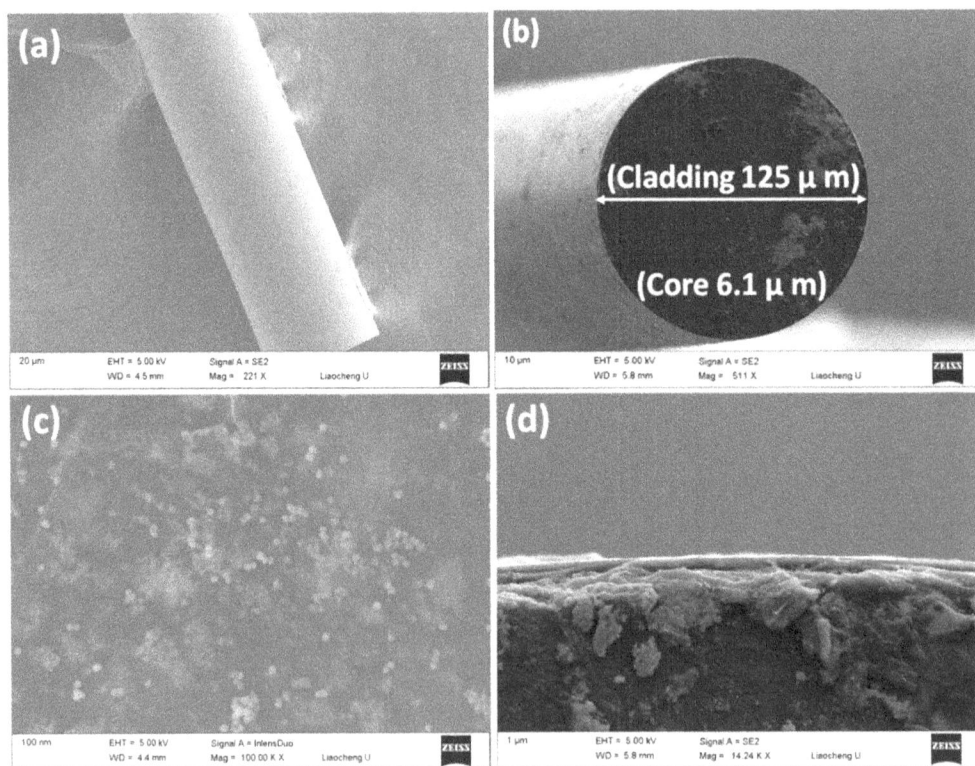

FIGURE 9.13   Scanning electron microscopic images of nonetched fiber with CuONFs/AuNPs/GO-NMs-coated—(a) SMF-MCF sensor structure (thickness 125 μm), (b) cross section of MCF, (c and d) CuONFs/AuNPs/GO-NMs over sensor structure.

Source: Reprinted with permission from *Biosensors & Bioelectronics.* Copyright, 2020, Elsevier (Singh et al. 2020).

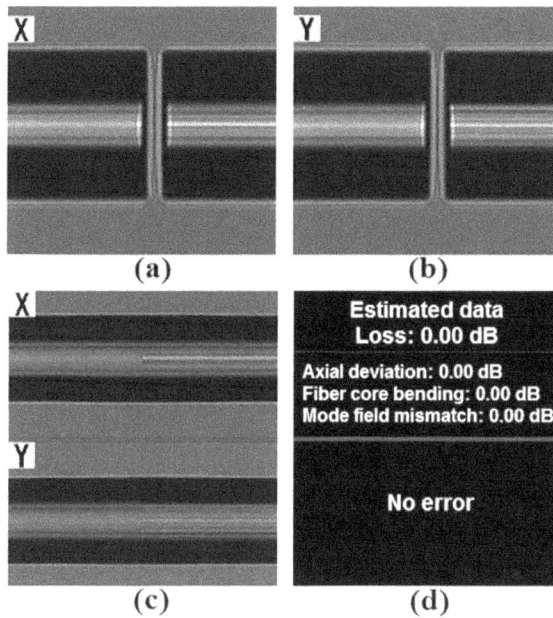

FIGURE 9.14 Spliced structure of SMF and MCF taken from splicer machine: (a) X-view before splicing, (b) Y-view before splicing, (c) after splicing, (d) estimated data of splicing.

Source: Reprinted with permission from *Biosensors & Bioelectronics.* Copyright, 2020, Elsevier (Singh et al. 2020).

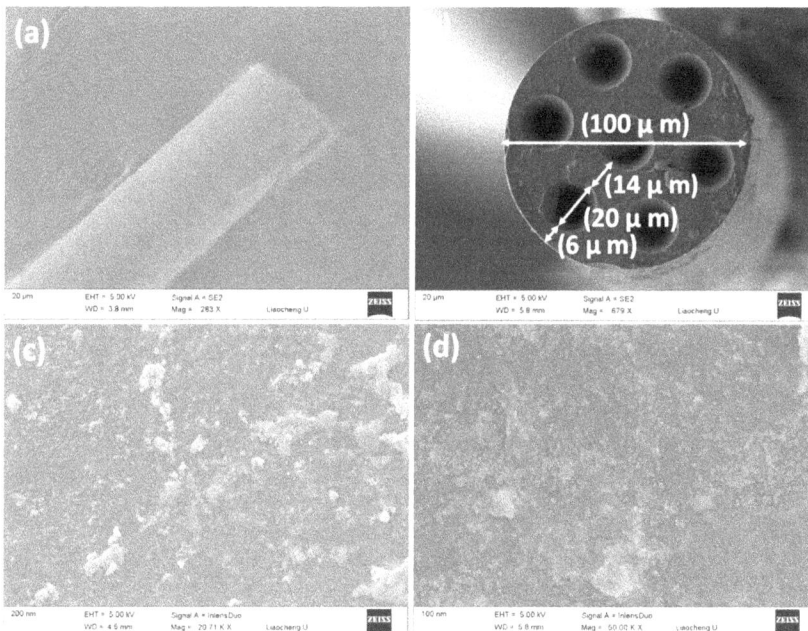

FIGURE 9.15 Scanning electron microscopic images of 10 minute-etched fiber with CuONFs/AuNPs/GO-NMs-coated: (a) SMF-MCF sensor structure (thickness 100 μm), (b) cross section of MCF, and (c and d) CuONFs/AuNPs/GO-NMs over sensor structure. (e) SEM-EDS of CuONFs/AuNPs/GO-NMs-coated SMF-MCF structure. Au, C, and Cu clearly show the presence of AuNPs, GO, and CuO-NFs nanomaterials on sensor structure.

Source: Reprinted with permission from *Biosensors & Bioelectronics.* Copyright, 2020, Elsevier (Singh et al. 2020).

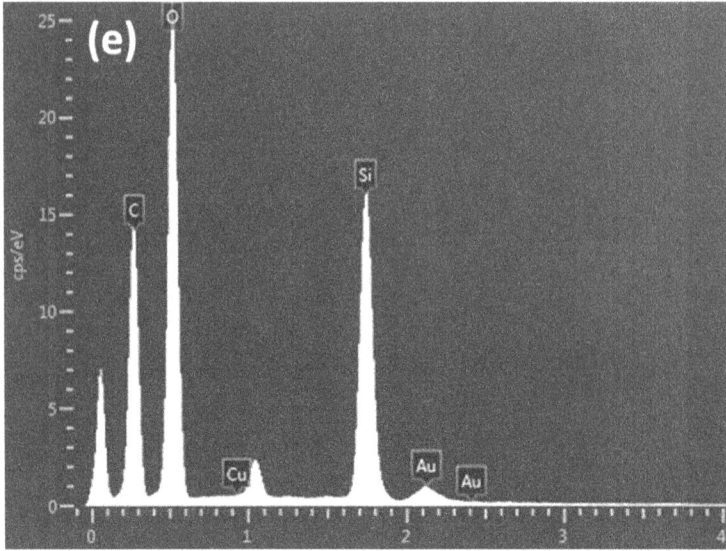

FIGURE 9.15 (Continued)

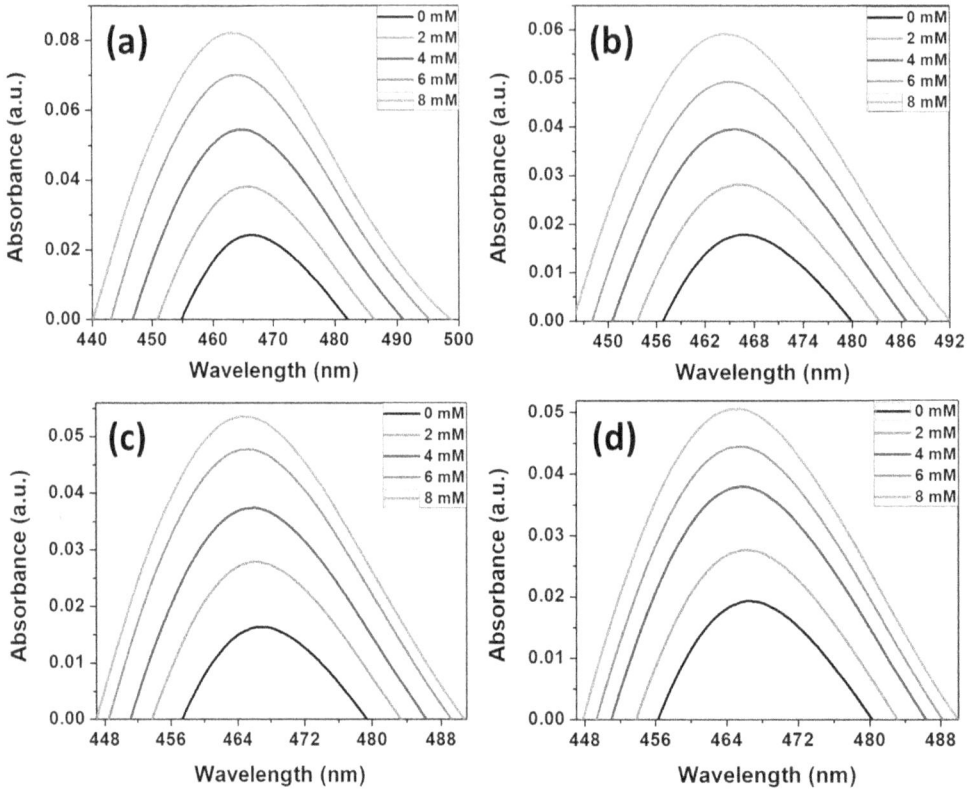

FIGURE 9.16 Detection of glucose using different sizes of gold nanoparticles-based glucose oxidase sensor probe (a) CuONFs/10 nm AuNPs/GO, (b) CuONFs/30 nm AuNPs/GO, (c) CuONFs/45 nm AuNPs/GO, (d) CuONFs/70 nm AuNPs/GO.

Source: Reprinted with permission from *Biosensors & Bioelectronics.* Copyright, 2020, Elsevier (Singh et al. 2020).

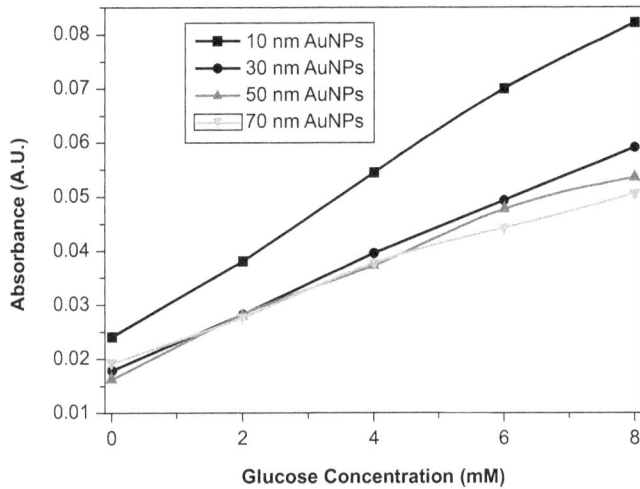

FIGURE 9.17 Analysis of the different sizes of gold nanoparticles and glucose oxidase-functionalized sensor probe, showing absorbance variation with 10 nm AuNPs is high.

Source: Reprinted with permission from *Biosensors & Bioelectronics.* Copyright, 2020, Elsevier (Singh et al. 2020).

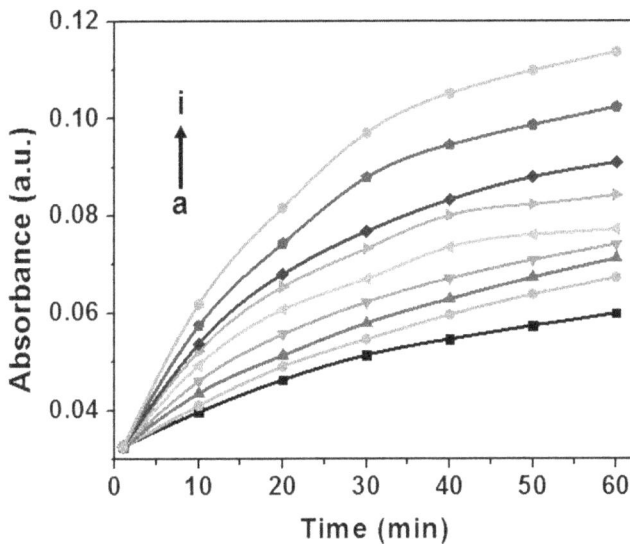

FIGURE 9.18 Detection of HePG$_2$ cells: (a–i): 1×10^2, 5×10^2, 1×10^3, 5×10^3, 1×10^4, 5×10^4, 1×10^5, 5×10^5, 1×10^6 cells/mL using CuONFs/AuNPs/GO-NMs coated etched fiber sensor for the duration of 60 minutes.

Source: Reprinted with permission from *Biosensors & Bioelectronics.* Copyright, 2020, Elsevier (Singh et al. 2020).

to investigate the effect of probe detection time on absorption efficiency as shown in Figure 9.18. The results demonstrate unequivocally that at this point in time, 60 minutes, samples of different cell numbers can be obtained for maximum light intensity differentiation. As a result, in order to minimize the loss of cell activity and test efficiency, it was decided to run all cyto-testing experiments for 60 minutes.

The abrupt fusion structure of SMF-MCF can enhance the stacking effect of the MCF isolated linear polarization mode, and etching of the MCF structure can amplify this effect even further. The results indicate that the etched fiber probes exhibit increased linearity that may be a result of the thinner cladding facilitating the coupling of surface signals back to the fiber core, thereby improving sensing performance (May-Arrioja and Guzman-Sepulveda 2017).

Because the CuONFs and GO have a large spacing volume ratio, they cover the entire surface of the probe, facilitating cancer cell adsorption. Additionally, it is compatible with AuNPs and provides an excellent platform for AuNPs to stimulate the specific LSPR phenomenon, thereby improving the stability and sensitivity of MCF etched optical fiber for cancer cell detection.

Compared to the results of Figure 9.19(a and b) and Figure 9.21(a and b), the etch-treated probes showed an obviously similar pattern in samples from HEPG2 cells and MCF-7 cells. That is, compared with the unetched probe in Figure 9.21(a and b), the sample with the cell concentration showed a lower absorbance. It can also be seen from these results that normally etched probes have a lower transmittance due to a decrease in their effective surface area, but the surface EWs and cancer cell have strong interaction on the probe surface, generating a numerically compensated absorbance. This indicates that the performance of the probe is not decreased due to the decrease of its effective surface area and the total amount of NMs coating, even if in the detection of HePG2 cells they have significantly enhanced sensing.

To explore performance behavior in the different cell samples, two kinds of normal cell samples (NCF and LO2) were selected, and the test results are demonstrated in Figure 9.22(a and b), respectively. As for this end, various types of cancerous cells are selected and compared as displayed in Figure 9.20. From these results, the absorbance of all the test concentrations was under 55%, which was lower than that of cancer cells. The explanation is that cancer cells have more GLUT receptors than normal cells, and these receptors can undergo specific binding to the coated 2-DG sensing region, causing strong RI perturbations that are sensed by the probe (Luo et al. 2019; Zhang et al. 2014).

Utilizing the sensor probe, the relationship between the absorption peak and the number of cancer cells can be described by the following formula in nine pre-set samples from the range of 100 to million cells (Figure 9.19[a]), peak absorbance $= 0.0323 + 0.0122\ x$, where x is the logarithmic scale of the number of cancer cells (cells/mL).

9.4.2.5   Analysis of Reusability, Selectivity, and Anti-Interference Ability

Reusability is a crucial index to evaluate the potential of biosensors. The absorbance of a sample with the same pre-set cell number is recorded after repeated detection. It is important to pay attention to the probe that should be carefully cleaned after each test with PBS to prevent any impact on results. Figure 9.23(a) reflects the results of two repeated tests of the same probe on two pre-set samples (100,000 and 500,000 cells). It was revealed that there is no remarkable change in the two data curves, which shows that the developed sensor probe has the potential for reusability.

Selectivity of the sensor probe is also crucial. As shown in Figure 9.23(b), HepG2 hepatoma cells of 5×10^6 cells/mL is selected as the blank group, and LO2 healthy hepatocytes of different concentrations (5×10^4, 1×10^5, and 5×10^5 cells/mL) are added as a control group. The results are clear that the change of the absorbance of the control group is not obvious (up to 1.7%), which shows that the sensor developed has good selectivity to LO2 cells.

For exploring the anti-interference ability of the sensor, the samples containing different concentrations of jamming were measured. Therefore, fetal bovine serum (FBS) was selected as the

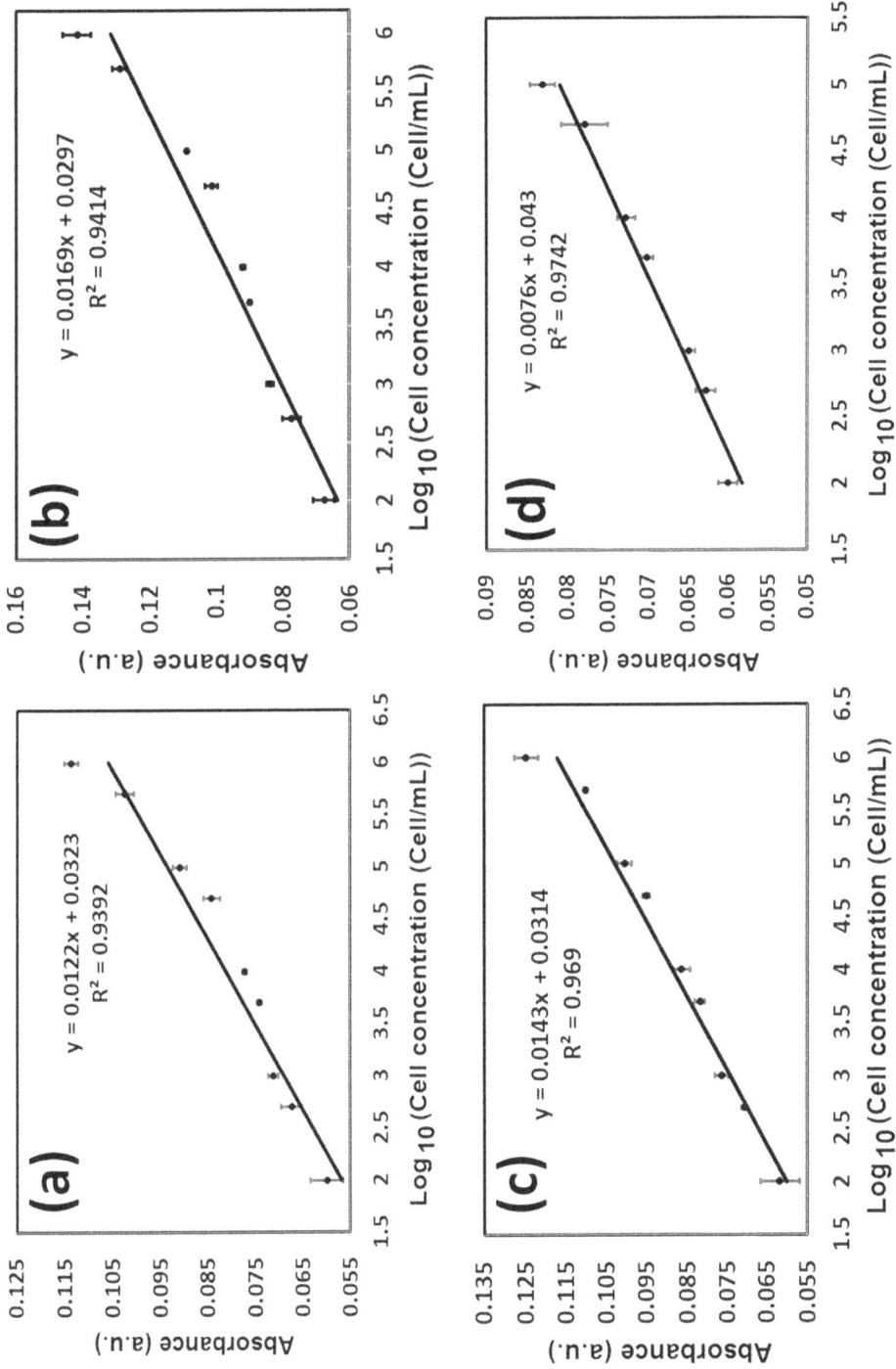

FIGURE 9.19 Linearity plot of cancerous cell detection by etched fiber (a) HepG2, (b) MCF 7, (c) Hepa1–6, and (d) A549.

Source: Reprinted with permission from *Biosensors & Bioelectronics.* Copyright, 2020, Elsevier (Singh et al. 2020).

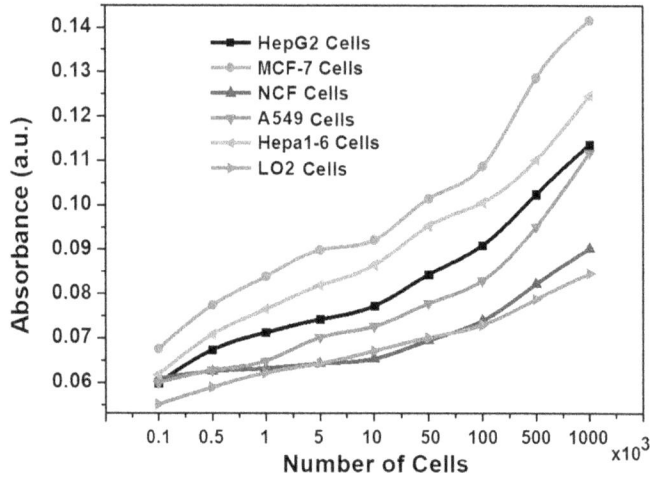

FIGURE 9.20 A comparative plot of sensing results of different types of cancer cells and normal cells using a proposed sensor.

Source: Reprinted with permission from *Biosensors & Bioelectronics.* Copyright, 2020, Elsevier (Singh et al. 2020).

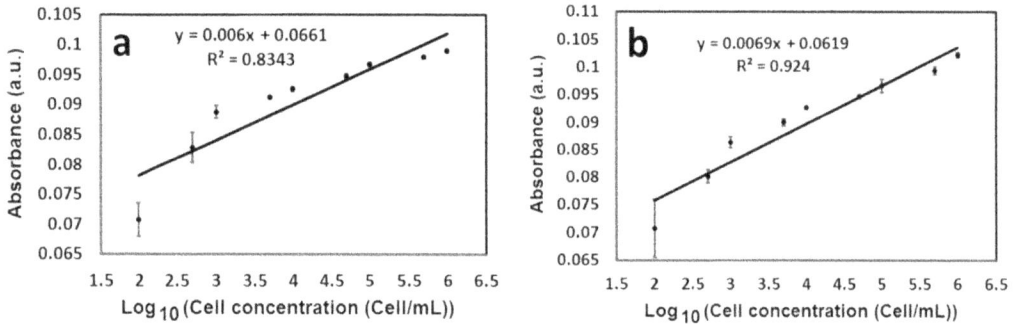

FIGURE 9.21 Linearity plot of cancerous cell detection by nonetched fiber: (a) HepG2 and (b) MCF 7.

Source: Reprinted with permission from *Biosensors & Bioelectronics.* Copyright, 2020, Elsevier (Singh et al. 2020).

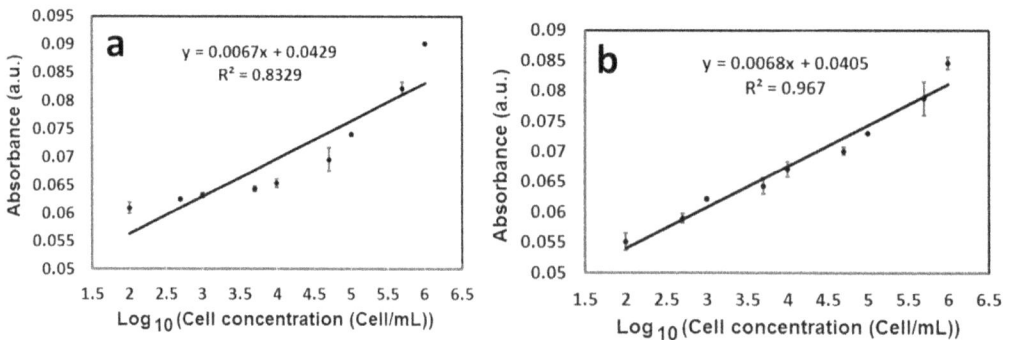

FIGURE 9.22 Linearity plot of normal cell detection: (a) NCF and (b) LO2.

Source: Reprinted with permission from *Biosensors & Bioelectronics.* Copyright, 2020, Elsevier (Singh et al. 2020).

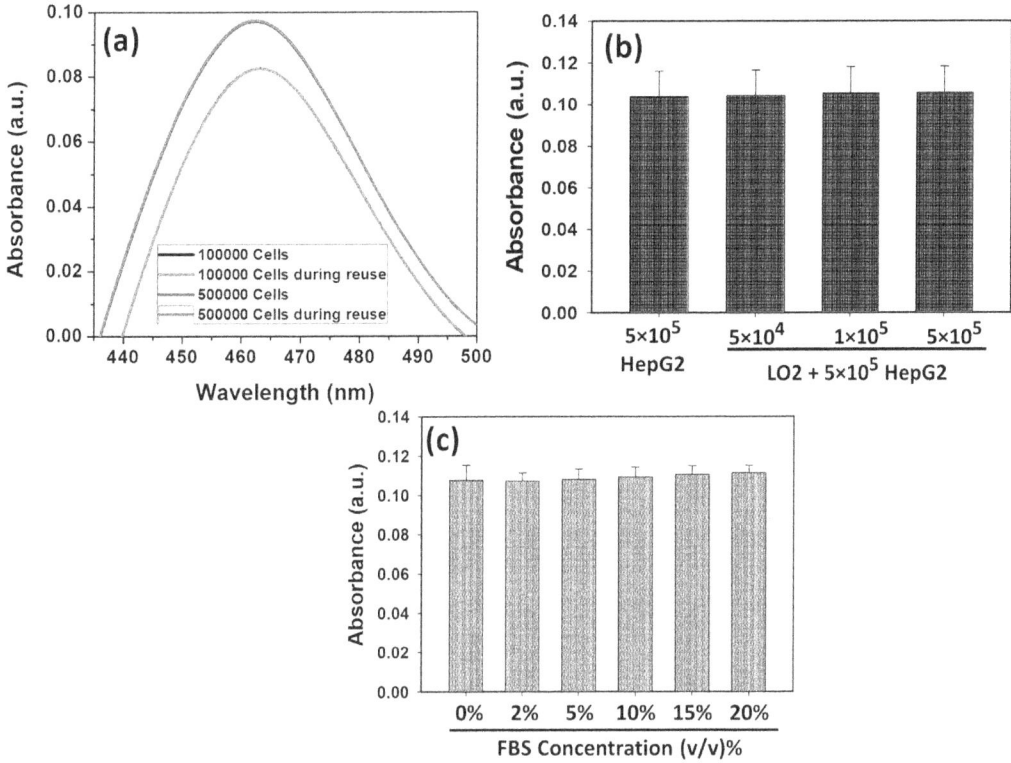

FIGURE 9.23 (a) Reusability result of developed probe using HepG2 (cells/mL), (b) selectivity result with HepG2 and LO2 cell lines, and (c) effect of FBS concentration on Hepa1–6 cells.

Source: Reprinted with permission from *Biosensors & Bioelectronics.* Copyright, 2020, Elsevier (Singh et al. 2020).

interfering substance, and a mixed sample containing 2%, 5%, 10%,15%, and 20% of FBS (v/v%) was prepared, respectively. The maximum relative measurement error is ~11.4%, which reflects that the anti-jamming ability of the sensor is excellent.

9.4.2.6 Performance Comparison

Prior to this work, various methods, such as potentiometry (Alizadeh et al. 2019; Huang et al. 2011), electrochemistry (Liu et al. 2016), and colorimetry (Tao et al. 2013) were proposed for the quantity test of various cancer cells by 2-DG binding NPs. These representative methods have been summarized and listed in Table 9.1 to facilitate comparison with the sensing performance and analytical parameters of the LSPR sensor developed for this test, so as to make a comprehensive evaluation of the developed sensor. After analysis from the results, the developed sensor has the merits of miniaturization, remote access, and compactness with higher sensitivity and selectivity. At the same time, the unique SMF-MCF structure coupled with supermodes is also a highlight of the sensor. The sensor proposed in this study will be a potential platform for rapid and real-time detection of various cancer cells, i.e., A549, A431, HeLa, HCT116, HepG2, and MDA MB 231 cells (Aydogan et al. 2010; Davidi et al. 2018; Shan et al. 2017; Suvarna et al. 2017).

TABLE 9.1

Different Methods and Properties of Prevailing Sensors

Nanomaterials	Method	Detection (cell line)	Linear range (cells/mL)	Detection limit (cells/mL)	Ref.
GO-Au NCs	Colorimetric	MCF-7[b], HeLa[c], NIH-3T3[d]	10^3–2×10^5	N.R.[a]	Tao et al. 2013
Gold NCs	Colorimetric	HER2[e]	5–1×10^3	5	Tao et al. 2017
CuO/WO$_3$-GO	Electrochemical	AGS[f], HEK 293[g]	50–1×10^5	18	Alizadeh et al. 2019
Graphene-hemin-Au NFs	Electrochemical	K562[h], HeLa[c], Romas[i]	10–5×10^4	10	Liu et al. 2016
Copper (II) oxide	Electrochemical	MCF-7[b]	50–7×10^3	27	Tian et al. 2018
AuNPs	LSPR	MDA-MB-231[b]	1×10^2–1×10^6	30	Luo et al. 2019
GO/AuNPs/ CuO-NFs	LSPR	HepG2[j]	1×10^2–1×10^6	3	Singh et al. 2020
		Hepa1 6[k]		2	
		A549[l]		2	
		MCF-7[b]		2	
		LO2[m]		4	
		NCF[n]		10	

Source: Reprinted with permission from *Biosensors & Bioelectronics*. Copyright, 2020, Elsevier (Singh et al. 2020).

[a] Not reported.
[b] Human cancer mammary cells.
[c] Human cervical cancer cells.
[d] Mouse fibroblasts normal cells.
[e] Human epidermal growth factor receptor-2 (SKBR3 and MCF7 breast cancer cells).
[f] Human Caucasian gastric adenocarcinoma (AGS).
[g] Human embryonic kidney normal cells.
[h] Human leukemic cells.
[i] Human lymphoma cells.
[j] Human liver cancer cells.
[k] Mouse liver cancer cells.
[l] Human hypotriploid alveolar basal epithelial cells (human lung cancer cells).
[m] Human normal liver cell line.
[n] Normal cancer cells.

9.5   MULTICORE FIBER PROBE FOR SELECTIVE DETECTION OF *SHIGELLA* BACTERIA

9.5.1 Materials and Methods

The same specifications of SMF and MCF are as discussed in Section 9.4. The reagents used for AuNPs in the lab are sodium citrate and hydrogen tetrachloroaurate (HAuCl$_4$), while N-methyl-2-pyrrolidone (NMP) and molybdenum disulfide (MoS$_2$) powders are used for the synthesis of MoS$_2$ solution. Other important reagents such as (3-mercaptopropyl) trimethoxysilane (MPTMS), n-hydroxysuccinimide (NHS) and N-(3-dimethylaminopropyl)-N-Ethyl carbodiimide hydrochloride (EDC), 11-mercaptodecanoic acid (11-MUA) are utilized in the immobilization and functionalization of the sensing probe. Other common chemicals and nutrients including beef extracts, agar, peptone, as well as sodium chloride (NaCl) can be used. Materials including bovine serum albumin (BSA), (3-aminopropyl) triethoxysilane (APTES), and streptavidin (SA) are used in the bacterial culture process. Total DNA oligonucleotide sequences (FC-TGT, 190916l87; 190916 L88 BPM-TGT; NC-TGT, 190916L89, IPA Probe, 190916A16) are used for selectivity experiments.

The large-scale precision instruments used in the experiment were used for characterization and observation of synthesized NMs and developed probe surfaces such as UV-Vis spectrophotometer, HRTEM, and field emission scanning electron microscope (FESEM). In addition, the large-scale equipment used for bacterial culture and experiment are the shaking incubator and the biological safety cabinet.

9.5.1.1 Fabrication of Sensor Probe

The basic structure of the probe used in this experiment is the SMF-MCF fused fiber structure. The specific fabrication process and parameters, such as the effective length of MCF, have been researched and discussed in detail in Section 9.4. For fabrication, the fusion splicing machine is used as shown in Figure 9.24 (Kumar, Guo et al. 2021; Singh et al. 2020). The running process of the machine is segmented into four parts: fiber end detection, automatic alignment, discharge fusion, and loss evaluation. First, FSM through the end detection function, the cutting angle of the optical fiber size, evaluates cutting surface cleanliness. Second, the fibers are aligned using the cladding alignment technique. Third, the electrodes prevent points clear of dust on the surface of the fiber, the main discharge for fusion splicing, and then discharge solid fusion point. Finally, the fusion loss, the shape of the splicing point, and the thermal imaging are detected and evaluated. As a result, a probe of SMF-MCF fiber structure with outstanding reconstruction is fabricated by this process. In addition, the same batch of fiber probes was immersed in 40% HF for 15 minutes to form etched SMF-MCF probes for comparison.

As demonstrated by the cross-sectional scan of MCF in Figure 9.24, it is a seven-core structure with a narrow diameter of 6.1 μm and six cores surrounding the center. After etching, the cladding

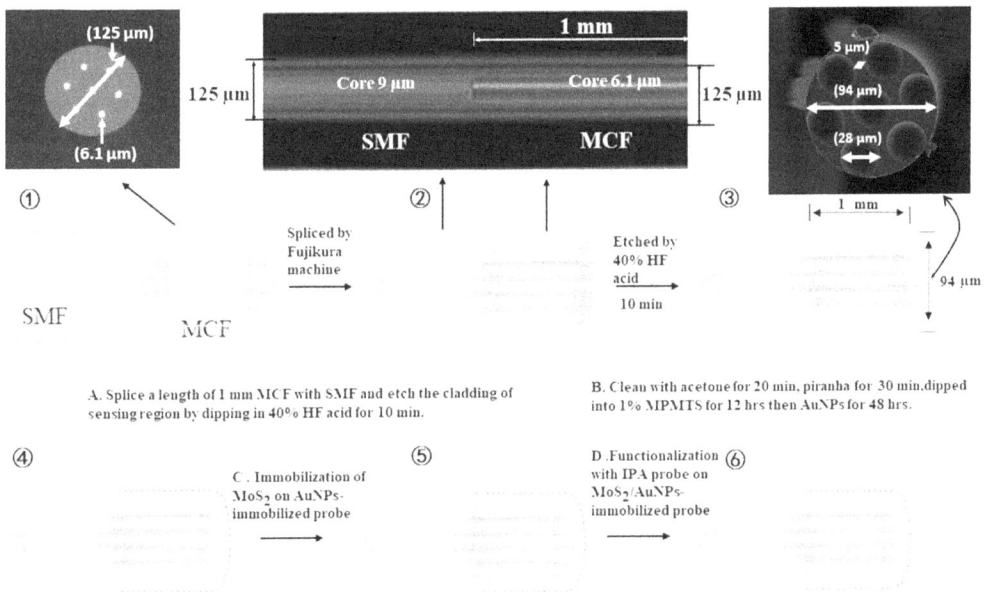

FIGURE 9.24 Development process of MoS$_2$/Au-NPs-immobilized SMF-MCF fiber sensor probe.

Source: Reprinted with permission from *Journal of Lightwave Technology.* Copyright, 2021, IEEE (Kumar, Guo et al. 2021).

layer is reduced from 125 to 94 μm, and the core diameter is increased to 28 μm, increasing the sensing probe's sensitivity.

9.5.1.2 Synthesis of AuNPs and MoS₂-NPs

Gold nanoparticles were chemo-synthesized by the classical Turkevich method. Here, the size of AuNPs can be adjusted by changing the ratio of $HAuCl_4$ (Kaur, Kumar, and Kaushik 2022). In this experiment, 10-nm AuNPs were used as the surface modifier of the probe. As another probe modifier, MoS₂-NPs were simply synthesized by adding 30 mg MoS_2 to 10 mL NMP to make a mixture, and then ultrasonic cracking was achieved at the power of 1000 W for 10 minutes. After 4000 rpm for 1 hour centrifugal treatment, then the MoS₂-NPs solution was taken from the supernatant solution and stored in 50-mL glass bottle for follow-up treatment.

9.5.1.3 Immobilization of AuNPs and MoS₂-NPs Over MCF-SMF Sensor Probe

Figure 9.24 illustrates the steps involved in immobilizing NMs such as MoS₂-NPs and AuNPs on the sensing probe's surface. It is critical to note that the MoS₂-NPs fixation process is based on the AuNPs fixation process, which was described in the preceding section. Additionally, the MoS₂-NPs fixation technique is based on the classic dip-coating technique described in Kaushik et al. (2019), that entails immersing the AuNPs immobilized sensing area for 20 seconds in a prepared 1 mL of MoS₂-NPs solution, followed by eight cycles of 2 minutes at 70°C in a drying oven. Finally, the probes were carefully placed in an oven set to 50°C for 2 hours to consolidate the results.

9.5.1.4 LSPR Measurements

Additionally, as the diameter of the core increases, the cladding decreases, which makes the leakage of EWs to the probe surface more powerful than the traditional single-core etched fiber to interaction with analytes (Li and Hayashi 2020). This makes this unique structure a platform for AuNPs (Turkevich, Stevenson, and Hillier 1951) and MoS₂-NPs (Kaushik et al. 2019) functional sensing platforms with the potential to stimulate a stronger LSPR. The detail of NMs immobilization method are discussed in Chapter 8 (Agrawal, Zhang et al. 2020). The detection device is identical to the one mentioned in Sharma et al. (Sharma, Semwal, and Gupta 2019). The HL-2000 halogen light source can generate optical signals in the wavelength range of 200–1000 nm for experiments. The USB2000 + spectrometer can accurately analyze the received signal in the range of 200–1100 nm. The probe is connected with a HL-2000 halogen light source and a USB2000 + spectrometer by a bifurcated optical fiber used before as shown in Figure 9.25. During the detection process, the probe is inserted into the sample solution, and the LSPR spectrum information produced by the probe is displayed and recorded in real time by the computer as shown in Figure 9.26.

9.5.1.5 Culture of *Shigella sonnei* Bacteria

This section discusses the culture of *Shigella sonnei* bacteria in detail. As illustrated in Figure 9.27, the first step is a conventional surface plate count method, which requires a DI water solution containing 1.25 g peptone, 0.75 g beef powder, and 1.25 g sodium chloride. *Shigella sonnei* bacteria were added to a flask containing medium using a tip probe, and the flask was gently placed in a shaker incubator at 37°C and 200 rpm for 12 hours. The sample solution containing the bacteria is then diluted to various concentrations and stored in a petri dish for 48 hours under aerobic conditions. Following that, the sample data were diluted to a predetermined standard concentration using the conventional plate counting method. Following that, 200 μL aptamer/oligonucleotide (Cy-5 labeled sequences) was added to the same batch of samples, and 1 mL *Shigella sonnei* was centrifuged at 4000 rpm for 5 minutes to prepare specific bacterial cell microspheres. Before testing, bacterial cell microsphere samples must be diluted with PBS buffer.

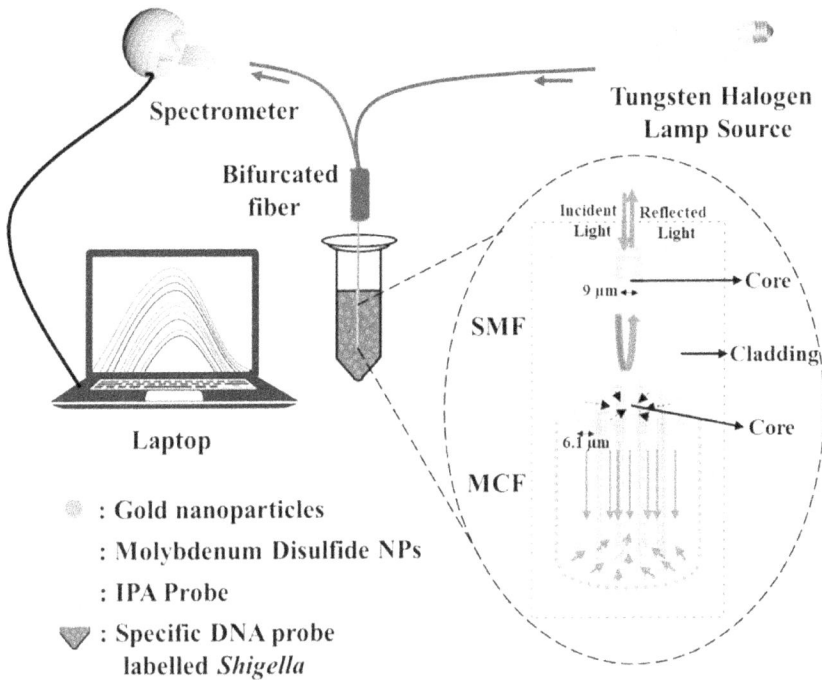

FIGURE 9.25 Experimental components for detection of *Shigella* bacteria by developed sensor probe.

Source: Reprinted with permission from *Journal of Lightwave Technology.* Copyright, 2021, IEEE (Kumar, Guo et al. 2021).

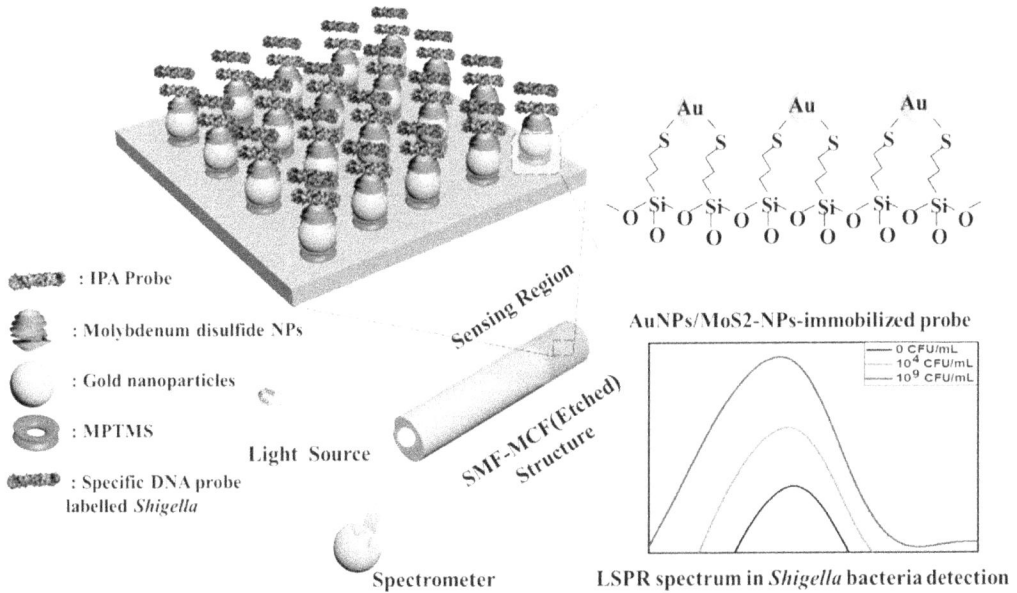

FIGURE 9.26 Detection of *Shigella* bacteria by developed sensor probe.

Source: Reprinted with permission from *Journal of Lightwave Technology.* Copyright, 2021, IEEE (Kumar, Guo et al. 2021).

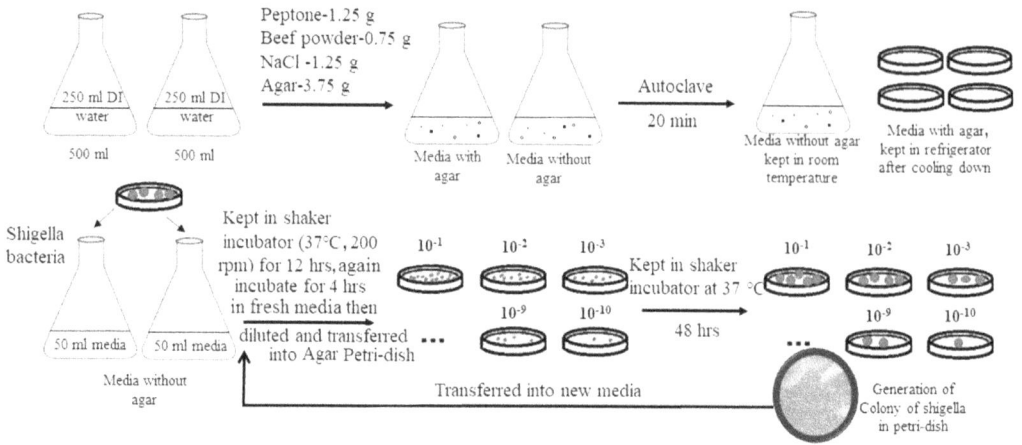

FIGURE 9.27 Culture steps of *Shigella sonnei* bacteria.

Source: Reprinted with permission from *Journal of Lightwave Technology.* Copyright, 2021, IEEE (Kumar, Guo et al. 2021).

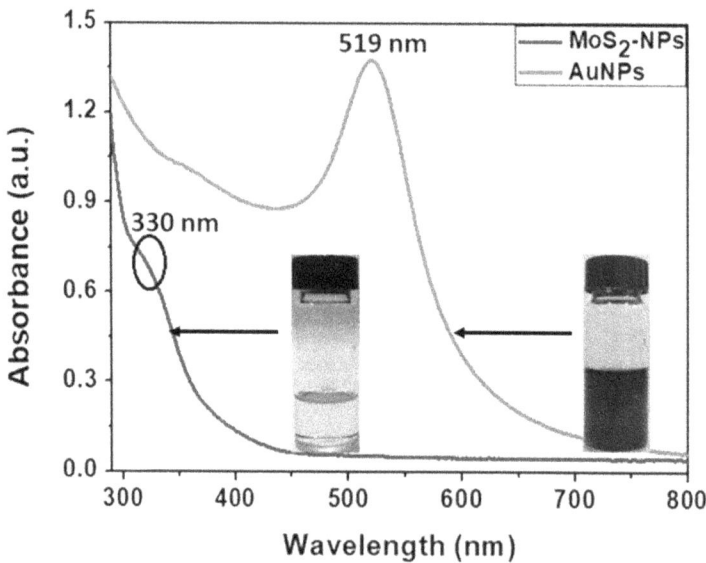

FIGURE 9.28 UV-Vis absorbance spectrum of AuNPs, and MoS$_2$-NPs solution along with their images.

Source: Reprinted with permission from *Journal of Lightwave Technology.* Copyright, 2021, IEEE (Kumar, Guo et al. 2021).

9.5.2 Results and Discussion

9.5.2.1 Characterization of Nanoparticles

The characteristic information of nanoparticles is significant for understanding the fabrication of biosensors. First, the characterization of NPs solution was researched with the help of UV-Vis spectrophotometer. From Figure 9.28, the absorption peaks of AuNPs and MoS$_2$-NPs were marked as 519 nm and 330 nm, respectively. Meanwhile, Figure 9.28 illustrates the AuNPs solution in red wine color, as well as transparent MoS$_2$-NPs solution in canary yellow.

9.5.2.2 Characterization of a Nanoparticles-Coated Sensor Probe

With the help of high-precision FESEM, the micromorphology of the etched probe surface can be observed. A uniform distribution of MoS_2-NPs/AuNPs in a thin coatings form on the sensing region can be observed by adjusting the appropriate power. The corresponding coating thicknesses are 13 nm and 2.3 nm, respectively.

9.5.2.3 LSPR Sensing Results

The process of sensor probe specificity processing at indoor temperature is as follows: 12 mL of ethanol solution (95%) mixed with 150 μL of APTES (98%) and 12 μL of 100% acetic acid are used. The MoS_2/AuNPs-immobilized probe was then immersed in the prepared medium for 30 minutes, and during this process, the surface of the probe was gradually aminated. Ethanol can be used to carefully clean unbound APTES molecules. Then, the dried treatment region was immersed in 10% glutaraldehyde solution for 1 hour and 0.05 mg/mL SA solution for 3 hours, which could fix a stable SA layer on the surface of the sensing region. Then, the probe was removed and rinsed carefully with PBST solution (PBS plus 0.05% Tween 20). The dried probe was then bio-labeled gradually and soaked carefully in TE buffer containing 1 mL IPA DNA for 1 hour. The TE buffer was prepared by adding 0.5 M $MgCl_2$ to 20 mM Tris-HCl at pH 8.0. Finally, to eliminate the non-specific absorption sites in the biomarker region, the sensing probe washed by PBST was carefully immersed in 1% BSA solution.

Table 9.2 shows the DNA oligonucleotide sequence used to detect *S. sonnei*. To compare the performance of the sensing probes, three oligonucleotide probes were ordered from high to low in order of their binding ability to the target, like fully complementary (FC) probes, single-base mismatch (BPM) probes, and noncomplementary (NC) probes were well fabricated. Before measurement, a group of *S. sonnei* bacterial samples was prepared with specific cell concentrations ranging from 1 to 10^9 CFU/mL. When the probe is inserted into the sample solution of *S. funiculus*, after 5 minutes of centrifugation according to the SELEX process (Feng et al. 2019), the *S. sonnei* bacteria cells with specific cell concentration in the sample will hybridize on the surface of the fiber, RI varied with the concentration of analyte cells. Before the next sample is tested, the probe is activated by soaking in 0.5% sodium dodecyl sulfate (SDS) solution for 1 minute, at pH 1.9, and then was carefully cleaned with PBST.

After the probes were inserted into the samples of the two concentrations (10 CFU/mL and 100 CFU/mL) for 5 minutes, the absorbance performance of FC-TGT/AuNPs/MoS_2-NPs-based non-etched sensor probe was close to the restriction of saturation. The absorbance value corresponding to $t = 0$ is regarded as the reference sample (PBS only) of 0 concentration of *S. sonnei* solution. Here, to explore the influence of PBS on the results of the experiment, the probes with PBS buffer only

---

TABLE 9.2

Different Oligonucleotides[a] Used for Sensing *Shigella sonnei*

Name	Sequence (5′—3′)
IPA Probe[b]	Biotin-TTTTTTTTTTTTTAGTCTTTCGCTGTTGCTGCTGATGCC
FC TGT[c]	Cy5.5-GGCATCAGCAGCAACAGCGAAAGACT
BPM TGT[c]	Cy5.5-GGCATCAGCA_C_CAACAGCGAAAGACT
NC TGT[c]	Cy5.5-TGGCAGAGCGGGTACTAACATGATT

Source: Reprinted with permission from *Journal of Lightwave Technology*. Copyright, 2021, IEEE (Kumar, Guo et al. 2021).

[a] BPM, base pair mismatched; FC, fully complementary; NC, noncomplementary; TGT, target.

[b] Receptor.

[c] Analyte.

were used as blank groups to eliminate the interference of PBS for the concentration-dependent absorbance of *S. sonnei.*

The characteristic curves of NC-TGT, BPM-TGT, and FC-TGT functional probes for detection of *S. sonnei* are shown in Figure 9.29(a), (c), and (e). The detection sequence of each group was from low to high in cell concentration, and the corresponding detection time was 5 minutes. The mentioned results demonstrated the absorbance intensity increased with the increase of *Shigella* concentration (CFU/mL). This may be that the electrostatic interaction between the metal NPs and the bacterial cell (Ragini Singh and Singh 2018) promotes the gradual blocking of active sites on the

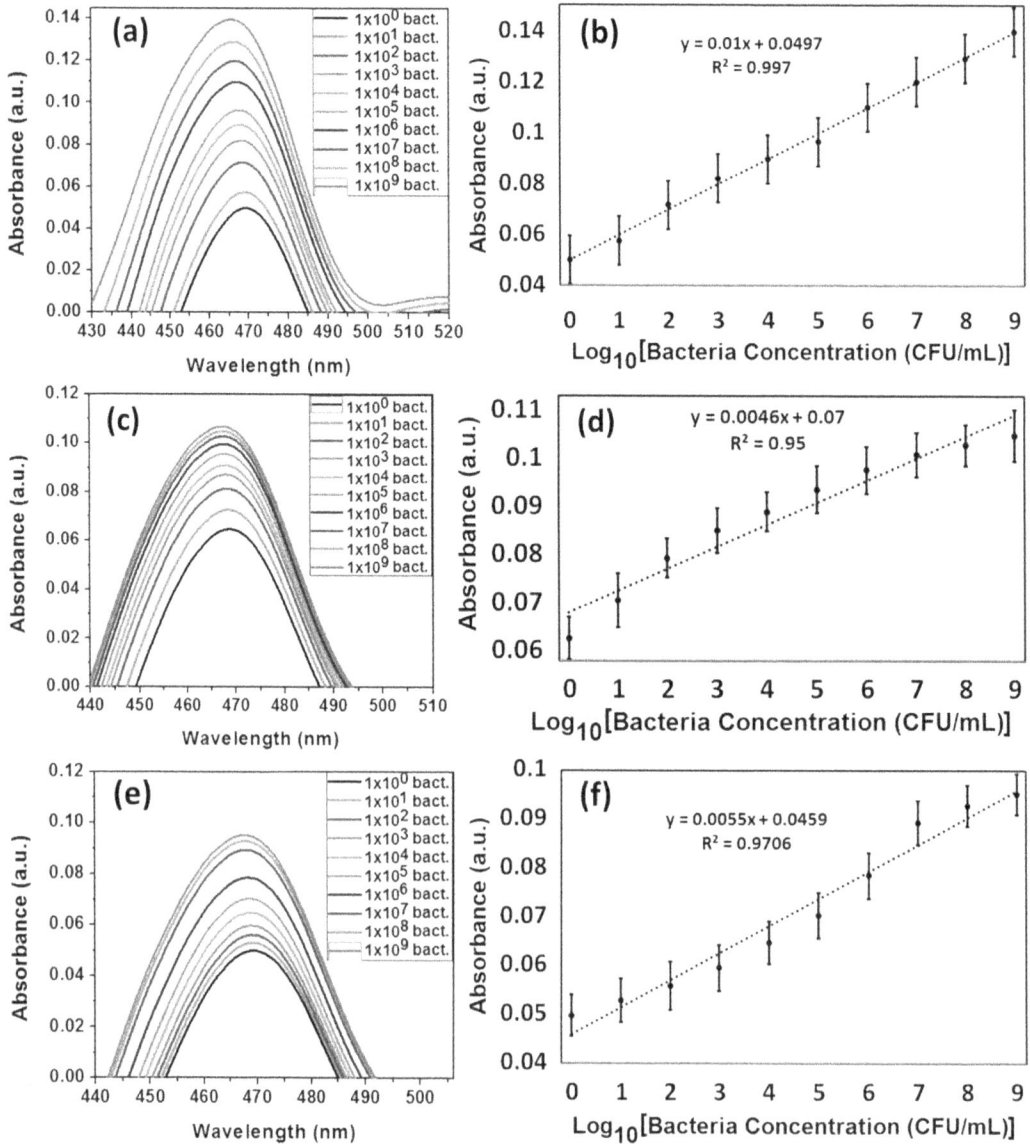

FIGURE 9.29 Bacterial sensing results and linearity plots of (a, b) FC-TGT; (c, d) BPM-TGT; (e, f) NC-TGT using AuNPs/MoS$_2$-NPs functionalized etched sensor probe.

Source: Reprinted with permission from *Journal of Lightwave Technology.* Copyright, 2021, IEEE (Kumar, Guo et al. 2021).

surface of the bacterial cell and the probe at a specific concentration nearby, causing more light to be absorbed. Results shown in Figure 9.29(b), (d) and (f) show the maximum linear range of the three nucleotides. The limits of detection (LoD) are 2.30 CFU/mL, 4.89 CFU/mL, and 5.59 CFU/mL, respectively, in the range of 1 to 1×10^9 CFU/mL. Here, the LoD may be calculated as three times the standard deviation of reference sample divided by calibration curve slope (Xiao et al. 2014).

From the results in Figure 9.29(a–f), it can be concluded that the complete complementary DNA probes exhibit the greatest range of absorbance variation that is caused by the most specific DNA hybridization, this also explains the reason for low LoD and high sensitivity. Detection of other types of DNA oligonucleotide, such as FC-TGT, NC-TGT, and BPM-TGT, may be relevant to probe specificity. The results show that the developed probe has a better selective response to FC-TGT than other DNA oligonucleotide, which proves its excellent specificity. From the summary information in Table 9.3, it can be concluded that FC-TGT, as a complete complementary DNA probe, has better accuracy and LoD, so it is more suitable for the detection of *Shigella*.

9.5.2.4 Comparison with Existing *Shigella* Biosensors

Table 9.4 demonstrates the reported representative works on the detection of *Shigella* including loop-mediated amplification technique, PCR, voltage control signals, amplification techniques, etc. At the same time, it is convenient to access the sensing property of the sensor developed in this work. The results clearly show that this sensor has an excellent advantage in LoD and can identify the bacteria concentration as low as 1.56 CFU/mL. Moreover, fiber-based LSPR biosensors are easy to operate, miniaturize, and fabricate, which makes them more useful for real-world applications.

TABLE 9.3

Comparison of Bacterial Sensors

Oligonucleotides	SMF-MCF fiber	Accuracy	Detection limit (CFU/mL)
FC-TGT	Nonetched	0.9732	2.30
BPM-TGT	Nonetched	0.9568	4.89
NC-TGT	Nonetched	0.9624	5.59
FC-TGT	Etched	0.997	1.56
BPM-TGT	Etched	0.95	3.40
NC-TGT	Etched	0.9706	2.85

Source: Reprinted with permission from *Journal of Lightwave Technology.* Copyright, 2021, IEEE (Kumar, Guo et al. 2021).

TABLE 9.4

Comparison of Existing Bacterial Biosensors

System	Method	Linear range (CFU/mL)	Detection limit	Detection time	Ref.
N.R.	A*	N.R.	5.8 CFU/vessel in milk	12 minutes	Wang et al. 2015
N.R.	B*	3×10^3–3×10^4	18 CFU/mL in blood	78 minutes	Luo et al. 2016
N.R.	PCR (Syber green)	1.5×10^6–1.5×10^2	1.5×10^3 CFU/g	N.R.	Mokhtari et al. 2013
N.R.	Evanescent wave	1–1×10^4	100 CFU/mL	5 minutes	Xiao et al. 2014
Au/MoS$_2$-NPs	LSPR	1–1×10^9	1.56 CFU/mL	5 minutes	Kumar et al. 2021

Source: Reprinted with permission from *Journal of Lightwave Technology.* Copyright, 2021, IEEE (Kumar, Guo et al. 2021).
Note: N.R., not reported; A*, real-time loop-mediated amplification technique; B*, voltage controlled signal amplification.

9.6 SUMMARY AND CONCLUSIONS

Researchers are focusing their efforts on developing high-sensitivity optical biomarker-based sensing technology for tumor cell detection. However, due to the lack of universal labeling methods, traditional biomarker-based sensors perform poorly in clinical settings and are unable to detect all types of cancer. Additionally, certain optical biosensors, such as interferometric biosensors, have packaging issues, with the limitation of transition efficiency acting as a technical bottleneck. Due to their advantages of miniaturization, label-free operation, rapid response time, simplicity of operation, high sensitivity, and remote access, optical fiber-based SPR and LSPR biosensors are expected to play a significant role in prospective clinical detection. Fiber-based biosensors can easily be inserted into the body for real-time detection, significantly reducing the difficulty of collecting fresh samples and economizing on diagnostic time.

Biosensors based on the SPR and LSPR have been commercialized. Unfortunately, their performance in clinical measurements has been unsatisfactory, with low specificity, narrow detection limits, and the presence of complex interferers, all of which undermine the results' credibility. As a result, the requirement to support large and complex equipment has more than compensated for the constraints. To address these issues, a novel LSPR biosensor based on a unique MCF/SMF splicing structure was developed for the quantitative detection of HepG2, Hepa 1–6, MCF-7, and A549. To enhance sensing properties, NMs such as gold nanoparticles, graphene oxide, and CuO-NFs were modified on the probe surface. Additionally, by etching the MCF and SMF joint structures, the coupling efficiency between the supermodes and the external NMs is significantly increased, as well as the LSPR phenomenon. To create a suitable and favorable stage for the specific detection of cancer cells, a 2-DG coating was chosen to functionalize NMs probes. Additionally, the developed probe was used to compare normal cells such as NCF and LO2 with the developed probe. The probe is more selective against tumor cell lines than it is against normal cells. The developed probe was then subjected to a more comprehensive performance test. The results indicate that the probe meets the required standards for reproducibility, selectivity, and anti-interference ability. It is worth noting, however, that during our research, we discovered that the GLUT receptors on cancer cells are tightly coupled to the probes. In conclusion, the developed sensor can bridge the gap between existing SPR and LSPR-based biosensors, which gives our future research work confidence.

Following that, sensing probes for *Shigella* detection using etched MCF-SMF probe and NMs such as AuNPs and MoS_2-NPs has been discussed. Similarly, IPA probes were functionally treated with a variety of DNA oligonucleotides, including NC-TGT, FC-TGT, and BPM-TGT, and quantitatively tested against *S. sonnei* bacteria. The results indicated that FC-TGT oligonucleotide was an effective functional material for detecting *S. sonnei*. FC-TGT had a detection limit of 1.56 CFU/mL and a linear range of 1 to 10^9 CFU/mL. In comparison to conventional detection methods in this field, the developed sensor achieves a significant improvement in the LoD, indicating that it has a greater potential for human dysentery diagnosis. The proposed sensing probe is intended to be used in the future to determine the concentration of biomolecules, toxic substances, and metal ions in a variety of marine life and aquaculture.

9.7 FUTURE PERSPECTIVE

At present, cancer detection technology is mainly through the specific identification of markers on single gene/protein, combined with the emerging nanotechnology, to achieve a function of single biosensor to produce multiple output excellence. At present, the high price of nanomaterials and the deficiency of biomolecular quality guarantee limit the commercialization of optical biosensors, and it is difficult to challenge the dominant position of traditional diagnostic techniques in cancer detection. Therefore, the optimization of nano-synthesis technology to enhance the stability of biomolecules has become eager to conquer the technical fortress. In recent years, the detection methods for diseases are becoming gradually diversified, and the study of the mechanisms of nanoparticles is gradually deepened. Multidisciplinary study is increasing. For example, it is said that magnetic nanostructures have great value to distinguish tumor cells from normal cells by coating the silicon dioxide with a diamagnetic particle that can form a large magnetic moment that helps bind to cancer cells. The continuous development of microfabrication technology of two-dimensional nanomaterials is also an important driving force in the growth of optical sensing technology. Various ranges of biocompatibility of two-dimensional materials and a larger surface volume ratio provide strong support for the specific binding of a large number of analytes. In addition, one of the practical problems facing the early clinical detection of cancer is the big challenge of distinguishing the classification of cancer in different organs of the body using a single protein as a biomarker. This will undoubtedly delay the golden time of early treatment. For this, DNA maintains longer activity and degrades less in tissue cells than protein and miRNA; therefore, the application of DNA in tumor detection opens the door for the growth of optical biosensing for clinical application. In addition, a protein called octamer binding transcription factor 4 (OCT4A) has been found in serum around embryonic-like stem cells and can change with the cancer stage. As a result, protein markers including OCT4A are expected to be a great success in liquid biopsies of cancer samples as well as a potential new high-sensitivity and selective sensing platform.

REFERENCES

Agrawal, N., C. Saha, C. Kumar, et al. 2020. "Detection of L-cysteine using silver nanoparticles and graphene oxide immobilized tapered SMS optical fiber structure." *IEEE Sensors Journal* 20 (19):11372–11379.

Agrawal, N., B. Zhang, C. Saha, C. Kumar, X. Pu, and S. Kumar. 2020. "Ultra-sensitive cholesterol sensor using gold and zinc-oxide nanoparticles immobilized core mismatch MPM/SPS probe." *Journal of Lightwave Technology* 38 (8):2523–2529.

Ahirwar, R., and P. Nahar. 2016. "Development of a label-free gold nanoparticle-based colorimetric aptasensor for detection of human estrogen receptor alpha." *Analytical and Bioanalytical Chemistry* 408 (1):327–332.

Alizadeh, Negar, Abdollah Salimi, Rahman Hallaj, Fardin Fathi, and Farzad Soleimani. 2019. "CuO/WO$_3$ nanoparticles decorated graphene oxide nanosheets with enhanced peroxidase-like activity for electrochemical cancer cell detection and targeted therapeutics." *Materials Science and Engineering: C* 99:1374–1383.

Arjmand, Mojtaba, Hossein Saghafifar, Mahdi Alijanianzadeh, and Mahmood Soltanolkotabi. 2017. "A sensitive tapered-fiber optic biosensor for the label-free detection of organophosphate pesticides." *Sensors and Actuators B: Chemical* 249:523–532.

Arumugam, Nandhini, and JongSung Kim. 2018. "Quantum dots attached to graphene oxide for sensitive detection of ascorbic acid in aqueous solutions." *Materials Science and Engineering: C* 92:720–725.

Aydogan, Bulent, Ji Li, Tijana Rajh, et al. 2010. "AuNP-DG: Deoxyglucose-labeled gold nanoparticles as X-ray computed tomography contrast agents for cancer imaging." *Molecular Imaging and Biology* 12 (5):463–467.

Ben Haddada, M., D. Hu, M. Salmain, et al. 2017. "Gold nanoparticle-based localized surface plasmon immunosensor for staphylococcal enterotoxin A (SEA) detection." *Analytical and Bioanalytical Chemistry* 409 (26):6227–6234.

Chang, C. Y., H. T. Lin, M. S. Lai, et al. 2018. "Flexible localized surface plasmon resonance sensor with metal-insulator-metal nanodisks on PDMS substrate." *Scientific Reports* 8 (1):11812.

Chocarro-Ruiz, Blanca, Adrián Fernández-Gavela, Sonia Herranz, and Laura M. Lechuga. 2017. "Nanophotonic label-free biosensors for environmental monitoring." *Current Opinion in Biotechnology* 45:175–183.

Davidi, E. S., T. Dreifuss, M. Motiei, et al. 2018. "Cisplatin-conjugated gold nanoparticles as a theranostic agent for head and neck cancer." *Head and Neck* 40 (1):70–78.

Dilsiz, N. 2020. "Role of exosomes and exosomal microRNAs in cancer." *Future Science OA* 6 (4):Fso465.

Duan, F., S. Zhang, L. Yang, Z. Zhang, L. He, and M. Wang. 2018. "Bifunctional aptasensor based on novel two-dimensional nanocomposite of MoS$_2$ quantum dots and g-C$_3$N$_4$ nanosheets decorated with chitosan-stabilized Au nanoparticles for selectively detecting prostate specific antigen." *Anal Chim Acta* 1036:121–132.

Feng, Junli, Qing Shen, Jiajia Wu, Zhiyuan Dai, and Yi Wang. 2019. "Naked-eyes detection of *Shigella flexneri* in food samples based on a novel gold nanoparticle-based colorimetric aptasensor." *Food Control* 98:333–341.

Fischer, E. G. 2020. "Nuclear morphology and the biology of cancer cells." *Acta Cytologica* 64 (6):511–519.

Guo, C., F. Su, Y. Song, et al. 2017. "Aptamer-templated silver nanoclusters embedded in zirconium metal-organic framework for bifunctional electrochemical and SPR aptasensors toward carcinoembryonic antigen." *ACS Applied Materials and Interfaces* 9 (47):41188–41199.

Hahn, Jungwoo, Eunghee Kim, Youngsang You, and Young Jin Choi. 2019. "Colorimetric switchable linker-based bioassay for ultrasensitive detection of prostate-specific antigen as a cancer biomarker." *Analyst* 144 (14):4439–4446.

Halkare, P., N. Punjabi, J. Wangchuk, K. Kondabagil, and S. Mukherji. 2015. "LSPR based fiber optic sensor for detection of *E. coli* using bacteriophage T4." Paper read at 2015 Workshop on Recent Advances in Photonics (WRAP), 16–17 December.

Hammond, Jules L., Nikhil Bhalla, Sarah D. Rafiee, and Pedro Estrela. 2014. "Localized surface plasmon resonance as a biosensing platform for developing countries." *Biosensors* 4 (2):172–188.

Hossain, Md Biplob, Md Muztahidul Islam, Lway Faisal Abdulrazak, Md Masud Rana, Tarik Bin Abdul Akib, and Mehedi Hassan. 2020. "Graphene-coated optical fiber SPR biosensor for BRCA1 and BRCA2 breast cancer biomarker detection: A numerical design-based analysis." *Photonic Sensors* 10 (1):67–79.

Huang, G. G., C. J. Lee, B. C. Tsai, J. Yang, M. Sathiyendiran, and K. L. Lu. 2011. "Gondola-shaped tetra-rhenium metallacycles modified evanescent wave infrared chemical sensors for selective determination of volatile organic compounds." *Talanta* 85 (1):63–69.

Janik, Monika, Marcin Koba, Anna Celebańska, Wojtek J. Bock, and Mateusz Śmietana. 2018. "Live *E. coli* bacteria label-free sensing using a microcavity in-line Mach-Zehnder interferometer." *Scientific Reports* 8 (1):1–8.

Jans, H., and Q. Huo. 2012. "Gold nanoparticle-enabled biological and chemical detection and analysis." *Chemical Society Reviews* 41 (7):2849–2866.

Jans, Hilde, and Qun Huo. 2012. "Gold nanoparticle-enabled biological and chemical detection and analysis." *Chemical Society Reviews* 41 (7):2849–2866.

Jayanthi, Vspksa, A. B. Das, and U. Saxena. 2017. "Recent advances in biosensor development for the detection of cancer biomarkers." *Biosensors and Bioelectronics* 91:15–23.

Kaur, Baljinder, Santosh Kumar, and Brajesh Kumar Kaushik. 2022. "Recent advancements in optical biosensors for cancer detection." *Biosensors and Bioelectronics* 197:113805.

Kaushik, Siddharth, Umesh K. Tiwari, Sudipta S. Pal, and Ravindra K. Sinha. 2019. "Rapid detection of *Escherichia coli* using fiber optic surface plasmon resonance immunosensor based on biofunctionalized molybdenum disulfide (MoS_2) nanosheets." *Biosensors and Bioelectronics* 126:501–509.

Kim, Hyeong-Min, Jae-Hyoung Park, and Seung-Ki Lee. 2019. "Fiber optic sensor based on ZnO nanowires decorated by Au nanoparticles for improved plasmonic biosensor." *Scientific Reports* 9 (1):15605.

Kim, Woo Hyun, Jong Uk Lee, Sojin Song, Soohyun Kim, Young Jae Choi, and Sang Jun Sim. 2019. "A label-free, ultra-highly sensitive and multiplexed SERS nanoplasmonic biosensor for miRNA detection using a head-flocked gold nanopillar." *Analyst* 144 (5):1768–1776.

Kumar, Santosh, Ragini Singh, Qinshan Yang, Shuang Cheng, Bingyuan Zhang, and Brajesh Kumar Kaushik. 2020. "Highly sensitive, selective and portable sensor probe using Germanium-doped photosensitive optical fiber for ascorbic acid detection." *IEEE Sensors Journal* 21 (1):62–70. 12 February. DOI: 10.1109/JSEN.2020.2973579.

Kumar, Santosh, Zhu Guo, Ragini Singh, et al. 2021. "MoS_2 functionalized multicore fiber probes for selective detection of *Shigella* bacteria based on localized plasmon." *Journal of Lightwave Technology* 39 (12):4069–4081.

Li, Ming-Jun, and Tetsuya Hayashi. 2020. "Chapter 1—Advances in low-loss, large-area, and multicore fibers." In *Optical Fiber Telecommunications VII*, edited by A. E. Willner. Cambridge, MA: Academic Press.

Li, Yuan, Yulong Zhang, Man Zhao, et al. 2016. "A simple aptamer-functionalized gold nanorods based biosensor for the sensitive detection of MCF-7 breast cancer cells." *Chemical Communications* 52 (20):3959–3961.

Lin, Haitao, Mengshi Li, Liyun Ding, and Jun Huang. 2019. "A fiber optic biosensor based on hydrogel-immobilized enzyme complex for continuous determination of cholesterol and glucose." *Applied Biochemistry and Biotechnology* 187 (4):1569–1580.

Liu, Jing, Meirong Cui, Li Niu, Hong Zhou, and Shusheng Zhang. 2016. "Enhanced peroxidase-like properties of graphene—hemin-composite decorated with Au nanoflowers as electrochemical aptamer biosensor for the detection of K562 leukemia cancer cells." *Chemistry—A European Journal* 22 (50):18001–18008.

Loyez, M., M. Lobry, E. M. Hassan, M. C. DeRosa, C. Caucheteur, and R. Wattiez. 2021. "HER2 breast cancer biomarker detection using a sandwich optical fiber assay." *Talanta* 221:121452.

Loyez, Médéric, Eman M. Hassan, Maxime Lobry, et al. 2020. "Rapid detection of circulating breast cancer cells using a multiresonant optical fiber aptasensor with plasmonic amplification." *ACS Sensors* 5 (2):454–463.

Luo, Jieling, Jiapeng Wang, Anup Mathew, and Siu-Tung Yau. 2016. "Ultrasensitive detection of *Shigella* species in blood and stool." *Analytical Chemistry* 88.

Luo, Zewei, Yimin Wang, Ya Xu, et al. 2019. "Ultrasensitive U-shaped fiber optic LSPR cytosensing for label-free and in situ evaluation of cell surface N-glycan expression." *Sensors and Actuators B: Chemical* 284:582–588.

Macfarlane, Leigh-Ann, and Paul R. Murphy. 2010. "MicroRNA: Biogenesis, function and role in cancer." *Current Genomics* 11 (7):537–561.

Maharana, Pradeep Kumar, Sriram Bharadwaj, and Rajan Jha. 2013. "Electric field enhancement in surface plasmon resonance bimetallic configuration based on chalcogenide prism." *Journal of Applied Physics* 114 (1):014304.

Maharana, Pradeep Kumar, Triranjita Srivastava, and Rajan Jha. 2014. "Low index dielectric mediated surface plasmon resonance sensor based on graphene for near infrared measurements." *Journal of Physics D: Applied Physics* 47 (38):385102.

Mao, X., L. Yang, X. L. Su, and Y. Li. 2006. "A nanoparticle amplification based quartz crystal microbalance DNA sensor for detection of *Escherichia coli* O157:H7." *Biosensors and Bioelectronics* 21 (7):1178–1185.

Martucci, Nicola M., Ilaria Rea, Immacolata Ruggiero, et al. 2015. "A new strategy for label-free detection of lymphoma cancer cells." *Biomedical Optics Express* 6 (4):1353–1362.

May-Arrioja, Daniel Alberto, and Jose Rafael Guzman-Sepulveda. 2017. "Highly sensitive fiber optic refractive index sensor using multicore coupled structures." *Journal of Lightwave Technology* 35 (13):2695–2701.

Mittal, Sunil, Hardeep Kaur, Nandini Gautam, and Anil K. Mantha. 2017. "Biosensors for breast cancer diagnosis: A review of bioreceptors, biotransducers and signal amplification strategies." *Biosensors and Bioelectronics* 88:217–231.

Mokhtari, W., S. Nsaibia, A. Gharbi, and M. Aouni. 2013. "Real-time PCR using SYBR green for the detection of *Shigella* spp. in food and stool samples." *Mol Cell Probes* 27 (1):53–59.

Nayak, Jeeban Kumar, Pradeep Kumar Maharana, and Rajan Jha. 2017. "Dielectric over-layer assisted graphene, its oxide and MoS₂-based fibre optic sensor with high field enhancement." *Journal of Physics D: Applied Physics* 50 (40):405112.

Nayak, Jeeban Kumar, Purnendu Parhi, and Rajan Jha. 2016. "Experimental and theoretical studies on localized surface plasmon resonance based fiber optic sensor using graphene oxide coated silver nanoparticles." *Journal of Physics D Applied Physics* 49:285101.

Punjabi, N., J. Satija, and S. Mukherji. 2015. "Evanescent wave absorption based fiber-optic sensor—Cascading of bend and tapered geometry for enhanced sensitivity." In *Sensing Technology: Current Status and Future Trends III*, edited by A. Mason, S. C. Mukhopadhyay, and K. P. Jayasundera. Cham: Springer International Publishing.

Ramanujam, Nambi R., I. S. Amiri, Sofyan A. Taya, et al. 2019. "Enhanced sensitivity of cancer cell using one dimensional nano composite material coated photonic crystal." *Microsystem Technologies* 25 (1):189–196.

Ravikumar, Raghunandhan, Li Han Chen, Premkumar Jayaraman, Chueh Loo Poh, and Chi Chiu Chan. 2018. "Chitosan-nickel film based interferometric optical fiber sensor for label-free detection of histidine tagged proteins." *Biosensors and Bioelectronics* 99:578–585.

Sasi, Simitha, Shinto Mundackal Francis, Jesly Jacob, and Vibin Ipe Thomas. 2021. "A tunable plasmonic refractive index sensor with ultrabroad sensing range for cancer detection." *Plasmonics* 16 (5):1705–1717.

Shah, Juhi, Rahul Purohit, Ragini Singh, Ajay Singh Karakoti, and Sanjay Singh. 2015. "ATP-enhanced peroxidase-like activity of gold nanoparticles." *Journal of Colloid and Interface Science* 456:100–107.

Shan, Xiu-Hong, Peng Wang, Fei Xiong, Hao-Yue Lu, and Hui Hu. 2017. "Detection of human breast cancer cells using a 2-deoxy-D-glucose-functionalized superparamagnetic iron oxide nanoparticles." *Cancer Biomarkers* 18 (4):367–374.

Sharma, Priyanka, Vivek Semwal, and Banshi D. Gupta. 2019. "A highly selective LSPR biosensor for the detection of taurine realized on optical fiber substrate and gold nanoparticles." *Optical Fiber Technology* 52:101962.

Singh, R., S. Kumar, F. Z. Liu, et al. 2020. "Etched multicore fiber sensor using copper oxide and gold nanoparticles decorated graphene oxide structure for cancer cells detection." *Biosensors and Bioelectronics* 168:112557.

Singh, Ragini, and Sanjay Singh. 2018. "Uptake and toxicity of different nanoparticles towards a tough bacterium." *Deinococcus Radiodurans Advanced Material Letters* 9 (7):531–537.

Srinivasan, R., S. Umesh, S. Murali, S. Asokan, and S. Siva Gorthi. 2017. "Bare fiber Bragg grating immunosensor for real-time detection of *Escherichia coli* bacteria." *Journal of Biophotonics* 10 (2):224–230.

Sun, Shaodong, Xiaozhe Zhang, Yuexia Sun, Shengchun Yang, Xiaoping Song, and Zhimao Yang. 2013. "Hierarchical CuO nanoflowers: Water-required synthesis and their application in a nonenzymatic glucose biosensor." *Physical Chemistry Chemical Physics* 15 (26):10904–10913.

Sung, H., J. Ferlay, R. L. Siegel, et al. 2021. "Global cancer statistics 2020: GLOBOCAN estimates of incidence and mortality worldwide for 36 cancers in 185 countries." *CA Cancer Journal for Clinicians* 71 (3):209–249.

Suvarna, S., U. Das, S. Kc, et al. 2017. "Synthesis of a novel glucose capped gold nanoparticle as a better theranostic candidate." *PLoS One* 12 (6):e0178202.

Tao, Y., Y. Lin, Z. Huang, J. Ren, and X. Qu. 2013. "Incorporating graphene oxide and gold nanoclusters: A synergistic catalyst with surprisingly high peroxidase-like activity over a broad pH range and its application for cancer cell detection." *Advanced Materials* 25 (18):2594–2599.

Tao, Yu, Mingqiang Li, Bumjun Kim, and Debra T. Auguste. 2017. "Incorporating gold nanoclusters and target-directed liposomes as a synergistic amplified colorimetric sensor for HER2-positive breast cancer cell detection." *Theranostics* 7 (4):899.

Tian, Liang, Jinxu Qi, Kun Qian, et al. 2018. "Copper (II) oxide nanozyme based electrochemical cytosensor for high sensitive detection of circulating tumor cells in breast cancer." *Journal of Electroanalytical Chemistry* 812:1–9.

Turkevich, John, Peter Cooper Stevenson, and James Hillier. 1951. "A study of the nucleation and growth processes in the synthesis of colloidal gold." *Discussions of the Faraday Society* 11 (0):55–75.

Underwood, J. J., R. S. Quadri, S. P. Kalva, et al. 2020. "Liquid biopsy for cancer: Review and implications for the radiologist." *Radiology* 294 (1):5–17.

Villatoro, Joel, Enrique Antonio-Lopez, Axel Schülzgen, and Rodrigo Amezcua-Correa. 2017. "Miniature multicore optical fiber vibration sensor." *Optics Letters* 42 (10):2022–2025.

Villatoro, Joel, Amy Van Newkirk, Enrique Antonio-Lopez, Joseba Zubia, Axel Schülzgen, and Rodrigo Amezcua-Correa. 2016. "Ultrasensitive vector bending sensor based on multicore optical fiber." *Optics Letters* 41 (4):832–835.

Wang, Q., Q. Li, X. Yang, et al. 2016. "Graphene oxide-gold nanoparticles hybrids-based surface plasmon resonance for sensitive detection of microRNA." *Biosensors and Bioelectronics* 77:1001–1007.

Wang, Songxue, Jiayu Tian, Qiao Wang, et al. 2019. "Development of CuO coated ceramic hollow fiber membrane for peroxymonosulfate activation: A highly efficient singlet oxygen-dominated oxidation process for bisphenol a degradation." *Applied Catalysis B: Environmental* 256:117783.

Wang, Y., Y. Wang, L. Luo, et al. 2015. "Rapid and sensitive detection of *Shigella* spp. and *Salmonella* spp. by multiple endonuclease restriction real-time loop-mediated isothermal amplification technique." *Front Microbiol* 6:1400.

Wu, Song, Wei Zhu, Patricia Thompson, and Yusuf A. Hannun. 2018. "Evaluating intrinsic and non-intrinsic cancer risk factors." *Nature Communications* 9 (1):3490.

Wu, W., J. Zhang, M. Zheng, et al. 2012. "An aptamer-based biosensor for colorimetric detection of *Escherichia coli* O157:H7." *PLoS One* 7 (11):e48999.

Xiao, Liangping, Aimei Zhu, Qingchi Xu, Ying Chen, Jun Xu, and Jian Weng. 2017. "Colorimetric biosensor for detection of cancer biomarker by Au nanoparticle-decorated Bi_2Se_3 nanosheets." *ACS Applied Materials and Interfaces* 9 (8):6931–6940.

Xiao, R., Z. Rong, F. Long, and Q. Liu. 2014. "Portable evanescent wave fiber biosensor for highly sensitive detection of *Shigella*." *Spectrochimica Acta A Molecular and Biomolecular Spectroscopy* 132:1–5.

Yang, G., Z. Xiao, C. Tang, Y. Deng, H. Huang, and Z. He. 2019. "Recent advances in biosensor for detection of lung cancer biomarkers." *Biosensors and Bioelectronics* 141:111416.

Yuan, Huizhen, Wei Ji, Shuwen Chu, et al. 2018. "Fiber-optic surface plasmon resonance glucose sensor enhanced with phenylboronic acid modified Au nanoparticles." *Biosensors and Bioelectronics* 117:637–643.

Zainuddin, N. H., H. Y. Chee, M. Z. Ahmad, M. A. Mahdi, M. H. Abu Bakar, and M. H. Yaacob. 2018. "Sensitive *Leptospira* DNA detection using tapered optical fiber sensor." *Journal of Biophotonics* 11 (8):e201700363.

Zeng, Shuwen, Siyi Hu, Jing Xia, et al. 2015. "Graphene—MoS$_2$ hybrid nanostructures enhanced surface plasmon resonance biosensors." *Sensors and Actuators B: Chemical* 207:801–810.

Zhang, Chuanbiao, Tigang Ning, Jing Li, Li Pei, Chao Li, and Heng Lin. 2017. "Refractive index sensor based on tapered multicore fiber." *Optical Fiber Technology* 33:71–76.

Zhang, Dongsheng, Juan Li, Fengzhen Wang, Jun Hu, Shuwei Wang, and Yueming Sun. 2014. "2-Deoxy-D-glucose targeting of glucose metabolism in cancer cells as a potential therapy." *Cancer Letters* 355 (2):176–183.

Zhou, Chen, Haimin Zou, Ming Li, Chengjun Sun, Dongxia Ren, and Yongxin Li. 2018. "Fiber optic surface plasmon resonance sensor for detection of *E. coli* O157: H7 based on antimicrobial peptides and AgNPs-rGO." *Biosensors and Bioelectronics* 117:347–353.

Index

Note: *Italic* page numbers denote references to illustrations.

A

absorbance, 28, 56, *57*, 75, *95*, 113–114, 118, *118–119*, 136–140, *137–140*, 142, *142–143*, 146–151, *146*, *148–151*, *153–154*, 169–184, *170–172*, *174–177*, *179–181*, *184*, 203–208, *202–208*, *251–252*, *257*, 258, *266*, 268–269
absorption, 3, 26, 31–32, 45, 47, 53, 59, 92, *94*, 113, 119, 120, *121*, 124, 127, 131, 139, 152, 167, 178, 200, 201–205, 211, 219, 233, 242–243, 247, 250, 257–258, 266
acute myocardial infarction, 198, 233
Ag, 167–193
agglomeration, 140, 162, 168
AgNPs, 47, 48, 52, 55, 74, 76, 113–127, 132, 162, 167–193, 201, 203–210, *205*, *207*, 227–228, *229*
alanine aminotransferase, 60, *61*, 102, 103, *104*, 197, *197*, 213–214
analyte, 1, 3, 14–15, 28, 32–33, 46, 76, 104–105, 114, 138, *138*, 142, **151**, 156, 158, 173, *176–176*, 177–178, 181–182, 241, 244, 254, 264
anti-interference ability, 258, 261
ascorbic acid, 157–162
atomic force microscopy (AFM), 59, 75, 97, 205
AuNPs, 97–99, 133, 200, 209, 210, 248–249, 264

B

bacteria, 78, 103–105, *see also Shigella*
bacterial cells, 241, 243, 264, 268–269
bacterial culture, 243, 263
beam propagation method (BPM), 16
biomolecules, 81, 124–125, 210–232
biosensing, 29–32
biosensors, 1–3, *2–4*, **5**
Brust method, 95
BSA, 131, *136*, 144–146, 149–151, 162, 262, 267

C

cancer, 53, 55, 75, 78–80, 123, 241–242, 244–245, 258, 270–271
cancer cells, 246–262
cancer detection, 246–262, 270
carbon nanotubes (CNTs), 47–48, 53, 96, 122
cardiac troponin I, 217–219
cardiovascular disease risk, 198
cells *see* bacterial cells; cancer cells; circulating tumor cells (CTCs); tumor cells
ceramic, 53
ceria nanoparticles (CeO$_2$-NPs), 60, 103, 201, *204*
characterization, 56–60, 74–75, 91–92, 115–122, 152–154, 202–207, *208*, 247, 250–254, 266–267
cholesterol, 76–77, *78*, 100–102, 223–227
cholesterol oxidase (ChOx), 98, 101, 114
circulating tumor cells (CTCs), 242

clinical diagnostics, 1, 7, 60, 69
collagen, 228–232
collagenase, 200, 229, 232
collagen-IV, 200, 229
combiner manufacturing system (CMS), 71
COMSOL Multiphysics, *181*, 186
copper oxide nanoflowers (CuO-NFs), 245–249, *253*
copper oxide nanoparticles (CuO-NPs), 202, 209
copper-oxide, 227
creatinine, 210–211
culture of *Shigella sonnei* bacteria, 264, *266*
cysteamine, 145–149, 162, 185–186, *187*

D

deoxyribonucleic acid (DNA), 81, 106–108
detection, 33, 76–81, 103–108, 124–125, 154–155, 158–162, 189–192, 210–232, 241–271
detection limit (LoD), 29, 33, 35, 45, 83, 113, 114, 124, 151, 154, 157, 161, 162, 214, 218, 223, 227, 228, 223, 234, 269–270
detection limit of sensor, 154, *155*
DNA, 81, 106–108
DNA oligonucleotide, 263, 267, 269–270
D-peak, 135, 170–171

E

electrochemical, 1, 46, 48, 52, 54–55, 69, 78, 114–115, 122, 131, 190, 199, 200, 201
electrochemical method, 96, 103, 115
electromagnetic, 6, 11, 13, 14, 21, 22, 26, 69, 71, 75–76, 200
energy-dispersive X-ray spectroscopy (EDS or XEDS), 75, 97
enzyme, 1, 54, 75, *94*, 99, 103, 113, 114, 120, 124, 197–198, 210, 211, 213–215, 231–233, 242
enzyme-linked immunosorbent assays (ELISA), 241
etched MCF, 219, *221*, 233, 270
evanescent fields, 10, 20, 71, 72, 211, 232
evanescent wave, 8–10
excitation, 20–27

F

FESEM, 97, 138, 144, 146–147, 173, *174*, *183*, 186, *187*, 188, 192, 263, 267
fiber Bragg grating (FBG), 7, 70, 80
fiber-optic, 6–14
field emission scanning electron microscope (FESEM), 97, 138, 144, 146–147, 173, *174*, *183*, 186, *187*, 188, 192, 263, 267
finite difference time-domain (FDTD), 15–16
functionalization, 34, 75, 81, 98–99, 124, 162, 174, 175, 186, 189, 211, 215, 249, 262
FWHM, 171–173

G

glucose, 76, 100
glutathione, 156, 189, 199
GO, 131–162, 167–193, 248–249, *252–253*
gold, 91–108, 131–162, 248
gold nanoparticles (AuNPs), 91–108, 131–162, 248
G-peak, 135
grapheme, 34, 45, 53, 56, 60, 107
graphene oxide (GO), 131–162, 167–193, 248–249, *252–253*
graphite flakes, 132, 246, 248

H

Hepa1 6 (mouse liver), 243, *259, 261*
HepG2 (human liver), 243, 249, 258, *259, 260, 261*, 270
hetero-core, 7, 34
hetero-core structure, 73, 76, 83, 192, 199
hetro-core fiber structure, 217–219, 232
HF solution, 219, 247
high-resolution transmission electron microscope (HRTEM), *57*, 75, 93, *95*, 97, 115, 140, *141*, 152, *154*, 170, *171–172*, 178, 202–208, 213, *251–253*, 263
hollow-core fiber (HCF), 70
HRTEM, *57*, 75, 93, *95*, 97, 115, 140, *141*, 152, *154*, 170, *171–172*, 178, 202–208, 213, *251–253*, 263
human serum, 156, *157*, 198, 199, 213, 223, 227
Hummer's method, 132, 144, 168, 186, 202, 246, 248

I

immobilization, 209–210, 248–249, 264
immunosensors, 1, 198–199, 243
intensity, 16
in vitro, 47, 73, 131, 200
in vivo, 47, 69, 73, 200

K

kidney disease, 197
Kretschmann's configuration, 14–15

L

label-free, 3, 20, 31–32, 69, 81, 83, 100, 109, 124, 127, 162, 198–199, 270
L-Cysteine, 189–192
limit of detection (LOD), 29, 33, 35, 45, 83, 113, 114, 124, 151, 154, 157, 161, 162, 214, 218, 223, 227, 228, 223, 234, 269–270
linearity, 33, 154
localized surface plasmon resonance (LSPR), 264
LoD, 29, 33, 35, 45, 83, 113, 114, 124, 151, 154, 157, 161, 162, 214, 218, 223, 227, 228, 223, 234, 269–270
LSPR, 264
LSPR based sensors, 21, 81, 228, 244–246
LSPR effect, 92, 157, 201, 210, 211, 223, 232
LSPR sensor, 27–29, 131–162, 167–193, 213–214
LSPR technique, 31–32, 244

M

Mach-Zehnder interferometer (MZI), 227, 228–232
MCF-7 (human breast), 243, 244, 249, 258, 270
metal enhanced fluorescence (MEF) technique, 113
metallic nanoparticles, 21–29
microorganism detection, 35, 241
microorganisms, 241–271
MMF, 20, *59*, 70, 107, 190, 199, 217
modified Hummer's method, 132, 186, 202, 248
molybdenum disulfide nanoparticles (MoS$_2$-NPs), 103, 201, 210, 243, 264
morphological, 56–57
MoS$_2$-NPs, 103, 201, 210, 243, 264
MPM fiber structure, 216–217
MPM probe, 73
MPTMS, 98, 209, 246, 262
multicore fibre (MCF), 70, 219, 233, 242–244, 246–247, 250, 254, *255*, 258, 262–264, 270
multicore fiber biosensor, 246–262
multimode fibre (MMF), 20, *59*, 70, 107, 190, 199, 217
multi-tapered fiber, 157, 158, 211–213
multiwalled carbon nanotubes (MWCNTs), 96, 122
MXene, 54–55, 201

N

nanocoating, 74–75
nanofibers, 48, 114
nanomaterials, 45–59, *60*, 197–234, 250, *250–253*
nanoparticles (NPs), 21–29, 48–55, 91–109, 113–126, 131–162, 190, 202–210, 248, 254, 266–267
nanoscale, 45–47, 52, 61, 75, 109, 199, 254
nanotechnology, 29, 32, 34, 45–47, 55, 60, 71, 74, 75, 124, 126, 242, 243, 244, 270
nanotubes, 45, 47, 55, 56, 96, 122
Nb$_2$CTx MXene, 232
numerical aperture, 139

O

optical fiber, *see* optical fiber sensors (OFSs); plasmonic-optical fiber sensors (P-OFSs); tapered optical fiber
optical fiber sensors (OFSs), 1, *6*, 60, 69, 91, 124, **125**, 132, 136, 162, 180, 200, 211, 233, 227, 231, 245
optical sensors, 241–271
organic, 46, 48, *51*, *53*, 98, 115, 120, 123, 126, 168, 244
oscillation, 12–13, 21–22, 31–32, 91, 132, 200

P

PBS solution, 99, 152, 154, 161, 213, 215, 220, 223, 249
p-cresol, 198, 214–215, 233
PCS, 134, 144, 183, 192
photocatalytic activity, 53, 61
photonic-crystal fibre (PCF), 34, 59, 70
photonics, 53, *59*, 167
photosensitive fibre (PSF), 34, 70, 228, 234
plasmonic optical sensing, 241
plasmonic-optical fiber sensors (P-OFSs), *6*, 45–61

plasmonics, 1–35
point-of-care (PoC), 69, 81, 83
polyvinyl alcohol (PVA), 120, *121*
polyvinyl alcohol stabilized AgNPs (PVA-AgNPs), 115, *118*, 120, 210, 229

R

reduced graphene oxide, 34, 56, 131
reflection mode, 132, 162
refractive index (RI), 28–29
reproducibility, 33
resolution, 101, 103, 171, 175, 189, 192
resonance peak, 29, 140, 213, 233
reusability, 258–261
rGO, 34, 56, 131
RI sensing, 27, 168
ribonucleic acid (RNA), 106–108

S

scanning electron microscope (SEM), 13, 119, 263
selectivity, 33, 156, 258–261
self-assembled monolayer (SAM), 186
sensitivity, 32–33, 154, *155*
sensors, 1–35, 45–61, 91–109, 113–127, 131–162, 167–193, 197–234, 241–271
shape, 21–22, 31–32, 34, 45, 47, 52–53, *70*, 72, 83, 95–98, *99*, 101, 105, *117*, **117**, 140, 157–158, 168, 173, 200, 203, 205, 241, 247, 250, 263
Shigella, 262–269
silane, 134, 144–146, 209, 246
silver, 167–193
silver nanoparticles, 47, 48, 52, 55, 74, 76, 113–127, 132, 162, 167–193, 201, 203–210, *205*, *207*, 227–228, *229*
single mode fiber (SMF), 70, 152, 157, 190, 199, 217, 246
SMF-MCF fiber structure, 247, 248–249, *250*
SMF-MCF-MMF-SMF structure, 210–211
SMSMS structure, 227–228
SNR, 173
sp^2 hybridization, 154
spectrometer, 21, 28, 113, 135–136, 139–140, 146, 152, 158, 170, 173, 185, 192, 211, 213, 215–216, 219, 220, 227, 231, 249–250, 264
spherical silver nanoparticles, 115, 118–119
SPR-based sensors, 244
SPS probe, 223–227
stability, 33

surface plasmon resonance (SPR), 30–32
surface plasmons, 10–14, 21–27
surface-enhanced Raman scattering (SERS), 21, 31, 34, 46, 53, 83, 113, 167
synthesis, 55–56, 91–97, 115–122, 132–134, 168, 190, 200–202, 248, 264

T

tapered fiber, 214–215, *216*
tapered MCF, *221*, 233
tapered optical fiber, 220–223
tapered probe structure, 223–228
taper-in-taper fiber structure, 213–214
TEM, 56, 92, *93*, *95*, 115, *117–118*, 120, *121*, *135*, 136, *137*, 140, 178, *178*, 180, *180*, 202, *202–203*, 207, 247, 250
tetraoctylammonium bromide (TOAB), 95
transferred matrix method (TMM), 15–20
transmission mode, 132, 134, 139, 232
triacylglycerides, 124, *125*
triangular silver nanoparticles, 119, *120*
tumor cells, 241, 242, 270, 271
tungsten-halogen light source, 136, 140, 152, 158, 211, 218
Turkevich protocol, 132
tyrosinase, 198, 215

U

ultraviolet–visible (UV-Vis), 31–32, 75, 97
uric acid, 151–156, *157*
uricase, 152, 154, *155*, 156, *157*, 227

V

virus, 78, **79**, *80*, 103–105

W

wet chemical method, 56

X

X-ray diffraction, 56, 135

Z

zinc-oxide, 244, *245*
zinc oxide nanoparticles (ZnO-NPs), *260*, 207, *208*, 209, 210

For Product Safety Concerns and Information please contact our EU
representative GPSR@taylorandfrancis.com
Taylor & Francis Verlag GmbH, Kaufingerstraße 24, 80331 München, Germany